ANNALS OF THE NEW YORK ACADEMY OF SCIENCES
Volume 1145

Learning, Skill Acquisition, Reading, and Dyslexia

Edited by
GUINEVERE F. EDEN

Georgetown University Medical Center
Washington, DC

D. LYNN FLOWERS

Wake Forest University Health Sciences
Winston-Salem, North Carolina

Published by Blackwell Publishing on behalf of the New York Academy of Sciences
Boston, Massachusetts
2008

Library of Congress Cataloging-in-Publication Data

International Rodin Remediation Conference (25th : 2006 : Georgetown University)

    Learning, skill acquisition, reading, and dyslexia/editors, Guinevere F. Eden, D. Lynn Flowers.

        p. ; cm.

    Includes bibliographical references.

    ISBN 978-1-57331-702-3

    1. Dyslexia–Congresses. 2. Reading ability–Congresses. 3. Learning ability–Congresses. I. Eden, Guinevere. II. Flowers, D. Lynn (Donna Lynn) III. Title. [DNLM: 1. Dyslexia–Congresses. 2. Learning–Congresses. 3. Reading–Congresses. WL 340.6 I612L 2008]
    RJ496.A5I58 2008
    616.85′53–dc22

                               2008041515

The *Annals of the New York Academy of Sciences* (ISSN: 0077-8923 [print]; ISSN: 1749-6632 [online]) is published 28 times a year on behalf of the New York Academy of Sciences by Wiley Periodicals, Inc., with offices at (US) 350 Main St., Malden, MA 02148-5020, (UK) 9600 Garsington Road, Oxford, OX4 2ZG, and (Asia) 165 Cremorne St., Richmond VIC 3121, Australia. Blackwell Publishing was acquired by John Wiley & Sons in February 2007. Blackwell's program has been merged with Wiley's global Scientific, Technical, and Medical business to form Wiley-Blackwell.

MAILING: The *ANNALS OF THE NEW YORK ACADEMY OF SCIENCES* (ISSN: 0077-8923), is published 28 times a year. The *Annals* is mailed standard rate. Mailing to rest of world by IMEX (International Mail Express). Canadian mail is sent by Canadian publications mail agreement number 40573520. POST-MASTER: Send all address changes to *ANNALS OF THE NEW YORK ACADEMY OF SCIENCES*, Journal Customer Services, John Wiley & Sons Inc., 350 Main St., Malden, MA 02148-5020.

Journal Customer Services: For ordering information, claims, and any inquiry concerning your subscription, please go to interscience.wiley.com/support or contact your nearest office:

Americas: Email: cs-journals@wiley.com; Tel: +1 781 388 8598 or 1 800 835 6770 (Toll free in the USA & Canada).

Europe, Middle East and Asia: Email: cs-journals@wiley.com; Tel: +44 (0) 1865 778315

Asia Pacific: Email: cs-journals@wiley.com; Tel: +65 6511 8000

Information for Subscribers: The *Annals* is published in 28 issues per year. Subscription prices for 2008 are:

Premium Institutional: US$4265 (The Americas), £2370 (Rest of World). Prices are exclusive of tax. Australian GST, Canadian GST and European VAT will be applied at the appropriate rates. For more information on current tax rates, please go to www.wiley.com, click on Help and follow the link through to Journal Subscriptions. The Premium institutional price also includes online access to the current and all online back files to January 1, 1997, where available. For other pricing options, including access information and terms and conditions, please visit www.interscience.wiley.com/journals.

Delivery Terms and Legal Title: Prices include delivery of print publications to the recipient's address. Delivery terms are Delivered Duty Unpaid (DDU); the recipient is responsible for paying any import duty or taxes. Legal title passes to the customer on despatch by our distributors.

Membership information: Members may order copies of *Annals* volumes directly from the Academy by visiting www.nyas.org/annals, emailing membership@nyas.org, faxing +1 212 298 3650, or calling 1 800 843 6927 (toll free in the USA), or +1 212 298 8640. For more information on becoming a member of the New York Academy of Sciences, please visit www.nyas.org/membership. Claims and inquiries on member orders should be directed to the Academy at email: membership@nyas.org or Tel: 1 800 843 6927 (toll free in the USA) or +1 212 298 8640.

Printed in the USA. Printed on acid-free paper.

The *Annals* is available to subscribers online at Wiley InterScience and the New York Academy of Sciences Web site. Visit www.interscience.wiley.com or www.annalsnyas.org to search the articles and register for table of contents e-mail alerts.

The paper used in this publication meets the minimum requirements of the National Standard for Information Sciences Permanence of Paper for Printed Library Materials, ANSI Z39.48 1984.

ISSN: 0077-8923 (print); 1749-6632 (online)
ISBN-10: 1-57331-702-0; ISBN-13: 978-1-57331-702-3

A catalogue record for this title is available from the British Library.

ANNALS OF THE NEW YORK ACADEMY OF SCIENCES

Volume 1145

Learning, Skill Acquisition, Reading, and Dyslexia

Editors
GUINEVERE F. EDEN AND D. LYNN FLOWERS

This volume is the expanded and updated proceedings of a conference entitled the **25th Rodin Remediation Conference,** held on October 11–13, 2006 at Georgetown University, Washington, DC.

CONTENTS

Introduction. *By* Guinevere F. Eden and D. Lynn Flowers ix

Part I. Reading and Reading Development: The Role of Language

The Development of Reading across Languages. *By* Usha Goswami 1

Development of Ventral Stream Representations for Single Letters. *By* Peter E. Turkeltaub, D. Lynn Flowers, Lynn G. Lyon, and Guinevere F. Eden 13

Neural Correlates of Nouns and Verbs in Early Bilinguals. *By* Alice H.D. Chan, Kang-Kwong Luke, Ping Li, Virginia Yip, Geng Li, Brendan Weekes, and Li Hai Tan 30

Logographic Kanji versus Phonographic Kana in Literacy Acquisition: How Important Are Visual and Phonological Skills? *By* Maki S. Koyama, Peter C. Hansen, and John F. Stein 41

Mapping Phonological Information from Auditory to Written Modality during Foreign Vocabulary Learning. *By* Margarita Kaushanskaya and Viorica Marian 56

Part II. Language and Reading: The Role of Language Modality

Visual Skills and Cross-Modal Plasticity in Deaf Readers: Possible Implications for Acquiring Meaning from Print. *By* Matthew W.G. Dye, Peter C. Hauser, and Daphne Bavelier 71

Phonological Awareness and Short-Term Memory in Hearing and Deaf Individuals of Different Communication Backgrounds. *By* Daniel Koo, Kelly Crain, Carol LaSasso, and Guinevere F. Eden 83

Signed Language and Human Action Processing: Evidence for Functional Constraints on the Human Mirror-Neuron System. *By* David P. Corina and Heather Patterson Knapp 100

Part III. Learning, Skill Acquisition, Language, and Dyslexia

Neurocognitive Basis of Implicit Learning of Sequential Structure and Its Relation to Language Processing. *By* Christopher M. Conway and David B. Pisoni . . .   113

Implicit Learning and Dyslexia. *By* Vasiliki Folia, Julia Uddén, Christian Forkstam, Martin Ingvar, Peter Hagoort, and Karl Magnus Petersson   132

Motor Sequence Learning and Developmental Dyslexia. *By* Pierre Orban, Ovidiu Lungu, and Julien Doyon   151

Implicit Learning in Control, Dyslexic, and Garden-Variety Poor Readers. *By* Catherine J. Stoodley, Nicola J. Ray, Anthea Jack, and John F. Stein   173

Two Forms of Implicit Learning in Young Adults with Dyslexia. *By* Ilana J. Bennett, Jennifer C. Romano, James H. Howard, Jr., and Darlene V. Howard   184

Impaired Serial Visual Search in Children with Developmental Dyslexia. *By* Ruxandra Sireteanu, Claudia Goebel, Ralf Goertz, Ingeborg Werner, Magdalena Nalewajko, and Aylin Thiel, ...   199

Structural Correlates of Implicit Learning Deficits in Subjects with Developmental Dyslexia. *By* Deny Menghini, Gisela E. Hagberg, Laura Petrosini, Marco Bozzali, Emiliano Macaluso, Carlo Caltagirone, and Stefano Vicari   212

Cerebellar Volume and Cerebellar Metabolic Characteristics in Adults with Dyslexia. *By* Suzanna K. Laycock, Iain D. Wilkinson, Lauren I. Wallis, Gail Darwent, Sarah H. Wonders, Angela J. Fawcett, Paul D. Griffiths, and Roderick I. Nicolson   222

A Meta-analysis of Functional Neuroimaging Studies of Dyslexia. *By* José M. Maisog, Erin R. Einbinder, D. Lynn Flowers, Peter E. Turkeltaub, and Guinevere F. Eden   237

Part IV. Speech, Communication, and Attention: Lessons from Other Disorders

Impact of Cerebellar Lesions on Reading and Phonological Processing. *By* Gal Ben-Yehudah and Julie A. Fiez   260

Morphosyntax and Phonological Awareness in Children with Speech Sound Disorders. *By* Jennifer Mortimer and Susan Rvachew   275

Brain Mechanisms for Social Perception: Lessons from Autism and Typical Development. *By* Kevin A. Pelphrey and Elizabeth J. Carter   283

From Loci to Networks and Back Again: Anomalies in the Study of Autism. *By* Ralph-Axel Müller   300

ADHD and Developmental Dyslexia: Two Pathways Leading to Impaired Learning. *By* Guinevere F. Eden and Chandan J. Vaidya   316

Index of Contributors   329

Introduction

This volume presents an international perspective on the current understanding of how reading is acquired by children and how the brain tackles this complex skill in a variety of languages, language modalities, and writing systems. It examines the reading disability developmental dyslexia through the lens of learning and skill acquisition, leaning heavily on research conducted on implicit learning processes that may support reading. The volume brings together contemporary expertise from the areas of neuropsychology, linguistics, psycholinguistics, cognitive neuroscience, education, and educational neuroscience and illustrates how these diverse disciplines unite to study reading and the mechanisms by which reading skills can be influenced, for worse or for better.

The first part of the volume focuses on reading and reading development, with particular emphasis on the role of language. Usha Goswami describes psycholinguistic grain size theory, which stresses the importance of language-specific characteristics that contribute to the development of phonological awareness and thereby to the acquisition of written language. Specifically, we learn from this work that variations in orthographic transparency and syllable structure determine the rate of decoding skill acquisition in a given language. We then turn to the brain correlates of skills that are known to be supportive of early reading acquisition. Turkeltaub *et al.* describe the functional anatomy supporting object and letter naming. Letter naming serves as the gateway to processing of words, and while its brain basis demonstrates a developmental trajectory, it is not differentiated for letters when considered in the context of naming other common objects. In another study employing functional brain imaging, Chan and colleagues examine cross-linguistic similarities and differences in the neural signature of word processing in logographic and alphabetic languages in bilingual subjects. They report how words in the two systems are differentially processed, suggesting that language-specific characteristics also influence the neural circuitry of written language. A further study of logographic languages is provided by Koyama and colleagues, who examined the relative contribution of phonological awareness and visual memory in predicting reading proficiency in Japanese children who learn to read in different scripts, one phonographic (Kana) and one logographic (Kanji). They report that phonological awareness skills are predictive of Kana proficiency and that visual memory predicts the acquisition of Kanji. These results suggest different systems for different aspects of reading and add further support to the importance of language-specific characteristics in reading acquisition. Finally, in this section we learn that language-specific characteristics become established during the learning of a language and that they are transferable. Kaushanskaya and Marian constructed artificial languages that varied in their similarity to the native language and showed that the more similar the "new" language is to the native language, the more accurately subjects recognize either spoken or written words in the novel language. Together this section speaks to the fact that the demands of a specific language will affect the requirements necessary for obtaining written language proficiency in that language and that the presence of multiple languages will influence how written language is organized in the brain.

Ann. N.Y. Acad. Sci. 1145: ix–xii (2008). © 2008 New York Academy of Sciences.
doi: 10.1196/annals.1416.027

The second part focuses on language modality, and here we are introduced to a series of studies that have emerged from current research in deaf populations. Opening with a review, Dye, Hauser, and Bavelier examine the influence of visual skills on reading acquisition by asking how the unique skills that deaf children bring to the task affect visual attention and visual perception of text. Koo and colleagues examine this question directly by studying the phonological awareness and verbal working memory skills in deaf and hearing young adults with a variety of language backgrounds. The results demonstrate that in skilled deaf readers, language experience has a specific influence on phonological awareness skills (stronger in users of cued speech and oral communication) and that retention of digits is influenced by the visual representation of language (shorter digit span in users of manual languages). In a closing review, Corina and Knapp explore behavioral, neurofunctional, and neuropsychological aspects of human communication by contrasting gestural language in deaf signers and human action perception mediated by a mirror neuron system. They argue that these two types of communication are dissociable. In sum, this section speaks to the importance of recognizing the significant impact of sensory and communication experience on language and reading acquisition and illustrates that models of reading acquisition can be strengthened by knowledge gained from populations whose language and learning occurs in the visual modality.

In the third part of the volume we turn to learning, skill acquisition, language, and dyslexia. Much investigation has been devoted to the causes of developmental dyslexia, with the most common finding being deficiencies related to phonological awareness and grapheme-phoneme correspondence. These skills rely on segmenting sound and mapping it to print. In their review, Conway and Pisoni point out that much of typical skill learning takes place unintentionally and automatically, but also that the data support stimulus-specific rather than domain-general learning mechanisms in implicit sequence learning. They argue effectively that implicit sequence learning and language processing likely share underlying neurocognitive mechanisms that rely on the encoding and representation of phonological sequences. A link between sequence learning and reading acquisition might be assumed simply on the bases that typical readers with good phonemic awareness are able to blend and segment sound sequences in words while persons with dyslexia must be taught this skill. Indeed, successful treatment for dyslexia relies on explicitly teaching sound sequences. Several studies have found implicit learning deficits in persons with dyslexia. Folia *et al.* review that literature and report on a study in typical readers of implicit sequence learning using a "mere exposure" paradigm of artificial grammar learning. Their findings support the hypothesis that knowledge about the rules of a complex system can be implicitly acquired simply by exposure. The paradigm holds promise for investigating how persons with dyslexia differ from typical readers in the ability to make use of this type of learning. A less investigated but promising avenue of inquiry concerns the learning of motor sequences. Pierre Orban and Julien Doyon review behavioral and brain imaging studies of this type of skill learning in poor readers, pointing out that persons with dyslexia are consistently found to underperform typical readers. On the basis of studies of the stages, processes, and mental representations of sequence learning acquisition in typical readers, they point out the importance of taking this motor skill learning into account when trying to understand the neural substrates of reading acquisition.

The next reports directly examine implicit learning in dyslexia. First, Stoodley *et al.* use an implicit serial reaction time task to investigate sequential skill learning. They report that dyslexic readers (poor readers who are IQ discrepant) performed more slowly than either typical readers or garden-variety poor readers (poor readers who are not IQ discrepant), implicating suboptimal cerebellar functioning in dyslexia. Like Orban and Doyon and Folia *et al.*, they propose that implicit sequential skill learning deficiencies may explain the deficits seen in developmental dyslexia. Understanding how persons with dyslexia process differently from garden-variety poor readers has implication for designing remediation programs as well as for defining study samples. Then Bennett and colleagues present further data in support of impaired implicit sequence learning in adults with dyslexia. They report that poor readers perform less well than good readers on a verbal task that does not involve the learning of a motor sequence. They argue, therefore, that impairment in implicit sequence learning in adults with dyslexia cannot be entirely accounted for by motor sequencing deficits. Another line of investigation into the causes and impairments of developmental dyslexia addresses visual search performance. Using a series of conjunction tasks, Sireteanu *et al.* found that dyslexic children performed less well than controls on complex serial visual search tasks requiring sustained visual attention. Differences were more apparent in the youngest children and tended to lessen with age.

Turning to studies using brain imaging technology, Menghini *et al.* performed a brain morphometric analysis to determine if there are structural abnormalities in cortical gray matter in the same regions that show abnormal activation in dyslexic readers during performance of an implicit learning task. They found smaller gray matter volumes in the right posterior superior parietal lobule, precuneus, and supplemental motor area in dyslexic subjects compared to typical readers. Importantly, greater gray matter volume in the parietal cortex was related to better implicit learning only within the typical reading group. The findings are interpreted as consistent with the notion that functional and structural deficiencies in the superior parietal lobe may be related to problems in reading acquisition. Others have focused on cerebellar function in developmental dyslexia. Laycock *et al.* report greater white matter volume in the cerebellum, bilaterally, and also differences in ratios of metabolic markers measured with spectroscopy. Finally, this section includes a meta-analysis by Maisog and colleagues, indicating brain regions where differences are most likely to exist between dyslexic and nondyslexic adolescents and adults during word processing paradigms. As a whole this section speaks to the role of implicit learning in reading acquisition and draws connections among this cognitive process, its neural underpinnings, and brain regions currently implicated in developmental dyslexia.

The final part gleams insights into speech, communication, and attention by examining other disorders of language and communication. Returning to the theme of cerebellar dysfunction and using a classical neurological approach, Ben-Yehudah and Fiez investigate a potential relationship between cerebellar dysfunction and reading skills. They found that the skills usually used to define developmental dyslexia (accuracy in single word and nonword naming, reading fluency and comprehension, phonological awareness, and phonological memory) did not differ between patients with cerebellar lesions and healthy adults, concluding that intact cerebellar function is not a requirement to maintain reading once it has been acquired. They leave the question open with respect to its function during reading acquisition. However, they also found that lesioned patients performed more poorly on visual rhyme judgment and verbal working tasks, suggesting cerebellar involvement in articulatory monitoring.

Important in early identification of children at risk is the ability to predict the acquisition of skills that support reading development. This is especially true for children with special needs. The findings from Mortimer and Rvachew's study hold promise for children with speech sound disorders as early as the pre-kindergarten year. For those pre-K children, finite verb morphology and inflectional suffix use significantly predicted phonological awareness in kindergarten. In other domains of communication impairment, Pelphrey and Carter summarize their studies in autism and the social brain. They investigate the neural substrates of social cognition and social perception, and their findings identify the superior temporal sulcus as an important part of a network that differentiates individuals with and without autism during the analysis of actions and intentions of others. This region has emerged from studies of children, adolescents, and adults with high-functioning autism. Staying within the field of autism, Müller discusses the importance in considering brain function through both localized function as well as network functioning. He illustrates this point using evidence from connectivity studies in autism that shows the interruption of long-range connectivity between cerebral regions. Finally, Eden and Vaidya also speak to the utility of functional brain imaging technology in the study of dyslexia and disorders of attention. Despite the common co-occurrence of developmental dyslexia and attention deficit disorder, the anatomical underpinnings of these disorders of learning are strikingly different; however, future studies on the functional correlates of successful intervention may shed insights into the etiologies of these common conditions. In sum, this section highlights some of the methodologies and theoretical frameworks that have served to advance areas of research in disorders of learning, language, and communication; these could inform future research in the field of developmental dyslexia.

Sadly, as this volume went to press we learned of the passing of Professor Sireteanu following a tragic accident. Our thoughts are with her family, friends and colleagues. Her death is a terrible loss to the research community.

Most of the contributions in this volume were initially presented at the Rodin Remediation Academy Conference held at Georgetown University in October 2006. The Rodin Remediation Academy, founded in 1984, was established as an interdisciplinary scientific roundtable for the exchange of information related to developmental dyslexia and dysphasia. During his lifetime, Dr. Per Uddén gave generously of his time and financial resources to promote the goals of the Academy through its conferences. Since his death, the continuation of these events have relied on other funding, and we acknowledge the following for their support of the conference: the National Institute of Child Health and Human Development; the National Institute of Deafness and Other Communication Disorders; the National Institute of Neurological Disorders and Stroke; the Nancy Lurie Marks Family Foundation; the Dana Alliance; Lindamood-Bell Learning Processes; Wilson Learning, the Swedish Embassy; and the Center for the Study of Learning, Georgetown University. Finally, we thank all of the authors for their stimulating contributions.

GUINEVERE F. EDEN
Georgetown University Medical Center
Washington, DC

D. LYNN FLOWERS
Wake Forest University Health Sciences
Winston-Salem, North Carolina

The Development of Reading across Languages

Usha Goswami

Centre for Neuroscience in Education, University of Cambridge,
Cambridge, England, United Kingdom

A selective review is presented of empirical evidence from different languages concerning phonological development and reading development in children. It is demonstrated that the development of reading depends on phonological awareness in all languages so far studied. However, because languages vary in syllable structure and in the consistency with which phonology is represented by the orthography, there are developmental differences in the grain size of lexical representations and in the reading strategies that develop across languages. It is argued that these cross-language data can be explained by a *psycholinguistic grain size* theory of reading and its development, as proposed by Ziegler and Goswami.

Key words: phonology; orthography; reading

Introduction

During the course of human development, a variety of symbolic systems have been invented to represent spoken language. These include alphabetic systems, character-based systems, and Braille. The efficient use of these systems is called reading. The acquisition of reading requires social transmission (e.g., by teachers), but some cognitive prerequisites on the part of the child are also necessary. These cognitive prerequisites are generally similar across languages because the "learning problem" faced by a child acquiring reading is also similar across languages. These cognitive factors are the focus of this chapter.

The Development of Reading across Languages

Orthographies are visual codes for spoken language. Meaning is communicated via printed symbols. Reading is thus in essence the cognitive process of understanding speech when it is written down. This suggests that factors affecting the development of speech processing will also affect the acquisition of reading. For example, awareness of the phonological structure of words (the sounds making up the words and the order in which they occur) is important for both language and reading acquisition. Skilled readers may appear to access meaning directly from visual codes, but, in fact, phonological activation is mandatory for them, too (Ziegler & Goswami, 2005). Visual codes differ across languages, however, in the units of sound that are represented by print. Ziegler and Goswami (2005) termed this a difference in psycholinguistic "grain size." For example, Japanese characters (called Kana) represent individual syllables, Chinese characters (called Kanji) represent whole words, and the alphabet represents small units of sound called "phonemes." Alphabets represent phonemes with more transparency in some languages than in others. For example, Italian, Greek, and Spanish are all highly consistent in their spelling-sound correspondences: one letter makes only one sound. English, Danish, and French are markedly less consistent: one letter can make multiple sounds. For example,

Address for correspondence: Usha Goswami, Centre for Neuroscience in Education, University of Cambridge, 184 Hills Road, Cambridge, CB2 8PQ, United Kingdom. ucg10@cam.ac.uk the letter *A* in English makes different sounds in the highly familiar words *man*, *make*, *car*, and *walk*. All of these factors matter in explaining cross-language differences in reading acquisition by children.

Early Phonological Development

Phonological development is an important part of language acquisition. Children need to learn the sounds and combinations of sounds that are permissible in the language that they are learning, so that their brains can develop "phonological representations" of the sound structures of individual words. Children also need to be able to produce these words themselves. Both processes require extensive development. Between the ages of 1 and 6 years, children acquire more than 14,000 words (Dollaghan, 1994). Powerful learning mechanisms are at work, such as statistical learning mechanisms. For example, babies need to learn the phonemes (individual sound elements) that make up words in their particular language. The physical changes in speech sounds where languages place phonetic boundaries are not random (Kuhl, 1986). This may explain why infants are sensitive to the acoustic boundaries that separate phonetic categories in all human languages from birth. Rapid token-based learning during the first year leads the infant brain to specialize in the phonemes particular to their language. The infants track the distributional properties of the sounds in the language that they hear and register the acoustic features that regularly co-occur. These relative distributional frequencies then yield phonetic categories (Kuhl, 2004).

Words are composed of sequences of phonemes, and so the infant also needs to group together the phonemes that make up individual words. The infant must learn which phonemes belong to one word and which phonemes belong to the next word. The rules that govern the sequences of phonemes used to make words in a particular language are called phonotactics. Infants also learn the phonotactics of their language during the first year of life, for example, by tracking the transitional probabilities between different phonemes (e.g., Jusczyk & Aslin, 1995). Furthermore, when caregivers talk to babies, they talk in a particular way (called "motherese" or "infant-directed speech"). Prosodic cues are exaggerated in infant-directed speech, and this also appears to have a learning function. The use of heightened pitch, increased duration, and exaggerated intonation appears to help babies to pick out words in the speech stream (e.g., Fernald & Mazzie, 1991). Prosodic cues also carry important information about how sounds are ordered into words when the words are multisyllabic. Therefore, by the end of the five year, infants are developing phonological representations of potential word forms that encode both lexical stress and segmental information.

The exponential increase in the number of words in the mental lexicon during the first 5 years of life poses additional challenges for phonological development. Each word has a unique phonological identity, and highly-similar words such as "back" and "bag" must be represented as distinct forms. Language-specific factors now begin to come into operation. For example, syllable structure, sonority profile, and phonological "neighborhood density" (the number of similar-sounding words to a particular target word) will all affect the development of phonological representations. These factors also affect the development of phonological awareness, which also emerges during the preschool period. Phonological awareness refers to a child's ability to detect and manipulate the component sounds that compose words at different grain sizes. For example, it is easier to become "phonologically aware" of the individual sound elements in syllables that have a simple structure (e.g., consonant-vowel or CV) than of sounds in syllables that have a complex structure (e.g., CCVCC). It is also easier to become phonologically aware of the constituent sounds in syllables when consonant phonemes are less sonorant (e.g., "at" is easier to segment than "am"). Other factors affecting the development of phonological representations are similar across languages. These include the age of acquisition of certain words, the speech-processing abilities of the child, and the "speech reading" abilities of the child (e.g., using lip-reading cues to help to distinguish sounds). As might be expected, there are some cross-language differences in the development of phonological awareness by children. There are also individual differences in the quality of the phonological representations developed by children. These individual differences turn out to be very important for the development of reading.

The Development of Phonological Awareness across Languages

The cognitive skills required for reading are usually described by the umbrella term "phonological awareness." Phonological awareness can occur at different "grain sizes." The primary linguistic processing unit is the syllable, and phonological awareness of syllables emerges first across languages. An important level of phonological awareness for literacy acquisition is awareness of "onset-rime" units. Onsets and rimes represent a grain size intermediate between syllables and phonemes. Each syllable making up a word can be decomposed into onsets, rimes, and phonemes in a hierarchical fashion. The onset-rime division of the syllable depends on dividing at the vowel. For English, words like *sing*, *sting*, and *spring* all share the same rime, the sound made by the letter string "ing." The onset of sing is /s/, the onset of sting is /st/, and the onset of spring is /spr/. These onsets make up one, two and three phonemes respectively. The rime can be divided into vowel and coda. The coda comprises any consonant sounds after the vowel. However, in many languages in the world, syllable structure is simple. Syllables are CV units. Hence for many languages, onsets, rimes, and phonemes are equivalent. Each onset and each rime in the syllable is also a single phoneme.

Prior to literacy instruction, the development of phonological awareness follows a similar developmental sequence across languages. Children first gain awareness of syllables. Syllabic awareness is usually present by around age three. Next, they gain awareness of onset-rime units. This emerges around the age of 3 to 4. Finally, children become aware of phonemes. Phoneme awareness emerges at different ages in different languages. This cross-language variation appears to depend on (1) the syllable structure of the language and (2) the transparency with which the orthography represents phonemes. It may also depend on morphology (Goswami & Ziegler, 2006).

Becoming Aware of Syllables

A number of different tasks are used across languages to measure the emergence of syllable awareness in children. Counting and tapping tasks are particularly frequent. For example, Liberman, Shankweiler, Fischer, and Carter (1974) gave American children aged from 4 to 6 years a wooden dowel and asked them to tap once for words that had one syllable (*dog*), twice for words that had two syllables (*dinner*), and three times for words that had three syllables (*president*). A criterion of six correct responses in a row was required in order for children to be accorded syllabic awareness. This criterion was passed by 46% of the 4-year-olds, 48% of the 5-year-olds, and 90% of the 6-year-olds. The 4- and 5-year-olds were prereaders, and the 6-year-olds had been learning to read for about a year.

A counting task was devised by the Russian psychologist Elkonin (1963). In this task, children are given plastic counters and are asked to use them to represent the number of syllables in words of increasing length. Treiman and Baron (1981) gave a syllable counting task to 5-year-old prereaders. For example, if the experimenter said "butter," the child had to set out two counters. Treiman and Baron (1981) also reported good syllable awareness in these prereaders. A less cognitively demanding task is the same–different judgment task. In this task, children have to decide whether two words share the same sound. Treiman and Zukowski (1991) gave children pairs of words like "hammer–hammock," and "compete–repeat," which share the first and second syllable, respectively. They found that 100% of 5-year-olds, 90% of 6-year-olds, and 100% of 7-year-olds succeeded in the same–different judgment task at the syllable level.

Similar performance levels are found in other languages. For example, Cossu, Shankweiler, Liberman, Katz, and Tola (1988) gave the tapping task to Italian prereaders aged 4 to 5 years, and to schoolchildren being taught to read aged 7 to 8 years. The children were asked to tap once for each syllable in words like "gatto," "melone," and "termometro." Syllable awareness was shown by 67% of the 4-year-olds, 80% of the 5-year-olds, and 100% of the school-age sample. Durgunoglu and Oney (1999) gave the tapping task to 6-year-old Turkish kindergartners, and performance was 94% correct at the syllable level. Hoien, Lundberg, Stanovich, and Bjaalid (1995) gave the syllable counting task to 128 Norwegian preschoolers aged 7 years. The children were asked to make pencil marks for each syllable in a word (e.g., "telephone" = 3 marks). They performed at an 83%-correct level. Counting tasks were also given to German preschoolers by Wimmer, Landerl, Linortner, and Hummer (1991) and to French kindergarteners by Demont and Gombert (1996). The German preschoolers performed at 81% correct in the syllable-counting task, and the French children performed at 69% correct. Clearly, prereading children across languages have good syllable awareness prior to receiving instruction in literacy.

Becoming Aware of Onsets and Rimes

The most widely used measure of onset-rime awareness in preschool children has been the oddity task (or odd-man-out task), which was devised by Bradley and Bryant (1978).

Children listen to an experimenter saying three or four words and are asked to select the "odd word out" on the basis of either the initial sound, the medial sound, or the final sound (e.g., *bus, bun, rug; pin, bun, gun; top, doll, hop*). When Bradley and Bryant (1983) gave the oddity task to around 400 preschool English children aged 4 to 5 years, average performance was 56% correct with onsets (initial sound task) and 71% correct with rimes (medial and final sounds tasks). Both performance levels were well above chance (33% correct). The same–different judgment task can also be used at the onset-rime level. For example, word pairs like "plank–plea" share the onset, and words like "spit–wit" share the rime. In the study mentioned earlier by Treiman and Zukowski (1991), 56% of the 5-year-olds, 74% of the 6-year-olds, and 100% of the 7-year-olds made accurate onset-rime judgments. Rime awareness can also be measured by asking children to complete nursery rhymes. Bryant, Bradley, Maclean, and Crossland (1989) asked 3-year-olds to complete familiar nursery rhymes by supplying missing rhyming words, such as "Jack and Jill went up the ? [hill]." The mean score for the group was 4.5 out of 10, and only one child out of 64 could complete no nursery rhymes. Hence onset-rime awareness is also well established in young children prior to schooling.

Again, a similar developmental picture is found in other languages. Chukovsky (1963) collected a large corpus of Russian children's language games and poems, and noted that the children were fascinated by rhymes. For example, Tania, aged 2.5 years, made up the following poem:

> Ilk, silk, tilk
> I eat Kasha with milk.
> Ilks, silks, tilks,
> I eat Kashas with milks.

The oddity task has been given to prereaders in a variety of languages. When Wimmer, Landerl, and Schneider (1994) tested German kindergartners, group performance was 44% correct with onsets and 73% correct with rimes. Wimmer *et al.* used sets of four words in order to increase task difficulty for these older children (German children do not go to school until age 6). Ho and Bryant (1997) gave Chinese 3-year-olds a rhyme-oddity task and found that performance was 68% correct. Hoien *et al.* (1995) gave their Norwegian preschoolers a match-to-sample rhyme task in which children had to select one picture out of three that rhymed with a target picture. Performance was 91% correct. Finally, Porpodas (1999) devised a Greek version of the oddity task. He reported that first-grade 7-year-old children in Greece scored 90% correct. As with syllables, therefore, cross-language data suggest that pre-reading children across languages have good onset-rime awareness prior to receiving instruction in literacy.

Becoming Aware of Phonemes

This developmental picture of cross-language consistency does not hold for the development of phoneme awareness (Ziegler & Goswami, 2005). This is not particularly surprising, as the phoneme is not a natural speech unit. The concept of a phoneme is an abstraction from the physical stimulus. For example, the "a" phoneme in "bag" and "back" is not exactly the same physical sound. In natural speech, acoustic features such as voicing determine phonetic differences (such as the difference between /p/ and /b/). Via prototype formation, the brain groups some similar but nonidentical sounds (called allophones) as the phoneme /b/ and many other similar but nonidentical sounds as the phoneme /p/. This grouping depends on acoustic features. The mechanism for learning about the abstract unit of the phoneme seems to be learning about letters. Letters are used to symbolize phonemes, even though the physical sounds corresponding, for example, to the vowel in "bag" and "back" are rather different. This means that the development of phoneme awareness depends in part on the consistency with which

letters symbolize phonemes. It also depends on the complexity of phonological syllable structure. Accordingly, there is cross-language divergence in the rate of development of phonemic awareness.

These cross-language differences in the development of phoneme awareness have been shown using a variety of cognitive tasks. One popular task has been phoneme counting. This is often used as a comparison task to syllable counting. For example, Wimmer *et al.* (1991) used a phoneme counting task in their German study, Demont and Gombert (1996) used a phoneme counting task in their French study, and Hoien *et al.* (1995) used a phoneme counting task in their Norwegian study. The German preschool children performed at 51% correct, the French preschool children performed at 2% correct, and the Norwegian kindergartners performed at 56% correct. Durgunoglu and Oney (1999) used a phoneme tapping task in their Turkish study, and the Turkish children performed at 67% correct. The Italian children studied by Cossu *et al.* (1988) were also given a phoneme tapping task. In their study, the criterion was reached by 13% of the 4-year-olds and 27% of the 5-year-olds. In English, as in French, phoneme counting tasks are typically performed rather poorly. For example, Liberman *et al.* (1974) reported levels of 0% correct for their 4-year-olds, and 17% correct for their 5-year-olds.

Clearly, the children in these different cross-language studies are already showing some language-specific variation in the ease with which they can identify individual phonemes in words. However, these different samples were not matched for any cognitive variables, and the words that they were asked to analyze were not matched either. Nevertheless, these differences by language become even more marked as children are taught to read. For example, in Cossu *et al.*'s Italian sample, 97% of the school-aged children were able to tap out phonemes. In contrast, in Liberman *et al.*'s American sample, phoneme tapping was at 70% correct when the children had been learning to read for about a year. Studies of English-speaking first-grade children by Tunmer and Nesdale (1985) and of second-grade children by Perfetti, Beck, Bell, and Hughes (1987) report comparable success levels (of 71% and 65%, respectively). Children learning to read other transparent languages typically score at levels more comparable to those of the Italian children. In studies using the phoneme counting measure, Turkish first-graders scored at 94% correct, Greek first-graders at 100% correct, and German first-graders at 92% correct (Durgunoglu & Oney, 1999; Harris & Giannouli, 1999; Wimmer *et al.*, 1991). In contrast, French children are more similar to English-speaking children. In their study, Demont and Gombert (1996) reported that by the end of first grade, group performance in the phoneme counting tasks was at 61% correct. Clearly, phoneme awareness develops at different rates in children who are learning to speak and read different languages.

Longitudinal Connections between Phonological Awareness and Reading

Despite this cross-language variability, preschool differences in phonological awareness predict reading and spelling development across languages. This has been shown most convincingly by longitudinal studies. These studies measure phonological awareness prior to school entry and then explore whether individual differences in phonological awareness predict children's performance in standardized tests of reading and spelling 2 to 3 years later. In order to measure whether there is a specific connection between phonological awareness and progress in literacy, other cognitive variables such as individual differences in intelligence or in memory must also be measured. These variables can then be controlled in longitudinal analyses seeking to establish a connection between phonological awareness and reading.

One of the first longitudinal studies of this nature was reported by Lundberg, Olofsson, and Wall (1980), who gave 143 Swedish children a range of phonological awareness tests in kindergarten. The tests used included syllable blending, syllable segmentation, rhyme production, phoneme blending, phoneme segmentation, and phoneme reversal. Predictive relationships between these tests and reading attainment were then measured in the second grade. Lundberg *et al.* reported that both the rhyme test and the phoneme tests were significant longitudinal predictors of reading. Another longitudinal study was reported by Bradley and Bryant (1983), using English children, who administered the oddity task to 400 preschool children at ages 4 and 5 years; they then tested the same children when they were aged (on average) 8 and 9 years. At follow-up, the children were given standardized tests of reading, spelling, and reading comprehension, and their performance was adjusted for age and I.Q. Bradley and Bryant reported significant correlations between performance on the oddity task at ages 4 and 5 and reading and spelling performance 3 years later. When the effects of I.Q. and memory were removed in multiple regression equations, the oddity task accounted for up to 10% of unique variance in reading. Similar results with English-speaking samples have been reported by a number of other research groups. For example, Baker, Fernandez-Fein, Scher, and Williams (1998) measured nursery rhyme knowledge in 39 kindergarten children and reported that it was the strongest predictor of nonword decoding and word identification skills measured in second grade. Rhyme knowledge at time 1 and at time 2 accounted for 36% and 48%, respectively, of unique variance in nonword decoding and word identification. The second strongest predictor of reading at time 2 was letter knowledge, which accounted for an additional 11% and 18% of the variance in each measure, respectively.

A German replication of Bradley and Bryant's study was reported by Wimmer *et al.* (1994). They followed up 183 German kindergartners who had received the oddity task at age 6 (in kindergarten) one year later (at first grade), and again 3 years later. When the German children were 7 to 8 years old (the same age as the English children in Bradley and Bryant's study), performance in the oddity task was only minimally related to reading and spelling progress. However, at the 3 year follow-up, when the children were aged (on average) 9 years 9 months, Wimmer *et al.* reported that rime awareness (although not onset awareness) was significantly related to both reading and spelling development. The Norwegian preschoolers studied by Hoien *et al.* (1995) were also followed longitudinally. When reading was tested in first grade, it was found that syllable, rhyme, and phoneme awareness all made independent contributions to variance in reading. The Chinese preschoolers studied by Ho and Bryant (1997) were also followed longitudinally. These 100 children were given the rime oddity task when they were 3 years old, and their progress in reading and spelling was assessed two years later. Phonological awareness was found to be a significant predictor of reading even after other factors such as age, I.Q., and mother's educational level had been controlled.

From this brief survey of studies, it is clear that individual differences in phonological awareness predict individual differences in reading attainment in all languages so far studied. Ho and Bryant's data show that this relationship between phonology and reading acquisition is equally strong for children who are learning to read nonalphabetic scripts (see also Siok & Fletcher, 2001). Because the children in these studies are preschoolers, the measures of phonological awareness used tend to be syllable, onset, and rime measures. However, once children are learning to read, individual differences in phoneme awareness also become predictive of individual differences in literacy attainment (Ziegler & Goswami, 2005). A similar cross-language picture emerges for developmental dyslexia. Deficits in phonological awareness predict developmental dyslexia across all languages so far studied, but the manifestation of developmental dyslexia varies with the language that the child is learning to read

(see Ziegler & Goswami, 2005, for a detailed cross-language survey). For example, in most European orthographies dyslexia is diagnosed on the basis of poor spelling rather than poor reading. Children with dyslexia who are learning to read transparent orthographies can become accurate decoders, although decoding remains very slow and effortful for these children, making them functionally dyslexic.

Phonological Awareness and Reading: Psycholinguistic Grain Size Theory

Theoretically, we (Ziegler & Goswami, 2005; 2006) have proposed that there are at least two language-dependent reasons for the cross-language variation that is found in reading acquisition and in developmental dyslexia. One is the phonological structure of the syllable. As noted earlier, syllables can be simple (CV) or complex (CCVCC). For many of the world's languages, the most frequent syllable type is CV. Languages like Spanish, Italian, Finnish, and Turkish contain predominantly CV syllables. In other languages, like English and German, syllable structure is more complex. The most frequent syllable type in English is CVC, with this structure accounting for 43% of monosyllables (e.g., "cat," "dog," "soap") (De Cara & Goswami, 2002). There are also many CCVC syllables (15% of monosyllables, e.g., "trip" and "spin"), CVCC syllables (21% of monosyllables, e.g., "fast" and "jump"), and some CCVCC syllables (6%, e.g., "trust"). Although a language like German has fewer monosyllables overall (approximately 1,400 compared to approximately 4,000 for English), phonological structure is similar. German has syllables with complex onsets, like "Pflaume" and syllables with complex codas like "Sand."

For languages like Italian and Spanish, onset-rime segmentation of the syllable is usually equivalent to phonemic segmentation. An Italian child who segments an early-acquired word like "Mamma" at the onset-rime level will also arrive at the phonemes comprising this word (e.g., /m/ /a/ /m/ /a/). Only 5% of English monosyllables follow the CV pattern (see De Cara & Goswami, 2002; examples are "go" and "see"). For languages like English and German, onset-rime segmentation is usually not equivalent to phoneme segmentation. For words like "dog," "spin," "jump," and "crust" both onsets and rimes can contain clusters of phonemes. Accordingly, another cognitive step is required to reach the phoneme level. Complex onsets like "sp" and complex rimes like "ust" must be segmented further. Other phonological factors will also contribute to the cross-language ease or difficulty of becoming aware of phonemes. For example, languages differ in the sonority profile of their syllables. Vowels are the most sonorant sounds, followed in decreasing order by glides (e.g., /w/), liquids (e.g., /l/), nasals (e.g., /n/), and obstruents or plosive sounds (e.g., /p/). Whereas the majority of syllables in English end with obstruents (almost 40%), the majority of syllables in French either end in liquids or have no coda at all (almost 50%).

The second important factor in explaining cross-language differences in phonemic awareness is orthographic transparency. Languages like Greek, German, Spanish, and Italian have a one-to-one mapping between letters and sounds. In these languages, letters correspond consistently to one phoneme. Languages like English have a one-to-many mapping between letters and sounds. Some letters or letter clusters can be pronounced in more than one way, for example, *O* in "go" and "to," *EA* in "speak" and "steak," and *G* in "magic" and "bag" (Berndt, Reggia & Mitchum, 1987; Ziegler, Stone & Jacobs, 1997). It is easier for a child to become aware of phonemes if one letter consistently maps to one and the same phoneme. It is relatively difficult to learn about phonemes if a letter can be pronounced in multiple ways (see Ziegler & Goswami, 2005, 2006, for more detailed arguments).

This theoretical analysis predicts that children learning to read in languages like Italian and Spanish should find it easiest to become aware of phonemes. They are learning languages with predominantly CV syllables, so

that onset-rime segmentation and phonemic segmentation are equivalent, and their written language consistently represents one phoneme by one letter. Children learning to read in languages like German should have a more difficult time, because spoken syllables are complex in structure. Nevertheless, German has a one-to-one mapping from letter to sound, facilitating the process of becoming aware of phonemes. Children who are learning to read in languages like English and French should have the most difficult time. These children are learning languages with a complex syllable structure and an inconsistent orthography. The cross-language comparisons discussed above confirm that it takes children longer to learn about phonemes in languages like English and French compared to languages like Italian and Spanish. As shall be discussed next, cross-language data on early reading acquisition also show that learning to decode efficiently takes longer in languages like English and French compared to languages like Spanish, German, and Italian.

Learning to Decode in Different Languages

These two factors of syllable structure and orthographic transparency also lead to cross-language differences in the rate at which children acquire reading skills. The children who acquire decoding skills most rapidly are those who are learning to read spoken languages with simple (CV) syllables and consistent letter-sound correspondences. Finnish, Italian, Greek, and Spanish children all learn to read very rapidly once they go to school and receive direct instruction in grapheme–phoneme correspondence. Graphemes are alphabetic units that make a single sound, for example, the phoneme /f/ can be represented by the grapheme "ph." Children who are learning to read spoken languages with more complex syllable structure, but nevertheless largely consistent letter-sound correspondences, also learn to read rapidly. German, Swedish, Dutch,

Norwegian, and Icelandic children provide good examples. Children who are learning to read spoken languages with phonologically complex syllables and with inconsistent letter–sound correspondences acquire decoding skills rather more slowly, such as Portuguese, Danish, and English children. English children make the slowest progress because English orthography has a rather high degree of inconsistency in symbol–sound mappings, and these inconsistencies occur for both reading and spelling (i.e., from orthography to phonology, and from phonology to orthography). Children who are learning to read English need to develop decoding strategies at a variety of grain sizes (e.g., whole-word strategies, rhyme analogy strategies and grapheme–phoneme recoding) (Ziegler & Goswami, 2005, 2006).

A striking illustration of the cross-language variability in the efficiency with which children acquire grapheme–phoneme recoding strategies during the first year of being taught to read comes from a study reported by Seymour, Aro, and Erskine (2003). They compared real word and nonword reading by children who were learning to read one of 14 European Union languages at the same time point during the first year of reading instruction. These first-grade children varied in age across the different E.U. countries, but they were chosen so that all were attending schools using "phonics" based (grapheme–phoneme based) instructional programs (Seymour *et al.*, 2003). The age differences were unavoidable, as (for example) children in England and Scotland begin school at age 5, whereas Scandanavian children begin school at age 7. The word and nonword items used were matched for difficulty across the languages, and the data are shown in Table 1. As can be seen, the efficiency of grapheme–phoneme recoding approached ceiling level during the first year of teaching for most of the European languages. Children learning to read languages like Finnish, German, Spanish, and Greek were decoding both words and nonwords with accuracy levels above 90%. In contrast, children learning to read French (79%

TABLE 1. Data (% Correct) from the Cross-Language Study of Grapheme–Phoneme Recoding Skills for Monosyllables in 14 European Languages

Language	Familiar Real Words	Nonwords
Greek	98	97
Finnish	98	98
German	98	98
Austrian German	97	97
Italian	95	92
Spanish	95	93
Swedish	95	91
Dutch	95	90
Icelandic	94	91
Norwegian	92	93
French	79	88
Portuguese	73	76
Danish	71	63
Scottish English	34	41

[a]Adapted from Seymour, Aro, and Erskine (2003).

and 88% correct), Danish (71% and 63% correct) and Portuguese (73% and 76% correct) were less-efficient readers, reflecting the reduced orthographic consistency of these languages. The children learning to read in English showed the slowest rates of acquisition, reading 34% of the simple words and 29% of the simple nonwords correctly. When followed up a year later, these children were achieving levels of 76% for real words and 63% for nonwords, still short of the early efficiency shown by the Finnish and Germans (Seymour *et al.*, 2003).

The problems experienced by the English children are not surprising in terms of the cross-language observations made earlier. The English children were learning a symbol system with inconsistent correspondences at the phoneme level, and they also had to match these symbols to phonemes that were embedded in complex syllables. In fact, the learning problem facing beginning readers across orthographies can be analyzed systematically using psycholinguistic grain size theory (see Ziegler & Goswami, 2005, 2006, for more detail). Ziegler and Goswami argue that, in general, there are more developmental similarities than differences across languages. Beginning readers across languages are faced with three problems: availability, consistency, and the granularity of symbol-to-sound mappings.

The availability problem reflects the fact that not all phonological units are accessible prior to reading. As we have seen, phonemes in particular may be inaccessible to prereaders. Furthermore, phonemic awareness develops at different rates in different languages, depending on orthographic consistency. The grain sizes that are most accessible prior to reading (syllables and onset-rimes) frequently do not correspond to the visual symbols used to represent phonology. Hence there may be a mismatch between the grain size represented by the orthography and the phonological grain sizes of which the child is aware. The severity of the mismatch will depend on the phonological and orthographic characteristics of the language. For example, a Japanese child, who is learning visual symbols that represent syllables (an early-developing grain size), should be at an advantage compared to an English child, who is learning letters that represent phonemes (a later-developing grain size, at least for languages where onset-rime units are not equivalent to phonemes).

Next, the consistency problem refers to the fact that the alphabet represents phonemes with more transparency in some languages than in others. As we have seen, Italian, Greek, and Spanish are all highly consistent in their spelling–sound correspondences. For these languages, one letter makes only one sound for reading. English, Danish and French are markedly less consistent in their spelling–sound correspondences, as, in reading, one letter can make multiple sounds. Although sound–spelling consistency can vary across languages as well (e.g., "feedback inconsistency," where one sound pattern has multiple spellings as in "hurt," "skirt," "Bert"), in terms of initial reading acquisition it is "feedforward inconsistency" (from spelling to sound) that appears to

be the most influential in slowing development. English has an unusually high degree of "feedforward" inconsistency. This creates problems for beginning readers in English, who have to decode words like "though," "cough," "through," and "bough."

Finally, the granularity problem refers to the fact that there are many more orthographic units to learn when access to the phonological system is based on bigger grain sizes as opposed to smaller grain sizes. That is, there are more words than there are syllables, there are more syllables than there are rimes, there are more rimes than there are graphemes, and there are more graphemes than there are letters. Ziegler and Goswami (2005, 2006) argued that reading proficiency in a particular language will depend on the resolution of all three of these problems. For example, children learning to read English must develop whole-word recognition strategies in order to read irregular words like "cough" and "yacht," they need to develop rhyme analogy strategies in order to read irregular words like "light," "night," and "fight," and they need to develop grapheme–phoneme recoding strategies in order to read regular words like "cat," "pen," and "big." In contrast, for many other languages, children only need to develop grapheme–phoneme recoding strategies in order to become highly skilled readers.

Conclusions

Learning to read in different languages depends on phonological awareness. During language acquisition, most children develop phonological awareness of syllables and of onset-rime units via the speech-processing skills that yield acoustic features and phonotactics and by processing prosodic cues such as duration and stress. However, there are variations between languages in syllable structure and in orthographic transparency which lead to cross-language divergence in the rate at which phonemic awareness is achieved and to cross-language divergence in the rate at which decoding skills develop. A way of describing the factors that determine the development of reading in different languages is offered by psycholinguistic grain size theory (Ziegler & Goswami, 2005, 2006).

Conflicts of Interest

The authors declare no conflicts of interest.

References

Baker, L., S. Fernandez-Fein, D. Scher & H. Williams. 1998. Home experiences related to the development of word recognition. In J. L. Metsala & L.C. Ehri (Eds.), *Word recognition in beginning literacy* (pp. 263–287). Mahwah, NJ: Erlbaum.

Berndt, R. S., J. A. Reggia & C. C. Mitchum. 1987. Empirically derived probabilities for grapheme-to-phoneme correspondences in English. *Behavior Research Methods, Instruments, & Computers* **19**: 1–9.

Bradley, L. & P. E. Bryant. 1983. Categorising sounds and learning to read: a causal connection. *Nature* **310**: 419–421.

Bryant, P. E., L. Bradley, M. MacLean & J. Crossland. 1989. Nursery rhymes, phonological skills and reading. *Journal of Child Language* **16**: 407–428.

Chukovsky, K. 1963. *From two to five*. Berkeley: University of California Press.

Cossu, G., D. Shankweiler, I. Y. Liberman, L. E. Katz & G. Tola. 1988. Awareness of phonological segments and reading ability in Italian children. *Applied Psycholinguistics* **9**: 1–16.

De Cara, B. & U. Goswami. 2002. Statistical analysis of similarity relations among spoken words: evidence for the special status of rimes in English. *Behavioural Research Methods and Instrumentation* **34**(3): 416–423.

Demont, E. & J. E. Gombert. 1996. Phonological awareness as a predictor of recoding skills and syntactic awareness as a predictor of comprehension skills. *British Journal of Educational Psychology* **66**: 315–332.

Dollaghan, C. A. 1994. Children's phonological neighbourhoods: half empty or half full? *Journal of Child Language* **21**: 257–271.

Durgunoglu, A. Y. & B. Oney. 1999. A cross-linguistic comparison of phonological awareness and word recognition. *Reading & Writing* **11**: 281–299.

Elkonin, D. B. 1963. The psychology of mastering the elements of reading. In B. Simon & J. Simon (Eds.), *Educational psychology in the USSR* (pp. 551–579). Stanford, CA: Stanford University Press.

Fernald, A. & C. Mazzie. 1991. Prosody and focus in speech to infants and adults. *Developmental Psychology* **2**: 209–221.

Goswami, U. & J. C. Ziegler. 2006. Fluency, phonology and morphology: a response to the commentaries on becoming literate in different languages. *Developmental Science* **9**: 451–453.

Harris, M. & V. Giannouli. 1999. Learning to read and spell in Greek: the importance of letter knowledge and morphological awareness. In M. Harris & G. Hatano (Eds.), *Learning to read and write: a cross-linguistic perspective* (pp. 51–70). Cambridge, UK: Cambridge University Press.

Ho, C. S.-H. & P. Bryant. 1997. Phonological skills are important in learning to read Chinese. *Developmental Psychology* **33**: 946–951.

Hoien, T., L. Lundberg, K. E. Stanovich & I. K. Bjaalid. 1995. Components of phonological awareness. *Reading & Writing* **7**: 171–188.

Jusczyk, P. W. & R. N. Aslin. 1995. Infants' detection of the sound patterns of words in fluent speech. *Cognitive Psychology* **29**: 1–23.

Kuhl, P. K. 1986. Reflections on infants' perception and representation of speech. In J. Perkell & D. Klatt (Eds.), *Invariance and variability in speech processes* (pp. 19–30). Norwood, NJ: Ablex.

Kuhl, P. K. 2004. Early language acquisition: cracking the speech code. *Nature Reviews Neuroscience* **5**: 831–843.

Liberman, I. Y., D. Shankweiler, F. W. Fischer & B. Carter. 1974. Explicit syllable and phoneme segmentation in the young child. *Journal of Experimental Child Psychology* **18**: 201–212.

Lundberg, I., A. Olofsson & S. Wall. 1980. Reading and spelling skills in the first school years predicted from phonemic awareness skills in kindergarten. *Scandinavian Journal of Psychology* **21**: 159–173.

Perfetti, C. A., I. Beck, L. Bell & C. Hughes. 1987. Phonemic knowledge and learning to read are reciprocal: a longitudinal study of first grade children. *Merrill-Palmer Quarterly* **33**: 283–319.

Porpodas, C. D. 1999. Patterns of phonological and memory processing in beginning readers and spellers of Greek. *Journal of Learning Disabilities* **32**: 406–416.

Seymour, P. H. K., M. Aro & J. M. Erskine. 2003. Foundation literacy acquisition in European orthographies. *British Journal of Psychology* **94**: 143–174.

Siok, W. T. & P. Fletcher. 2001. The role of phonological awareness and visual-orthographic skills in Chinese reading acquisition. *Developmental Psychology* **37**: 886–899.

Treiman, R. & J. Baron. 1981. Segmental analysis: developmental and relation to reading ability. In G. C.

MacKinnon & T. G. Waller (Eds.), *Reading research: advances in theory and practice* (Vol III, pp. 159–198). New York: Academic Press.

Treiman, R. & A. Zukowski. 1991. Levels of phonological awareness. In S. Brady & D. Shankweiler (Eds.), *Phonological processes in literacy* (pp. 67–83). Hillsdale, NJ: Erlbaum.

Tunmer, W. E. & A. R. Nesdale. 1985. Phonemic segmentation skill and beginning reading. *Journal of Educational Psychology* **77:** 417–427.

Wimmer, H., K. Landerl, R. Linortner & P. Hummer. 1991. The relationship of phonemic awareness to reading acquisition: more consequence than precondition but still important. *Cognition* **40:** 219–249.

Wimmer, H., K. Landerl & W. Schneider. 1994. The role of rhyme awareness in learning to read a regular orthography. *British Journal of Developmental Psychology* **12:** 469–484.

Ziegler, J. C. & U. Goswami. 2005. Reading acquisition, developmental dyslexia and skilled reading across languages: a psycholinguistic grain size theory. *Psychological Bulletin* **131**(1): 3–29.

Ziegler, J. C. & U. Goswami. 2006. Becoming literate in different languages: similar problems, different solutions. *Developmental Science* **9:** 429–453.

Ziegler, J. C., G. O. Stone & A. M. Jacobs. 1997. What's the pronunciation for -OUGH and the spelling for /u/? A database for computing feedforward and feedback inconsistency in English. *Behavior Research Methods, Instruments, & Computers* **29:** 600–618.

Development of Ventral Stream Representations for Single Letters

Peter E. Turkeltaub,[a,b] **D. Lynn Flowers,**[c] **Lynn G. Lyon,**[a] **and Guinevere F. Eden**[a]

[a] *Center for the Study of Learning, Department of Pediatrics, Georgetown University, Washington, DC, USA*

[b] *Department of Neurology, University of Pennsylvania Health System, Philadelphia, Pennsylvania, USA*

[c] *Wake Forest University School of Medicine, Winston-Salem, North Carolina, USA*

Visual form recognition is mediated by the ventral extrastriate processing stream. Some regions of ventral stream cortex show preferential activity for specific stimulus categories, but little is known about how this regional specialization develops. Acquisition of letter-naming skill is of particular interest because letter recognition serves as the gateway to visual processing of words, and fluent letter naming predicts children's reading success. For this reason, we examined the school-age development of visual letter processing using fMRI. In a 2 x 2 design, we compared ventral stream BOLD activity in two groups, children ($n = 22$, age 6–11) and adults ($n = 15$, age 20–22), during two tasks: naming of single letters and naming of simple line drawings of objects. We hypothesized that, based on adults' greater experience with letters, the posterior left fusiform gyrus would be activated more in adults for letter naming than it would be in children. We found that bilateral areas of ventral stream cortex during letter naming were activated in both children and adults and that the midposterior areas of the fusiform gyrus in both hemispheres were activated to a greater degree in adults than in children. There were no areas within the ventral stream in either hemisphere that were activated preferentially for letters over line drawings, nor were there any significant differences in the developmental changes observed for letter naming compared to object naming. These findings indicate that visual processing of single letters continues to develop in both hemispheres during grade school. However, we found no evidence for development of areas specialized for single letter processing. Rather, our findings suggest that letter recognition is performed using the same general form recognition systems as are used to process other visually similar stimuli.

Key words: letter-naming development; ventral stream; single letters

Introduction

Visual recognition of objects in human and nonhuman primates is mediated by the ventral extrastriate processing stream (Aggleton & Mishkin, 1983; Haxby *et al.*, 1991). In adults, the ventral stream neural representations of specific categories of visual stimuli such as faces, body parts, letter strings, and words have been characterized using functional neuroimaging (Clark *et al.*, 1996; Cuenod *et al.*, 1995; D'Esposito, Ballard, Aguirre, & Zarahn, 1998; Haxby *et al.*, 1994; Kanwisher, McDermott, & Chun, 1997; Polk & Farah, 2002; Puce, Allison, Asgari, Gore, & McCarthy, 1996). While the degree of domain specificity in these regions is debated (Haxby *et al.*, 2001),

Address for correspondence: Guinevere Eden, D.Phil., Center for the Study of Learning, Georgetown University Medical Center, Box 571406, Suite 150, Building D, 4000 Reservoir Road, NW, Washington, DC 20057. edeng@georgetown.edu
[b]Current address: Department of Neurology, University of Pennsylvania Health System, 3400 Spruce Street, 3W Gates Building, Philadelphia, PA 19104, USA.

Ann. N.Y. Acad. Sci. 1145: 13–29 (2008). © 2008 New York Academy of Sciences.
doi: 10.1196/annals.1416.026

evidence of localized preferential activation for specific categories of stimuli is well established (e.g., faces vs. houses). The question of how this differentiation occurs remains a matter of debate. The relative roles of genetic predetermination and environmental influence, the attributes of visual stimuli and their context that drive experiential specification, and the time course of development all remain active areas of investigation.

The development of ventral stream representations of linguistic stimuli is of particular interest. Written language is an invention of modern humans, and thus the extrastriate encoding of this class of stimuli cannot be genetically predetermined. Furthermore, rapid automatic identification of words, thought to be mediated by ventral stream processing, is vital to fluent reading. Typical adult readers consistently activate left midfusiform gyrus when presented with single words or pseudowords. The functional properties of this area in neuroimaging studies and its role in disorders of reading have lead some to refer to it as the "visual word form area" (VWFA) (Cohen *et al.*, 2004; Cohen *et al.*, 2000; Price & Devlin, 2003; see also Price & Devlin, 2004). Despite this moniker, recent neuroimaging studies of reading acquisition in unimpaired children have yielded inconsistent results in the development of ventral stream representations of words. While some have identified increases in left fusiform activity associated with increasing reading skill (Shaywitz *et al.*, 2002; Simos *et al.*, 2001), others have not (Schlaggar *et al.*, 2002; Turkeltaub, Gareau, Flowers, Zeffiro, & Eden, 2003). Conversely, some studies have identified areas of decreasing word-reading activity in right hemisphere ventral stream cortex over the course of schooling (Simos *et al.*, 2001; Turkeltaub *et al.*, 2003), while others have not (Schlaggar *et al.*, 2002; Shaywitz *et al.*, 2002). Neuroimaging and electrophysiological studies of learning novel writing systems in adult subjects have generally demonstrated changes in temporoparietal and frontal activity associated with learning, rather than changes in ventral stream activity (Bitan,

Manor, Morocz, & Karni, 2005; Lee *et al.*, 2003).

Reading is a complex skill involving several interacting cognitive processes that could make delineating the development of visual word recognition units difficult. Access to the identity of a word may be achieved through one of multiple proposed routes (e.g., letter-by-letter decoding vs. holistic orthographic access) (Coltheart, Curtis, Atkins, & Haller, 1993; Jobard, Crivello, & Tzourio-Mazoyer, 2003), and hence the strategy of the reader may affect the localization of activity (Cohen, Jobert, Le Bihan, & Dehaene, 2004). While a consistent change in strategy across readers may be part of the developmental course of reading acquisition (Ehri, 1999; Turkeltaub *et al.*, 2003), these strategic shifts may also alter the relative contributions of different aspects of visual recognition, making it difficult to decipher whether true developmental changes in visual representations of words have occurred. Likewise, interconnections of phonological and semantic processing systems have been implicated in feedback and top-down modulation of visual orthographic representations of words (Bokde, Tagamets, Friedman, & Horwitz, 2001; Ishai, Ungerleider, & Haxby, 2000; Pecher, 2001). Thus, differences between adults and children in the number of phonological or semantic neighbors of selected words or the complexity of semantic or phonological representations of words may distort localization of true visual developmental effects in extrastriate cortex.

Because of these interactions, it is important to first ask how single letters are recognized and whether visual representations of single letters change over the course of reading acquisition. Letter recognition serves as the initial gateway for access to abstract representations of words (Pelli, Farell, & Moore, 2003), and knowledge of letter identity and fluency of rapid letter naming are predictors of later reading ability when measured in young children (Badian, 1998; Neuhaus, Foorman, Francis, & Carlson, 2001; Neuhaus & Swank, 2002; Wolf, 1986). As letters are unitary symbols, no serial decoding mechanisms are available as they are for word reading, and so no developmental shifts in strategic approach to letter naming are expected. Likewise, because letters have no semantic representations and far simpler phonological representations compared to words, they are subject to less top-down and feedback modulation of visual processes by frontal and temporoparietal systems. Hence, identification of letters is a more purely visual task, and observed developmental effects in visual cortex are relatively interpretable. Additionally, children typically begin to learn the identity of letters at a very young age and hence can participate in experiments using naturalistic naming tasks rather than decision tasks, which require additional processes that may alter localization within the ventral stream (Cohen *et al.*, 2004).

Psychometric studies have provided some evidence that visual processing of single letters changes over the course of schooling (Nazir, Ben-Boutayab, Decoppet, Deutsch, & Frost, 2004). To further address the localization of single-letter visual processing and its development, we performed an fMRI study examining these processes in primary school–age children and adults. Depending on the timing of maturation of letter-form processing systems we anticipated two opposite patterns of age-related differences in ventral stream activity. If circuitry for letter recognition is established prior to age 6, when children are first gaining familiarity with letters, then both groups in our study would perform the letter naming task using the same neural processing system. However, within this ventral stream area, we would expect less activity for adults compared to children during letter naming because automaticity of performance is associated with a decreased level of activity in mature systems. This inverse relationship between activity and task performance was demonstrated specifically for ventral extrastriate single-letter recognition activity in a PET study of normal adult readers (Garrett *et al.*, 2000). In contrast, if mature letter-form processors are not established early, but continue to develop as children gain exposure to print in late childhood, we would expect greater ventral stream activity for adults during letter naming compared to children on account of the engagement of new processing systems. If multiple distributed systems are utilized for letter identification, the timing of maturation might occur differentially in distinct regions of the ventral stream, such that adults would activate some areas more than children and some areas less.

The precise localization of these developmental changes is somewhat more difficult to predict. Variable findings in studies of adults cannot be used to support a specific hypothesis of localization. Visual and orthographic processing of letter strings has been studied frequently in adults (Polk & Farah, 1998, 2002; Puce *et al.*, 1996; Pugh *et al.*, 1996), but these results are not likely to generalize to single-letter recognition given previous evidence for differential activation to single letters and strings (James, James, Jobard, Wong, & Gauthier, 2005). Because single letters are relatively simple shapes composed of few edges and angles and recognition of single letters is a preliminary step in recognition of whole words, we hypothesized that letter identification would localize to an area earlier than the VWFA in the ventral processing stream, that is, the left fusiform gyrus posterior to the VWFA.

We used a simple overt single-letter naming task as our activation condition. Although silent viewing or naming has been used in some of the studies of single-letter processing in adults, we required overt responses in order to monitor our subjects' performance of the task. We also examined naming of simple line drawings of objects for comparison of developmental changes in ventral stream activity. Objects were selected because they have previously been contrasted with single letters in a neuroimaging study of adults (Joseph, Gathers, & Piper, 2003), and children do not gain repeated exposure to every member of their class during school, as they do for both letters and digits. We generated a ROI of ventral stream cortex in each hemisphere to maximize statistical power and looked for effects of age, task, and hemisphere in the regions as a whole and on a voxel-wise basis within the ROI.

Methods

Subjects

We studied 22 healthy children (age range, 6.4–11.6 years [mean = 8.7]; 11 female) and 15 healthy adults (age range 20.0–22.1 [mean = 20.7]; 8 female). All subjects were monolingual, right-handed native English speakers with no personal or family history of neurological or learning disorders. Subjects were recruited through flyers distributed to Washington, DC–area private schools and posted at Georgetown University. The Georgetown University Institutional Review Board approved all experimental procedures, and written informed consent was obtained from each participant and a legal guardian. Each subject completed the experimental protocol in three sessions over a 3-week span. Subjects participated in fMRI tasks examining single-word processing and simple motor processing in addition to the experiments presented here (Turkeltaub, Weisberg, Flowers, Basu, & Eden, 2005). Adult subjects were paid for their participation, whereas children received small prizes, stamps, and stickers.

All subjects completed a behavioral battery including standardized measures of I.Q., confrontation picture naming, rapid automatized naming, word reading, novel word decoding, passage-reading fluency, verbal fluency, reading and oral comprehension, receptive and expressive language, working memory, phonological processing, and gross and fine motor coordination (Turkeltaub *et al.*, 2005). A clinical neuropsychologist (D.L.F.) evaluated scores on behavioral measures to rule out previously undiagnosed learning disorders. The children in this study could identify all 26 English letters, and all but the youngest subject could name the sound associated with each letter. Right-

handedness was confirmed by the Edinburgh Handedness Inventory (Oldfield, 1971).

fMRI Methods

fMRI Task

We used a simple block design overt naming paradigm to assess brain activity during identification of letters and objects. Individual stimuli were presented and subjects were instructed to name each item aloud as quickly and as accurately as possible. Ten letter stimuli (a, b, c, d, e, o, p, r, s, x) were selected on the basis of their early age of acquisition to ensure maximal performance by even the youngest subjects. Letters were presented in lowercase Arial font. Visually simple line drawings of objects with single-syllable names and early age of acquisition (key, heart, box, spoon, star, sun, nail, cup, sock, moon) were selected to match letter stimuli as best possible for visual and phonological complexity (Snodgrass & Vanderwart, 1980). In some cases, lines were thickened or thinned to better match the visual density of letter stimuli. All stimuli were presented in black on a white background for 1 second, followed by a response period in which a black crosshair appeared on a white background for 1.65 seconds. Task performance was interleaved with fMRI volume acquisition so that three stimuli were presented serially in this manner, followed by a 4-second period of fMRI gradient noise during which the crosshair appeared. Subjects completed two runs with two 60-second epochs of letter naming and two 60-second epochs of object naming interleaved with five 24-second epochs of visual fixation. Fifteen items were presented in random order during each task epoch. Each item was repeated six times over the two runs. Vocalized responses were recorded when possible for scoring accuracy and reaction time.

Subjects were shown the list of possible stimuli prior to scanning to ensure that they knew their identity. Occasionally, subjects used an alternate name for object items (e.g., mug instead of cup). In these cases, they were not corrected to avoid inhibition and self-correction during scanning. Subjects then completed an abbreviated computer-administered practice run outside the scanner.

fMRI Data Acquisition

To minimize head motion and improve compliance, we trained children extensively on an MRI simulator prior to scanning, used foam pads to restrict head movement during scanning, and limited children's time in the scanner to 25 minutes per session. Functional MRI data presented here were collected during a single session lasting approximately 20 minutes. Children then received a 20-minute break outside the scanner prior to collection of anatomical data and additional fMRI data not considered here. Adults remained in the scanner prior to collection of these additional data. Anatomical data consisted of two MPRAGE 3-D T1-weighted images.

We acquired whole-brain echo-planar images (EPI; TR = 4 s, TE = 40 ms, 64 × 64 matrix, 230 mm FOV, 46 axial slices, 3.6 mm cubic voxels) on a 1.5 Tesla Siemens Vision Magnetom scanner with a circularly polarized head coil. To minimize susceptibility artifacts associated with spoken responses and acoustic contamination from gradient noise, we used the "behavior-interleaved gradient" (BIG) technique, in which fMRI data are acquired during periods between task performance (Eden & Zeffiro, 1999). Subjects named three items presented during an 8-second period of gradient silence, followed by a 4-second interval of no task performance during which one whole-head volume was acquired. In this way, subjects are able to give spoken responses without interference from gradient noise and jaw motion occurred between scan acquisitions, thereby minimizing artifact. The acquisition of images immediately after an 8-second period of task performance assures that BOLD signal is measured after the initiation and maximization of the hemodynamic response (Eden & Zeffiro, 1999). Further, this method allows a greater number of volumes to be acquired in a given time relative to event-related paradigms. This factor is important in order to maximize statistical power within the limited time that children tolerate the MRI environment. Two runs were collected, each lasting 6.5 minutes, and consisting of 32 EPI volumes. Each run began with an acclimation period of two volumes (24 seconds) to allow for longitudinal magnetization equilibration. A total of 20 volumes per condition (letters, objects, fixation) was acquired across the two runs.

Data Postprocessing

Imaging data were analyzed using MEDx (Sensor Systems, Sterling, VA, USA). Each run from each subject underwent the following processing steps: head motion detection and correction (automated image registration (AIR) six-parameter rigid body realignment algorithm) (Woods, Grafton, Holmes, Cherry, & Mazziotta, 1998; Woods, Grafton, Watson, Sicotte, & Mazziotta, 1998), global intensity normalization, gaussian spatial filtering (10.8 mm FWHM), high-pass temporal filtering (Butterworth 243.5 second cutoff). Mean difference, percent change, and Z-maps were calculated for each subject for each run. These statistical maps were aligned with the SPM99 Talairach template using an AIR 12 parameter linear affine transformation. Individual subject mean-difference and percent-change maps (letter versus fixation, object versus fixation) were created by averaging the two spatially normalized single-run maps for each subject. Individual subject Z-maps were created by combining Z-maps from both runs ($Z = (Z_1 + Z_2)/\sqrt{2}$) (Turkeltaub *et al.*, 2005). Images were checked for head motion and artifact to ensure the quality of data. Subjects were excluded if they had greater than 0.7 mm peak-to-peak head motion in any dimension on either run after motion correction, or if the combined unthresholded Z-map received an artifact rating (based mainly on rimming) of five or greater on a seven-point scale, as assessed by two blinded experts. After motion correction, there were no significant differences between adults and children in head motion as measured by the

TABLE 1. Performance of Naming Tasks

	Accuracy (%)	Response time (ms)
Children		
Letters	98.4 (3.2)	911 (130)
Objects	94.8 (6.0)	1165 (153)
Adults		
Letters	100.0 (0.0)	753 (65)
Objects	99.8 (0.6)	931 (67)

mean 3D pathlength per volume of the image center of intensity (children 0.07 mm/volume, adults 0.06 mm/volume, $P = 0.28$). Group-level voxel-wise statistics were calculated as random effects analyses using a single mean-difference image for each task comparison (letters versus fixation, objects versus fixation) for each subject.

Results

Task Performance

All subjects' responses were monitored at the time of scanning for compliance with task instructions. Responses were recorded for 17 children and nine adults. Accuracy of naming was calculated for all of these subjects, and response times were measured for 16 children and eight adults (Table 1). All subjects performed the task with greater than 80% accuracy.

Performance scores were entered into a 2 × 2 ANOVA with age (children vs. adults) and task (letter naming vs. object naming) as fixed factors, and response time and accuracy as dependent variables. Despite efforts to make the tasks as simple as possible for young children and reassuring pilot data, a significant main effect of age was observed for naming accuracy, $F(1,22) = 8.38$, $P = 0.006$. Post-hoc t-tests demonstrated that adults named objects more accurately than did children, $t(25) = 3.42$, $P = 0.003$. The difference in letter-naming accuracy did not achieve significance, $t(25) = 2.08$, $P = 0.054$. There was no effect of task on accuracy, $F(1,22) = 2.67$, $P = 0.11$. For response time, main effects of

both task, $F(1,22) = 32.89$, $P < 0.001$ and age, $F(1,22) = 27.1$, $P < 0.001$ were significant. Post-hoc t-tests demonstrated that both children and adults named letters more quickly than objects, children $t(25) = 18.4$; adults $t(25) = 11.7$, both $P < 0.001$, and adults performed both tasks more quickly than children, letters $t(25) = 3.98$, objects $t(25) = 5.18$, both $P < 0.001$. No age × task interactions were observed for either accuracy, $F(1,22) = 2.16$, $P = 0.15$, or response time, $F(1,22) = 0.99$, $P = 0.33$.

fMRI Results

To address questions of ventral stream development for naming of objects and letters, we developed regions of interest defining the ventral occipitotemporal areas activated during letter and object naming regardless of age. A main effect of naming Z-map was generated using a single group t-test combining both letter-naming-versus-fixation and object-naming-versus-fixation mean-difference images for all 37 subjects. This statistical map was thresholded at $P < 0.05$, resel-corrected for multiple comparisons. Clusters within the ventral occipitotemporal cortex were identified and converted to masks. Because the resultant clusters were contiguous with nearby cerebellar activations, cerebellar voxels were eliminated on the basis of anatomical boundaries in an averaged T-1 weighted image of adults and children. This process resulted in one ROI in each hemisphere representing areas within the ventral stream that were active during naming regardless of task and regardless of age (Fig. 1: *Left*: 600 voxels, *center:* −42 −61 −17, bounding box × −27 to −52, y −41 to −82, z 0 to −31; *Right*: 832 voxels, *center:* 41 −61 −24, bounding box × 14 to 53, y −39 to −85, z −8 to −35). These ROI encompassed large segments of the fusiform gyri in both hemispheres, and parts of the inferior occipital gyri, middle occipital gyri, and the inferior temporal gyri. Most voxels lay within Brodmann's areas 37 and 19, with fewer within area 18.

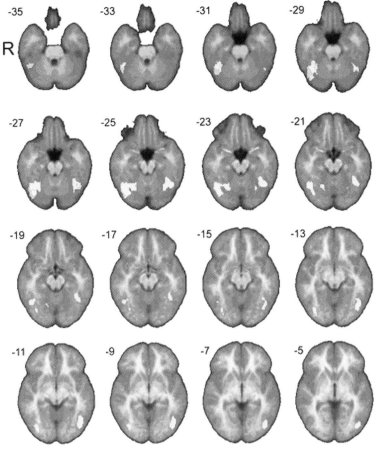

Figure 1. Main effect of naming region-of-interest (ROI). Axial slices demonstrate ventral occipitotemporal voxels achieving a corrected significance of $P < .05$ in the main effect of naming analysis. Voxels in the cerebellum were removed on the basis of anatomic boundaries to create one VOI in each hemisphere. These two VOIs were used to constrain hypothesis testing in all further analyses.

Analysis of the fMRI data was restricted to the voxels in these two ROI in order to constrain our hypothesis testing to ventral occipitotemporal cortex and to increase the sensitivity of our analyses by reducing the number of comparisons performed for voxel-wise analyses. Results of these ROI analyses are organized as follows: First we present the results of single-group analyses to demonstrate areas activated by each group of subjects for each of the naming tasks. Next, we present results of a 2×2 voxel-wise ANOVA comparing activity between groups and between tasks. Finally, we present results of similar ANOVA performed on mean activity within the ROI in order to identify hemispheric differences in development of visual activity.

Single-Group Analyses

We first examined the group-level activity within the ventral stream ROI of the adults and children for letter naming and object naming compared to fixation. The critical threshold for these comparisons was a two-tailed $P < 0.05$, resel-corrected for multiple comparisons. Both groups activated several areas of ventral occipitotemporal cortex for both stimulus types, including Brodmann's areas (BA) 18, 19, and 37 (Fig. 2; Table 2). Adults activated large areas of cortex both anteriorly and posteriorly, medially

TABLE 2. Significant Foci of Activity in Naming Tasks versus Fixation

Gyrus	BA	Adults				Chidren			
		x	y	z	Z-score	x	y	z	Z-score
Letters versus Fixation									
Left Fusiform	37					−40	−44	−16	2.86
Fusiform	37	−38	−48	−28	3.17				
Fusiform	37	−50	−58	−24	3.56	−44	−54	−22	4.09
Fusiform	19	−30	−60	−24	3.59				
Fusiform	19	−36	−64	−26	3.60				
Fusiform	19	−50	−66	−10	3.66				
Inferior/middle occipital	18	−44	−74	−8	3.98	−44	−76	−8	3.46
Inferior/middle occipital	18	−42	−74	−12	3.78				
Right Fusiform	37	40	−40	−28	3.03				
Fusiform	37					38	−52	−30	3.09
Fusiform	37	50	−60	−24	3.55				
Fusiform	19	30	−60	−22	5.38				
Fusiform	19	18	−64	−18	4.08				
Fusiform	19	38	−70	−28	3.77				
Fusiform	18	42	−74	−20	4.09				
Inferior/middle occipital	18	40	−76	−10	2.84	40	−80	−10	3.31
Objects versus Fixation									
Left Fusiform	37	−34	−44	−24	3.28	−36	−44	−22	4.53
Fusiform	37	−42	−52	−28	4.58	−36	−52	−22	4.47
Fusiform	37	−40	−56	−12	2.97				
Fusiform	37	−32	−56	−24	4.37				
Fusiform	37	−46	−62	−24	4.31				
Inferior temporal	37					−46	−64	−12	4.11
Inferior/middle occipital	18	−40	−72	−12	4.70	−44	−76	−8	4.05
Right Fusiform	37	42	−48	−30	4.35	44	−46	−34	3.57
Fusiform	37	50	−56	−26	4.63	48	−60	−16	4.34
Fusiform	37	32	−58	−24	4.73	30	−58	−26	3.15
Fusiform	37					46	−60	−24	3.84
Fusiform	19	18	−64	−18	3.98				
Fusiform	19	42	−74	−20	4.43	46	−76	−26	4.40
Inferior/middle occipital	18	42	−74	−12	3.76				
Fusiform	18	38	−84	−12	3.27				

and laterally for both tasks. The number and distribution of significant maxima were qualitatively similar between adults and children for object naming, but the children activated only a few areas during letter naming: one mid BA 37 and one posterior BA 18 locus in the right hemisphere, and one anterior BA 37, one mid BA 37, and one posterior BA 18 locus in the left hemisphere.

Comparisons between Groups and Tasks Using Voxel-Wise ANOVA

We next examined the magnitude and location of between-group differences in ventral

TABLE 3. Significant Activation Foci from the ANOVA

	Gyrus	BA	x	y	z	Z-score	Post-hoc test Z-scores			
							Children O > L	Adults O > L	Objects A > C	Letters A > C
Main Effects										
Objects > letters	Fusiform	37	−34	−48	−22	2.84	3.66*	1.96		
Letters > objects						n.s.				
Adults > children	Fusiform	37	−30	−58	−24	2.91			1.34	2.84*
	Fusiform	37	−48	−60	−28	3.00			2.40	1.99
	Inferior occipital	37	−50	−66	−12	3.43			1.59	3.28*
	Fusiform	37	34	−56	−28	3.92			2.49	2.71*
	Fusiform	37	50	−56	−32	3.30			2.23	2.21
	Fusiform	19	40	−64	−28	4.00			2.07	3.18*
Children > adults						n.s.				
Interaction										
Age × task						n.s.				

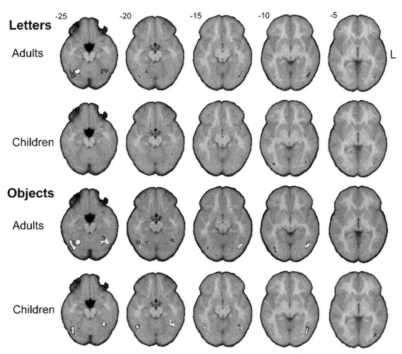

Figure 2. Single-group analyses. Axial slices show ventral occipitotemporal voxels achieving a corrected significance of $P < 0.05$ in the within-group comparisons of letter naming versus fixation and object naming versus fixation.

stream naming activity with a voxel-wise 2×2 ANOVA of BOLD activity within the ROIs using age and task as factors (Table 3). The critical threshold for these comparisons was a two-tailed $P < 0.05$, resel-corrected for multiple comparisons. Areas of the mid/posterior fusiform gyrus in BA 37 and 19 in both hemispheres demonstrated main effects of age with greater activity for adults than children. No areas were identified with greater activity for

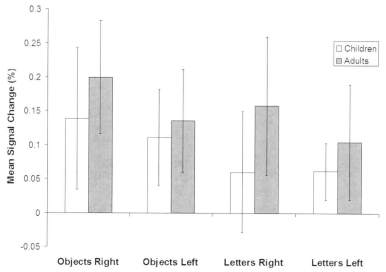

Figure 3. ROI mean activity ANOVA. An ANOVA of mean signal change for letter naming versus fixation and object naming versus fixation comparisons revealed significant main effects of age, hemisphere, and task. Post-hoc analyses showed significantly greater letter-naming activity for adults in the right hemisphere compared to children, and greater object naming activity compared to letter naming in both hemispheres for children and in the right hemisphere for adults.

children than adults. Post-hoc tests demonstrated that in most cases effects of age were driven by significant differences between adults and children in letter-naming activity. In no cases did the post-hoc tests reveal significantly greater object-naming activity for adults compared to children. The main effect of task revealed a single left hemisphere locus in the fusiform gyrus BA 37 anterior to those identified above which activated preferentially for objects over letters. Post-hoc testing revealed significantly greater object-naming activity for children, but not for adults. No voxels demonstrated significant interactions of age and task.

ROI Mean Activity ANOVA

To evaluate global ventral stream activity in adults and children for object and letter naming and to compare left and right hemisphere activity, we next performed an ANOVA of the mean BOLD signal in the ventral stream ROI using age, hemisphere, and task as factors (Fig. 3). This analysis revealed significant main effects of all three factors: age, $F(1,32) = 16.8$,

$P < 0.001$; hemisphere $F(1,32) = 6.597$, $P = 0.01$; task $F(1,32) = 13.0$, $P < 0.001$; but no significant interactions: task × hemisphere $F(1,32) = 0.51$, $P = 0.48$; task × age $F(1,32) = 0.99$, $P = 0.32$; hemisphere × age $F(1,32) = 2.68$, $P = 0.10$; task × age × hemisphere $F(1,32) = 0.10$, $P = 0.75$. Post-hoc t-tests for the main effect of age demonstrated significantly higher activity for adults compared to children only in the right hemisphere for letter naming, $t(36) = 3.01$, $P = 0.006$. There were also trends towards greater activity for adults in the left hemisphere for letter naming, $t(36) = 1.84$, $P = 0.08$, and in the right hemisphere for object naming, $t(36) = 1.98$, $P = 0.06$. Post-hoc t-tests for the effect of hemisphere showed trends towards greater object-naming activity in the right hemisphere compared to the left for both adults, $t(36) = 2.10$, $P = 0.054$, and children $t(36) = 1.89$, $P = 0.07$. No significant or near-significant hemispheric difference was found for letter-naming activity in either age group. Post-hoc tests for the effect of task revealed greater activity for object naming compared to letter naming in both hemispheres for children, right hemisphere $t(36) = 3.61$, $P = 0.002$; left hemisphere $t(36) = 3.66$, $P = 0.001$, and in the right hemisphere for adults, $t(36) = 2.74$, $P = 0.02$. There was also a trend toward greater object-naming activity compared to letter naming in the left hemisphere for adults, $t(36) = 1.96$, $P = 0.07$.

Discussion

The main findings of this study are threefold: (1) letter naming in both children and adults occurred bilaterally with no left hemisphere dominance; (2) adults activated midposterior areas of the fusiform gyrus in both hemispheres to a greater degree than children during letter naming; and (3) there were no areas within the ventral stream in either hemisphere that were activated preferentially for letters over objects, nor were there any significant differences in the developmental patterns for letters compared to objects.

Lateralization of Visual Letter Processing

Given the link between letters and the sounds of speech, one might expect visual processing of single letters to be left-lateralized as it is for words. Indeed, adults activate the left hemisphere more than the right in neuroimaging studies of letter-string processing (Polk & Farah, 1998, 2002; Puce *et al.*, 1996; Pugh *et al.*, 1996). However, these results do not necessarily generalize to single-letter recognition, given evidence for differential activation to single letters and strings (James *et al.*, 2005). Prior imaging studies of single-letter specific processing in adults have isolated right hemisphere areas of letter-selective activity as often as left (Table 4). Likewise, tachistoscopic studies of visual field effects in letter naming have not consistently shown right visual field (left hemisphere) advantage for single letters, nor developmental shifts in laterality of letter processing. For example, Wagner and Harris (Torgesen, Wagner, & Rashotte,

1994) examined the impact of font complexity on visual field effects for letter naming in fourth graders, ninth graders, and adults. None of the three groups showed a significant right visual field advantage for letter naming irrespective of font, and there was no effect of age on the calculated laterality index. Thus, neuroimaging and psychometric data have converged to indicate bilateral visual processing of single letters. Our findings extend these results to include neuroimaging data in children.

The bilateral pattern of activity and development we observed for letter naming in this study contrasts with published studies of word reading. Studies of word reading in adults show left lateralized ventral temporal activity (Turkeltaub, Eden, Jones, & Zeffiro, 2002), and studies of reading development have shown either specific left hemisphere increases in ventral stream cortex or decreasing activity in right hemisphere areas (Schlaggar *et al.*, 2002; Shaywitz *et al.*, 2002; Simos *et al.*, 2001; Turkeltaub *et al.*, 2003). Despite the association between letters and sounds of speech and the improvement in phonological processing skills that occurs coincident with learning to read, letter recognition requires no serial decoding or sequencing of speech sounds, and as such little interaction with left hemisphere phonological systems is expected. This difference in linguistic processing explains why letter recognition is relatively spared compared to word reading in pure alexia, a disorder caused by lesions disconnecting ventral visual cortex from left temporoparietal language areas (McCandliss, Cohen, & Dehaene, 2003). Interactions with these linguistic processing systems may drive lateralization of visual word, pseudoword, and letter-string processing, while not affecting the laterality of single-letter recognition. Alternatively, the task of serial processing and sequencing itself may stimulate left lateralization independent of linguistic or phonological interactions. Because letters are unitary symbols that require no serial decoding, they would remain bilaterally represented in this case.

TABLE 4. Foci of Single-Letter Preferential Activity in Previous Studies

Study	Task	x	y	z
Gauthier *et al.* (2000)	One-back location judgment letters versus faces	50	−59	3
		−53	−62	3
Joseph *et al.* (2003)	Silent naming letters versus line drawings, visual noise, and fixation	–	–	–
Longcamp *et al.* (2003)	Silent viewing letters versus false-font characters (right-handed subjects)	2	−92	29
		8	−83	4
Flowers *et al.* (2004)	Letter judgment versus symbol judgment and color judgment (using the same stimuli)	−62	−57	−6
James *et al.* (2005)	One-back matching letters versus digits and letters versus Chinese characters	−42	−37	−3
Longcamp *et al.* (2005)	Silent viewing letters versus false-font characters (left-handed subjects)	59	−28	−10
Joseph *et al.* (2006)	Silent naming and perceptual matching of letters versus objects	–	–	–

Development of Visual Letter Processing

Our results indicate that adults activate ventral stream cortex bilaterally to a greater degree than children during simple letter-naming tasks. Greater activity in the adults associated with better letter-recognition skill indicates that children were utilizing immature letter-recognition systems, while adults utilized mature ones. As demonstrated in a prior study of letter recognition in adults, if a mature form recognition system is already in place, improved performance on letter-recognition measures is associated with decreased activity in ventral stream cortex, representing automaticity (Garrett *et al.*, 2000). Thus, had the two groups used identical mature recognition systems, the adults would have activated ventral stream cortex less than children did. Increased activity in the adult group here indicates ongoing development of an efficient system for letter recognition in ventral stream cortex during schooling.

This finding supports psychometric evidence that the visual experience of learning to read text influences visual processing of single letters. A tachistoscopic study comparing English and Hebrew letter detection demonstrated that the left-right scanning orientation of a script has an impact on visual processing of even single letters in experienced readers (Nazir

et al., 2004). This indicates that the process of learning to read a given script influences the experience-dependent learning in perception of single letters. While other studies have not found changes in laterality of single-letter processing between children and adults (Wagner & Harris, 1994), none would be expected if development occurs bilaterally, as our data indicate.

Even though explicit instruction on single-letter identification ends very early in schooling, ongoing development of letter-recognition systems later in grade school is not surprising given the accelerating rate at which children are exposed to print during this period. Reading ability and rate of print exposure interact in a feed-forward fashion during grade school; in unimpaired children reading ability increases as a function of print exposure, and in turn the rate of print exposure increases as children become more fluent readers. This increasing rate of print exposure is likely key in the consolidation of efficient form recognition systems used to rapidly identify letters as well as words.

Localization and Specificity of Visual Letter Processing

Letters are relatively simple objects composed of a few edges and angles, typically viewed in high contrast relative to their background. Identification of letters requires processing of first-order characteristics only (e.g., two vertical lines with a horizontal line between is an "H"). Second-order characteristics that vary with size and font are disregarded so that a given stimulus can be identified based on first-order characteristics (Gauthier *et al.*, 2000). Given these processing demands and that identification of letters is a necessary preliminary step leading to word reading (Pelli *et al.*, 2003), one might anticipate that letter recognition would primarily engage areas somewhat earlier in the processing stream compared to words, that is, posterior and medial to the midfusiform gyrus VWFA. Indeed, the left hemisphere regions we identified showing developmental changes in letter-naming activity lie just medial and posterior to the typical peaks for the VWFA (as compared to mean coordinates −43, −54, −12 for the VWFA; Cohen *et al.*, 2000). The right hemisphere regions showing development of letter processing lie in the homologous areas contralaterally. However, our results also reveal large areas of bilateral ventral stream activity for letter naming in comparison with fixation, consistent with a distributed network subserving visual letter processing.

While all complex stimuli seem to engage distributed areas of extrastriate cortex (Haxby *et al.*, 2001), other commonly encountered classes of objects elicit activity in specific ventral stream areas that respond preferentially to that stimulus class over others (e.g., faces, houses, words), and are consistently localized across subjects (e.g., fusiform face area, parahippocampal place area, visual word form area) (Cohen *et al.*, 2004; Haxby *et al.*, 1994; Ishai, Ungerleider, Martin, Schouten, & Haxby, 1999; Kanwisher *et al.*, 1997). Given the frequency with which literate adults encounter letters in daily life, one might also expect that a cortical area would develop to specifically or preferentially process letters. However, the few studies contrasting single-letter processing with processing of other stimulus categories have yielded mixed results in both localization

and specialization of letter processing (Table 4). Gauthier (Gauthier *et al.*, 2000) used a one-back location matching task to compare activation for viewing single letters and faces. They identified bilateral regions in the fusiform gyri that responded preferentially to letters. The left hemisphere region was near the posterior edge of the VWFA, and the right hemisphere region was in a homologous location. These regions also showed habituation in that activity was greater when the font varied between stimuli compared to when the font of all stimuli was the same. Longcamp and colleagues. (Longcamp, Anton, Roth, & Velay, 2003) compared letter viewing to false font character viewing in a group of right-handed adults and identified early medial visual areas in the right cuneus and posterior lingual gyrus which responded preferentially to letters. However, when the experiment was repeated in a group of left-handed adults, a different region, in the right posterior middle temporal gyrus (BA 21) responded preferentially to letters (Longcamp, Anton, Roth, & Velay, 2005). Flowers (Flowers *et al.*, 2004) utilized different decision tasks to direct subjects' attention to specific attributes of the same stimuli (letters and symbols displayed in two colors), and isolated a lateral middle occipital gyrus region of BA 37 specifically activated by attention to letter identity. This area lay anterior and lateral to a midposterior fusiform region, which was active regardless of the attentional focus of the task. James (James *et al.*, 2005) used a one-back matching task comparing Roman letters, digits, and unfamiliar Chinese characters both individually and embedded within strings. They localized an area selective for individual letters anterior and medial to the VWFA, which was identified using a pseudoword versus letter-string contrast. This was differentiated from an area just posterior to the VWFA that was responsive to Roman letters strings. Joseph (Joseph *et al.*, 2003) compared silent naming of single letters and objects and found conjoined areas of activity for the two tasks, but no area that responded specifically to letters. The logically based analysis technique used in this study may have precluded localization of areas responsive to both stimulus types but preferential for letters. Using both silent naming and a perceptual matching task, Joseph, Cerullo, Farley, Steinmetz, and Mier (2006) identified areas of common activity in ventral stream cortex for letters and objects, but no area specialized for letters in comparison to objects for both naming and matching tasks.

Even though most of the studies above identified at least one area that responded preferentially to letters, given the inconsistency in localization of these findings, these reports cannot be used to support a domain-specific region for letter processing. In the absence of a specialized area, the comparison chosen by a given imaging study likely highlights regions involved in processing the attributes that are maximally different between letters and the particular control condition. Additionally, differing task demands may affect the degree of activation in various parts of the distributed system, altering the areas activated by each study.

Likewise, we found no clear evidence for progressive specialization of any area for letter recognition in comparison to recognition of objects. No areas were identified as a main effect or in either age group individually that responded preferentially to letters over drawings. While the developmental effects in ventral stream activity observed in the main effect of age analysis were primarily driven by differences between the groups in letter-naming activity, there were no significant interactions between task and age. It is possible that greater effort and duty cycle required for naming objects, as evidenced by lower accuracy and longer response times compared to letter naming, artificially increased object-naming activity and hence masked letter-preferential areas. It is also possible that a study with the statistical power to support single subject analyses would have revealed letter-specific activations that were relatively co-localized across subjects, but too disparate to result in group-level activity. However, given our findings, along with those of Joseph and colleagues in adults (Joseph *et al.*, 2003) and children (Joseph *et al.*, 2006), and the variability in the results of other studies of single-letter processing, it is likely that single letters are processed using the same distributed form recognition circuits as other simple high-contrast stimuli. Further support of this theory comes from a behavioral study of literate and illiterate Portuguese women that found that formal schooling improved accuracy and reaction time for naming line drawings of objects (taken from the same collection as our stimuli; Snodgrass & Vanderwart, 1980), but not the actual corresponding three-dimensional objects (Reis, Petersson, Castro-Caldas, & Ingvar, 2001). This effect was interpreted as generalization of improving letter-recognition systems as a consequence of learning to read, implying that visual processing of letters and line drawings might rely on overlapping cortical networks. Imaging studies of letter naming using longitudinal designs with sufficient statistical power to support single subject analyses will be needed to further test this theory.

Conclusions

Aloud naming of letters activated bilateral areas of ventral stream cortex in children and adults. Task-related signal change was greater in the adult group compared to children in bilateral midposterior areas of the fusiform gyrus. However, we found no evidence of preferential brain activity for the naming of letters compared to the naming of objects within the ventral stream nor did we observe any differences in their developmental patterns. We conclude from this study that letter naming matures during schooling and that this development occurs in the ventral stream of both the left and right hemispheres. Finally, we did not see a differentiation in the development between letters and objects, suggesting that letter processing relies on the same general form recognition systems as that used to process other visually similar stimuli.

Acknowledgments

This work was supported by NICHD Grant HD40095, NIMH Grant F31 MH6500, and by the General Clinical Research Center Program of the National Center for Research Resources (MO1-RR13297). We wish to thank Martha Miranda, Meagan Lansdale, Sarah Baron, Alyssa Verbalis, Lauren Penniman, Carol Montgomery, and Katherine Cappell for contributing to data collection. We also thank our subjects for their participation.

Conflicts of Interest

The authors declare no conflicts of interest.

References

Aggleton, J. P., & Mishkin, M. 1983. Visual recognition impairment following medial thalamic lesions in monkeys. *Neuropsychologia* **21**(3): 189–197.

Badian, N. A. 1998. A validation of the role of preschool phonological and orthographic skills in the prediction of reading. *Journal of Learning Disabilities* **31**(5): 472–481.

Bitan, T., Manor, D., Morocz, I. A., & Karni, A. 2005. Effects of alphabeticality, practice and type of instruction on reading an artificial script: an fMRI study. *Brain Research. Cognitive Brain Research* **25**(1): 90–106.

Bokde, A. L., Tagamets, M. A., Friedman, R. B., & Horwitz, B. 2001. Functional interactions of the inferior frontal cortex during the processing of words and word-like stimuli. *Neuron* **30**(2): 609–617.

Clark, V. P., Keil, K., Maisog, J. M., Courtney, S., Ungerleider, L. G., & Haxby, J. V. 1996. Functional magnetic resonance imaging of human visual cortex during face matching: a comparison with positron emission tomography. *NeuroImage* **4**(1): 1–15.

Cohen, L., Dehaene, S., Naccache, L., Lehericy, S., Dehaene-Lambertz, G., Henaff, M. A., *et al.* 2000. The visual word form area: spatial and temporal characterization of an initial stage of reading in normal subjects and posterior split-brain patients. *Brain* **123**(Pt 2): 291–307.

Cohen, L., Jobert, A., Le Bihan, D., & Dehaene, S. 2004. Distinct unimodal and multimodal regions for word processing in the left temporal cortex. *NeuroImage* **23**(4): 1256–1270.

Coltheart, M., Curtis, B., Atkins, P., & Haller, M. 1993. Models of reading aloud: dual-route and parallel-distributed-processing approaches. *Psychological Review* **100**(4): 589–608.

Cuenod, C. A., Bookheimer, S. Y., Hertz-Pannier, L., Zeffiro, T. A., Theodore, W. H., & Le Bihan, D. 1995. Functional MRI during word generation, using conventional equipment: a potential tool for language localization in the clinical environment. *Neurology* **45**(10): 1821–1827.

D'Esposito, M., Ballard, D., Aguirre, G. K., & Zarahn, E. 1998. Human prefrontal cortex is not specific for working memory: a functional MRI study. *NeuroImage* **8**(3): 274–282.

Eden, G., & Zeffiro, T. 1999. The possible relationship between visual deficits and dyslexia. *Journal of Learning Disabilities* **32**(5): 378.

Ehri, L. C. 1999. Phases of development in learning to read words. In J. Oakhill & R. Beard (Eds.), *Reading development and the teaching of reading* (pp. 79–108). Oxford: Blackwell.

Flowers, D. L., Jones, K., Noble, K., VanMeter, J., Zeffiro, T. A., Wood, F. B., *et al.* 2004. Attention to single letters activates left extrastriate cortex. *NeuroImage* **21**(3): 829–839.

Garrett, A. S., Flowers, D. L., Absher, J. R., Fahey, F. H., Gage, H. D., Keyes, J. W., *et al.* 2000. Cortical activity related to accuracy of letter recognition. *NeuroImage* **11**(2): 111–123.

Gauthier, I., Tarr, M. J., Moylan, J., Skudlarski, P., Gore, J. C., & Anderson, A. W. 2000. The fusiform "face area" is part of a network that processes faces at the individual level. [erratum appears in *Journal of Cognitive Neuroscience* 2000 Sep;12(5):912]. *Journal of Cognitive Neuroscience* **12**(3): 495–504.

Haxby, J. V., Gobbini, M. I., Furey, M. L., Ishai, A., Schouten, J. L., & Pietrini, P. 2001. Distributed and overlapping representations of faces and objects in ventral temporal cortex. *Science* **293**(5539): 2425–2430.

Haxby, J. V., Grady, C. L., Horwitz, B., Ungerleider, L. G., Mishkin, M., Carson, R. E., *et al.* 1991. Dissociation of object and spatial visual processing pathways in human extrastriate cortex. *Proceedings of the National Academy of Sciences of the United Sates of America* **88**(5): 1621–1625.

Haxby, J. V., Horwitz, B., Ungerleider, L. G., Maisog, J. M., Pietrini, P., & Grady, C. L. 1994. The functional organization of human extrastriate cortex: a PET-rCBF study of selective attention to faces and locations. *Journal of Neuroscience* **14**(11 Pt 1): 6336–6353.

Ishai, A., Ungerleider, L. G., & Haxby, J. V. 2000. Distributed neural systems for the generation of visual images. *Neuron* **28**(3): 979–990.

Ishai, A., Ungerleider, L. G., Martin, A., Schouten, J. L., & Haxby, J. V. 1999. Distributed representation of objects in the human ventral visual pathway. *Proceedings of the National Academy of Sciences of the United Sates of America* **96**(16): 9379–9384.

James, K. H., James, T. W., Jobard, G., Wong, A. C., & Gauthier, I. 2005. Letter processing in the visual system: different activation patterns for single letters and strings. *Cognitive, Affective & Behavioral Neuroscience* **5**(4): 452–466.

Jobard, G., Crivello, F., & Tzourio-Mazoyer, N. 2003. Evaluation of the dual route theory of reading: a metanalysis of 35 neuroimaging studies. *NeuroImage* **20**(2): 693–712.

Joseph, J. E., Cerullo, M. A., Farley, A. B., Steinmetz, N. A., & Mier, C. R. 2006. fMRI correlates of cortical specialization and generalization for letter processing. *NeuroImage* **32**(2): 806–820.

Joseph, J. E., Gathers, A. D., & Piper, G. A. 2003. Shared and dissociated cortical regions for object and letter processing. *Brain Research. Cognitive Brain Research* **17**(1): 56–67.

Kanwisher, N., McDermott, J., & Chun, M. M. 1997. The fusiform face area: a module in human extrastriate cortex specialized for face perception. *Journal of Neuroscience* **17**(11): 4302–4311.

Lee, J. S., Narayana, S., Lancaster, J., Jerabek, P., Lee, D. S., & Fox, P. 2003. Positron emission tomography during transcranial magnetic stimulation does not require micro-metal shielding. *NeuroImage* **19**(4): 1812–1819.

Longcamp, M., Anton, J. L., Roth, M., & Velay, J. L. 2003. Visual presentation of single letters activates a premotor area involved in writing. *Neuroimage* **19**(4): 1492–1500.

Longcamp, M., Anton, J. L., Roth, M., & Velay, J. L. 2005. Premotor activations in response to visually presented single letters depend on the hand used to write: a study on left-handers. *Neuropsychologia* **43**(12): 1801–1809.

McCandliss, B. D., Cohen, L., & Dehaene, S. 2003. The visual word form area: expertise for reading in the fusiform gyrus. *Trends in Cognitive Sciences* **7**(7): 293–299.

Nazir, T. A., Ben-Boutayab, N., Decoppet, N., Deutsch, A., & Frost, R. 2004. Reading habits, perceptual learning, and recognition of printed words. *Brain and Language* **88**(3): 294–311.

Neuhaus, G., Foorman, B. R., Francis, D. J., & Carlson, C. D. 2001. Measures of information processing in rapid automatized naming (RAN) and their relation to reading. *Journal of Experimental Child Psychology* **78**(4): 359–373.

Neuhaus, G. E., & Swank, P. R. 2002. Understanding the relations between RAN letter subtest components and word reading in first-grade students. *Journal of Learning Disabilities* **35**(2): 158–174.

Oldfield, R. C. 1971. The assessment and analysis of handedness: the Edinburgh inventory. *Neuropsychologia* **9**(1): 97–113.

Pecher, D. 2001. Perception is a two-way junction: feedback semantics in word recognition. *Psychonomic Bulletin & Review* **8**(3): 545–551.

Pelli, D. G., Farell, B., & Moore, D. C. 2003. The remarkable inefficiency of word recognition. *Nature* **423**(6941): 752–756.

Polk, T. A., & Farah, M. J. 1998. The neural development and organization of letter recognition: evidence from functional neuroimaging, computational modeling, and behavioral studies. *Proceedings of the National Academy of Sciences of the United Sates of America* **95**(3): 847–852.

Polk, T. A., & Farah, M. J. 2002. Functional MRI evidence for an abstract, not perceptual, word-form area. *J Exp Psychol Gen* **131**(1): 65–72.

Price, C. J., & Devlin, J. T. 2003. The myth of the visual word form area. *NeuroImage* **19**(3): 473–481.

Price, C. J., & Devlin, J. T. 2004. The pro and cons of labelling a left occipitotemporal region: the visual word form area. *NeuroImage* **22**(1): 477–499.

Puce, A., Allison, T., Asgari, M., Gore, J. C., & McCarthy, G. 1996. Differential sensitivity of human visual cortex to faces, letterstrings, and textures: a functional magnetic resonance imaging study. *Journal of Neuroscience* **16**(16): 5205–5215.

Pugh, K. R., Shaywitz, B. A., Shaywitz, S. E., Constable, R. T., Skudlarski, P., Fulbright, R. K., *et al.* 1996. Cerebral organization of component processes in reading. *Brain* **119**(Pt 4): 1221–1238.

Reis, A., Petersson, K. M., Castro-Caldas, A., & Ingvar, M. 2001. Formal schooling influences two- but not three-dimensional naming skills. *Brain and Cognition* **47**(3): 397–411.

Schlaggar, B. L., Brown, T. T., Lugar, H. M., Visscher, K. M., Miezin, F. M., & Petersen, S. E. 2002. Functional neuroanatomical differences between adults and school-age children in the processing of single words. *Science* **296**(5572): 1476–1479.

Shaywitz, B. A., Shaywitz, S. E., Pugh, K. R., Mencl, W. E., Fulbright, R. K., Skudlarski, P., *et al.* 2002. Disruption of posterior brain systems for reading in children with developmental dyslexia. *Biological Psychiatry* **52**(2): 101–110.

Simos, P. G., Breier, J. I., Fletcher, J. M., Foorman, B. R., Mouzaki, A., & Papanicolaou, A. C. 2001. Age-related changes in regional brain activation during phonological decoding and printed word recognition. *Developmental Neuropsychology* **19**(2): 191–210.

Snodgrass, J. G., & Vanderwart, M. 1980. A standardized set of 260 pictures: norms for name agreement, image agreement, familiarity, and visual complexity. *Journal of Experimental Psychology. Human Learning* **6**(2): 174–215.

Torgesen, J. K., Wagner, R. K., & Rashotte, C. A. 1994. Longitudinal studies of phonological processing and reading. *Journal of Learning Disabilities* **27**(5): 276–286; discussion 287–291.

Turkeltaub, P. E., Eden, G. F., Jones, K. M., & Zeffiro, T. A. 2002. Meta-analysis of the functional neuroanatomy of single-word reading: method and validation. *NeuroImage* **16**(3 Pt 1): 765–780.

Turkeltaub, P. E., Gareau, L., Flowers, D. L., Zeffiro, T. A., & Eden, G. F. 2003. Development of neural mechanisms for reading. *Nature Neuroscience* **6**(7): 767–773.

Turkeltaub, P. E., Weisberg, J., Flowers, D. L., Basu, D., & Eden, G. F. 2005. The neurobiological basis of reading: a special case of skill acquisition. In H. Catts & A. Kamhi (Eds.), *The connection between language and reading disabilities* (pp. 105–130). Mahwah, NJ: Lawrence Erlbaum.

Wagner, N. M., & Harris, L. J. 1994. Effects of typeface characteristics on visual field asymmetries for letter identification in children and adults. *Brain and Language* **46**(1): 41–58.

Wolf, M. 1986. Rapid alternating stimulus naming in the developmental dyslexias. *Brain and Language* **27**: 360–379.

Woods, R. P., Grafton, S. T., Holmes, C. J., Cherry, S. R., & Mazziotta, J. C. 1998. Automated image registration: I. General methods and intrasubject, intramodality validation. *Journal of Computer Assisted Tomography* **22**(1): 139–152.

Woods, R. P., Grafton, S. T., Watson, J. D., Sicotte, N. L., & Mazziotta, J. C. 1998. Automated image registration: II. Intersubject validation of linear and nonlinear models. *Journal of Computer Assisted Tomography* **22**(1): 153–165.

Neural Correlates of Nouns and Verbs in Early Bilinguals

Alice H.D. Chan,[a,b] Kang-Kwong Luke,[a,b] Ping Li,[c] Virginia Yip,[d] Geng Li,[e] Brendan Weekes,[f] and Li Hai Tan[a,b]

[a]State Key Laboratory of Brain and Cognitive Sciences

[b]Department of Linguistics, University of Hong Kong, Hong Kong, China

[c]Department of Psychology, University of Richmond, Richmond, Virginia, USA

[d]Department of Linguistics and Modern Languages, Chinese University of Hong Kong, Hong Kong, China

[e]Faculty of Medicine, University of Hong Kong, Hong Kong, China

[f]Department of Psychology, University of Sussex, Brighton, United Kingdom

Previous neuroimaging research indicates that English verbs and nouns are represented in frontal and posterior brain regions, respectively. For Chinese monolinguals, however, nouns and verbs are found to be associated with a wide range of overlapping areas without significant differences in neural signatures. This different pattern of findings led us to ask the question of where nouns and verbs of two different languages are represented in various areas in the brain in Chinese–English bilinguals. In this study, we utilized functional magnetic resonance imaging (fMRI) and a lexical decision paradigm involving Chinese and English verbs and nouns to address this question. We found that while Chinese nouns and verbs involved activation of common brain areas, the processing of English verbs engaged many more regions than did the processing of English nouns. Specifically, compared to English nouns, English verb presentation was associated with stronger activation of the left putamen and cerebellum, which are responsible for motor function, suggesting the involvement of the motor system in the processing of English verbs. Our findings are consistent with the theory that neural circuits for linguistic dimensions are weighted and modulated by the characteristics of a language.

Key words: nouns and verbs; bilingualism; fMRI; reading; language; Chinese–English bilinguals; putamen; cerebellum

Introduction

How do bilinguals process and organize two languages in the brain? Are the distinctive features of two languages differentially weighted in cortical representations? Research on these questions is important for advancing our understanding of how one brain supports separate languages. While recent brain imaging studies have investigated neural circuits underlying language organization and language selection in bilinguals who speak similar (e.g., both languages are alphabetic) (Crinion *et al.*, 2006; Kim, Relkin, Lee, & Hirsch, 1997; Klein, Milner, Zatorre, Meyer, & Evans, 1995; Mahendra, Plante, Magloire, Milman, & Trouard, 2003; Mechelli *et al.*, 2004; Perani *et al.*, 1998; Price, Green, & Studnitz, 1999; Rodriguez-Fornells, Rotte, Heinze, Nösselt, &

Address for correspondence: Li Hai Tan or K.K. Luke, State Key Laboratory of Brain and Cognitive Sciences, University of Hong Kong, Pokfulam Road, Hong Kong, China. Voice: +852-2859-1109. tanlh@hku.hk or kkluke@hkusua.hku.hk

Ann. N.Y. Acad. Sci. 1145: 30–40 (2008). © 2008 New York Academy of Sciences.
doi: 10.1196/annals.1416.000

Münte, 2002; Wartenburger *et al.*, 2003) or different languages (Chee, Tan, & Thiel, 1999; Crinion *et al.*, 2006; Gandour *et al.*, 2007; Liu, Dunlap, Fiez, & Perfetti, 2007; Liu & Perfetti, 2003; Luke, Liu, Wai, Wan, & Tan 2002; Tan *et al.*, 2003; Weber-Fox & Neville, 1996), little is known about whether the linguistic distance between the two languages influences neural signatures in the bilingual brain (Jeong *et al.*, 2007).

In the more extreme case, English and Chinese represent languages that vary in numerous aspects, and these linguistic features of each language may make differential demands on the neural circuitry that supports them. This can be extrapolated from studies of monolinguals in these languages (e.g., Gandour *et al.*, 2000; Siok, Perfetti, Jin, & Tan, 2004; Turkeltaub, Gareau, Flowers, Zeffiro, & Eden, 2003). In the Chinese and English languages the two writing systems present sharp contrasts in several dimensions, including orthography, phonology, semantics, and grammar. With respect to grammatical categories, some linguists have gone so far as to argue that grammatical classes like nouns and verbs cannot be properly distinguished as such in Chinese because of the lack of inflectional morphology and the multiple grammatical roles that words can play in this language (Kao, 1990; see also Hu, 1996, for a review of the debates on Chinese lexical classes). In many Indo-European languages, nouns are marked for gender, number, and definiteness, while verbs are marked for aspect, tense, and number. In Chinese, most of these grammatical markers for nouns and verbs are absent (with the exception of aspect markers). In addition, many Chinese verbs can occur freely as subjects and nouns as predicates involving no morphological change (Mo & Shan, 1985). Furthermore, Chinese has a large number of class-ambiguous words that can be used as nouns and as verbs (like *paint* in English); unlike their counterparts in English or other languages, these ambiguous words involve no morphological changes when used in the sentence (Li, Jin, & Tan, 2004). Although such

ambiguous words are also possible in other languages, they may not occur as frequently and may involve morphological changes.

Past research with English has shown that verbs are represented in the left prefrontal cortex, whereas nouns are stored in the posterior brain systems encompassing temporal-occipital regions. This conclusion is supported by both reports from patients of selective dysfunction of word classes (Baxter & Warrington, 1985; Caramazza & Hillis, 1991; Corina *et al.*, 2005; McCarthy & Warrington, 1985; Miceli, Silveri, Villa, & Caramazza, 1984; Zingeser & Berndt, 1988) as well as by neuroimaging studies conducted in normal adults (Damasio & Tranel, 1993; Hauk & Pulvermüller, 2004; Martin, Haxby, Lalonde, Wiggs, & Ungerleider, 1995; Petersen, Fox, Posner, Mintun, & Raichle, 1989; Pulvermuller, 1999; Shapiro, Moo, & Caramazza, 2006; Wise *et al.*, 1991). However, a recent fMRI study examining monolingual Chinese adults in our own laboratory indicated that Chinese nouns and verbs activate a wide range of overlapping brain areas (without a significantly different network) than those reported in the English studies cited above (Li *et al.*, 2004). Relatively fewer distinctive grammatical features of nouns and verbs at the lexical level are likely to be responsible for this finding, but the question may be addressed more directly by employing bilingual individuals.

Hence, in the current study we asked whether for those Chinese-English bilinguals who have acquired the two languages early in life, nouns and verbs of the Chinese and the English language are processed separately. We used functional magnetic resonance imaging (fMRI) while subjects were asked to perform a lexical decision task on nouns and verbs in both Chinese and English. On the basis of the common neural system theory of early bilingualism (Kim *et al.*, 1997; Klein *et al.*, 1995; Mahendra *et al.*, 2003; Wartenburger et al., 2003), one would predict that the pattern of brain activity evoked by nouns and verbs in the two languages is identical.

Methods

Subjects

We carried out functional magnetic resonance imaging (fMRI) in 11 undergraduate students of the University of Hong Kong, whose ages ranged from 21 to 32 years. They gave informed consent in accordance with guidelines set by the Ethics Committee at the University of Hong Kong. All subjects were early Chinese–English bilinguals who started to learn English and Chinese (Cantonese) at age 3 to age 5 (formally through preschool). All were strongly right-handed as judged by the handedness inventory devised by Snyder and Harris (1993). We used nine items involving tasks typically done by only one hand. A 5-point Liket-type scale was used, with "1" representing exclusive left-hand use, and "5" representing exclusive right-hand use. The items were writing a letter, drawing a picture, throwing a ball, holding chopsticks, hammering a nail, brushing teeth, cutting with scissors, striking a match, and opening a door. The scores on the nine items were summed for each subject, with the lowest score (9) indicating exclusive left-hand use for all tasks, and the highest score (45) indicating exclusive right-hand use. All subjects had scores higher than 40.

A first- and second-language proficiency questionnaire was devised to obtain measures of self-reported current abilities in English and Chinese for the bilingual subjects (Tan *et al.*, 2003). On average, subjects began reading English at 3 years of age and received a minimum of 16 years of formal training in English throughout primary school, high school, and university in Hong Kong. The questionnaire also contained a rating scale to assess subjects' self-reported language skills in speaking and reading. Item scores ranged from 1 (*not fluent at all*) to 7 (*very fluent*). The average rating scores of fluency in subjects' English were 5.18 (speaking, SD = 0.75), 5.73 (reading, SD = 0.47). Subjects' scores in Chinese were 6.27 (speaking, SD = 0.90) and 6.36 (reading,

SD = 0.92). There was no significant difference between subjects' rating scores in English and Chinese reading ($t = 1.89$, $P = 0.09$), although their ratings in Chinese speaking was significantly superior to that in English speaking ($t = 3.46$, $P < 0.01$). Thus, the subjects' Chinese-speaking performance was better than the English-speaking performance, despite the early age of acquisition of both languages for Hong Kong students, as has previously been reported (Bolton & Luke, 1999; Luke, 1997).

MRI Data Acquisition

The experiment was performed with a 1.5T scanner (Signa Horizon EchoSpeed with version 8.2 software, General Electric Medical Systems, Milwaukee, WI, USA) at the Queen Mary Hospital, University of Hong Kong. All subjects were visually familiarized with the entire procedure and the experimental conditions before the fMRI scans. A T2*-weighted gradient-echo EPI sequence was used, with the slice thickness = 5 mm, in-plane resolution = 4.3 mm × 4.3 mm, and TR/TE/FA = 3000 ms/60 ms/90 degree. Twenty-four contiguous axial slices were acquired to cover the whole brain. One hundred eighty (180) images were acquired in a single run. The anatomic brain MR images ($1.09 \times 1.09 \times 5$ mm^3) were acquired using a T1-weighted, spin-echo sequence.

fMRI Paradigm

There were four types of stimuli, English verbs, English nouns, Chinese verbs, and Chinese nouns. A total of 66 two-character Chinese words and 66 English words were used. Chinese disyllabic (two-character) words had a frequency of occurrence of no less than 23 per million according to the *Modern Chinese Frequency Dictionary* (1986). English words were of relatively high frequency and had a frequency of occurrence no less than 21 per million (Francis & Kucera, 1982). Within the two language categories, the visual complexity of the stimuli was controlled by the number of strokes in the two characters for Chinese (mean number of strokes for nouns was 20.9, for verbs 19.8), and by the number of letters for English (mean number of letters was 5.9 both for nouns and verbs). Separate sets of 66 disyllabic Chinese pseudowords and English pseudowords were selected to serve as distractors. The Chinese pseudowords were made by the juxtaposition of two legal characters that do not form legal words. English pseudowords were orthographically legal and pronounceable, but had no meanings (e.g., *thove*). The visual complexity of these nonwords was comparable to that of the word stimuli (mean number of strokes was 21.8 for Chinese; mean number of letters was 5.4 for English).

The stimuli were shown through an LCD projector system. Subjects were asked to perform two runs separately, namely, in Chinese and English. Each experimental condition consisted of 33 real words and 33 pseudowords. A block design was used, with three blocks for each experimental condition and six blocks for the baseline condition. Blocks of experimental condition were separated by the baseline condition. Each block in one experimental condition had 22 trials. In each trial, a word (or pseudoword) was exposed for 600 ms, followed by a 1400-ms blank screen. Subjects performed a lexical decision task in which they judged whether or not a visually presented stimulus was a real word. Subjects indicated a positive response by pressing a key with the index finger of their right hand. They were asked to perform the task as quickly and as accurately as possible. A fixation baseline was used, and during this time subjects maintained fixation on a crosshair for 45 seconds.

Data Analysis

Processing of fMRI data was performed using the MATLAB software (Version 6.1; Math Works Inc., Natick, MA, USA) and the SPM99 software package (Wellcome Department of Cognitive Neurology, Institute of Neurology, Queen Square, London, UK). Images were corrected for motion across all runs by using sinc interpolation (Friston *et al.*, 1995). They were then spatially normalized to an EPI template based on the ICBM152 stereotactic space (Cocosco, Kollokian, Kwan, & Evans, 1997), an approximation of canonical space (Talairach & Tournoux, 1988). Images were resampled into $2 \times 2 \times 2$ mm cubic voxels and then spatially smoothed with an isotropic Gaussian kernel (8 mm full width at half-maximum).

Functional images were grouped into English verb, English noun, Chinese verb, and Chinese noun sets. Images from first 6 seconds of each condition were excluded from data processing to minimize the transit effects of hemodynamic responses. Activation maps were generated by using a cross-correction method (Friston *et al.*, 1995), where the activity of each pixel was correlated to a boxcar function that was convolved with the canonical hemodynamic response function. Low-frequency signal components were treated as nuisance covariates. Intersubject variability in global intensity was corrected by the use of proportional scaling to a common mean. Subject-specific linear contrasts for each of the effects of interest were assessed, including noun versus baseline, verb versus baseline, noun versus verb, and verb versus noun, within the same language. These contrasts were then entered into a second-level analysis treating subjects as a random effect, using a one-sample Student's t test against a contrast value of zero at each voxel. Only activations that fell within clusters of fifteen or more contiguous voxels exceeding the uncorrected statistical threshold of $P < 0.005$ were considered significant.

Results

Images of group maps (11 subjects) for nouns versus baseline (fixation) and verbs versus baseline (fixation) in both languages are shown in Figures 1 and 2 and significant areas of

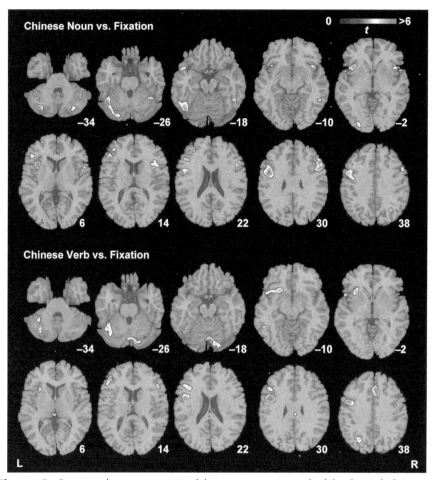

Figure 1. Functional maps: averaged brain activation evoked by lexical decision on Chinese words. The functional maps (*in color*) are overlaid on the corresponding T1 images (*in grayscale*). Planes are axial sections, labeled with the height (mm) relative to the bicommissural line. L = the left hemisphere; R = the right hemisphere.

activation for these comparisons are summarized in Table 1.

Chinese: Chinese nouns and verbs activated a wide range of brain areas, distributed in the frontal, parietal, and occipital areas as well as the cerebellum. Particularly strongly activated by both Chinese nouns and verbs were left middle frontal gyrus (BA 9), left inferior frontal cortex (BAs 44/45/46/47), left medial frontal gyrus (BA 6), left insula, left inferior parietal (BAs 40), left precentral gyrus (BA 4), and bilateral cerebellar regions. Right middle (BAs 9/6) and inferior frontal (BAs 44/45) gyri and left fusiform gyrus also mediated the process-

ing of both kinds of Chinese words. Importantly, a direct comparison of Chinese verbs and nouns did not show significant differences for either direction (i.e., nouns > verbs, or verbs > nouns).

English: Relative to fixation, English nouns and verbs both showed brain activity in left inferior frontal gyrus, left inferior parietal gyrus (BA 40), left medial frontal gyrus, and left cerebellum. Direct comparisons between English verbs and nouns were performed. There was no significant difference for the noun > verb comparison. However, English verbs evoked stronger activation in the left putamen,

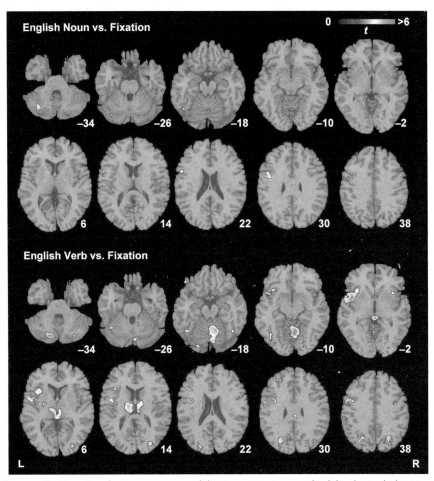

Figure 2. Functional maps: averaged brain activation evoked by lexical decision on English words. The functional maps (*in color*) are overlaid on the corresponding T1 images (*in grayscale*). Planes are axial sections, labeled with the height (mm) relative to the bicommissural line. L = the left hemisphere; R = the right hemisphere.

cerebellum, bilateral medial frontal gyri (BA 6), bilateral precentral gyri (BAs 4 and 6), left fusiform gyrus (BA 37), left precuneus (BA 7), right cuneus (BA 19), and right middle occipital areas (BA 18) (Table 2). Figure 3 illustrates blood-oxygen-level dependent (BOLD) signal changes in two selected regions.

Discussion

This fMRI study used nouns and verbs as stimuli to investigate how bilinguals represent categorical information of words from two different types of written languages. It has demon-strated that, in the early Chinese–English bilinguals' brain, Chinese nouns and verbs showed a largely overlapping pattern of cortical activity. In contrast, English verbs activated more brain regions compared to English nouns. Specifically, the processing of English verbs evoked stronger activities of left putamen, left fusiform gyrus, cerebellum, right cuneus, right middle occipital areas, and supplementary motor area. The recognition of English nouns did not evoke stronger activities in any cortical regions.

Overlapping neural representations for Chinese nouns and verbs may be explained by the ambiguous classification of these two word

TABLE 1. Regions Showing Significant Activations

Regions activated	Noun versus fixation			Verb versus fixation		
	BA	Coordinate	*t*	BA	Coordinate	*t*
Chinese						
Frontal						
L. middle frontal gyrus	9	−45, 18, 32	4.7	9	−43, 20, 27	5.19
	10	−32, 39, 14	4.0			
L. inferior frontal gyrus	45/46	−40, 22, 17	9.50	44	−40, 1, 23	9.34
	44	−40, −5, 21	7.58	46	−41, 32, 10	6.39
				47	−18, 16, −10	5.25
L. medial frontal gyrus	6/8	−4, −1, 54	5.29	6	−3, 14, 55	10.82
L. insula	–	−32, 10, 4	8.55	–	−45, 10, −3	5.76
L. precentral gyrus	4	−34, −11, 45	3.75	4	−27, −9, 50	4.64
R. middle frontal gyrus	9	48, 21, 30	5.80	46	40, 34, 21	4.87
R. inferior frontal gyrus	44	45, 18, 24	6.80	45	41, 24, 15	3.95
R. medial frontal gyrus				8	1, 20, 47	14.49
R. insula	–	38, 10, −5	5.57			
R. precentral gyrus				6	38, −5, 35	3.58
Temporal						
L. superior temporal gyrus	38	−43, 8, −16	4.60			
Parietal						
L. inferior parietal gyrus	40	−43, −48, 38	7.56	40	−38, −54, 44	4.69
				40/7	−34, −46, 50	5.95
L. precuneus	19	−25, −65, 39	6.65	19	−24, −67, 42	9.50
Occipital						
L. inferior occipital gyrus	18	−22, −91, −3	5.22			
L. fusiform gyrus	37	−50, −55, −16	3.25	37	−45, −52, −10	4.11
R.. superior occipital gyrus	19	27, −65, 32	7.14			
Other areas						
Cingulate				32	3, 22, 40	16.14
Thalamas				–	−8, −23, 7	4.57
Cerebellum	–	−32, −75, −34	6.78	–	−32, −75, −34	5.88
		36, −52, −24	7.40		4, −73, −18	5.38
English						
Frontal						
L. superior frontal gyrus				9	−29, 37, 28	3.95
L. inferior frontal gyrus	44	−47, 3, 26	6.05	44	−40, 1, 28	10.23
				45	−36, −1, 19	7.77
L. medial frontal gyrus	6	−3, 10, 50	4.69	6	−1, −9, 56	4.74
L. precentral gyrus				4	−29, −15, 43	4.57
L. putamen				–	−30, −15, −2	5.91
R. inferior frontal gyrus				44	48, 4, 23	4.23
R. medial frontal gyrus				6	3, 1, 49	6.93
R. precentral gyrus				6	36, −5, 33	3.96
Parietal						
L. inferior parietal gyrus	40	−43, −44, 47	4.00	40	−41, −48, 40	4.26
Occipital						
L. superior occipital gyrus				19	−22, −73, 31	12.9
L. fusiform gyrus				19/37	−36, −67, −14	5.67
L. precuneus				7	−22, −71, 42	4.49
L. cuneus				18	−20, −89, 13	4.94
R. middle occipital gyrus				18	22, −77, 19	4.52
				19	26, −83, 8	4.36
R. inferior occipital gyrus				18	24, −91, −3	3.51
R. fusiform gyrus				37	40, −60, −17	4.65
R. cuneus				19	22, −75, 36	9.31
R. precuneus				19	26, −67, 37	6.81
Cerebellum	–	−31, −73, −34	4.59	–	−13, −81, −33	5.96
		−40, −63, −28	3.83		3, −63, −9	6.53

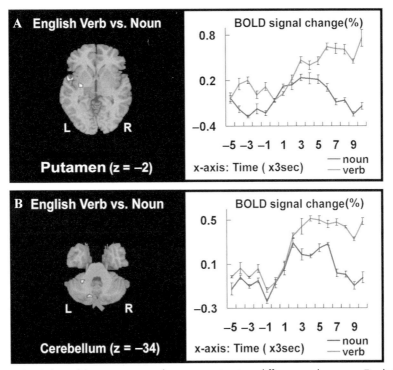

Figure 3. Selected brain regions showing activation differences between English verbs and English nouns. Presented are time course and activation maps in left putamen (**A**) and cerebellum (**B**).

TABLE 2. Regions Showing Significant Activations for English Verbs Compared with English Nouns

Regions activated	English verb versus noun		
	BA	Coordinate	t
Frontal			
L. medial frontal gyrus	6	−20, −5, 58	4.34
L. precentral gyrus	4/6	−40, −1, 14	5.83
L. putamen	–	−30, −14, −2	3.55
R. medial frontal gyrus	6	15, −7, 54	3.52
R. precentral gyrus	4	24, −19, 45	4.42
Occipital			
L. fusiform gyrus	37	−31, −23, −16	4.85
L. precuneus	7	−3, −63, 44	7.87
		−4, −71, 40	7.36
R. middle occipital gyrus	18	24, −81, 10	3.69
R. cuneus	19	4, −69, 37	10.41
Cerebellum	–	−15, −73, −34	5.70

types in Chinese (Li *et al.*, 2004). Hu (1996) suggested that a major portion of the class-ambiguous words were cases whose noun uses were derived from their verb uses, and many nouns in Chinese can be used as verbs (Chan & Tai, 1994). While word classes could hardly be distinguished from each other in Chinese, one can much more easily draw a line to separate English nouns and verbs. In the present study, using fixation as a baseline, English nouns and verbs showed similar patterns of activation in left inferior frontal cortex and left medial frontal gyrus. Importantly, more brain activity was found for English verbs relative to nouns in the left insula, left putamen, left fusiform gyrus, left cerebellum, supplementary motor area (SMA), and right visual cortex. The present pattern of results from our bilingual subjects seems at odds with previous studies with native English speakers, which showed distinct sites for noun processing (Martin *et al.*, 1995; Pulvermuller, 1999; Shapiro *et al.*, 2006), except for one report by Perani and colleagues (1999) who showed that no areas were more active for nouns than for verbs. Thus, verbs seem to be an extremely complex word category, as argued by Pinker (1989).

The involvement of the cerebellum in lexical processing of English verbs is consistent with the recent views that the cerebellum, in addition to its traditionally held motor functions, may play a crucial role in cognitive operations such as sensory acquisition and discrimination (Gao *et al.*, 1996), semantic association in word generation tasks (Martin *et al.*, 1995; Petersen *et al.*, 1989), semantic discrimination (Xiang *et al.*, 2003), verbal learning (Fiez & Raichle, 1997) and reading (Ben-Yehuda & Fiez, this volume). Hypothetically, cerebellar activation for English action words may arise from the action and movement valence denoted by verbs. The strong activity in processing English verbs was also seen in left putamen/insula, and SMA, regions known to formulate motor programming and coordinate speech articulation (Dronkers, 1996; Price, 2000; Wise, Greene, Büchel, & Scott, 1999; Xu *et al.*, 2001), suggesting their particular role in mediating motor-related functions of verbs. Left fusiform gyrus, right cuneus, and left precuneus all exhibited stronger activation in the processing of English verbs. Their function remains to be investigated.

Conclusions

The present findings lend support to the proposal that under specific conditions bilingual learners may deal with word-categorical information of the two languages separately. Specifically, when word class is an important semantic/syntactic marker of language development, such as in English, early bilinguals are able to acquire such category-specific information swiftly. This can be the case even when the other of the two native languages, Chinese, is impoverished in providing morphological devices to distinguish nouns and verbs and does not manifest the same neuronal differentiation. Thus, the bilingual brain is highly plastic in that it handles two language systems in ways that reflect their different design principles.

Acknowledgments

This research was supported by the Hong Kong Research Grants Council Grant HKU 7275/03H (to L.H.T.), the University of Hong Kong Grant 200607176135 (to A.C.), and a 973 Grant (2005CB522802) from the Ministry of Science and Technology of China (to L.H.T.).

Conflicts of Interest

The authors declare no conflicts of interest.

References

Baxter, D. M. & E. K. Warrington. 1985. Category specific phonological dysgraphia. *Neuropsychologia* **23:** 653–666.

Ben-Yehuda, G. & J. A. Fiez. 2008. Impact of cerebellar lesions on reading and phonological processes. Annals of the New York Academy of Sciences, this volume.

Bolton, K. & K. K. Luke. 1999. *Language and society in Hong Kong: The social survey of languages in the 1980s.* Hong Kong: Social Sciences Research Centre, University of Hong Kong.

Caramazza, A. & A. E. Hillis. 1991. Lexical organization of nouns and verbs in the brain. *Nature* **349:** 788–790.

Chan, M. K. M. & J. H. -Y. Tai. 1994. From nouns to verbs: verbalization in Chinese dialects and East Asian languages. In J. Camacho & L. Choueiri (Eds.), *Sixth North American conference on Chinese linguistics* (pp. 49–74). Los Angeles: USC Graduate students in Linguistics (GSIL).

Chee, M. W., E. W. Tan & T. Thiel. 1999. Mandarin and English single word processing studied with functional magnetic resonance imaging. *Journal of Neuroscience* **19:** 3050–3056.

Cocosco, C. A., V. Kollokian, R. K. S. Kwan & A. C. Evans. 1997. Brainweb: online interface to a 3D MRI simulated brain database. *NeuroImage* **5:** 425.

Corina, D. P., E. K. Gibson, R. Martin, A. Poliakov, J. Brinkley & G. A. Ojemann. 2005. Dissociation of action and object naming: evidence from cortical stimulation mapping. *Human Brain Mapping* **24:** 1–10.

Crinion, J., R. Turner, A. Grogan, T. Hanakawa, U. Noppeney, J. T. Devlin, *et al.* 2006. Language control in the bilingual brain. *Science* **312:** 1537–1539.

Damasio, A. R. & D. Tranel. 1993. Nouns and verbs are retrieved with differently distributed neural systems.

Proceedings of the National Academy of Sciences USA **90:** 4957–4960.

Dronkers, N. F. 1996. A new brain region for co-ordinating speech articulation. *Nature* **384:** 159–161.

Fiez, J. A. & M. E. Raichle. 1997. Linguistic processing. In J. D. Schmahmann (Ed.), *The cerebellum and cognition* (pp. 233–254). San Diego: Academic Press.

Francis, W. N. & H. Kucera. 1982. *Frequency analysis of English usage*. Boston: Houghton Mifflin.

Friston, K. J., A. P. Holmes, K. J. Worsley, J. P. Poline, C. D. Frith & R. S. J. Frackowiak. 1995. Statistical parametric maps in functional imaging: a general linear approach. *Human Brain Mapping* **2:** 189–210.

Gandour, J., D. Wong, L. Hsieh, B. Weinzapfel, D. Van Lancker & G. D. Hutchins. 2000. A crosslinguistic PET study of tone perception. *Journal of Cognitive Neuroscience* **12**(1): 207–222.

Gandour, J., Y. Tong, T. Talavage, D. Wong, M. Dzemidzic, Y. Xu, *et al*. 2007. Neural basis of first and second language processing of sentence-level linguistic prosody. *Human Brain Mapping* **28**(2): 94–108.

Gao, J. H., L. M. Parsons, J. M. Bower, J. Xiong, J. Li & P. T. Fox. 1996. Cerebellum implicated in sensory acquisition and discrimination rather than motor control. *Science* **272:** 545–547.

Hauk, O. & F. Pulvermüller. 2004. Neurophysiological distinction of action words in the fronto-central cortex. *Human Brain Mapping* **21:** 191–201.

Hu, M. Y. 1996. *Cilei wenti kaocha [A study of lexical categories]*. Beijing: Institute Press.

Jeong, H., M. Sugiura, Y. Sassa, T. Haji, N. Usui, M. Taira, *et al*. 2007. Effect of syntactic similarity on cortical activation during second language processing: a comparison of English and Japanese among native Korean trilinguals. *Human Brain Mapping* **28**(3): 194–204.

Kao, M. K. 1990. Guanyu hanyu de cilei fenbei [On the differentiation of lexical classes in Chinese]. In M. K. Kao (Ed.), *Kao MK yuyanxue lunwenji [Linguistic essays of Kao Ming Kai]* (pp. 262–272). Beijing: Commercial Press.

Kim, K. H., N. R. Relkin, K. M. Lee & J. Hirsch. 1997. Distinct cortical areas associated with native and second languages. *Nature* **388:** 171–174.

Klein, D., B. Milner, R. J. Zatorre, E. Meyer & A. C. Evans. 1995. The neural substrates underlying word generation: a bilingual functional-imaging study. *Proceedings of the National Academy of Sciences USA* **92:** 2899–2903.

Li, P., Z. Jin & L. H. Tan. 2004. Neural representations of nouns and verbs in Chinese: an fMRI study. *NeuroImage* **21:** 1533–1541.

Liu, Y. & C.A. Perfetti. 2003. The time course of brain activity in reading English and Chinese: an ERP study of Chinese bilinguals. *Human Brain Mapping* **18:** 167–175.

Liu, Y., S. Dunlap, J. Fiez & C. Perfetti. 2007. Evidence for neural accommodation to a writing system following learning. *Human Brain Mapping* **28**(11): 1223–1234.

Luke, K. K., H. L. Liu, W. W. Wai, W. L. Wan & L. H. Tan. 2002. The functional anatomy of syntactic and semantic processing in language comprehension. *Human Brain Mapping* **16:** 133–145.

Luke, K. K. 1997. Why two languages might be better than one: motivations of language mixing in Hong Kong. In M. C. Pennington (Ed.), *Language in Hong Kong at century's end* (pp. 145–160). Hong Kong: Hong Kong University Press.

Mahendra, N., E. Plante, J. Magloire, L. Milman & T. P. Trouard. 2003. FMRI variability and the localization of languages in the bilingual brain. *Neuroreport* **14:** 1225–1228.

Martin, A., J. V. Haxby, F. M. Lalonde, C. L. Wiggs & L. G. Ungerleider. 1995. Discrete cortical regions associated with knowledge of color and knowledge of action. *Science* **270:** 102–105.

McCarthy, R. & E. K. Warrington. 1985. Category specificity in an agrammatic patient: the relative impairment of verb retrieval and comprehension. *Neuropsychologia* **23:** 709–727.

Mechelli, A., J. T. Crinion, U. Noppeney, J. O'Doherty, J. Ashburner, R. S Frackowiak, *et al*. 2004. Neurolinguistics: structural plasticity in the bilingual brain. *Nature* **431:** 757.

Miceli, G., M. C. Silveri, G. Villa & A. Caramazza. 1984. On the basis for the agrammatics difficulty in producing main verbs. *Cortex* **20:** 207–220.

Mo, P. L. & Q. Shan. 1985. Sandalei shici jufa gongleng de tongji fenxi [A statistical analysis of the syntactic functions of three major content word categories]. *Journal of the Nanjing Normal University [Social Science Edition]* **3:** 55–61.

Modern Chinese frequency dictionary. 1986. Beijing, China: Beijing Language Institute.

Perani, D., S. F. Cappa, T. Schnur, M. Tettamanti, S. Collina, M. M. Rosa, *et al*. 1999. The neural correlates of verb and noun processing: a PET study. *Brain* **122:** 2337–2344.

Perani, D., E. Paulesu, N. S. Galles, E. Dupoux, S. Dehaene, V. Bettinardi, *et al*. 1998. The bilingual brain: proficiency and age of acquisition of the second language. *Brain* **121:** 1841–1852.

Petersen, S., P. Fox, M. Posner, M. Mintun & M. Raichle. 1989. Positron emission tomography studies of the processing of single words. *Journal of Cognitive Neuroscience* **1:** 153–170.

Pinker, S. 1989. *Learnability and cognition the acquisition of argument structure*. Cambridge, MA: MIT Press.

Price, C. J. 2000. The anatomy of language: contributions from functional neuroimaging. *Journal of Anatomy* **197:** 335–359.

Price, C. J., D. W. Green & R. Studnitz. 1999. A functional imaging study of translation and language switching. *Brain* **122:** 2221–2235.

Pulvermuller, F. 1999. Words in the brain's language. *Behavioral and Brain Sciences* **22:** 253–279.

Rodriguez-Fornells, A., M. Rotte, H. J. Heinze, T. Nösselt & T. F. Münte. 2002. Brain potential and functional MRI evidence for how to handle two languages with one brain. *Nature* **415:** 1026–1029.

Shapiro, K. A., L. R. Moo & A. Caramazza. 2006. Cortical signatures of noun and verb production. *Proceedings of the National Academy of Sciences USA* **103:** 1644–1649.

Siok, W. T., C. A. Perfetti, Z. Jin & L. H. Tan. 2004. Biological abnormality of impaired reading is constrained by culture. *Nature* **431:** 71–76.

Snyder, P. J. & L. J. Harris. 1993. Handedness, sex, and familial sinistrality effects on spatial tasks. *Cortex* **29:** 115–134.

Talairach, J. & P. Tournoux. 1988. *Co-planar stereotactic atlas of the human brain.* New York: Thieme Medical.

Tan, L. H., J. A. Spinks, C. M. Feng, W. T. Siok, C. A Perfetti, J. Xiong, *et al*. 2003. Neural systems of second language reading are shaped by native language. *Human Brain Mapping* **18:** 158–166.

Turkeltaub, P. E., L. Gareau, D. L. Flowers, T. A. Zeffiro & G. F. Eden. 2003. Development of neural mechanisms for reading. *Nature Neuroscience* **6:** 767–773.

Wartenburger, I., H. R. Heekeren, J. Abutalebi, S. F. Cappa, A. Villringer & D. Perani. 2003. Early setting of grammatical processing in the bilingual brain. *Neuron* **37:** 159–170.

Weber-Fox, C. M. & H. J. Neville. 1996. Maturational constraints on functional specializations for language processing: ERP and behavioral evidence in bilingual speakers. *Journal of Cognitive Neuroscience* **8:** 231–256.

Wise, R. J., J. Greene, C. Büchel & S. K. Scott. 1999. Brain regions involved in articulation. *Lancet* **353:** 1057–1061.

Wise, R., F. Chollet, U. Hadar, K. Friston, E. Hoffner & R. Frackowiak. 1991. Distribution of cortical neural networks involved in word comprehension and word retrieval. *Brain* **114:** 1803–1817.

Xiang, H., C. Lin, X. Ma, Z. Zhang, J. M. Bower, X. Weng, *et al*. 2003. Involvement of the cerebellum in semantic discrimination: an fMRI study. *Human Brain Mapping* **18:** 208–214.

Xu, B., J. Grafman, W. D. Gaillard, K. Ishii, F. Vega-Bermudez, P. Pietrini, *et al*. 2001. Conjoint and extended neural networks for the computation of speech codes: the neural basis of selective impairment in reading words and pseudowords. *Cerebral Cortex* **11:** 267–277.

Zingeser, L. B. & R. S. Berndt. 1988. Grammatical class and context effects in a case of pure anomia: implications for models of language production. *Cognitive Neuropsychology* **5:** 473–516.

Logographic Kanji versus Phonographic Kana in Literacy Acquisition

How Important Are Visual and Phonological Skills?

Maki S. Koyama,[a] **Peter C. Hansen,**[b] **and John F. Stein**[a]

[a]*University of Oxford, Oxford, United Kingdom*

[b]*University of Birmingham, Birmingham, United Kingdom*

It is well-established that phonological skills are important for literacy acquisition in all scripts. However, the role of visual skills is less well understood. For logographic scripts in which a symbol represents a whole word or a meaningful unit, the importance of visual memory in literacy acquisition might be expected to be high because of the visual complexity of logographic characters, but in fact its role remains poorly understood. The Japanese writing system uses both phonographic "Kana" and logographic "Kanji" scripts concurrently and thus allows for the assessment of the contribution of phonological and visual processing to literacy acquisition in these two different scripts in the same language. We tested 74 Japanese children (39 second graders and 35 fourth graders) on a range of literacy, sensory, and cognitive tasks. We found that Kana literacy performance was significantly predicted by low-level sensory processing (both auditory frequency modulation sensitivity and visual motion sensitivity) as well as phonological awareness, but not by visual memory. This result is largely consistent with previous studies in other phonographic scripts such as English. In contrast, Kanji literacy performance was strongly predicted by visual memory (particularly visual long-term memory), but not by either low-level sensory processing or phonological awareness. Our results show differences in the skills that predict literacy performance in phonographic Kana and logographic Kanji, as well as providing experimental evidence that visual memory is important when learning Kanji. Therefore, children's literacy problems and remediation programs should be considered in the context of the script in which children are learning to read and write.

Key words: logographic versus phonographic; visual long-term memory; phonological awareness; low-level sensory processing; reading and writing; Japanese

Introduction

The acquisition of literacy skills varies according to writing systems. These can be broadly divided into phonographic and logographic scripts, and the Japanese writing system uses both scripts concurrently (Fig. 1). Phonographic systems, in which a symbol is mapped onto a sound unit, use alphabetic or syllabic scripts, such as English or Japanese

"Kana," respectively. Logographic systems in which a symbol is mapped onto either a word or morpheme (a meaningful unit) are exemplified by Chinese and by Japanese "Kanji" scripts. There is now a general consensus that phonological skills, such as phonological awareness and phonological short-term memory, play essential roles in reading acquisition in both phonographic (Bradley & Bryant, 1983; Bryant, Maclean, Bradley, & Crossland, 1990; Gathercole, Hitch, Service, & Martin, 1997; Muter, Hulme, Snowling, & Stevenson, 2004) and Chinese logographic writing systems (Ho & Bryant, 1997; Siok & Fletcher,

Address for correspondence: Maki S. Koyama, Department of Physiology, Anatomy and Genetics, University of Oxford, Sherrington Bldg., Parks Road, Oxford, OX1 3PT, UK. maki.koyama@dpag.ox.ac.uk

Ann. N.Y. Acad. Sci. 1145: 41–55 (2008). © 2008 New York Academy of Sciences.
doi: 10.1196/annals.1416.005

私は猫が大好きです。

Figure 1. An example of Japanese sentence. Underlined characters are logographic Kanji and the rest are phonographic Kana (= I like cats very much).

2001). However, phonological awareness seems to contribute to literacy performance to a lesser extent in logographic scripts (McBride-Chang, Bialystok, Chong, & Li, 2004; McBride-Chang *et al.*, 2005; Tan, Spinks, Eden, Perfetti, & Siok, 2005). In contrast, the importance of visual skills in learning to read logographic scripts is still debated. Inconsistent results have been obtained about correlations between visual skills & Chinese reading performance (evidence *for* is provided by Everatt, Jeffries, Elbeheri, Smythe, & Veii, 2006; Ho, Chan, Lee, Tsang, & Luan, 2004; Huang & Hanley, 1995; and evidence *against* is provided by Hu & Catts, 1998; McBride-Chang & Kail, 2002). Therefore, in this study we aimed to clarify the contribution(s) of phonological and visual skills (particularly those involving visual memory) to literacy acquisition by comparing Japanese phonographic Kana and logographic Kanji.

Each Japanese Kana letter represents one mora, which is a subsyllabic unit of sound in Japanese. A mora usually consists of a consonant and a vowel (e.g., "か" represents the mora /ka/). The letter-to-sound correspondence is highly regular and consistent, nearly one-to-one, with minor exceptions. Kana is subdivided into Hiragana and Katakana; Hiragana is usually used for morphological endings and function words, while Katakana is used to write loan words, which are words taken directly into Japanese from another language with very little translation. At school, all 92 Kana letters (46 letters for Hiragana and 46 for Katakana) are introduced to children before Kanji, usually at the beginning of first grade (at the age of 6–7 years). Since Kana has a highly regular orthography, most Japanese children master Kana reading quickly even before the onset of the formal education, but Kana writing is not acquired so fast (Shimamura & Mikami, 1994).

Unlike Kana, Kanji characters are visually complex and usually have multiple pronunciations depending on the context. Although a word can be represented by a single Kanji character, most Kanji words comprise more than two characters, forming so-called compound Kanji words. Thus, the correct pronunciations of Kanji words, especially compound Kanji words, are determined at the whole-word level in a similar fashion to learning to read English exception words such as *yacht*. This unique linguistic property in Kanji differentiates Japanese Kanji from the Chinese logographic system, in which each character has only one or two pronunciations.

Japanese children normally start learning Kanji after having learnt Kana. They are expected to learn 80 Kanji characters by the end of first grade, and by the end of sixth grade they should have mastered 1006 Kanji characters along with 2005 possible pronunciations for these characters (Kess & Miyamoto, 1999). Thus learning Kanji makes intensive demands on memory capacity in both the visual and phonological domains. This is reflected in the higher prevalence of literacy problems in Kanji than in Kana among Japanese children (Uno, 2004).

Consistent with studies in other phonographic scripts, phonological awareness (Hara, 1998) and phonological short-term memory (Kobayashi, Haynes, Macaruso, Hook, & Kato, 2005) are important in learning to read Kana. However, few studies have attempted to elucidate the relationship between phonological skills and literacy development in Kanji. Clearly, the multiple possible pronunciations of each Kanji character demand a retentive phonological memory. As to auditory sensory processing, its contribution to the acquisition of Kana or Kanji remains unknown. However, in phonographic scripts children's sensitivity to auditory frequency modulations (Talcott *et al.*, 2002; Witton, Stein, Stoodley, Rosner, & Talcott, 2002), auditory amplitude modulations (Goswami *et al.*, 2002) and rhythm (Anvari, Trainor, Woodside, & Levy, 2002) are related to their phonological and literacy skills. Similarly, reading performance in logographic Chinese is predicted by auditory frequency and tone discrimination tasks (Meng *et al.*, 2005). However, Chinese is a far more tonal language than Japanese, and thus basic auditory processing may be more important for literacy acquisition in Chinese than in Japanese. To date, no study has investigated the relationship between auditory processing and literacy development in Japanese.

Because of the visual complexity of Kanji, it is likely that visual memory plays an important role in literacy acquisition of this logographic writing system. Yet results of previous studies of logographic reading in Chinese have been inconsistent (Siok & Fletcher, 2001). In phonographic scripts, only a few studies have shown a close relationship between visual memory and reading English (Watson *et al.*, 2003). Recent research, however, has shown that Japanese (Uno, Kaneko, Haruhara, & Kaga, 2000) and Chinese (Ho, Chan, Tsang, Lee, & Chung, 2006) dyslexic children seem to have problems with visual long-term memory. In addition, visual-orthographic skills are impaired in Chinese individuals with dyslexia (Ho, Chan, Lee, Tsang, & Luan, 2004). Unlike letters in phonographic systems, most logographic characters can be visually decomposed into a semantic radical on the left and a phonetic radical on the right, and this sublexicality is thought of as orthography in logographic systems. But phonetic radicals do not always provide reliable information about the pronunciation of logographic characters in either Chinese or Japanese (Saito, Kawakami, & Masuda, 1995). For this reason, it is most likely that skilled Japanese readers showed negative priming effects in phonological and visual-orthographic modalities during a semantic judgment task of Kanji words (Sakuma, Sasanuma, Tatsumi, & Masaki, 1998). These results suggest the strong involvement of visual-orthographic processing in reading logographic Kanji.

One specific measure of low-level visual sensory processing, namely visual motion sensitivity, has been shown to correlate with orthographic skills in both phonographic (Boets, Wouters, van Wieringen, & Ghesquiere, 2006; Talcott *et al.*, 2002) and logographic writing systems (Meng, Zhou, Zeng, Kong, & Zhuang, 2002). Visual motion sensitivity is thought to be a function of the visual magnocellular system, and it may play a role in focusing visual attention and controlling eye movements during reading for sequences of letters and words (Stein, 2003). Although it is controversial as to what extent visual motion sensitivity is causally related to literacy performance in phonographic scripts such as English (Hutzler, Kronbichler, Jacobs, & Wimmer, 2006), little is known about whether low-level visual sensory processing is important for the acquisition of orthographic and literacy skills in phonographic Kana with its extremely regular orthography or in logographic Kanji.

The present study therefore aimed to investigate the contribution of auditory-phonological and visual-orthographic skills to the acquisition of phonographic Kana and logographic Kanji in Japanese children. Our main hypothesis is that, like other phonographic scripts, Kana acquisition will depend on auditory-phonological skills whereas Kanji acquisition will be more affected by visual-orthographic skills, particularly visual long-term memory. Although previous studies using the Rey–Osterrieth Complex Figure test (ROCF) have shown the importance of visual long-term memory for literacy skills in Kanji (Uno, Kaneko, Haruhara, & Kaga, 2000), this test measures many different cognitive abilities in children, such as visuospatial perception, visuospatial construction, and visuospatial memory as well as executive functions (planning and organizational skill) (Watanabe *et al.*, 2005). Hence, the ROCF does not clearly identify which visual-cognitive components contribute to learning Kanji. We have therefore developed a novel recognition task that focuses on the capacity to store visual information in long-term memory and retrieve it in order to understand its specific contribution to Kanji acquisition. In addition, our results should increase our understanding of which abilities are universally important for the development of literacy skills, irrespective of the script or writing system.

Methods

Participants

Seventy-four (74) Japanese children in a state primary school were tested, of whom 39 were second graders (7–8 years of age) and 35 were fourth graders (9–10 years of age). This primary school was located in a middle-class suburban community in Shizuoka prefecture. All children were native Japanese speakers and had no history of neurobiological disorders. Informed parental consent was obtained prior to testing. They had not started learning English reading (or other languages) at the time this study was conducted.

Measures

An extensive battery of intelligence, literacy, sensory, and cognitive tasks was administered to each child individually. None of the tasks in this study have been standardized on a large number of children; thus, we used raw scores and partialled out the effects of age in the analyses.

Nonverbal Intelligence

Raven's Colored Progressive Matrices (Raven, Raven, & Court, 1998) were used to index nonverbal intelligence. The children's nonverbal IQ performance fell within the average range using age-referenced norms at a cutoff level of 1.5 standard deviations (Uno, Shinya, Haruhara, & Kaneko, 2005). Originally, 77 children participated in this study, but 3 children who did not meet this criterion were removed from the data set, resulting in a sample size of 74 children.

Reading and Writing Tasks

Because of the lack of standardized tests for reading and writing in Japanese, new reading and writing tasks were developed to measure children's literacy skills in Kana and Kanji. For reading, the children were asked to read words aloud as accurately and quickly as possible. The writing task was to write down words dictated to them by the experimenter. For each reading and writing task, 20 Kana words were selected from official textbooks used at state primary schools in Japan for first to sixth graders. These included several sounds which are specific to Japanese, such as contracted, double consonant, and long vowel sounds. Likewise, the Kanji words were chosen from the national survey on the "acquisition of Kanji at each grade level" (Japan Foundation for Educational and Cultural Research, 1998). For these Kanji tasks, 60 words were used for the reading task and 40 words for the writing task. Both one-character Kanji words and two-character (compound) Kanji words were arranged in such a way that the difficulty level increased from first to sixth grade. In addition, each set of Kanji words included both visually simple and complex characters, whose complexity was defined by the number of strokes composing the character. Because the number of characters to be mastered for Kanji (640 characters up to the end of fourth grade) is far greater than that for Kana (only 92 characters for Kana), the Kanji tasks included more words than did the Kana tasks.

To measure children's sensory abilities, we used auditory frequency modulation, visual coherent motion, and visual form tasks. All sensory tasks used a 1-up, 2-down adaptive staire procedure.

Auditory Frequency Modulation Task

The frequency modulation task was designed to measure low-level auditory processing (Witton *et al.*, 1998). Children were asked to discriminate between a pure 1-kHz tone and a 1-kHz tone that was frequency modulated at a rate of 2 Hz; the stimuli lasted 1000 ms and the interstimulus interval (ISI) was 500 ms. On each trial, two birds on a computer screen sang the tones one after the other. The children, wearing headphones at a comfortable hearing level (60 dB) in a quiet room, were asked to report verbally which bird, the first or second, had a wobbly voice (the frequency-modulated tone). The detection threshold was estimated as the mean of 16 reversals.

Visual Coherent Motion and Visual Form Tasks

The two low-level visual sensory tasks, the visual motion and visual form tasks, were designed to measure dynamic and static visual processing, respectively (Hansen, Stein, Orde, Winter, & Talcott, 2001). For the visual motion task, children viewed two rectangular patches, each of which contained 300 moving dots. In one patch, the dots moved randomly; in the other, a proportion of the dots moved in the same direction coherently. The children were asked to press the key on the side corresponding to the patch that contained the dots that were moving coherently. Coherent motion was varied to each child's motion-detection threshold by the 1-up, 2-down adaptive staircase procedure, with a constant starting value of 80% coherence. The coherence threshold, indexing the children's visual motion sensitivity, was estimated from the geometric mean of 12 reversals.

For the visual form task, the children viewed two rectangular patches, each of which contained 300 randomly oriented stationary short lines. They were asked to press the key on the side where a subset of the oriented lines formed concentric circles. This subset was then reduced in number according to the 1-up, 2-down staircase. The form threshold was estimated as the mean of 12 reversals.

To measure children's cognitive abilities, we used a battery of phonological, orthographic, and visual tasks. All of these tasks, except for the visual short-term memory task, were developed specially for this study.

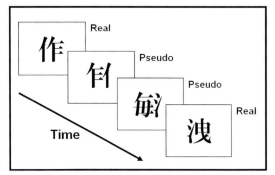

Figure 2. The radical position task (orthographic processing). Children were asked to judge whether a presented character was real or not by pressing the appropriate key. Pseudocharacters were made by reversing radicals between left and right, as shown by the second and third stimuli from the top.

Phonological Tasks

Two phonological tasks were used. The mora deletion task, using "mora" as a subsyllabic unit of sound in Japanese, was a measure of phonological awareness. The nonword repetition task, modified from the original version by Saito (Saito, Saito, & Yoshimura, 2000), was designed to measure children's phonological short-term memory. In the mora deletion task, a set of 25 nonwords, whose length varied from 2 to 6 moras, were presented auditorily. The children were asked to delete one mora (e.g., /ka/) from the spoken nonword (e.g., /sa-ka-jo/). In the nonword repetition task, the children were asked to repeat the nonword immediately after they listened to it. Nonword repetition (Gathercole, Baddeley, & Emslie, 1994) has been used intensively in studying reading in English and is closely related to children's reading performance (Hulslander *et al.*, 2004). For both tasks, the difficulty was increased by increasing the number of mora. The number of correct nonwords repeated by the child was recorded for each task.

Orthographic Task

To measure children's orthographic knowledge, as indicated by their awareness of the internal structure of Kanji, we developed the radical position task (Fig. 2). A randomly mixed

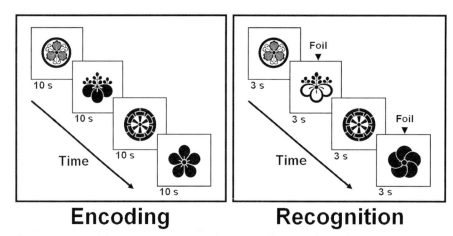

Encoding   Recognition

Figure 3. Visual long-term memory task. During the encoding phase, 20 target stimuli were presented successively (10 sec for each) on a computer screen. For the recognition test (2 hr later), the target stimuli and visually similar foils were randomly and repeatedly presented (3 sec for each), and children were asked to press a key when they thought they had seen the stimulus 2 hr earlier.

set of 40 real Kanji characters and 43 pseudo Kanji characters was presented sequentially on a computer. The pseudocharacters were constructed by reversing the position of the radicals between the left and right. The children were asked to judge whether a presented character was real or not by pressing the appropriate key. Although the real Kanji characters in this task had not been explicitly taught to either group of children, all the left radicals used in this task were familiar to both groups. This was possible because there are only 214 radical elements in Kanji characters and different combinations of these radicals generate an enormous number of Kanji characters. Hence, children theoretically ought to be able to recognize real Kanji characters merely by detecting a left radical on the left side. The task was self-paced by the children, although they were encouraged to proceed as quickly as possible. To perform this task well, the children needed both to understand the internal structure of radicals and to efficiently encode the radical position visually.

Short-Term and Long-Term Visual Memory Tasks

Children's visual memory capacity was measured using both short-term and long-term memory tasks. As a visual short-term memory task, the Visual Patterns Test, which involves no sequencing processing, was used (Della Sala, Gray, Baddeley, Allamano, & Wilson, 1999). Children were presented with a matrix in which half of the squares were black and half white for 3 sec. They were then asked to reproduce the pattern of black squares on the answer sheet by ticking them off with a pen. The difficulty was increased by increasing the number of both black and white squares in the matrix.

To measure visual long-term memory, we developed a new visual long-term memory task (Fig. 3), which used Japanese crests, "Kamon," as visual stimuli. At the beginning of the testing session, the children were instructed to memorize 20 target stimuli that would be presented successively (10 sec for each stimulus) on a computer screen for the later recognition test. At the end of the testing session (approximately 2 hr later), 20 target stimuli and 20 foils, which were visually similar to the target stimuli, were presented for 3 sec per stimulus, and the children were asked to press a key if they thought they had seen the stimulus 2 hr ago. The stimuli were randomly presented and repeated twice in order to reduce false alarms to an acceptable level. To perform this recognition task

TABLE 1. Descriptive Statistics for the Second and Fourth Graders

Measures	Second graders ($N = 39$)		Fourth graders ($N = 35$)	
	Mean	(SD)	Mean	(SD)
Age (months)	96.53	(5.48)	119.49	(3.97)
Literacy				
Kana reading (%)	98.13	(2.93)	99.71	(1.69)
Kana writing (%)	94.75	(5.06)	99.43	(2.65)
Kanji reading (%)	45.12	(10.37)	92.76	(7.40)
Kanji writing (%)	34.17	(11.49)	72.86	(11.60)
Nonverbal IQ				
Raven's Progressive Matrices (max = 36)	27.67	(4.32)	32.76	(1.97)
Sensory				
Frequency modulation (%)[a]	1.49	(0.49)	1.41	(0.86)
Visual motion (%)[a]	9.68	(2.44)	9.22	(3.30)
Visual form (%)[a]	31.55	(4.96)	23.80	(5.69)
Cognitive				
Mora deletion (max = 25)	15.02	(4.41)	20.54	(2.47)
Nonword repetition (max = 40)	20.00	(3.97)	26.40	(4.53)
Radical position (%)	56.99	(10.87)	85.84	(7.21)
Visual Patterns Test (max = 42)	12.33	(3.11)	16.91	(2.51)
Visual LTM (%)	49.42	(12.01)	69.07	(8.83)

Abbreviation: LTM = long-term memory.
[a](%) threshold (%) acuracy.

successfully, the children needed to memorize both global and local (detailed) information about each crest. Of importance, this type of information processing is essential for learning Kanji characters, which often have a strong visual resemblance to each other.

Results

Table 1 shows the descriptive statistics for the Japanese children (second and fourth graders). Even in the second graders, Kana reading performance was very high (at ceiling), confirming that reading Kana is mastered before formal school education starts (Shimamura & Mikami, 1994). Therefore, we did not further analyze the Kana reading data but used only three dependent variables: Kana writing (only for second graders), Kanji reading, and Kanji writing.

Partial correlation analysis controlling for age (Table 2) showed that Kana writing significantly correlated with performance on the Raven's matrices, frequency modulation, vi-

sual motion, mora deletion, nonword repetition, and radical position tasks, but not with the visual memory tasks. Like Kana writing performance, both Kanji reading and Kanji writing correlated with the Raven's matrices, mora deletion, nonword repetition, and radical position tasks, but unlike Kana, strong and significant correlations were found with the visual short-term and long-term memory tasks.

Which Processing Skills Predict Kana Acquisition?

The Kana writing data were negatively skewed, so the data were power transformed; this showed that the data were dichotomous. Therefore we used logistic regression analysis. The second graders were subgrouped into good ($N = 24$) or poor ($N = 15$) Kana writing groups. Poor Kana writers' accuracy rates were 1 standard deviation below the mean of the second graders' performance. These subgroups significantly differed from

TABLE 2. Correlation Analyses between Literacy Measures and Sensory/Cognitive Measures (Controlling for Age)

Measures	Kana writing ($N = 39$)	Kanji reading ($N = 74$)	Kanji writing ($N = 74$)
Raven's matrices	0.58**	0.43**	0.40**
Frequency modulation	−0.63**	0.02	−0.27
Visual motion	−0.52**	−0.02	−0.19
Visual form	−0.17	−0.12	−0.23
Mora deletion	0.60**	0.38*	0.34*
Nonword repetition	0.61**	0.50**	0.37*
Radical position	0.74**	0.59**	0.57**
Visual Patterns	0.19	0.43**	0.60**
Visual LTM	0.14	0.51**	0.78**

Note: The Kana writing data are based on only the second graders' performance ($N = 39$), and nonparametric correlation analysis was performed.

Abbreviation: LTM = long-term memory.

*$P < 0.05$; **$P < 0.01$ (2-tailed).

each other in their performance on the Kana writing task ($P < 0.01$, as determined by the Mann–Whitney U test).

In the logistic regression analyses, we tested five models, each of which controlled for nonverbal IQ (Raven's matrices) and included one of the other independent measures, which showed significant correlations with Kana writing; these included the frequency modulation, visual motion, mora deletion, nonword repetition, and radical position tasks. The co-linearity diagnostics showed a low variance inflation factor (VIF) for each measure in each model (VIFs < 1.3), indicating that there was no problem of multicollinearity in these five models (Allison, 1999). Table 3 shows the descriptive statistics for the good and poor Kana writers and the results of the logistic regression analyses with odds ratios and 95% confidence intervals of the odds ratios. In logistic regression analyses, if there is group difference on the measure concerned, the odds ratio will be significantly larger or smaller than 1.0 (indicating no group difference). After controlling for the Raven's scores, the frequency modulation, visual motion, and mora deletion tasks strongly differentiated the two groups, with odds ratios of 8.64, 3.59, and 0.69, respectively. In other words, when the detection threshold in these low-level sensory processing tasks increased (i.e., the sensitivity to low-level sensory stimuli decreased), the likelihood of being a poor writer in Kana increased significantly. Similarly, when the score in the mora deletion task increased, the likelihood of being a poor writer in Kana decreased significantly (Note: the odds ratio was smaller than 1). The nonword repetition and radical position task predicted Kana writing less strongly.

Which Processing Skills Predict Kanji Reading and Writing Acquisition?

Our main interest in this study was to highlight the similarities and differences in literacy acquisition between phonographic Kana and logographic Kanji. So we combined the data for the Kanji performance of the second and fourth graders and removed the effect of age using multiple regression analyses. The children's age and their Raven's matrices scores were entered as Step 1 and Step 2, respectively, and then one of the other independent measures that correlated with Kanji measures was entered as the final step (Table 4). As would be expected, the child's age or grade was important for both Kanji reading and Kanji writing, accounting for 84.4% ($\Delta F = 388.13, P < 0.01$) and 78.4% ($\Delta F = 260.88, P < 0.01$) of the variance, respectively. This can be partially

TABLE 3. Descriptive Statistics for Good and Poor Kana Writers and the Logistic Regression Analyses Predicting the Success of Kana Writing

Models	Mean (SD)			Odds ratio (95% C.I.)	$P<$
	Good ($N = 24$)	Poor ($N = 15$)	$P<$		
Model 1					
Raven	28.87 (3.06)	26.96 (4.07)	0.01	0.88 (0.79–0.98)	0.05
FM	1.25 (0.45)	1.92 (0.40)	0.01	8.64 (1.59–47.10)	0.01
Model 2					
Raven				0.87 (0.79–0.97)	0.05
Visual motion	8.99 (2.02)	12.54 (3.29)	0.01	3.59 (1.34–9.65)	0.01
Model 3					
Raven				0.90 (0.83–0.98)	0.05
Mora deletion	17.04 (4.07)	13.20 (3.59)	0.01	0.69 (0.68–0.89)	0.01
Model 4					
Raven				0.89 (0.81–0.97)	0.05
Nonword repetition	21.13 (3.88)	18.33 (3.60)	0.01	0.82 (0.66–0.96)	0.05
Model 5					
Raven				0.92 (0.84–1.02)	NS
Radical position	62.21 (8.96)	48.24 (11.98)	0.01	0.88 (0.79–0.97)	0.05

Note: Units are as in Table 1.
Abbreviations: FM = frequency modulation; NS = nonsignificant.

TABLE 4. Summary of Multiple Regressions Predicting Literacy Measures in Kanji (Controlling for Age and Raven Score)

Step	Measures	Literacy measures (ΔR^2)	
		Kanji reading ($N = 74$)	Kanji writing ($N = 74$)
1	Age	0.844**	0.784**
2	Raven score	0.028**	0.024*
3	Mora deletion	0.006	0.008
	Nonword repetition	0.029**	0.025*
	Radical position	0.032**	0.054**
	Visual patterns	0.016*	0.059**
	Visual long term-memory	0.021*	0.097**

*$P < 0.05$; **$P < 0.01$ (two-tailed).

attributed to the Japanese national curriculum: children continue to learn new Kanji characters systematically throughout their primary school education. Nonverbal IQ as measured by Raven's matrices explained an additional 2.8% ($\Delta F = 13.60$, $P < 0.01$) and 2.4% ($\Delta F = 8.77$, $P < 0.05$) of the variance in Kanji reading and Kanji writing, respectively.

After controlling for age and nonverbal IQ, Kanji reading was best predicted by the radical position task, which accounted for an additional 3.2% ($\Delta F = 23.21$, $P < 0.01$) of the variance, followed by the nonword repetition, visual long-term memory, and visual pattern tasks; these accounted for an additional 2.9% ($\Delta F = 19.91$, $P < 0.01$), 2.1% ($\Delta F = 12.98$, $P < 0.05$), and 1.6% ($\Delta F = 9.89$, $P < 0.05$) of the variance, respectively. Kanji writing was best predicted by the visual long-term memory task, which accounted for an additional 9.7% ($\Delta F = 71.39$, $P < 0.01$) of the variance, followed by the visual pattern, radical position, and nonword repetition tasks; these accounted for 5.9% ($\Delta F = 30.67$, $P < 0.01$), 5.4% ($\Delta F = 27.33$, $P < 0.01$), and 2.5% ($\Delta F = 8.87$, $P < 0.05$) of the variance, respectively. Although the mora deletion task was correlated with both Kanji reading and Kanji writing, it was not a significant predictor of Kanji performance when the effect of nonverbal IQ was removed.

Discussion

Our main aim in this study was to investigate similarities and differences in the skills that predict reading and writing in phonographic Kana and logographic Kanji. Our results showed that Kana writing was strongly predicted by low-level sensory processing (in both auditory and visual modalities) and phonological awareness, but not by visual memory, whereas Kanji measures were strongly predicted by visual memory measures, particularly visual long-term memory, but not by either low-level sensory processing or phonological awareness. Another important finding was that both orthographic processing and phonological short-term memory predicted literacy skills in both Kana and Kanji. The results for phonographic Kana are largely consistent with previous studies on reading in other phonographic scripts. But for learning logographic Kanji, visual memory is clearly most important.

Our behavioral results are corroborated by a recent functional magnetic resonance imaging (fMRI) study, which demonstrated that reading Kana and Kanji rely upon some common neural circuits, but differences between the scripts are reflected in greater activation of the left inferior parietal cortex for Kana and in greater activation of the right fusiform area for Kanji (Nakamura, Dehaene, Jobert, Bihan, & Kouider, 2005). The left inferior parietal cortex especially the left supramarginal gyrus, is thought to be involved in phonological storage (Pugh *et al.*, 2000) and the right fusiform gyrus is specifically activated by face perception (Kanwisher, McDermott, & Chun, 1997) and object identification (Vandenbulcke, Peeters, Fannes, & Vandenberghe, 2006). Thus, phonographic Kana may require more phonological processing than logographic Kanji, whereas Kanji may place more visual processing demand than Kana or other phonographic scripts.

Visual-Orthographic Skills

Children's visual long-term memory ability appears to be a robust and unique predictor of their Kanji performance, particularly of Kanji writing. This result is not surprising on account of the visual complexity of Kanji characters, but this study was the first to test children's visual long-term (i.e., recognition) memory experimentally. The results suggest that visual long-term memory is very important for reading and writing logographic characters.

Visual long-term memory has previously been shown to be impaired in dyslexics when learning logographic scripts. For example, some Chinese dyslexic children show problems in retrieval of visual information from long-term memory when writing their names in logographic form even though they were familiar with the sound of their names (Ho, Chan, Tsang, Lee, & Chung, 2006). Similarly, Japanese dyslexic children are poor at delayed recall of the Rey–Osterrieth Complex Figure test (ROCF) (Uno, Kaneko, Haruhara, & Kaga, 2000), which taps a component of visual long-term memory. However, our visual long-term memory task minimized the involvement of executive functions (i.e., organization and planning), which are required for the ROCF, thus demonstrating that visual long-term recognition memory is indeed important in reading and writing logographic Kanji.

The involvement of visual long-term memory in learning to write Kanji should be considered in the light of the close relationship that has been shown between visual long-term memory and sensory-motor representation. A study by Sasaki and Watanabe (1983) demonstrated that the retrieval of familiar Kanji characters was disturbed when finger movements to trace Kanji symbols was prohibited. Furthermore, fMRI studies have shown that both retrieval and writing of well-learned Kanji activated the premotor cortex (Kato *et al.*, 1999), which was also activated by the perception of visually presented Kanji characters (Matsuo *et al.*, 2000) and alphabetic letters (Longcamp, Anton, Roth, & Velay, 2003). These findings suggest that visual representations of characters that are stored in long-term memory may be intimately connected with specific movements that are required for writing them. In fact, Japanese children typically learn to write Kanji characters by repeatedly copying them according to specific stroke orders. Taken together, visual-motor interaction may facilitate memory consolidation for the visual features of Kanji characters and make a specific contribution to learning to write Kanji.

In addition to visual long-term memory, visual short-term memory was a significant predictor of Kanji, but not Kana, performance. This result is in accordance with cross-linguistic studies that show that visual short-term memory is more important for reading in logographic scripts than in phonographic scripts (Everatt, Jeffries, Elbeheri, Smythe, & Veii, 2006; Huang & Hanley, 1995). Although some studies claim that short-term memory and long-term memory are dissociable (Sullivan & Sagar, 1991), the successful transfer of information from short-term memory into long-term memory is crucial for learning in all cognitive modalities. A recent fMRI study has demonstrated a close functional relationship between short-term memory and long-term memory in the visual modality (Ranganath, Cohen, & Brozinsky, 2005): the brain activation in the dorsolateral prefrontal cortex and hippocampus when holding visual information in short-term memory was predictive of successful long-term memory formation. Therefore, good visual short-term memory may lead to good visual long-term memory, which appears to be essential for learning logographic Kanji.

Another important finding was that orthographic processing, measured by the radical position task, was a significant predictor of both Kana and Kanji acquisition. This task was designed to measure children's orthographic knowledge and their visual efficiency for encoding radical position, thus being more visual-orthographic than phonological-orthographic in nature. Similar tasks also predict Chinese reading (Ho, Chan, Lee, Tsang, & Luan, 2004), confirming the importance of visual-orthographic processing in literacy skills in logographic scripts. However, this task used radicals as stimuli, which are constituent elements of Kanji, thus raising the question of its close relationship with Kana writing performance. A possible answer to this question is children's Kana writing was related to their capacity to visually determine the position of the radical within a given character (or pseudocharacter). Indeed, the radical position task was significantly correlated with the visual motion task ($r = -0.47$, $P < 0.01$ from the second graders data and $r = -0.37$, $P < 0.01$ from the full set of data). This is consistent with previous studies, demonstrating that visual motion sensitivity is correlated with orthographic processing in both phonographic (Talcott *et al.*, 2002) and logographic reading (Meng, Zhou, Zeng, Kong, & Zhuang, 2002) as well as with the accurate encoding of letter position (Cornelissen, Hansen, Hutton, Evangelinou, & Stein, 1998). Visual motion sensitivity is a function of the visual magnocellular system, which is thought to be involved in the control of eye movements and attention while reading letters and words sequentially (Stein, 2003). Hence, the visual magnocellular system may contribute to the development of orthographic processing. Although we found no significant correlation between visual motion sensitivity and literacy measures in logographic Kanji, motion sensitivity was a significant predictor of orthographic processing measured by the radical position task, which was the strongest predictor of Kanji reading.

Auditory-Phonological Skills

Our results also revealed relationships between auditory-phonological skills and literacy performance in Kana and Kanji: low-level auditory processing and phonological awareness predicted only Kana writing, whereas phonological short-term memory predicted all the literacy measures (i.e., Kana writing, Kanji reading, and Kanji writing). Low-level auditory processing is closely related to reading in languages with both regular and irregular orthographies such as Norwegian (Talcott *et al.*, 2003) and English (Talcott *et al.*, 2000), respectively. Similarly, phonological awareness predicts literacy performance, irrespective of the level of orthographic regularity (al Mannai & Everatt, 2005; Caravolas & Volin, 2001; Di Filippo *et al.*, 2005; Nikolopoulos, Goulandris, Hulme, & Snowling, 2006). Kana has an extremely regular orthography, and thus children's typical errors in Kana writing were restricted to the sounds which are specific to Japanese, such as double consonants and contractions, as well as to a few Kana letters with exceptional letter-sound correspondences (i.e., letters with more than two pronunciations). To write these sounds successfully, the children needed to be sensitive to the auditory representations being recognized, to be aware of the phonological representations and then to transcribe them into their visual forms. This error trend in Kana confirms that low-level auditory processing and phonological awareness are important in the acquisition of phonographic scripts, irrespective of the level of orthographic regularity. Educationally, our phonological awareness task, which is based on

mora and involves sounds unique to Japanese, may be a sensitive measure to detect children's literacy problems in Kana.

For Kanji performance, phonological short-term memory was a strong predictor, particularly for reading. Because each Kanji character has different pronunciations depending on the context, it is plausible that the memory capacity to store phonological representations of each Kanji character or word plays an important role in learning to read and write Kanji. In contrast, Kanji performance was neither correlated with the auditory processing task (frequency modulation) nor predicted by phonological awareness. This result is different from previous studies on Chinese acquisition, demonstrating that auditory processing (Meng *et al.*, 2005) and phonological awareness (Ho & Bryant, 1997; Siok & Fletcher, 2001) are related to logographic reading in Chinese. This difference between Chinese and Kanji may be attributed to linguistic differences between Chinese and Japanese. First, Chinese is very tonal, but Japanese is not; hence, sensitivity to auditory stimuli, particularly tones, may be more important for Chinese than for Kanji reading. Secondly, Chinese children use "pinyin," a Romanized phonetic system for learning standard Mandarin Chinese. Pinyin seems to improve phonological awareness in Chinese children, as they performed better at phonological awareness tasks than did Hong Kong Chinese children without pinyin training (McBride-Chang, Bialystok, Chong, & Li, 2004). Hence, phonological awareness is often found to be a significant predictor of Chinese reading. Although further investigation directly comparing Chinese and Japanese Kanji may be necessary, our results for Kanji suggest that phonological awareness has a different significance for different logographic writing systems.

Conclusions

There appear to be differences in the skills that predict literacy performance in phonographic Kanji and logographic Kanji. Visual memory, particularly long-term memory, makes a strong contribution to the acquisition of logographic Kanji, but not to the learning of phonographic Kana. In contrast, low-level sensory processing (in both auditory and visual modalities) and phonological awareness play important roles in Kana but not in Kanji acquisition. In addition, phonological short-term memory and orthographic processing may be essential for literacy acquisition, regardless of the script or language. Educationally, our results suggest that children's literacy problems and remediation programs should be considered in the context of the script in which children are learning to read and write.

Conflicts of Interest

The authors declare no conflicts of interest.

References

al Mannai, H., & Everatt, J. 2005. Phonological processing skills as predictors of literacy amongst Arabic speaking Bahraini children. *Dyslexia*, **11**(4): 269–291.

Allison, P. 1999. *Logistic Regression Using the SAS System*; Theory and Application. Cary, NC: SAS Publishing, Wiley InterScience.

Anvari, S. H., Trainor, L. J., Woodside, J., & Levy, B. A. 2002. Relations among musical skills, phonological processing, and early reading ability in preschool children. *Journal of Experimental Child Psychology*, **83**(2): 111–130.

Boets, B., Wouters, J., van Wieringen, A., & Ghesquiere, P. 2006. Coherent motion detection in preschool children at family risk for dyslexia. *Vision Research*, **46**(4): 527–535.

Bradley, L., & Bryant, P. E. 1983. Categorizing sounds and learning to read: causal connection. *Nature*, **301:** 419–421.

Bryant, P. E., Maclean, M., Bradley, L., & Crossland, J. 1990. Rhyme and alliteration, phoneme detection and learning to read. *British Journal of Developmental Psychology*, **26:** 429–438.

Caravolas, M., & Volin, J. 2001. Phonological spelling errors among dyslexic children learning a transparent orthography: the case of Czech. *Dyslexia*, **7**(4): 229–245.

Cornelissen, P. L., Hansen, P. C., Hutton, J. L., Evangelinou, V., & Stein, J. F. 1998. Magnocellular visual function and children's single word reading. *Vision Research*, **38**(3): 471–482.

Della Sala, S., Gray, C., Baddeley, A., Allamano, N., & Wilson, L. 1999. Pattern span: a tool for unwelding visuo-spatial memory. *Neuropsychologia*, **37**(10): 1189–1199.

Di Filippo, G., Brizzolara, D., Chilosi, A., De Luca, M., Judica, A., Pecini, C., et al. 2005. Rapid naming, not cancellation speed or articulation rate, predicts reading in an orthographically regular language (Italian). *Child Neuropsychology*, **11**(4): 349–361.

Everatt, J., Jeffries, S., Elbeheri, G., Smythe, I., & Veii, K. 2006. Cross language learning disabilities and verbal versus spatial memory. *Cognitive Processing*, **7:** 32.

Gathercole, S. E., Baddeley, A. D., & Emslie, H. 1994. The Children's Test of Nonword Repetition: a test of phonological working memory. *Memory*, **2**(2): 103–127.

Gathercole, S. E., Hitch, G. J., Service, E., & Martin, A. 1997. Phonological short-term memory and new word learning in children. *Developmental Psychology*, **33**(6): 966–979.

Goswami, U., Thomson, J., Richardson, U., Stainthorp, R., Hughes, D., Rosen, S., et al. 2002. Amplitude envelope onsets and developmental dyslexia: a new hypothesis. *Proceedings of the National Academy of Sciences of the United States of America*, **99**(16): 10911–10916.

Hansen, P., Stein, J., Orde, S., Winter, J., & Talcott, J. 2001. Are dyslexics' visual deficits limited to measures of dorsal stream function? *Neuroreport*, **12**(7): 1527–1530.

Hara, K. 1998. The development of phonological awareness in normally developing children. In *The Report of Comparative Study in Japan & the U.S. Children with Learning Disabilities* (pp. 117–124). Kanagawa, Japan: Kanagawa Research Institute of Learning Disabilities.

Ho, C. S.-H., & Bryant, P. 1997. Phonological skills are important in learning to read Chinese. *Developmental Psychology*, **33**(6): 946–951.

Ho, C. S.-H., Chan, D. W.-O., Lee, S.-H., Tsang, S.-M., & Luan, V. H. 2004. Cognitive profiling and preliminary subtyping in Chinese developmental dyslexia. *Cognition*, **91**(1): 43–75.

Ho, C. S.-H., Chan, D. W., Tsang, S. M., Lee, S. H., & Chung, K. K. 2006. Word learning deficit among Chinese dyslexic children. *Journal of Child Language*, **33**(1): 145–161.

Hu, C. F., & Catts, H. W. 1998. The role of phonological processing in reading abilities: what we can learn from Chinese. *Scientific Studies of Reading*, **2**(1): 55–79.

Huang, H. S., & Hanley, J. R. 1995. Phonological awareness and visual skills in learning to read Chinese and English. *Cognition*, **54**(1): 73–98.

Hulslander, J., Talcott, J., Witton, C., DeFries, J., Pennington, B., Wadsworth, S., *et al*. 2004. Sensory processing, reading, IQ, and attention. *Journal of Experimental Child Psychology*, **88**(3): 274–295.

Hutzler, F., Kronbichler, M., Jacobs, A. M., & Wimmer, H. 2006. Perhaps correlational but not causal: no effect of dyslexic readers' magnocellular system on their eye movements during reading. *Neuropsychologia*, **44**(4): 637–648.

Japan Foundation for Educational and Cultural Research. 1998. *Kanji Mastery Levels for Each Graders at Japanese Elementary School*. www.jfecr.or.jp/kanji/index.html.

Kanwisher, N., McDermott, J., & Chun, M. M. 1997. The fusiform face area: a module in human extrastriate cortex specialized for face perception. *J. Neurosci.*, **17**(11): 4302–4311.

Kato, C., Isoda, H., Takehara, Y., Matsuo, K., Moriya, T., & Nakai, T. 1999. Involvement of motor cortices in retrieval of kanji studied by functional MRI. *Neuroreport*, **10**(6): 1335–1339.

Kess, J. F., & Miyamoto, T. 1999. *The Japanese Mental Lexicon: Psycholinguistic Studies of Kana and Kanji Processing*. Amsterdam: John Benjamins.

Kobayashi, M. S., Haynes, C. W., Macaruso, P., Hook, P. E., & Kato, J. 2005. Effects of mora deletion, nonword repetition, rapid naming, and visual search performance on beginning reading in Japanese. *Annals of Dyslexia*, **55**(1): 105–128.

Longcamp, M., Anton, J.-L., Roth, M., & Velay, J.-L. 2003. Visual presentation of single letters activates a premotor area involved in writing. *NeuroImage*, **19**(4): 1492–1500.

Matsuo, K., Nakai, T., Kato, C., Moriya, T., Isoda, H., Takehara, Y., *et al*. 2000. Dissociation of writing processes: functional magnetic resonance imaging during writing of Japanese ideographic characters. *Cognitive Brain Research*, **9**(3): 281–286.

McBride-Chang, C., Bialystok, E., Chong, K. K. Y., & Li, Y. 2004. Levels of phonological awareness in three cultures. *Journal of Experimental Child Psychology*, **89**(2): 93–111.

McBride-Chang, C., Cho, J.-R., Liu, H., Wagner, R. K., Shu, H., Zhou, A., *et al*. 2005. Changing models across cultures: associations of phonological awareness and morphological structure awareness with vocabulary and word recognition in second graders from Beijing, Hong Kong, Korea, and the United States. *Journal of Experimental Child Psychology*, **92**(2): 140–160.

McBride-Chang, C., & Kail, R. V. 2002. Cross-cultural similarities in the predictors of reading acquisition. *Child Development*, **73**(5): 1392–1407.

Meng, X., Sai, X., Wang, C., Wang, J., Sha, S., & Zhou, X. 2005. Auditory and speech processing and reading development in Chinese school children: behavioural and ERP evidence. *Dyslexia*, **11**(4): 292–310.

Meng, X., Zhou, X., Zeng, B., Kong, R., & Zhuang, J. 2002. [Visual perceptual skills and reading abilities in Chinese-speaking children.] *Acta Psychologica Sinica*, **34**(1): 16–22.

Muter, V., Hulme, C., Snowling, M. J., & Stevenson, J. 2004. Phonemes, rimes, vocabulary, and grammatical skills as foundations of early reading development: evidence from a longitudinal study. *Developmental Psychology*, **40**(5): 665–681.

Nakamura, K., Dehaene, S., Jobert, A., Bihan, D. L., & Kouider, S. 2005. Subliminal convergence of kanji and kana words: further evidence for functional parcellation of the posterior temporal cortex in visual word perception. *Journal of Cognitive Neuroscience*, **17**(6): 954–968.

Nikolopoulos, D., Goulandris, N., Hulme, C., & Snowling, M. J. 2006. The cognitive bases of learning to read and spell in Greek: evidence from a longitudinal study. *Journal of Experimental Child Psychology*, **94**(1): 1–17.

Pugh, K., Mencl, W., Jenner, A., Katz, L., Frost, S., Lee, J., *et al*. 2000. Functional neuroimaging studies of reading and reading disability (developmental dyslexia). *Mental Retardation and Developmental Disabilities Research Reviews*, **6**(3): 207–213.

Ranganath, C., Cohen, M. X., & Brozinsky, C. J. 2005. Working memory maintenance contributes to long-term memory formation: neural and behavioral evidence. *Journal of Cognitive Neuroscience*, **17**(7): 994–1010.

Raven, J., Raven, J., & Court, J. 1998. *Coloured Progressive Matrices*. Oxford: Oxford Psychologists Press.

Saito, H., Kawakami, M., & Masuda, H. 1995. Table of phonetic correspondences for radical components in complex kanji. *Bulletin of the Nagoya University Graduate School of Infomatics and Science*, **2:** 89–115.

Saito, S., Saito, A., & Yoshimura, T. 2000. Wordlikeness values of 120 nonwords. *Education, Psychology, Special Education and Physical Education (Memoirs of Osaka Kyoiku University Series IV)*, **48**(2).

Sakuma, N., Sasanuma, S., Tatsumi, I., & Masaki, S. 1998. Orthography and phonology in reading Japanese kanji words: evidence from the semantic decision task with homophones. *Memory & Cognition*, **26**(1): 75–87.

Sasaki, M., & Watanabe, A. 1983. An experimental study of spontaneous writing-like behaviour ("Kusho") in Japanese. *The Japanese Journal of Educational Psychology*, **31**(4): 1–10.

Shimamura, N., & Mikami, H. 1994. Acquisition of Hiragana letters by pre-school children: a comparison with the 1967 survey by the National Language Research Institute *Kyoiku Shinrigaku Kenkyu*, **42:** 70–76.

Siok, W., & Fletcher, P. 2001. The role of phonological awareness and visual-orthographic skills in Chinese reading acquisition. *Developmental Psychology*, **37**(6): 886–899.

Stein, J. F. 2003. Visual motion sensitivity and reading. *Neuropsychologia*, **41**(13): 1785–1793.

Sullivan, E. V., & Sagar, H. J. 1991. Double dissociation of short-term and long-term memory for nonverbal material in Parkinson's disease and global amnesia: a further analysis. *Brain*, **114**(2): 893–906.

Talcott, J. B., Gram, A., Van Ingelghem, M., Witton, C., Stein, J. F., & Toennessen, F. E. 2003. Impaired sensitivity to dynamic stimuli in poor readers of a regular orthography. *Brain and Language*, **87**(2): 259–266.

Talcott, J. B., Witton, C., Hebb, G., Stoodley, C., Westwood, E., France, S., *et al.* 2002. On the relationship between dynamic visual and auditory processing and literacy skills: results from a large primary-school study. *Dyslexia*, **8**(4): 204–205.

Talcott, J. B., Witton, C., McLean, M. F., Hansen, P. C., Rees, A., Green, G. G. R., *et al.* 2000. Dynamic sensory sensitivity and children's word decoding skills. *Proceedings of the National Academy of Sciences of the United States of America*, **97**(6): 2952–2957.

Tan, L. H., Spinks, J. A., Eden, G. F., Perfetti, C. A., & Siok, W. T. 2005. Reading depends on writing, in Chinese. *Proceedings of the National Academy of Sciences of the United States of America*, **102**(24): 8781–8785.

Uno, A. 2004. Developmental dyslexia. *Molecular Medicine*, **41**(5): 601–603.

Uno, A., Kaneko, M., Haruhara, N., & Kaga, M. 2000. Disability of phonological and visual information processing in Japanese dyslexic children. *International Conference on Spoken Language Processing*, **2:** 42–45.

Uno, A., Shinya, N., Haruhara, N., & Kaneko, M. 2005. Raven's Coloured Progressive Matrices in Japanese children as a screening intelligence test for children with learning disorder and acquired childhood aphasia. *Japan Journal of Logopedics and Phoniatrics*, **46:** 185–189.

Vandenbulcke, M., Peeters, R., Fannes, K., & Vandenberghe, R. 2006. Knowledge of visual attributes in the right hemisphere. *Nature Neuroscience*, **9**(7): 964–970.

Watanabe, K., Ogino, T., Nakano, K., Hattori, J., Kado, Y., Sanada, S., *et al.* 2005. The Rey-Osterrieth Complex Figure as a measure of executive function in childhood. *Brain and Development*, **27**(8): 564–569.

Watson, C., Kidd, G., Homer, D., Connell, P., Lowther, A., Eddins, D., *et al.* 2003. Sensory, cognitive, and linguistic factors in the early academic performance of elementary school children: The Benton-IU project. *Journal of Learning Disabilities*, **36**(2): 165–197.

Witton, C., Stein, J. F., Stoodley, C., Rosner, B., & Talcott. J. B. 2002. Separate influences of acoustic AM and FM sensitivity on the phonological decoding skills of impaired and normal readers. *Journal of Cognitive Neuroscience*, **14**(6): 866–874.

Witton, Talcott, J. B., Hansen, P. C., Richardson, A. J., Griffiths, T. D., Rees, A., *et al.* 1998. Sensitivity to dynamic auditory and visual stimuli predicts nonword reading ability in both dyslexic and normal readers. *Current Biology*, **8**(14): 791–797.

Mapping Phonological Information from Auditory to Written Modality during Foreign Vocabulary Learning

Margarita Kaushanskaya[a] and Viorica Marian[b]

[a]*Department of Communicative Disorders and the Waisman Center, University of Wisconsin–Madison, Madison, Wisconsin, USA*

[b]*Department of Communication Sciences and Disorders, Northwestern University, Evanston, Illinois, USA*

Learning to read in a foreign language often entails recognizing the printed form of words learned by sound. In the current study, the ability to map novel phonological information from the auditory modality onto the written modality was examined at different levels of overlap between the native language and an artificially constructed foreign language. In this study, monolingual English-speaking adults learned novel foreign words in the auditory modality. Recognition testing was first conducted in the auditory modality and then in the written modality. Participants who learned foreign words that matched English phonology showed similar accuracy rates when tested in either modality. Participants who learned foreign words that mismatched English phonology showed decreased recognition accuracy when tested in the written modality. Results indicate that cross-linguistic matching in phonology facilitated mapping of phonological information to the written modality. In addition, at different levels of cross-linguistic overlap, specific cognitive skills were found to correlate with the ability to map phonological information across modalities. This finding suggests that the cognitive skills required for acquisition of a foreign language may vary depending upon degree of cross-linguistic similarity.

Key words: phonology; orthography; cross-linguistic overlap; foreign vocabulary learning; reading acquisition

Introduction

Cross-linguistic similarity is an important variable in second-language acquisition, modulating the critical period phenomenon (De Keyeser, 2000) as well as the metacognitive advantage associated with knowing two languages (Bialystok, Majumder, & Martin, 2003). The ease of learning in situations in which the foreign linguistic system is similar to the native linguistic system is ascribed to the learner's reliance on L1 (first language) long-term memory representations. When the foreign phonological inventory is similar to the native language phonological inventory, a learner can rely on the established phonemic categories associated with the native language to process and integrate foreign language information. Studies examining the effect of cross-linguistic similarity on foreign vocabulary acquisition consistently demonstrate that phonological similarity across languages facilitates learning (Ellis & Beaton, 1993a; Gathercole, Willis, Emslie, & Baddeley, 1991). In addition, orthographic similarity across languages has been shown to facilitate foreign vocabulary acquisition (Ellis & Beaton, 1993b). For instance, Ellis and Beaton (1993a) demonstrated that the degree to which the foreign

Address for correspondence: Margarita Kaushanskaya, Ph.D., Assistant Professor, Dept. of Communicative Disorders, University of Wisconsin–Madison, 1975 Willow Drive, Madison, WI 53706. kaushanskaya@wisc.edu

Ann. N.Y. Acad. Sci. 1145: 56–70 (2008). © 2008 New York Academy of Sciences.
doi: 10.1196/annals.1416.008

word conformed to the phonotactic patterns of the native language correlated highly with its "learnability." Similarly, Gathercole *et al.* (1991) found that nonwords that were structured in accordance with native-language phonotactic rules were more accurately repeated than nonwords that were not consistent with the native phonotactic system. Phonological similarity between the foreign and the native languages can facilitate acquisition because the learner can rely on long-term phonological knowledge to support learning (Gathercole & Baddeley, 1990; De Jong, Seveke, & Van Veen, 2000; Gathercole & Baddeley, 1990; Masoura & Gathercole, 1999; Papagno, Valentine, & Baddeley, 1991).

Because learning to read in a foreign language requires integration of novel phonological and orthographic information, it is likely that similarity in phonological and orthographic properties across L1 and L2 would facilitate reading acquisition in the second language. In situations in which the foreign language is similar to the native language, learners would be able to rely on long-term knowledge of orthography and phonology to support learning. Therefore, the first objective of the present study was to examine the effect of cross-linguistic similarity on acquisition of early reading in a foreign language. Early reading in a foreign language was operationally defined as participants' ability to map phonological information acquired in the auditory modality onto the written modality. It was hypothesized that cross-linguistic similarity would facilitate adults' ability to map phonological information from the auditory onto the written modality because it would enable reliance on native-language phonological and orthographic knowledge.

In addition to testing the effect of cross-linguistic similarity, we were also interested in cognitive skills that may underlie acquisition of early literacy in adults. Two general types of cognitive skills were considered: phonological capacity and vocabulary knowledge. Phonological abilities and vocabulary skills have consis-

tently been identified as necessary for acquisition of reading in children (Corneau, Cormier, Grandmaison, & Lacroix, 1999) and adults (Cisero & Royer, 1995; Majeres, 2005) as well as for acquisition of foreign vocabulary (e.g., Cheung, 1996; Gathercole & Baddeley, 1990; Service, 1992; Service & Kohonen, 1995). For acquisition of reading by children, it has consistently been demonstrated that the more words a child knows, the easier it is for him or her to learn to read, since a greater number of words can be phonologically mapped and recognized. In fact, children's vocabulary skills are highly predictive of their ability to acquire print knowledge (Stahl & Fairbanks, 2006). Equally, if not more, important for acquisition of reading, are the child's phonological skills (Corneau *et al.*, 1999). Children who demonstrate superior phonological awareness tend to acquire the alphabetic reading principles with greater efficiency, since they are better able to rely on their phonological skills in mapping orthographic forms onto their phonological representations. For acquisition of reading in adults, it has also been shown that poor phonological skills result in less-accurate and less-efficient reading performance (e.g., Majeres, 2005).

For foreign word learning, research consistently demonstrates that higher scores on various phonological measures (e.g., nonword repetition, phoneme manipulation, etc.) are associated with increased retention of foreign vocabulary in both children (Gathercole & Baddeley, 1990; Service, 1992) and adults (Gupta, 2003; Papagno & Vallar, 1992, 1995; Speciale, Ellis, & Bywater, 2004). For instance, children with good nonword repetition skills are consistently found to outperform their poor nonword repetition peers when learning novel words (Cheung, 1996; Gathercole & Baddeley, 1990; Service, 1992; Service & Kohonen, 1995). In primary school students, repetition accuracy for nonwords in a second language predicts learning of vocabulary of the second language (Service, 1992). Similarly, Gathercole and Baddeley (1989) found that children's short-term memory span (e.g., the ability to repeat nonwords) is highly predictive of their vocabulary size one year later.

Phonological short-term memory also contributes to foreign language learning in adults. For instance, the role of phonological short-term memory in adult word learning has been supported by findings of Gupta (2003), Papagno and Vallar (1995), and Speciale *et al.* (2004), but results of the three studies did not completely converge. Papagno and Vallar (1995) demonstrated that nonword repetition correlated highly with participants' word learning performance. Gupta (2003) also demonstrated a correlation between nonword repetition performance and word learning in adults; however, when digit span performance was partialed out, correlations between nonword repetition and word learning failed to reach significance. In contrast, Speciale *et al.* (2004) found that nonword repetition correlated with participants' ability to learn L2 words, but only when participants produced the novel word in response to its native-language translation. When the direction of testing changed (i.e., participants had to produce native-language translations for novel words), nonword repetition scores were not related to performance. The role of phonological memory in adult word learning may also vary across age groups. For instance, Service and Craik (1993) examined word learning in younger and older participants and found that older, but not younger, adults showed a strong relationship between repetition performance for unfamiliar words (indexing phonological short-term memory) and word learning.

While phonological short-term memory skills are fundamental for acquisition of foreign-language vocabulary, vocabulary abilities in the native language have also been linked with second-language acquisition. For children, Masoura and Gathercole (1999) showed that the ease of L2 vocabulary learning is strongly influenced by the stability and extent of representations in L1 vocabulary. For adults, recent studies have found that adults who acquired the second language after the critical period are capable of achieving near-native performance in the foreign language if they possess high verbal ability in their native language (De Keyeser, 2002).

Given the role of phonological memory and vocabulary knowledge in acquisition of a foreign language and in acquisition of reading, it is likely that the same skills would underlie acquisition of early literacy in the foreign language. However, the extent of involvement of phonological memory and vocabulary knowledge in the learning process may vary according to how much L1 and L2 overlap. For instance, previous work suggests that phonological capacity may be especially important for learning phonologically unfamiliar foreign words (De Jong, Seveke, & Van Veen, 2000; Papagno *et al.*, 1991). Children with poor nonword repetition skills were shown to be slower at learning phonologically unfamiliar names for toys, but not at learning familiar names for them (Gathercole & Baddeley, 1990). Similarly, in children older than 5 years of age, phonological sensitivity (i.e., the ability to detect and manipulate sound units in words) contributed to learning novel names with unfamiliar phonological structure, but not to learning familiar names (De Jong, Seveke, & Van Veen, 2000). Further, nonword repetition scores predicted knowledge of foreign, but not of native vocabulary (Masoura & Gathercole, 1999). Together, these findings suggest that phonological skills and L1 vocabulary influence L2 acquisition and affect foreign word learning differently, depending on the extent of cross-linguistic overlap between the native and the foreign languages.

In the current research, acquisition of early reading skills in a foreign language was examined within the context of a foreign vocabulary learning task. The objective of the present study was to examine adults' ability to map phonological information from the auditory modality onto the written modality at different levels of cross-linguistic overlap. It was expected that cross-linguistic similarity would modulate participants' ability to map phonological information across modalities. It was also expected that phonological short-term memory and vocabulary knowledge would influence adults' ability to map phonological information across modalities. Since the ability to map phonological information onto the written modality is an important component of literacy acquisition in the second language, we were also interested in the role of native-language reading skills. Therefore, three types of cognitive measures were considered: phonological short-term memory (as measured by digit span and nonword repetition), native-language vocabulary knowledge (as measured by receptive and expressive vocabulary), and reading skills in the native language (as measured by a reading fluency test).

Cross-linguistic overlap was manipulated by creating four artificial languages that shared different degrees of phonemic and alphabetic overlap with English. Four versions of artificial vocabulary items were constructed to (1) match both the phonological system and the orthographic systems of English (+P+O); (2) mismatch the phonological, but match the orthographic system of English (−P+O); (3) match the phonological, but mismatch the orthographic system of English (+P−O); and (4) mismatch both the phonological and the orthographic systems of English (−P−O). English-speaking monolingual adults were assigned to one of four groups, with participants in each group learning a different version of the foreign vocabulary using the Paired Associate Learning (PAL) paradigm (Van Hell & Mahn, 1997), in which a novel word is paired with its native-language translation. Participants in each of the four groups learned vocabulary items in the auditory modality. Retention of novel vocabulary items was first tested in the auditory modality and then in the written modality.

It was hypothesized that cross-linguistic overlap, phonological skills, and vocabulary abilities would be associated with adults' ability to map phonological information across modalities. It was predicted that:

(1) Cross-linguistic similarity would facilitate participants' ability to map phonological information from the auditory modality onto the written modality;

(2) Better performance on cognitive measures of phonological memory and L1 vocabulary would lead to improved ability to map phonological information onto the written modality; and

(3) Mapping of phonological information onto the written modality would be supported by phonological memory and L1 vocabulary differently, depending on the extent of cross-linguistic overlap between the native and the foreign language.

Methods

The study followed a three-way mixed design in which the within-subjects independent variables were modality of testing (auditory versus written) and testing session(immediate versus delayed), and the between-subjects independent variable was group (+P+O, −P+O, +P−O, and −P−O). Dependent variables intended to capture the success of vocabulary learning included both accuracy and reaction time (RT) measures. Accuracy of recognition was defined as proportion correct in selecting the appropriate response out of five available choices. Efficiency of recognition (reaction times) was defined as the response latency for selection of the correct translation.

Participants

Ninety-six monolingual speakers of English (mean age = 23 years, 11 months; SD = 0.83 years) were randomly assigned to one of four groups (+P+O; −P+O; +P−O; and −P−O). Groups did not differ in age, education level, gender distribution, vocabulary knowledge (Peabody Picture Vocabulary Test, 3rd edition, Dunn & Dunn, 1997; Expressive Vocabulary Test, Williams, 1997), or performance on standardized measures of short-term phonological memory (digit span and nonword repetition sub-test of the Comprehensive Test of Phonological Processing (Wagner, Torgesen, & Rashotte, 1999).

Materials

Four versions of artificial foreign vocabulary items were constructed. Each of the versions consisted of eight sounds (and their associated letters). Four sounds and letters corresponded to English (in order to ease the vocabulary learning process), and four varied across vocabulary versions in their similarity to English (in order to test the effect of cross-linguistic overlap). The four English phonemes included two vowels (/ˆ/-A and /e/-E) and two consonants (/f/-F and /n/-N). The remaining four phonemes, two vowels and two consonants, were manipulated across the four vocabulary versions, so that in versions +P+O and +P−O they remained English (/i/, /u/, /t/, /g/), but in versions −P+O and −P−O they were replaced with non-English phonemes. The non-English phonemes were selected to be perceptually different from all existing English phonemes and yet to be pronounceable by native speakers of English. In order to rule out confounds associated with articulatory difficulties, the non-English phonemes shared place of articulation with the English phonemes. The non-English phonemes in the stimuli for −P conditions were taken from languages other than English (French, Russian, Urdu, and Hebrew). The vowels /i/ and /u/ were replaced by the non-English vowels /I/ and /y/, respectively, while the consonants /t/ and /g/ were replaced by the non-English consonants /T/ and /χ^2/, respectively. Further, four English letters were manipulated across vocabulary versions, so that they remained English for versions +P+O and −P+O, but were replaced with non-English symbols for versions +P−O and −P−O. The non-English letters used to spell foreign words in −O conditions were selected on the basis of their similarities (in terms of number of elements) to the English letters

they replaced. For instance, the letter T and the corresponding non-English symbol both consist of two crossing strokes. The non-English letter symbols were drawn from rare languages (Bassa, Albanian, N'Ko) in order to rule out familiarity effects. None of the participants reported familiarity with these letters.

Twenty-four monosyllabic and disyllabic nonwords corresponding to both English phonology and English orthography were constructed. All nonwords were recorded by a native English-speaking male audiologist, who was extensively trained on the nonwords' pronunciation prior to the recording session. Each nonword was paired with its English "translation." All 24 English translations referred to concrete, highly imageable objects with frequent English names. The English words were on average 4.51 (SE = 0.52) letters in length with an average of 47.79 (SE = 56.24) words/million frequency of use, 578.38 (SE = 35.71) concreteness rating, 593.58 (SE = 30.15) imageability rating, and 547.50 (SE = 35.84) familiarity rating. Frequency ratings (Francis & Kucera, 1982) as well as concreteness, imageability, and familiarity ratings (Gilhooly & Logie, 1980; Paivio, Yuille, & Madigan, 1968; Toglia & Battig, 1978) for English words were obtained using the MRC Psycholinguistic Database. The nonwords were three to five phonemes in length, with an average phoneme frequency of 1.14 (SE = 0.06), an average biphone frequency of 1.00 (SE = 0.003), an average bigram frequency of 4951.92 (SE = 2925.51), and had an average 1.04 (SE = 1.99) orthographic neighbors.

Procedure

Alphabet Learning

At the beginning of the experimental session, each participant was taught the sounds and the corresponding letters of the foreign language. Each letter appeared on the computer screen, and the corresponding sound was played twice over the headphones. The participant was instructed to repeat the sound out loud three times. After all letters and sounds had been presented, the participant was asked to match each sound to the appropriate letter and to pronounce each sound when presented with a letter. All participants were 100% accurate in producing the correct sounds for the letters at the end of the alphabet-learning sequence.

Vocabulary Learning

Participants heard the novel word pronounced twice over the headphones and saw its written English translation on the right side of the computer screen. The participants were instructed to repeat the novel word and its English translation out loud three times. Each pair was presented twice during the learning phase. Learning was self-paced.

Immediate Vocabulary Testing

After the vocabulary-learning phase, the participant's memory for presented items was tested using both an auditory and a written recognition task. During auditory recognition, participants heard foreign words over headphones and chose the correct English translations from five alternatives listed on the computer screen as fast as possible. Of the five alternatives, one answer was correct, two answers were translations of foreign words from the same list, one answer was an English word that was semantically related to the correct answer, and one answer was an unrelated English word not previously presented. Immediately after completing the auditory recognition test, participants completed the written recognition test. During the written recognition test, participants saw foreign words spelled out on the computer screen and chose the correct English translation from five alternatives. The alternatives were the same choices offered to the participants during auditory testing and they were presented in the same order as during the auditory testing. Therefore, performance on the written test indicated the accuracy and the speed with which participants

could map newly learned phonological information onto the written modality.

Delayed Vocabulary Testing

One week after the initial learning session, participants returned to the laboratory and were tested on long-term retention of the learned vocabulary. Participants completed both the auditory and the written recognition tasks in the same manner as during immediate testing.

Standardized Assessment of Short-Term Memory and Vocabulary Knowledge

After delayed testing was completed, participants were given standardized assessment measures of vocabulary knowledge and phonological short-term memory. Phonological short-term memory was measured using two tests: the digit span test and the nonword repetition test (Comprehensive Test of Phonological Processing; Wagner, Torgesen, & Rashotte, 1999). Native-language vocabulary knowledge was measured using two standardized tests, the Peabody Picture Vocabulary Test, 3rd edition (PPVT; Dunn & Dunn, 1997), which measured receptive vocabulary, and the Expressive Vocabulary Test (EVT; Williams, 1997), which measured expressive vocabulary. In addition, a reading fluency test was administered that required participants to read sentences and judge their content for veracity (Woodcock–Johnson Tests of Achievement). Tests were administered in the following order: (1) PPVT, (2) EVT, (3) reading fluency, (4) digit span, and (5) nonword repetition.

Data Analyses

For each measure, univariate analyses of variance (ANOVAs) were conducted, with group (+P+O,−P+O,+P−O,−P−O) as a between-subjects independent variable. Next, accuracy and reaction time data for each group were analyzed using repeated-measures ANOVAs, comparing performance on the written recognition test to performance on the

---

auditory recognition test, both immediately after learning and during delayed testing.

In addition, a difference score between performance on the written test and performance on the auditory test was determined for each group (score on written testing minus score on auditory testing). This difference score reflected the gain or drop in accuracy rates or reaction times with repeated testing in a different modality. For accuracy rates, a score above zero reflected higher accuracy rates on the written testing than on the auditory testing, and a score below zero reflected lower accuracy rates on the written testing than on the auditory testing. For reaction times, a lower difference score reflected shorter reaction times on written testing in relation to auditory testing. Therefore, a successful learner capable of transferring phonological information from the auditory modality into the written modality would receive a higher difference score for accuracy and a lower difference score for RT. Correlation analyses between cognitive measures and difference scores were conducted in order to examine which cognitive skills might underlie the ability to transfer phonological information across modalities at different levels of cross-linguistic overlap.

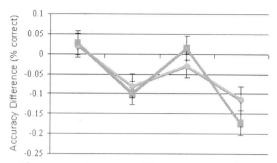

Figure 1. Accuracy difference scores (written testing minus auditory testing) for each group (+P+O; −P+O; +P−O; −P−O), during immediate (*solid circle*) and delayed (*solid square*) testing.

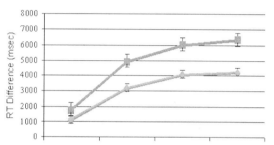

Figure 2. RT difference scores (written testing minus auditory testing) for each group (+P+O; −P+O; +P−O; −P−O), during immediate (*solid circle*) and delayed (*solid square*) testing.

Results

Between-Group Differences in Recognition Performance

To examine between-group differences in recognition performance as a function of cross-linguistic overlap, accuracy rates and reaction times were examined using univariate analyses of variance with group (+P+O;−P+O;+P−O;−P−O) as a between-subjects independent variable. Table 1 shows the accuracy rates (means and standard deviations) for each group and testing condition. Table 2 shows the reaction times (means and standard deviations) for each group and testing condition.

During written testing, significant between-group differences were observed for accuracy rates during both immediate $F(3, 89) = 5.30$, $P < 0.01$, $\eta_p^2 = 0.15$ and delayed testing, $F(3, 86) = 3.95$, $P < 0.05$, $\eta_p^2 = 0.12$. Post-hoc analyses revealed that participants in the +P+O group were more accurate than participants in the −P+O group and than participants in the −P−O group, all least-significant P values < 0.05 (Table 1). Similarly, participants in the +P−O group were more accurate than participants in the −P+O group and than participants in the −P−O group, all least-significant P values < 0.05. These findings indicate that participants were more accurate at mapping phonology onto orthography in a new language if the foreign-language phonology matched native-language phonology.

TABLE 1. Recognition Accuracy Rates for Written and Auditory Testing

Group	Auditory testing mean (SE)	Written testing mean (SE)	Between-group comparisons (for difference scores)		
			+P+O	−P+O	+P−O
+P+O	0.77 (0.03)	0.79 (0.03)	—		
−P+O	0.71 (0.04)	0.63 (0.04)*	$P < 0.05$	—	
+P−O	0.78 (0.04)	0.75 (0.05)	n.s.	n.s.	—
−P−O	0.71 (0.03)	0.60 (0.04)*	$P < 0.05$	n.s.	$P < 0.05$
			+P+O	−P+O	+P−O
+P+O	0.66 (0.04)	0.66 (0.04)	—		
−P+O	0.55 (0.04)	0.54 (0.04)	n.s.	—	
+P−O	0.63 (0.04)	0.67 (0.03)	n.s.	n.s.	—
−P−O	0.61 (0.04)	0.55 (0.03)	n.s.	n.s.	$P < 0.05$

Note: A significant difference between written and auditory recognition accuracy is marked by an asterisk next to the written testing mean (SE)*, indicating a $P < 0.05$.

TABLE 2. Recognition Reaction Times for Written and Auditory Testing

Group	Auditory testing mean (SE)	Written testing mean (SE)	Between-group comparisons (for difference scores)		
			+P+O	−P+O	+P−O
+P+O	3305.48 (215.79)	4420.92 (229.90)*	—		
−P+O	3320.45 (277.27)	6531.72 (471.64)*	$P < 0.05$	—	
+P−O	3105.93 (166.21)	7217.44 (733.68)*	$P < 0.05$	n.s.	—
−P−O	2964.17 (128.60)	7216.96 (515.01)*	$P < 0.05$	n.s.	n.s.
			+P+O	−P+O	+P−O
+P+O	3431.80 (182.27)	4095.69 (252.50)*	—		
−P+O	3238.67 (234.24)	4982.54 (352.15)*	$P < 0.05$	—	
+P−O	3607.07 (261.63)	5530.68 (364.45)*	$P < 0.05$	n.s.	—
−P−O	3430.06 (203.92)	5538.95 (339.56)*	$P < 0.05$	n.s.	n.s.

Note. A significant difference between written and auditory recognition RT is marked by an asterisk next to the Written Testing Mean (SE)*, indicating a $P < 0.05$.

In addition to accuracy differences, significant between-group differences were also observed for *reaction times*, both during immediate written testing, $F(3, 89) = 6.74$, $P < 0.001$, $\eta_p^2 = 0.19$ and during delayed written testing, $F(3, 86) = 4.35$, $P < 0.01$, $\eta_p^2 = .43$. Participants in the +P+O group were faster than participants in the −P+O group, +P−O group, and −P−O group, all least significant P values < 0.01 (Table 2).

During auditory testing, results revealed comparable *accuracy* and *reaction time* rates across the four groups for both immediate and delayed testing, $P > 0.1$.

Within-Group Differences in Recognition Performance

To examine within-group differences in recognition performance as a function of testing modality, accuracy, and reaction time measures were analyzed using repeated-measures ANOVAs. For the +P+O group, repeated-measures ANOVAs revealed comparable accuracy rates for auditory and written testing, both immediately after learning, $F(1, 23) = 0.82$, $P = 0.37$, $\eta_p^2 = 0.04$, and during delayed testing, $F(1, 22) = 0.06$, $P = 0.82$, $\eta_p^2 = 0.003$. Conversely, analyses revealed longer reaction times during written than during auditory testing, both immediately after learning, $F(1, 23) = 56.32$, $P < 0.001$, $\eta_p^2 = 0.71$, and at delayed testing, $F(1, 22) = 16.81$, $P < 0.001$, $\eta_p^2 = 0.43$. Thus, participants in the +P+O group were slower, but not less accurate, when tested in the written modality than when tested in the auditory modality.

For the −P+O group, repeated-measures ANOVAs revealed that when tested immediately after learning, participants were less accurate when tested in the written modality than in the auditory modality, $F(1, 22) = 12.89$, $P < 0.01$, $\eta_p^2 = 0.37$. However, testing-modality differences disappeared with delayed testing, $F(1, 20) = 0.37$, $P = 0.55$, $\eta_p^2 = 0.02$, and participants were just as accurate during written as during auditory testing. RT analyses revealed longer reaction times during written than during auditory testing, both immediately after learning, $F(1, 22) = 91.80$, $P < 0.001$, $\eta_p^2 = 0.81$, and at delayed testing, $F(1, 20) = 31.42$, $P < 0.001$, $\eta_p^2 = 0.61$. Thus, participants in the −P+O group were slower, and less accurate, when tested in the written modality than when tested in the auditory modality.

For the +P−O group, repeated-measures ANOVAs revealed comparable accuracy rates for the auditory and the written testing, both immediately after learning, $F(1, 22) = 1.67$, $P = 0.21$, $\eta_p^2 = 0.07$, and during delayed testing, $F(1, 22) = 2.19$, $P = 0.15$, $\eta_p^2 = 0.09$. Conversely, analyses revealed longer reaction times during written than during auditory testing, both immediately after learning, $F(1, 22) = 40.82$, $P < 0.001$, $\eta_p^2 = 0.65$, and at delayed testing, $F(1, 22) = 66.87$, $P < 0.001$,

$\eta_p^2 = 0.75$. Thus, similar to participants in the +P+O group, participants in the +P−O group were slower, but not less accurate, when tested in the written modality than when tested in the auditory modality.

For the −P−O group, repeated-measures ANOVAs revealed that when tested immediately after learning, participants were less accurate when tested in the written modality than in the auditory modality, $F(1, 22) = 11.76$, $P < 0.01$, $\eta_p^2 = 0.35$. This testing-modality difference attenuated and became marginal with delayed testing, $F(1, 22) = 3.57$, $P = 0.07$, $\eta_p^2 = 0.14$, but participants remained less accurate at written than at auditory testing. Similarly, analyses revealed longer reaction times during written than during auditory testing, both immediately after learning, $F(1, 22) = 91.85$, $P < 0.001$, $\eta_p^2 = 0.81$, and at delayed testing, $F(1, 22) = 72.30$, $P < 0.001$, $\eta_p^2 = 0.77$. Thus, participants in the −P−O group were slower, and less accurate when tested in the written modality than when tested in the auditory modality.

Relating Cognitive Abilities and Recognition Performance

Correlation analyses were used to examine which cognitive skills would be associated with the ability to map phonological information from the auditory modality onto the written modality. Participants' performance on cognitive measures was correlated with the difference scores between the written and the auditory testing modalities. Because a higher difference score for accuracy would indicate better performance on written compared to auditory testing, positive correlations between cognitive measures and accuracy difference would indicate that better performance on the cognitive test was associated with a better ability to map phonological information across modalities. Conversely, because a higher difference score for RT would indicate less efficient performance on written testing, positive correlations between cognitive measures and RT difference would indicate that better performance on cognitive measures was associated with a lower ability to map phonological information across modalities.

In the +P+O group, no significant correlations were observed among any of the cognitive measures and difference scores obtained immediately after learning for accuracy or RTs. For delayed testing, RT difference correlated negatively with expressive vocabulary (EVT $R = -0.39$, $P = 0.06$), indicating that higher vocabulary knowledge was associated with more efficient mapping of phonological information onto the written modality. RT difference also correlated positively with performance on the digit span measure of phonological memory ($R = 0.40$, $P = 0.05$), indicating that a larger digit span was associated with less efficient mapping of phonological information onto the written modality. Difference scores between written and auditory testing for each group are presented in Figure 1 (accuracy) and Figure 2 (reaction times).

In the −P+O group, significant correlations were observed between the digit span measure of phonological memory and accuracy difference scores, both immediately after learning ($R = -0.46$, $P < 0.05$) and during delayed testing ($R = -0.45$, $P < 0.05$), indicating that a larger digit span was associated with less accurate mapping of phonological information from the auditory modality onto the written modality. A similar inverse relationship was observed between the accuracy difference score and the reading fluency measure during delayed testing ($R = -0.70$, $P < 0.01$), suggesting that participants with higher reading fluency scores were less accurate at mapping phonological information onto the written modality. Interestingly, the nonword repetition measure of phonological memory correlated positively with accuracy difference scores during delayed testing ($R = 0.52$, $P < 0.05$), suggesting that participants with a higher phonological short-term memory span tended to be more successful at mapping newly learned phonological information onto the written modality.

For the +P−O group, RTdiff-erence scores during delayed testing correlated negatively with expressive vocabulary (EVT $R = -0.42$, $P < 0.05$) and with nonword repetition ($R = -0.48$, $P < 0.05$); no other significant correlations were observed. This suggests that better vocabulary knowledge and phonological short-term memory skills were associated with more efficient mapping of phonological information from the auditory onto the written modality.

For the −P−O group, only one marginally significant correlation was observed between reading fluency and RT difference scores immediately after learning ($R = -0.50$, $P = 0.059$), suggesting that higher reading fluency scores were associated with more efficient mapping of phonological information onto the written modality.

Discussion

Learning to read in a foreign language often entails recognition of printed words originally acquired in the auditory modality. This recognition relies on the ability to map phonological representations across modalities (auditory to written). In the current research, adults' ability to map phonological information from the auditory onto the written modality was examined within the context of a foreign-word learning task. We aimed to explore whether the underlying cognitive skills that may support mapping of phonological information from the auditory onto the written modality would vary, depending on the degree of cross-linguistic similarity between the native and the foreign language.

Cross-Linguistic Similarity in Foreign Vocabulary Learning

Results revealed that cross-linguistic overlap mediated adults' ability to map phonological information across modalities. Specifically, adults found it easier to map phonological information onto the written modality when it matched the phonology of their native language (+P+O and +P−O groups) than when it mismatched the phonology of their native language (−P+O and −P−O groups). Switching modalities at testing carried efficiency costs for all participants, but accuracy costs were observed only for participants who acquired a phonologically mismatching foreign language (−P+O and −P−O).

The role of cross-linguistic similarity in foreign vocabulary acquisition has been substantiated by previous research (Ellis & Beaton, 1993a; Gathercole *et al.*, 1991). The current work suggests that cross-linguistic similarity also plays an important role in participants' ability to transfer phonological information across modalities (auditory to written). This ability is fundamental for literacy acquisition in a foreign language, and the results of this research suggest that phonological similarity between L1 and the foreign language makes this task easier. Interestingly, phonological, but not orthographic similarity across languages facilitated participants' performance. Thus, participants who acquired a foreign language that mismatched L1 in orthography, yet matched it in phonology (+P−O), maintained their accuracy of mapping a foreign word to its English translation when tested in the written modality. Conversely, participants who acquired a phonologically mismatching foreign language showed accuracy costs when testing modality switched from auditory to written. It is possible that this is due to the initial weak encoding of phonologically mismatching information and not to difficulty mapping phonological information onto a different modality. However, the fact that all four groups of participants demonstrated comparable accuracy rates on auditory testing indicates that participants retained comparably strong phonological representations across the four groups. Thus, it is more likely that the difficulty observed during written testing for participants in the −P+O and −P−O groups was due to a more effortful mapping of phonologically unfamiliar information onto the corresponding orthography and not to the less-robust representation of phonological information.

The Relationship between Measures of Cognitive Function and Foreign Vocabulary Learning

Results revealed that different sets of cognitive skills were associated with adults' ability to map phonological information across modalities, and patterns of correlation depended on the degree of cross-linguistic overlap between the native and the foreign languages. Specifically, better vocabulary knowledge in L1 led to better ability to map phonological information across modalities, but only when L1 and the foreign language shared phonology (+P+O and +P−O groups). Interestingly, we found distinct correlation patterns between word-learning performance and the two phonological memory measures (the digit span and the nonword repetition). Higher performance on the digit span measure led to less efficient and/or less accurate mapping of phonological information across modalities in cases in which participants learned a foreign language that matched L1 in orthography (+P+O and −P+O groups). Conversely, higher nonword repetition performance was positively associated with adults' ability to map phonological information across modalities, but only for groups who learned a foreign language that mismatched L1 in either phonology (−P+O) or orthography (+P−O).

The finding that better L1 vocabulary skills led to better recognition performance is consistent with previous studies showing that native-language vocabulary becomes an important predictor of foreign word learning (Masoura & Gathercole, 1999). Better vocabulary skills in the native language can support further word learning, since new words can be incorporated into the existing system with greater ease. Note that vocabulary skills were associated with performance only by participants who acquired foreign languages that matched L1 in phonology and were not associated with performance by participants in phonologically mismatching groups. This pattern is likely due to the fact that L1 vocabulary knowledge is indicative of the strength of lexical-level phonological representations. When a foreign word fits the phonology of the native language, the native-language phonological lexicon can support learning; however, when the foreign word does not fit the phonology of the native language, the native-language phonological lexicon cannot support learning. This differential impact of L1 vocabulary on participants' ability to map phonology across modalities suggests that native-language vocabulary can support further language learning, but only when the phonological systems of the two languages are aligned.

The finding that higher nonword repetition scores led to better performance for the −P+O and the +P−O groups is consistent with a number of previous studies showing that phonological short-term memory skills are predictive of foreign word-learning performance (Gathercole & Baddeley, 1990; Gupta, 2003; Speciale *et al.*, 2004). In the current study, better ability to maintain the phonological shape of the foreign word in working memory (nonword repetition score) led to better ability to map this phonological representation onto a different modality. Interestingly, this relationship was observed only for situations when the foreign language mismatched the native language in one of the parameters—phonology or orthography. The finding that nonword repetition scores predicted learning in the phonological mismatch condition is consistent with previous studies showing stronger contribution of phonological short-term memory to learning unfamiliar foreign words than to learning familiar foreign words (De Jong, Seveke, & Van Veen, 2000; Papagno *et al.*, 1991). While acquisition of phonologically familiar foreign words is supported by long-term phonological knowledge, acquisition of phonologically unfamiliar foreign words must rely entirely on one's phonological short-term memory (Papagno *et al.*, 1991). Moreover, in the current study, nonword repetition scores were also associated with learning in the orthographic mismatch condition. It is possible that in situations of

mismatch (phonological or orthographic), one's capacity for maintaining phonological information in short-term memory is especially important for mapping across modalities. However, when both foreign phonology and orthography match that of the native language, it may be unnecessary to maintain the phonological shape of the word in working memory, since it can be easily reconstructed online when presented with the orthographic shape of the word. In a situation when neither foreign phonology nor orthography match that of the native language, one's skill in maintaining the phonological shape of the word in working memory may not be sufficient to facilitate mapping onto the novel orthography. The task of mapping unfamiliar phonology onto unfamiliar orthography may draw upon a set of skills that is distinct from those relied on when the two languages overlap in at least one dimension. Lack of significant correlations between recognition performance and cognitive skills for the −P−O group supports this notion and suggests the need to explore cognitive skills other than those tested here.

In contrast to nonword repetition performance, digit span performance correlated negatively with participants' ability to map phonological information across modalities, but only for foreign languages that matched L1 in orthography (+P+O and −P+O). It is possible that the inverse relationship between the digit span and performance accuracy is driven by the mismatch between phonological information maintained in working memory and the phonological information activated during written testing. In both the +P+O and the −P+O conditions, orthographic information presented during written testing consisted of familiar English letters. Because of the firm bidirectional connections that exist between letters and phonemes in the native-language (Seidenberg & McClelland, 1989; Van Orden & Goldinger, 1994), it is likely that orthographic information presented at testing activated native-language phonology. This phonology was likely to conflict with phonology remembered by participants (since the foreign words in the −P+O condition contained non-English phonemes). Participants with high digit span may have been more capable of remembering phonological information associated with auditorily learned foreign words than participants with low digit span. This high phonological capacity may have led high digit span participants to activate the remembered phonological representation during testing. However, the remembered phonology would conflict with phonological representations activated during written testing, resulting in less-successful written recognition performance in high digit span participants. While this account can explain the findings in the −P+O group, it is less clear why an inverse relationship between digit span and reaction times would be obtained in the +P+O condition. The ability to maintain phonological information in the working memory should help participants map phonological information onto the written modality, not hinder it. One explanation for this observed pattern is a possibility that phonological information activated via orthography did not exactly match phonological information acquired during auditory learning. In the +P+O foreign language constructed for the present study, the mappings between letters and phonemes were always consistent. For example, the vowel /a/ was always pronounced as /ˆ/. This is not the case in English, however, where the closed-syllable /a/ often maps onto the phoneme /æ/. It is possible that such inconsistencies in mappings between letters and phonemes of L1 and the foreign language led to the observed negative correlation between the digit span and the recognition performance in the +P+O group.

The distinct correlation patterns between participants' ability to map phonological information across modalities, on the one hand, and nonword repetition and digit span, on the other hand, suggests that nonword repetition and digit span performance may reflect different sub-components of working memory. It is possible that nonword repetition is more reflective of sublexical phonological abilities, while digit span is more reflective of lexically based phonological memory. It is also possible that digit span incorporates a sizable sequencing component with performance reflective not only of one's ability to maintain phonological information in short-term memory, but also one's ability to maintain it in a very specific order (Gupta, 2003). By this logic, successful performance on a nonword repetition task requires less of a sequencing ability than successful performance on a digit span task. This difference between the tasks cannot explain, however, why the two load differently and inversely onto participants' ability to map phonological information across modalities, and future studies may examine this question.

Conclusions

In sum, results of the current study suggest a pattern of complex interactions between adults' ability to map phonological representations across modalities, cross-linguistic similarity, and underlying cognitive skills. It appears that phonological similarity across the native and the foreign languages facilitates one's ability to map phonological information onto a new modality and that vocabulary knowledge in the native language supports this ability. In general, the findings of the current study suggest that adult acquisition of early literacy in different foreign language systems is associated with distinct sets of skills and depends, to a large extent, on the overlap between the phonological and the orthographic inventories in the native and the foreign languages.

Future work may examine more closely the developmental course of the interplay between cross-linguistic similarity and cognitive skills. For that, language learning would have to be examined in a long-term fashion (i.e., retention over longer periods of time) as well as for other linguistic structures (e.g., morphology, syntax). A more immediate goal may be to perform a large-scale study that would employ factor analysis to examine whether word learning would cluster with the digit span measure of phonological memory or with the nonword repetition measure of phonological memory as well as whether the clustering patterns would depend on the degree of cross-linguistic overlap between the native language and the foreign language.

This research has implications for clinical and education practices with second-language learners and bilingual populations as well as with adult speakers who have difficulty reading in their native language. Findings suggest that a core set of cognitive skills may underlie reading acquisition. It is possible that improving those skills may indirectly affect reading. For instance, improving an English as a second language (ESL)-speaker's native-language vocabulary may facilitate his or her reading acquisition. However, results indicate that the link between reading acquisition and L1 vocabulary knowledge relies on shared phonology between L1 and L2. Therefore, improvement in vocabulary skills may be less helpful for literacy acquisition in a phonologically mismatching language. Instead, improving one's phonological memory may carry greater benefits in situations in which the foreign language mismatches the native language in phonology.

To conclude, foreign language learning and acquisition of reading need to be considered within a larger, interactive framework. For instance, previous work showed that while vocabulary skills influence acquisition of early literacy, as reading becomes automatic, reading skills predict vocabulary growth. Similarly, while phonological skills influence one's ability to acquire foreign words, as foreign language knowledge progresses, bilinguals' phonological capacity increases. The present study shows that phonological capacity, vocabulary knowledge, and cross-linguistic similarity are three variables that not only influence learning outcomes, but also mutually influence each other. Together, these findings support an interactive, dynamic account of vocabulary and literacy acquisition in a second language.

Acknowledgments

This research was supported in part by NSF Grant BCS0617455 and by the Joseph Levin Foundation Scholarship to Margarita Kaushanskaya and by Grants NSF BCS0418495 and NICHD 1R03HD046952-01A1 to Viorica Marian. We would like to thank Henrike Blumenfeld, James Booth, Doris Johnson, Karla McGregor, and members of the Bilingualism and Psycholinguistics Laboratory for helpful discussions of this work; Bronwyn Woods for help with data collection; and Tina Yao, Swapna Musunuru, and Erica Meeks for help with data coding.

Conflicts of Interest

The authors declare no conflicts of interest.

References

Bialystok, E., S. Majumder & M. M. Martin. 2003. Developing phonological awareness: is there a bilingual advantage? *Applied Psycholinguistics* **24:** 27–44.

Cheung, H. 1996. Nonword span as a unique predictor of second-language vocabulary learning. *Developmental Psychology* **32:** 867–873.

Cisero, C. A. & J. M. Royer. 1995. The development and cross-language transfer of phonological awareness. *Contemporary Educational Psychology* **20:** 275–303.

Corneau, L., P. Cormier, E. Grandmaison & D. Lacroix. 1999. A longitudinal study of phonological processing skills in children learning to read in a second language. *Journal of Educational Psychology* **91:** 29–43.

De Jong, P. F., M-J. Seveke & M. van Veen. 2000. Phonological sensitivity and the acquisition of new words in children. *Journal of Experimental Child Psychology* **76:** 275–301.

De Keyeser, R. M. 2000. The robustness of the critical period effects in second language acquisition. *Studies in Second Language Acquisition* **22:** 499–533.

Dunn, L. M. & L. M. Dunn. 1997. *Peabody picture vocabulary test* (3rd ed.). Circle Pines, MN: American Guidance Service.

Ellis, N. C. & A. Beaton. 1993a. Psycholinguistic determinants of foreign language vocabulary learning. *Language Learning* **43**(4): 559–617.

Ellis, N. & A. Beaton. 1993b. Factors affecting the learning of foreign language vocabulary: Imagery keyword mediators and phonological short-term memory. *Quarterly Journal of Experimental Psychology* **46A**(3): 533–558.

Francis, W. N. & H. Kucera. 1982. *Frequency analysis of English usage: lexicon and grammar*. Boston: Houghton Mifflin.

Gathercole, S. E. & A. D. Baddeley. 1989. Evaluation of the role of phonological STM in the development of vocabulary in children: a longitudinal study. *Journal of Memory & Language* **28**: 200–213.

Gathercole, S. E. & A. D. Baddeley. 1990. The role of phonological memory in vocabulary acquisition: a study of young children learning new names. *British Journal of Psychology* **81**: 439–454.

Gathercole, S. E., C. Willis, H. Emslie & A. D. Baddeley. 1991. The influences of number of syllables and wordlikeness on children's repetition of nonwords. *Applied Psycholinguistics* **12**: 349–367.

Gilhooly, K. J. & R. H. Logie. 1980. Age of acquisition, imagery, concreteness, familiarity and ambiguity measures for 1944 words. *Behavior Research Methods and Instrumentation* **12**: 395–427.

Gupta, P. 2003. Examining the relationship between word learning, nonword repetition, and immediate serial recall in adults. *Quarterly Journal of Experimental Psychology* **56A**: 1213–1236.

Majeres, R. L. 2005. Phonological and orthographic coding skills in adult readers. *Journal of General Psychology* **132**(3): 267–280.

Masoura, E.V. & S. E. Gathercole. 1999. Phonological short-term memory and foreign language learning. *International Journal of Psychology* **34**(5/6): 383–388.

Paivio, A., J. C. Yuille & S. A. Madigan. 1968. Concreteness imagery and meaningfulness values for 925 words. *Journal of Experimental Psychology Monograph Supplement* **76**: 1–25.

Papagno, C., T. Valentine & A. Baddeley. 1991. Phonological short-term memory and foreign-language vocabulary learning. *Journal of Memory and Language* **30**: 331–347.

Papagno, C. & G. Vallar. 1992. Phonological short-term memory and the learning of novel words: the effects of phonological similarity and item length. *Quarterly Journal of Experimental Psychology* **44A**: 44–67.

Papagno, C. & G. Vallar. 1995. Verbal short-term memory and vocabulary learning in polyglots. *Quarterly Journal of Experimental Psychology* **48A**: 98–107.

Service, E. 1992. Phonology, working memory, and foreign-language learning. *Quarterly Journal of Experimental Psychology* **45A**(3): 21–50.

Service, E. & F. I. M. Craik. 1993. Differences between young and older adults in learning a foreign vocabulary. *Journal of Memory and Language* **32**: 608–623.

Service, E. & V. Kohonen. 1995. Is the relationship between phonological memory and foreign language learning accounted for by vocabulary acquisition? *Applied Psycholinguistics* **16**: 155–172.

Seidenberg, M. S. & J. McClelland. 1989. A distributed, developmental model of word recognition and naming. *Psychological Review* **96**: 523–568.

Speciale, G., N. C. Ellis & T. Bywater. 2004. Phonological sequence learning and short-term store capacity determine second language vocabulary acquisition. *Applied Psycholinguistics* **25**: 293–321.

Stahl, S. A. & M. M. Fairbanks. 2006. The Effects of vocabulary Instruction: A model-based meta-analysis. In K. A. Dougherty Stahl & M. C. McKenna, (Eds.) *Reading research at work: foundations of effective practice* (pp. 226–261). New York: Guilford Press.

Toglia, M. P. & W. F. Battig. 1978. *Handbook of semantic word norms*. Hillsdale, NJ: Erlbaum.

Van Hell, J. G. & A. C. Mahn. 1997. Keyword mnemonics versus rote rehearsal: Learning concrete and abstract foreign words by experienced and inexperienced learners. *Language Learning* **47**: 507–546.

Van Orden, G. C. & S. D. Goldinger. 1994. Interdependence of form and function in cognitive systems explains perception of printed words. *Journal of Experimental Psychology: Human Perception and Performance* **20**: 1269–1291.

Wagner, R. K., J. K. Torgesen & C. A. Rashotte. 1999. *Comprehensive test of phonological processing*. Austin, TX: Pro-Ed, Inc.

Williams, K. T. 1997. *Expressive vocabulary test*. Circle Pines, MN: American Guidance Service.

Visual Skills and Cross-Modal Plasticity in Deaf Readers

Possible Implications for Acquiring Meaning from Print

Matthew W.G. Dye,[a] Peter C. Hauser,[b] and Daphne Bavelier[a]

[a]*University of Rochester, Rochester, New York, USA*

[b]*National Technical Institute for the Deaf, Rochester Institute of Technology, Rochester, New York, USA*

Most research on reading skill acquisition in deaf individuals has been conducted from the perspective of a hearing child learning to read. This approach may limit our understanding of how a deaf child approaches the task of learning to read and successfully acquires reading skills. An alternative approach is to consider how the cognitive skills that a deaf child brings to the reading task may influence the route by which he or she achieves reading fluency. A review of the literature on visual spatial attention suggests that deaf individuals are more distracted by visual information in the parafovea and periphery. We discuss how this may have an influence upon the perceptual processing of written text in deaf students.

Key words: **deaf; reading; visual attention; distractibility; cross-modal plasticity**

Every one of us is different in some way, but for those of us who are more different, we have to put more effort into convincing the less different that we can do the same thing they can, just differently.

—Marlee Matlin

Introduction

Communication in a Visual World

The ability to read successfully requires extracting meaning from print. In hearing children, this is thought to involve the development of phonological awareness and the acquisition of grapheme–phoneme correspondences, both of which are related to the child's preexisting acquisition of the spoken language that

corresponds to the printed medium (Brady & Shankweiler, 1991). For deaf children, this "typical" pattern of literacy acquisition is not available. Specifically, these children have little or no access to a spoken language. For many deaf children, their access to the world of shared meanings is through the visual sense. They rely upon visual communication strategies whether by speechreading, a manually coded form of the spoken language (such as Signed Exact English), or the use of a natural visual language such as American Sign Language (ASL). Can these deaf children then achieve literacy? The lack of linguistic structures corresponding to acoustic properties of spoken language, in particular phonology, would seem to inhibit this "typical" pattern of development. Indeed, many deaf children seem to have problems with literacy acquisition. Over the past 100 years, deaf high school graduates' average reading levels have remained around the fourth-grade level (Holt, Traxler, & Allen, 1997; Pintner &

Address for correspondence: Matthew W.G. Dye, Department of Brain and Cognitive Sciences, University of Rochester, Rochester NY 14627. Voice: +1-585-275-0759; fax: +1-585-442-9216. mdye@bcs.rochester.edu

Ann. N.Y. Acad. Sci. 1145: 71–82 (2008). © 2008 New York Academy of Sciences.
doi: 10.1196/annals.1416.013

Patterson, 1916). Importantly, however, inter-individual variability in reading achievement is quite large and a significant number of deaf students do achieve age-appropriate or better reading skills. What distinguishes these individuals? A host of factors may contribute. Have they been deaf from birth? How much residual hearing is available? In what kind of program were they educated? Do they have good speech reception and intelligibility? Of particular interest in this regard are profoundly deaf individuals (those with hearing losses of 90 dB or greater within the speech range), educated within bilingual–bicultural programs that promote the use of ASL, who have little or no competence in the spoken language domain. For good readers from within this population, which cognitive skills are recruited or acquired in order to read succesfully?

Heterogeneity of the Deaf Population

It is important to note that deaf individuals in general vary greatly with regard to the etiology of their deafness, its severity, and the age of onset. According to the National Institute on Deafness and Other Communication Disorders, approximately 127 in 1,000 children under the age of 18 years in the United States, have some hearing loss. The etiology of hearing loss can be hereditary ($\sim$50%) or acquired by several causes which include prenatal or perinatal infections (cytomegalovirus, rubella, and herpes simplex), postnatal infections (meningitis), premature birth, anoxia, trauma, or it can occur as a result of ototoxic drugs administered during pregnancy. Many of these causes have been associated with other, sometimes severe, neurological sequelae that affect behavioral, cognitive, and psychosocial functioning (Hauser, Wills, & Isquith, 2006; King, Hauser, & Isquith, 2006). Hereditary deafness is associated with more than 350 genetic conditions (Martini, Mazzoli, & Kimberling, 1997), and about a third of these genetic conditions are associated with syndromes (Petit, 1996). Although not all hereditary cases of deafness are

nonsyndromic, hereditarily deafened individuals are more likely to have unremarkable neurologic and psychiatric histories. In the United States, many individuals who have severe to profound hearing loss before the age of 3 years acquire ASL as their first language. This group relies on visual routes for learning and language access and has similar values, beliefs, and behaviors that reflect deaf culture. The community of ASL users is often referred to in the literature as a linguistic minority community because of the similarities it has with other minority communities in terms of language and culture (Ladd, 2003; Padden & Humphries, 2005). The National Association of the Deaf estimates that there are 250,000 to 500,000 ASL users in the United States and Canada. The group often referred to as "deaf native signers" are those born deaf to at least one deaf parent from whom they acquired ASL as a first language in infancy. Such individuals were reported to represent only 4.4% of the 6–19-year-old deaf students in the United States in 1999–2000 (Mitchell & Karchmer, 2004).

Cognition and Literacy Acquisition

A new approach to considering the development of literacy proposes a different way of thinking about the acquisition process that may suggest answers to this apparent conundrum. Usually, we think of children trying to link the printed word to their preexisting knowledge of spoken language. The problem is one of mapping from print-to-sound—dyslexic individuals are thought by some to have problems in this domain (Rack, Snowling, & Olson, 1992). But what if this mapping is one of many possible mechanisms by which a child can achieve literacy? For example, a different approach for examining the acquisition of a written language is the study of a nonalphabetic writing system such as Chinese. Studies of how that logographic writing system is learned suggest that orthographic awareness may be of more importance (Tan, Spinks, Eden, Perfetti, & Siok, 2005) and involve right hemisphere areas to a greater extent (Tan *et al.*, 2001). This raises the possibility that deaf readers with little access to spoken phonology may have alternative routes available to them for the extraction of meaning from words. That is, for deaf readers, words may function similarly to logographs, bypassing the need for grapheme–phoneme conversion skills. What little data are available concerning the brain areas involved in reading in deaf individuals suggests that the right hemisphere also plays a role in English reading for deaf individuals, whereas the left hemisphere is predominant for hearing individuals (Neville *et al.*, 1998).

To better understand the routes by which a deaf child may achieve literacy in an alphabetic script such as English, one approach that has been advocated is to think of the printed word as the starting point (Kuntze, 1998). The child's task is to extract some meaning from this visual pattern. In order to do this, he or she can use a range of cognitive skills (memory, attention, pattern matching, etc.) and knowledge bases (such as metalinguistic knowledge of written English and contextual information that will help decode the text). The "typical" child may use print-to-sound mappings and a spoken language lexicon to perform the task. A deaf child may rely on visual grapheme recognition strategies and either conceptual knowledge or an ASL lexicon. When considering the development of literacy in deaf children from this perspective, the question changes. It becomes, "which cognitive skills and knowledge bases best allow deaf children to extract meaning from print in an automatic and fluent manner?" Importantly, these mechanisms may be very different from those employed by hearing children. It is only by reformulating the question in this way that we will be led to consider several different reading acquisition mechanisms rather than just one. Similarly, it does not make sense to talk of an "optimal" mechanism for reading acquisition. Which mechanism is optimal for any individual will depend upon the nature of the language being read, the cognitive skills and knowledge bases that the individual brings to the task of reading, and, crucially, the act of reading itself. Through experience with text and attempting to extract meaning from it with the resources at their disposal, a child will move toward the acquisition of fluent literacy.

Whereas studies that determine the cognitive factors that lead to successful literacy acquisition in deaf students are still rare, much work has been conducted examining the perceptual and attentional processes of vision. A large body of work is now accumulating that focuses on the development of visual skills of deaf children, but their role with regards to achieving literacy has not been widely discussed. In this brief article, we will review that literature and make suggestions about the possible implications of this work for literacy in this population. Our emphasis will be on factors influencing adult reading skill, rather than the process of literacy acquisition per se. First, we will present what is known about the deployment of visual attention across space in deaf individuals. We will then suggest how differences in visual attention between deaf and hearing individuals may affect reading skill in the deaf learner. Finally, we will suggest what we believe to be fruitful avenues of future research that will help elucidate the mechanisms by which deaf individuals master literacy. More broadly, we hope to demonstrate that an understanding of reading skill in deaf individuals can be fostered by an understanding of the preexisting cognitive skills that these individuals bring to the task of reading. We believe this will complement more traditional approaches in which reading skill in deaf individuals is interpreted in terms of the mechanisms relied upon by hearing individuals. It is not our aim to provide a review of the literature on deafness and literacy acquisition (see Musselman, 2000, for a recent such review). Rather, we will focus upon an aspect of cognition that deaf readers are likely to rely upon heavily—visual cognition, and visual attention in particular—and explore what implications that may have for their reading skills.

Visual Skills in Deaf Individuals

Behavioral Studies of Visual Spatial Attention in Deaf Individuals

Deficiencies

The earliest work looking at the development of visual skills in deaf children suggested that the effect of early auditory deprivation was an associated deficiency in visual function. One early study (Myklebust & Brutten, 1953) reported that deaf children had low-level visual deficits, as measured by the Keystone Visual Survey, as well as poor levels of performance on visual pattern-matching tasks such as the Marble Boards test. Deficits in a visual continuous performance task (CPT) have also been reported in deaf children (Quittner, Leibach, & Marciel, 2004; Quittner, Smith, Osberger, Mitchell, & Katz, 1994; Smith, Quittner, Osberger, & Miyamoto, 1998). In this task, a rapid series of digits is presented, and children are required to make a response to a "9" only when it is preceded by a "1" but otherwise to withhold responding. They observed that deaf children were delayed in the development of this ability, never attaining the level of even the youngest hearing children tested. Furthermore, their data suggest that cochlear implantation (CI) enhances the development of this skill although, again, those children with CIs did not achieve the performance levels of hearing controls. The authors suggest that this represents a deficit in visual selective attention, although it could also represent difficulties integrating visual information over time or just a problem dealing with numerals. Taken together, these findings have been used in support of the deficiency hypothesis. Generally stated, this hypothesis states that integration of information from the different senses is an essential component to the development of normal function in each individual sense. For the deaf child, then, the lack of audition impairs the development of multisensory integration and therefore the development of typical visual skills.

It is important to note some of the shortcomings of these studies and to acknowledge the populations from which the data were drawn. For example, the results that Myklebust obtained using the Marble Boards test have been difficult to replicate (Hayes, 1955; Larr, 1956), suggesting either experimenter error or small effect sizes in the original published work. Also, differences between deaf and hearing children have not always been observed using CPT tasks (Tharpe, Ashmead, & Rothpletz, 2002). So there are issues of replicability that need to be considered when interpreting these data. In addition, much of the work that has suggested visual deficits in deaf children has used extremely heterogeneous samples, bringing into question the role that deafness per se has in the effect reported and questioning the generalizability of those results to all deaf children. For example, an examination of the demographics of the deaf children used in the CPT studies suggests differences between those who had CIs and those who did not. The CI group was more likely to have received an education using oral methods as opposed to Total Communication (a combination of auditory and visual communication modes), and less likely to have viral meningitis as a cause of their deafness. Moreover, the cause of deafness for most children in those studies was unknown.

Benefits

In contrast to those studies reporting visual deficits, different results are obtained when homogenous samples of deaf participants are used. Those born to deaf parents with mostly genetic etiologies who learn a signed language from an early age have demonstrated differences in visual function compared to hearing controls that could be considered adaptive by showing a compensation in the visual modality for the lack of auditory input. Using deaf native signers such as these, a selective enhancement in deaf individuals for stimuli that are peripheral or in motion and require attentional selection has been demonstrated using a variety of paradigms. In a task employing a flanker compatibility paradigm, enhanced processing has been reported of peripheral distractors located at 4.2 degrees of visual angle from a concurrent target combined with decreased processing of central distractors located at 0.5 degrees (Proksch & Bavelier, 2002). Subsequently, another study demonstrated that the responses of deaf individuals were more influenced by distractor letters positioned at ∼1.5 degrees from a letter target than were responses of hearing controls (Sladen, Tharpe, Ashmead, Wesley Grantham, & Chun, 2005). Most recently, some researchers have shown that as nonletter distractors (arrows) are positioned at increasing eccentricities (1.0, 2.0 and 3.0 degrees), their effect on deaf individuals increases relative to how these distractors affect hearing individuals (Dye, Baril, & Bavelier, 2007). Finally, using peripheral kinetic and foveal static perimetry, deaf individuals were reported to be better than hearing controls at detecting moving lights in the periphery (manifested as a difference in field of view) and not different in their sensitivity to points of light presented foveally (Stevens & Neville, 2006). What all of these "compensation" studies have in common is that they focus upon visual attention skills, that is, how deaf individuals allocate limited processing resources to the visual scene. In terms of adaptation to the environment, the change observed in deaf individuals makes intuitive sense: a redistribution of visual attention to the periphery in order to compensate for the lack of peripheral auditory cues provided by the environment, such as the sound of an approaching vehicle or the creak of an opening door.

In contrast to these changes in visual attention in which the onset and location of stimuli are unknown, attempts to demonstrate changes in basic visual skills using psychophysical methods (and where target location and onset are known *a priori*) have been unsuccessful (Bosworth & Dobkins, 1999, 2002a, 2002b; Bross, 1979; Bross & Sauerwein, 1980; Brozinsky & Bavelier, 2004; Finney & Dobkins, 2001; Mills, 1985; Poizner & Tallal,

1987). Thus it appears that low-level visual processing is unaffected by early auditory impairment. One working hypothesis is that a sensory loss leads to changes in higher-level attentional processing, especially in domains in which information from multiple senses is integrated (Bavelier, Dye, & Hauser, 2006; Bavelier & Neville, 2002). Multisensory integration is most important in situations where no one sense dominates; accordingly, the largest behavioral differences between deaf and hearing persons have been observed during the processing of the visual periphery. In particular, early deafness results in a redistribution of attentional resources to the periphery, most commonly observed when input from peripheral and central space competes for privileged access to processing resources (Bavelier *et al.*, 2006).

Studies of the Functional Anatomy of Cross-Modal Plasticity in Deaf Individuals

Given these changes in visual function that have been observed behaviorally, it makes sense to ask whether we can observe associated neuronal changes. There is now a substantial body of work looking at compensatory changes in brain activation following early auditory deprivation. One well-studied area is MT/MST, an area of visual cortex involved in the detection and analysis of movement whose activity is known to be modulated by attentional processes (O'Craven, Rosen, Kwong, Treisman, & Savoy, 1997). When viewing unattended moving stimuli, deaf and hearing participants do not differ in their recruitment of MT/MST cortex. However, when required to attend to peripheral movement and ignore concurrent central motion, enhanced recruitment of MT/MST is observed relative to hearing controls (Bavelier *et al.*, 2001; Fine, Finney, Boynton, & Dobkins, 2005). This pattern echoes a general trend in the literature, whereby the greatest population differences have been reported for motion stimuli in the visual periphery under conditions that engage selective attention, such as when the location or time of arrival of the stimulus is unknown or when the stimulus has to be selected from among distractors (Bavelier *et al.*, 2006).

There are several potential ways in which cross-modal reorganization could support the changes observed in the spatial distribution of visual attention in deaf individuals. One possibility is that there is an expansion in the representation of the peripheral visual field in early visual cortex. However, there is currently little data to support this hypothesis (Fine *et al.*, 2005). Recent studies in the macaque (Falchier, Clavagnier, Barone, & Kennedy, 2002; Rockland & Ojima, 2003) have highlighted projections from auditory cortex to early visual areas (V1 and V2). This raises the possibility that in the absence of auditory input these pathways are susceptible to the attentional modulations observed in deaf individuals, although this remains an open question. Another possibility is that the multimodal associative cortex may display a greater sensitivity to input from remaining modalities such as vision and touch. Evidence for this hypothesis comes from studies reporting changes in the posterior parietal cortex of deaf individuals (Bavelier *et al.*, 2001), an area known to be involved in the integration of information from different sensory modalities. Finally, it is possible that in deaf individuals, the lack of input from audition causes the auditory cortex—which is multimodal in nature—to reorganize and process visual information. Indeed, there is some evidence that auditory areas in the superior temporal sulcus show greater recruitment in deaf than in hearing individuals for visual, tactile, and signed input (Bavelier *et al.*, 2001; Fine *et al.*, 2005; Finney, Clementz, Hickok, & Dobkins, 2003; Levanen, Jousmaki, & Hari, 1998; Neville *et al.*, 1998; Pettito *et al.*, 2000). This may or may not be the case for primary auditory cortex (A1) with brain averaging studies (where data from several individuals are combined and analyzed as a group), suggesting recruitment of

areas adjacent to and overlapping the posterior part of A1 (Fine *et al.*, 2005; Finney, Fine, & Dobkins, 2001; Lambertz, Gizewski, de Greiff, & Forsting, 2005; Levanen *et al.*, 1998), and studies in which A1 is delineated on a subject-by-subject basis (without averaging across individuals in a group), suggesting little functional change except in the adjacent secondary auditory region (Bavelier *et al.*, 2001; Kral, Hartmann, Tillein, Heid, & Klinke, 2001; Nishimura *et al.*, 1999).

To summarize, behavioral studies suggest that there is redistribution of attentional resources in deaf individuals with an enhancement of representations from peripheral space. This behavioral difference appears to be accompanied by neural changes suggesting cross-modal reorganization in areas that integrate information from different modalities and possible recruitment of multimodal cortex in auditory regions for the processing of visual information.

Deafness, Visual Cognition, and Reading

We noted in the introduction that literacy can be regarded as the reader's attempt to acquire meaning from the printed word. Insight from deaf readers (Hofsteater, 1959; Kuntze, 1998) suggests that for many deaf individuals this acquisition is a predominantly visual process, building upon their world knowledge and linguistic skills in English and/or ASL. If this is the case (and it may be for some if not all deaf readers), then it is important to investigate the visual skills that the deaf individual brings to the task if we are to understand how literacy can be acquired exclusively through the visual domain. Differences in visual processing in the deaf reader may result in different perceptual processes involved in reading as compared to those of hearing readers. Below we discuss how visual skill differences between deaf and hearing readers may have an impact on reading skills.

Visual Attention and Perceptual Processes in Reading

The proposal that changes in visual skills are likely to alter reading strategies is not new. A recent review by Boden and Giaschi (2007) discusses various ways in which changes in the magnocellular stream may be implicated in the reading problems experienced by those with developmental dyslexia. While the focus of their review is not upon reading in deaf populations, two aspects of visual processing they discuss have implications for individuals with a different spatial distribution of visual attention: parafoveal-on-foveal interactions and covert spatial attention.

We begin by observing that a reader must fixate upon and pay attention to printed words in order to extract meaning from a text. Much is now known about the perceptual processes involved in reading, especially about how eye movements (saccades) and fixations on text are planned and executed, to the extent that there exist computational models that provide good fits to the data (e.g., the E-Z Reader model; Reichle, Rayner, & Pollatsek, 2003). It is becoming clear that low-level visual properties of words exert a large influence upon where readers look in a text and how long they fixate upon a word (Radach, Kennedy, & Rayner, 2004). One of the properties that influences where a reader will fixate in a word is the length of that word and of neighboring words (to the right of the fixated word in a left-to-right language like English). These "parafoveal-on-foveal" effects can be defined as the effect of a not-yet fixated word on the processing of a currently fixated word (Kennedy & Pynte, 2005). If deaf readers have a spatial distribution of attention which biases them toward processing parafoveal input, then parafoveal-on-foveal effects may be stronger in deaf than in hearing readers, resulting in qualitatively different scanning patterns over written texts and differences in the amount and type of information extracted from the parafoveal region. Greater availability of parafoveal information may slow down foveal processing, resulting in longer fixations and slowing down the reading process. One knock-on effect of these changes in how text is processed at a perceptual level may be a greater demand on memory on account of longer processing times, causing problems in interpreting complex syntactic structures or making appropriate references within a sentence or passage. Interestingly, a case study of a hearing individual (S.J.) has been reported in which reading problems were attributed to an inability to selectively attend to the fixated word and suppress processing of information in the parafovea (Rayner, Murphy, Henderson, & Pollatsek, 1989), resulting in reasonable word recognition performance, but poor comprehension of passages of text. It is possible that deaf readers may consistently demonstrate this pattern and benefit from a "windowed reading" remediation program, which was successful for S.J., whereby only limited amounts of text are made available at any one time, limiting the amount of distracting information that occupies the parafovea.

Another aspect of visual attention likely to affect reading skills is visual selective attention. For example, Facoetti and colleagues (Facoetti & Molteni, 2001; Lorusso et al., 2004) suggest that as the reader makes a series of successive saccades across written text, it is important that he or she both spatially disambiguate proximal letters and temporally integrate that spatial arrangement of letters over the series of saccades. Thus an alteration in how visual selective attention is deployed will alter how a series of visual events is integrated over time and may lead to confusions both in identifying the letters of a word and in creating representations that preserve both the correct letters and their correct spatial arrangements. Facoetti has proposed that such deficits in visual selective attention, possibly resulting from deficits in posterior parietal cortex, may play a role in some of the difficulties experienced by dyslexic readers (Facoetti, 2005). In the case of deaf readers, this may be instantiated as enhanced processing of parafoveal letters at the expense of the fixated letters. In addition, given possible problems in temporally integrating rapid serial visual presentations (Quittner *et al.*, 1994, 2004; Smith *et al.*, 1998), further difficulties in constructing representations on the basis of successive saccades across written text are also possible. In support of this, recent work by Valdois and colleagues has suggested that problems in selective visual attention (a narrower attentional window in which graphemes are available for processing) play a functional role in reading problems observed in some developmental dyslexics, separately from problems that are phonological in nature (Bosse, Tainturier, & Valdois, 2006; Valdois, Bosse, & Tainturier, 2004). We are not suggesting, however, that deaf readers should be considered *a priori* as dyslexics. Not only is the selective attention account of dyslexia controversial, but there is also evidence that magnocellular visual functions differ between deaf and dyslexic individuals (Stevens & Neville, 2006). However, considering this line of investigation provides a way to theorize about how the visual cognitive skills of deaf readers may interact with the integration of visual information during the reading process. Indeed, differences in the deployment of visual attention may be just one of several factors that influence the acquisition pathway of literacy in deaf readers.

Conclusions and Avenues for Future Research

Although the literature on literacy in deaf individuals is extensive, there is still much that we do not know. What are the mechanisms by which deaf individuals can learn to read, and how are these influenced by changes in visual cognition? Studies are needed that explore the neuroanatomical underpinnings of fluent and dysfluent reading in deaf readers (as well as in "typical" readers) with assessments of how deafness, language history, and educational methods influence the development of reading networks in deaf brains. The question of whether

or not deaf individuals differ in their perceptual processing of text remains open and is susceptible to empirical inquiry. The knowledge gained by such studies will allow us to begin to understand how the peculiar cognitive skills of deaf children influence their acquisition of reading skills and will, it is hoped, lead to remediation techniques and instructional protocols that will allow more deaf children to excel and become literate.

To our knowledge, no work has yet looked at saccades and fixations of deaf readers in a rigorous or systematic manner. Some work has looked at viewing position effects (VPE; O'Regan, 1981), whereby the ability to correctly identify a word varies as a function of where in a word the reader fixates. Aghababian and colleagues report that the VPE curves for a young deaf girl (A.H.) were flat, indicating that her ability to identify a word did not vary as a function of the fixated letter within the word (Aghababian, Nazir, Lançon, & Tardy, 2001). They report that training in grapheme–phoneme correspondence skills resulted in A.H.'s exhibiting more "normal" VPE curves, such as those typically acquired by hearing children after only 7–8 months of reading instruction (Aghababian & Nazir, 2000). Given our knowledge of how textual information in the periphery of the reading window influences the programming of saccades during reading (Kennedy & Pynte, 2005; Rayner *et al.*, 1989), it makes sense to ask whether a redistribution of attention in deaf readers actually results in qualitatively different scanning of text. That is, the target of a saccade by deaf readers may have quantitatively different determinants, resulting in a qualitatively different pattern of saccades and fixations. The frameworks provided by Facoetti (2005) and Bosse *et al.* (2006) provide a means by which studies can investigate the possible interaction between the deployment of spatial attention in deaf readers and the acquisition of reading skill. It also remains possible, however, that a strategic allocation of attention by deaf readers allows them to overcome these attentional constraints. Studies on the automaticity of attentional distribution across space in deaf individuals will help elucidate this question.

As well as behavioral explorations of reading performance in deaf readers, more studies are needed that examine the neuroanatomical underpinnings of fluent reading. Some work has suggested that the right hemisphere may have a greater involvement than it does for hearing readers (Neville *et al.*, 1998). These studies will need to dissociate carefully the effects of hearing loss, language background, education, and reading skill in determining which neural pathways are available to support fluent reading skill.

In conclusion, we have reported on a range of studies that suggest a different distribution of attentional resources in deaf individuals associated with cross-modal plasticity in higher visual and attentional areas of cortex. These modulations of visual processing may hold one key to understanding the difficulties faced by deaf readers beyond access to the phonology of the spoken language being expressed in written form. We acknowledge that the amount of residual hearing available to a deaf individual will be a major predictor of reading skill among other important factors (Perfetti & Sandak, 2000). Our consideration here is for the deaf child for whom this is not a viable option. While some deaf children will be able to acquire literacy via the traditional route and demonstrate good phonological awareness and grapheme–phoneme correspondence skills, there are many others who will not be able to do so. If an approach focusing upon cognitive skills and knowledge bases, rather than print-to-sound mapping per se, is successful in explaining literacy acquisition in these deaf children, it may help in the development of appropriate instructional strategies that can be tailored to the needs of an individual deaf child. It may also, by extension, help us to understand the issues faced by other children who have difficulties in this most crucial of skills.

We propose that trying to understand reading skill acquisition in a deaf child from the perspective of what works for hearing children may at best provide a limited understanding and at worst be misleading. In contrast, we argue that understanding reading skill acquisition from the perspective of the visual cognitive skills that a deaf child brings to the task may provide fruitful insights that both guide our understanding of the human capacity for learning and provide concrete and research-grounded strategies for the teaching of literacy to deaf children.

Acknowledgments

This work was supported by National Institutes of Health Grant DC-04418 to Daphne Bavelier, and by NSF Grant SBE-0541953 to Peter Hauser under Gallaudet University's Science of Learning Center on Visual Language and Visual Learning. We are grateful to the editors for their comments and suggestions for improving the initial draft of this manuscript.

Conflicts of Interest

The authors declare no conflicts of interest.

References

Aghababian, V. & T. Nazir. 2000. Developing normal reading skills: aspects of the visual processes underlying word recognition. *Journal of Experimental Child Psychology* **76:** 123–150.

Aghababian, V., T. A. Nazir, C. Lançon & M. Tardy. 2001. From "logographic" to normal reading: the case of a deaf beginning reader. *Brain and Language* **78**(2): 212–223.

Bavelier, D. & H. J. Neville. 2002. Cross-modal plasticity: Where and how? *Nature Reviews Neuroscience* **3**(6): 443–452.

Bavelier, D., C. Brozinsky, A. Tomann, T. Mitchell, H. Neville & G. Liu. 2001. Impact of early deafness and early exposure to sign language on the cerebral organization for motion processing. *Journal of Neuroscience* **21**(22): 8931–8942.

Bavelier, D., M. Dye & P. Hauser. 2006. Do deaf individuals see better? *Trends in Cognitive Sciences* **10**(11): 512–518.

Boden, C. & D. Giaschi. 2007. M-stream deficits and reading-related visual processes in developmental dyslexia. *Psychological Bulletin* **133**(2): 346–366.

Bosse, M.-L., M. J. Tainturier & S. Valdois. 2006. Developmental dyslexia: the visual span deficit hypothesis. *Cognition* **104**(2): 198–230.

Bosworth, R. G. & K. R. Dobkins. 1999. Left-hemisphere dominance for motion processing in deaf signers. *Psychological Science* **10**(3): 256–262.

Bosworth, R. G. & K. R. Dobkins. 2002a. The effects of spatial attention on motion processing in deaf signers, hearing signers, and hearing nonsigners. *Brain and Cognition* **49**(1): 152–169.

Bosworth, R. G. & K. R. Dobkins. 2002b. Visual field asymmetries for motion processing in deaf and hearing signers. *Brain and Cognition* **49**(1): 170–181.

Brady, S. A. & D. P. Shankweiler, (Eds.). 1991. *Phonological processes in literacy: A tribute to Isabelle Y. Liberman.* Hillsdale, NJ: Lawrence Erlbaum.

Bross, M. & H. Sauerwein. 1980. Signal detection analysis of visual flicker in deaf and hearing individuals. *Perceptual and Motor Skills* **51**: 839–843.

Bross, M. 1979. Residual sensory capacities of the deaf: A signal detection analysis of a visual discrimination task. *Perceptual and Motor Skills* **48**: 187–194.

Brozinsky, C. J. & D. Bavelier. 2004. Motion velocity thresholds in deaf signers: Changes in lateralization but not in overall sensitivity. *Cognitive Brain Research* **21**(1): 1–10.

Dye, M. W. G., D. E. Baril & D. Bavelier. 2007. Which aspects of visual attention are changed by deafness? The case of the Attentional Network Test. *Neuropsychologia* **45**(8):1801 1811.

Facoetti, A. & M. Molteni. 2001. The gradient of visual attention in developmental dyslexia. *Neuropsychologia* **39**: 352–357.

Facoetti, A. 2005. Reading and selective spatial attention: evidence from behavioral studies in dyslexic children. In H. D. Tobias (Ed.), *Trends in dyslexia research* (pp. 35–71). Hauppauge, NY: Nova Science Publishers.

Falchier, A., S. Clavagnier, P. Barone & H. Kennedy. 2002. Anatomical evidence of multimodal integration in primate striate cortex. *Journal of Neuroscience* **22**: 5749–5759.

Fine, I., E. M. Finney, G. M. Boynton & K. R. Dobkins. 2005. Comparing the effects of auditory deprivation and sign language within the auditory and visual cortex. *Journal of Cognitive Neuroscience* **17**(10): 1621–1637.

Finney, E. M. & K. R. Dobkins. 2001. Visual contrast sensitivity in deaf versus hearing populations: exploring the perceptual consequences of auditory deprivation and experience with a visual language. *Cognitive Brain Research* **11**(1): 171–183.

Finney, E. M., B. A. Clementz, G. Hickok & K. R. Dobkins. 2003. Visual stimuli activate auditory cortex in deaf subjects: evidence from MEG. *Neuroreport* **14**(11): 1425–1427.

Finney, E. M., I. Fine & K. R. Dobkins. 2001. Visual stimuli activate auditory cortex in the deaf. *Nature Neuroscience* **4**(12): 1171–1173.

Hauser, P. C., K. Wills & P. K. Isquith. 2005. Hard of hearing, deafness, and being deaf. In J. D. J. E. Farmer & S. Warschausky (Eds.), *Neurodevelopmental disabilities: Clinical research and practice* (pp. 119–131). New York: Guilford Press.

Hayes, G. M. 1955. *A study of the visual perception of orally educated deaf children.* M.S. thesis, University of Massachusetts, Amherst, MA.

Hofsteater, H. T. 1959. An experiment in preschool education: An autobiographical case study. *Gallaudet College Bulletin* **3**(8): 1–17.

Holt, J. A., C. B. Traxler & T. E. Allen. 1997. *Interpreting the scores: A user's guide to the 9th edition Stanford Achievement Test for educators of deaf and hard-of-hearing students.* (Gallaudet Research Institute Technical Report No. 97–1). Washington, DC: Gallaudet University.

Kennedy, A. & J. Pynte. 2005. Parafoveal-on-foveal effects in normal reading. *Vision Research* **45**: 153–168.

King, B. H., P. C. Hauser & P. K. Isquith. 2006. Psychiatric aspects of blindness and severe visual impairment, and deafness and severe hearing loss in children. In C. E. Coffey & R. A. Brumback (Eds.), *Textbook of pediatric neuropsychiatry* (pp. 397–423). Washington, DC: American Psychiatric Association.

Kral, A., R. Hartmann, J. Tillein, S. Heid & R. Klinke. 2001. Delayed maturation and sensitive periods in the auditory cortex. *Audiological Neurootology* **6**(6): 346–362.

Kuntze, M. 1998. Literacy and deaf children: the language question. *Topics in Language Disorders* **18**(4): 1–15.

Ladd, N. P. 2003. *In search of deafhood.* Clevedon, UK: Multilingual Matters.

Lambertz, N., E. R. Gizewski, A. de Greiff & M. Forsting. 2005. Cross-modal plasticity in deaf subjects dependent on the extent of hearing loss. *Cognitive Brain Research* **25**(3): 884–890.

Larr, A. L. 1956. Perceptual and conceptual ability of residential school deaf children. *Exceptional Children* **23**: 63–66, 88.

Levanen, S., V. Jousmaki & R. Hari. 1998. Vibration-induced auditory-cortex activation in a congenitally deaf adult. *Current Biology* **8**(15): 869–872.

Lorusso, M. L., A. Facoetti, S. Pesenti, C. Cattaneo, M. Molteni & G. Geiger. 2004. Wider recognition in peripheral vision common to different subtypes of dyslexia. *Vision Research* **44**: 2413–2424.

Martini, A., M. Mazzoli & W. Kimberling. 1997. An introduction to genetics of normal and defective hearing. *Annals of the New York Academy of Sciences* **830**: 361–374.

Mills, C. 1985. Perception of visual temporal patterns by deaf and hearing adults. *Bulletin of the Psychonomic Society* **23**: 483–486.

Mitchell, R. E. & M. A. Karchmer. 2004. Chasing the mythical ten percent: parental hearing status of deaf and hard of hearing students in the United States. *Sign Language Studies* **4**(2): 138–163.

Musselman, C. 2000. How do children who can't hear learn to read an alphabetic script? A review of the literature on reading and deafness. *Journal of Deaf Studies and Deaf Education* **5**: 9–31.

Myklebust, H. R. & M. A. Brutten. 1953. A study of the visual perception of deaf children. *Acta Otolaryngologia Supplement* **105**: 1–126.

Neville, H. J., D. Bavelier, D. P. Corina, J. P. Rauschecker, A. Karni, A. Lalwani, *et al.* 1998. Cerebral organization for language in deaf and hearing subjects: biological constraints and effects of experience. *Proceedings of the National Academy of Science USA* **95**(3): 922–929.

Nishimura, H., K. Hashidawa, K. Doi, T. Iwaki, Y. Watanabe, H. Kusuoka, *et al.* 1999. Sign language 'heard' in the auditory cortex. *Nature* **397**: 116.

O'Craven, K. M., B. R. Rosen, K. K. Kwong, A. Treisman & R. L. Savoy. 1997. Voluntary attention modulates fMRI activity in human MT-MST. *Neuron* **18**(4): 591–598.

O'Regan, J. K. 1981. The convenient viewing hypothesis. In D. F. Fisher, R. A. Monty, & J. W. Senders (Eds.), *Eye movements: Cognition and visual perception* (pp. 289–298). New York: Wiley.

Padden, C. & T. Humphries. 2005. *Inside deaf culture*. Cambridge, MA: Harvard University Press.

Perfetti, C. A. & R. Sandak. 2000. Reading optimally builds on spoken language. *Journal of Deaf Studies and Deaf Education* **5**(1): 32–50.

Petit, C. 1996. Genes responsible for human hereditary deafness: symphony of a thousand. *Nature Genetics* **14**: 385–391.

Pettito, L. A., R. J. Zatorre, K. Gauna, E. J. Nikelski, D. Dostie & A. C. Evans. 2000. Speech-like cerebral activity in profoundly deaf people processing signed languages: implications for the neural basis of human language. *Proceedings of the National Academy of Sciences USA* **97**(25): 13961–13966.

Pintner, R. & D. Patterson. 1916. A measure of the language ability of deaf children. *Psychological Review* **23**: 413–436.

Poizner, H. & P. Tallal. 1987. Temporal processing in deaf signers. *Brain and Language* **30**: 52–62.

Proksch, J. & D. Bavelier. 2002. Changes in the spatial distribution of visual attention after early deafness. *Journal of Cognitive Neuroscience* **14**(5): 687–701.

Quittner, A. L., L. B. Smith, M. J. Osberger, T. V. Mitchell & D. B. Katz. 1994. The impact of audition on the development of visual attention. *Psychological Science* **5**(6): 347–353.

Quittner, A. L., P. Leibach & K. Marciel. 2004. The impact of cochlear implants on young deaf children: new methods to assess cognitive and behavioral development. *Archives of Otolaryngology: Head and Neck Surgery* **130**(5): 547–554.

Rack, J. P., M. J. Snowling & R. K. Olson. 1992. The nonword reading deficit in developmental dyslexia: a review. *Reading Research Quarterly* **27**(1): 28–53.

Radach, R., A. Kennedy & K. Rayner (Eds.). 2004. *Eye movements and information processing during reading*. New York: Psychology Press.

Rayner, K., L. A. Murphy, J. M. Henderson & A. Pollatsek. 1989. Selective attentional dyslexia. *Cognitive Neuropsychology* **6**(4): 357–378.

Reichle, E. D., K. Rayner & A. Pollatsek. 2003. The E-Z Reader model of eye movement control in reading: comparisons to other models. *Behavioral and Brain Sciences* **26**: 445–476.

Rockland, K. S. & H. Ojima. 2003. Multisensory convergence in calcarine visual areas in macaque monkey. *International Journal of Psychophysiology* **50**: 19–26.

Sladen, D. P., A. M. Tharpe, D. H. Ashmead, D. Wesley Grantham & M. M. Chun. 2005. Visual attention in deaf and normal hearing adults: effects of stimulus compatibility. *Journal of Speech, Language and Hearing Research* **48**(6): 1529–1537.

Smith, L. B., A. L. Quittner, M. J. Osberger & R. Miyamoto. 1998. Audition and visual attention: the developmental trajectory in deaf and hearing populations. *Developmental Psychology* **34**(5): 840–850.

Stevens, C. & H. Neville. 2006. Neuroplasticity as a double-edged sword: deaf enhancements and dyslexic deficits in motion processing. *Journal of Cognitive Neuroscience* **18**(5): 701–714.

Tan, L. H., H. L. Liu, C. A. Perfetti, J. A. Spinks, P. T. Fox & J. H. Gao. 2001. The neural system underlying Chinese logograph reading. *NeuroImage* **13**(5): 836–846.

Tan, L. H., J. A. Spinks, G. F. Eden, C. A. Perfetti & W. T. Siok. 2005. Reading depends on writing, in Chinese. *Proceedings of the National Academy of Sciences USA* **102:** 8781–8785.

Tharpe, A. M., D. H. Ashmead & A. M. Rothpletz. 2002. Visual attention in children with normal hearing, children with hearing aids, and children with cochlear implants. *Journal of Speech, Language and Hearing Research* **45:** 403–413.

Valdois, S., M.-L. Bosse & M.-J. Tainturier. 2004. The cognitive deficits responsible for developmental dyslexia: review of evidence for a selective visual attentional disorder. *Dyslexia* **10:** 339–363.

Phonological Awareness and Short-Term Memory in Hearing and Deaf Individuals of Different Communication Backgrounds

Daniel Koo,[a,b] **Kelly Crain,**[c] **Carol LaSasso,**[a,b,c] **and Guinevere F. Eden**[a,b]

[a] Center for the Study of Learning, Georgetown University Medical Center, Washington, DC, USA

[b] Center for Visual Learning and Visual Language and [c] Department of Hearing, Speech, and Language Sciences, Gallaudet University, Washington, DC, USA

Previous work in deaf populations on phonological coding and working memory, two skills thought to play an important role in the acquisition of written language skills, have focused primarily on signers or did not clearly identify the subjects' native language and communication mode. In the present study, we examined the effect of sensory experience, early language experience, and communication mode on the phonological awareness skills and serial recall of linguistic items in deaf and hearing individuals of different communicative and linguistic backgrounds: hearing nonsigning controls, hearing users of ASL, deaf users of ASL, deaf oral users of English, and deaf users of cued speech. Since many current measures of phonological awareness skills are inappropriate for deaf populations on account of the verbal demands in the stimuli or response, we devised a nonverbal phonological measure that addresses this limitation. The Phoneme Detection Test revealed that deaf cuers and oral users, but not deaf signers, performed as well as their hearing peers when detecting phonemes not transparent in the orthography. The second focus of the study examined short-term memory skills and found that in response to the traditional digit span as well as an experimental visual version, digit-span performance was similar across the three deaf groups, yet deaf subjects' retrieval was lower than that of hearing subjects. Our results support the claim (Bavelier *et al.*, 2006) that lexical items processed in the visual-spatial modality are not as well retained as information processed in the auditory channel. Together these findings show that the relationship between working memory, phonological coding, and reading may not be as tightly interwoven in deaf students as would have been predicted from work conducted in hearing students.

Key words: phonological awareness; deaf individuals; ASL

Introduction

In languages with alphabetic writing systems, individuals typically acquire reading by matching knowledge of the phonological content of their spoken language to the corresponding orthographic representation. This process of applying the alphabetic principle, combined with phonemic awareness and rules of phonics, allows for decoding of words, which eventually leads to reading fluency and comprehension of text (Juel, 1988). Phonological coding or phonological awareness (PA), which is the ability to recognize that words in spoken languages are composed of a set of meaningless discrete segments called phonemes (Scarborough & Brady, 2002) has been shown in hearing children to be a powerful predictor of subsequent reading achievement (Bradley & Bryant, 1985; Adams, 1990; Ehri & Sweet, 1991; Goswami & Bryant,

Address for correspondence: Guinevere Eden, D.Phil, 4000 Reservoir Road, NW Building D, Suite 150, Washington, DC 20057. edeng@georgetown.edu

1992; Snow, Burns, & Griffin, 1998; Wagner & Torgeson, 1987; Olson, Forsberg, Wise, & Rack, 1994; Torgeson, Wagner, & Rashotte, 1994; Schatschneider *et al.*, 2002). In addition, investigations into the relation between early oral language proficiency and later reading outcome have repeatedly shown that comprehension of oral language is a strong predictor of reading ability (Catts *et al.*, 2003; Bishop & Adams, 1990; Scarborough, 1989).

In contrast, congenitally deaf children generally do not have sufficient auditory access to spoken languages and for them learning to read is an entirely different endeavor. Many studies have consistently shown that profoundly and prelingually deaf individuals lag significantly behind their hearing peers in standardized measures of reading achievement (Furth, 1966; Karchmer, Milone, & Wolk, 1979; Conrad, 1979; Karchmer & Mitchell, 2003; Traxler, 2000). Their reading abilities vary widely, but national surveys indicate an average of third- or fourth-grade reading level (Furth, 1966; Trybus & Karchmer, 1977; Quigley & Paul, 1986; Allen, 1986; Traxler, 2000). One explanation for this performance deficit is that deafness prevents access to spoken phonology (Shankweiler, Liberman, Mark, Fowler, & Fischer, 1979; Perfetti & Sandak, 2000) and, by extension, the use of phonetic coding in working memory, phonological awareness, and phonetic recoding in lexical access, which are considered to be interdependent hallmarks of successful reading development in hearing children (Wagner & Torgeson, 1987; Tractenberg, 2002). This claim, however, is not without dispute as certain deaf individuals demonstrate evidence of phonological coding (Hanson, 1989; Hanson & Lichtenstein, 1990; Hanson & Fowler, 1987; Leybeart, 1993; Conrad, 1979; LaSasso, Crain, & Leybaert, 2003). Still, others have argued that the reason for limited reading achievement among many deaf students is the lack of higher-order language skills, not phonological decoding, (Chamberlain & Mayberry, 2000), and that levels of comprehension required at the higher grade levels presents an obstacle to reading

development. To complicate matters further, there is considerable variability in the use of communication systems among deaf students and their use is usually determined by whether they are born into families of deaf or hearing parents. Unfortunately, many early studies on reading outcomes have not taken into consideration the role of the various communication systems available to the deaf population, each of which may independently influence the degree to which deaf students access written English.

Communication Choices

Generally, deaf and hard-of-hearing individuals living in the United States have three visually based communication choices available to them: (1) sign communication (e.g., American Sign Language); (2) oral/aural communication (the exclusive use of audition, speech/lip-reading, and speech production); and (3) cued speech (CS), which is a communication system designed to visually convey the phonology of spoken languages.

American Sign Language (ASL) is a widely used manual form of communication in the North American deaf community and is recognized by linguists as a fully autonomous natural language, because it contains the same complex linguistic elements as spoken languages: phonology, morphology, syntax, semantics, and prosody (Klima & Bellugi, 1979; Lane & Grosjean, 1980; Wilbur, 1987; Lucas, 1990). In ASL, signs are produced by a combination of parameters (e.g., handshape, place of articulation, movement, and orientation; Stokoe, Casterline, & Croneberg, 1965; Bellugi, Klima, & Siple, 1975). ASL is one of a class of signed languages indigenous to deaf communities around the globe (other languages include British Sign Language and French Sign Language among others) that has evolved independently and are structurally distinct from one another.

Oral/aural communication (sometimes referred to as "lip reading" or "speech reading") is an approach that places great emphasis and training on the use of speech, residual hearing, and speech reading with the goal of developing intelligible speech, optimal use of residual hearing (generally with the assistance of a hearing aid or cochlear implant), and communicative independence. A national survey reported that 47.8% of more than 37,000 American deaf and hard-of-hearing children use "speech only" as a primary mode of communication (Gallaudet Research Institute, 2005). However, the amount of linguistic information conveyed using the oral method is extremely limited. Research has shown that lip reading single words is only 30% accurate, even in contextual sentences or phrases (Nicholls & Ling, 1982; Clarke & Ling, 1976). Skilled speech-readers often use their grammatical and semantic knowledge to infer messages when the information seen on the lips is ambiguous; this is often referred to in the reading literature as top-down processing (Goodman, 1985).

A much smaller subgroup of deaf individuals uses a communication system commonly known as *cued speech*. This manual system utilizes a set of handshapes to indicate and distinguish (receptively and expressively) the consonants that appear similar on the lips of the "speaker" and a set of hand locations to distinguish vowels that are visibly similar on the mouth of the speaker (Cornett, 1967). For instance, the consonant phonemes /b/, /p/, and /m/ are visually indistinguishable when articulated without the benefit of sound but are fully specified, or differentiated in cued speech via different handshapes for each phoneme. Similarly, the vowel phonemes /I/ and /E/ are easily misperceived in the absence of sound, but are fully distinguished in cued speech via different hand placements. Cued speech is designed to provide the deaf or hard-of-hearing person with clear and unambiguous visual access to the phonemic information of spoken language by combining the different handshapes and locations with natural mouth movements inherent in speech. As a result, deaf children who are exposed to cued speech from an early age have demonstrated comparable phonological knowledge to their hearing counterparts (LaSasso, Crain, & Leybeart, 2003). The national survey reports that 0.3% of more than 37,000 deaf and hard-of-hearing students use cued speech (Gallaudet Research Institute, 2005).

Phonology, Reading, and Deafness

Because of the predictive power of phonological skills in determining reading outcome in hearing students, the role of phonology in deaf students vis-à-vis reading has been a subject of great interest. Historically, the definition of phonemes has often been characterized as sound-based units, in part because much of the literature on phonology has focused on spoken languages (e.g., Wagner & Torgeson, 1987). In reality, phonemes are abstract cognitive units whose physical (or phonetic) forms are typically manifested via speech or cued gestures (Scarborough & Brady, 2002; Hanson, 1989; Fleetwood & Metzger, 1998).

Studies investigating the role of phonology and reading in deaf individuals have focused largely on the recognition or generation of rhymes (as rhyming is seen as an indicator of PA). For example, in a UK-based study of orally raised deaf students, Conrad (1979) found better readers recalled fewer items from rhyming lists of printed letters than from corresponding nonrhyming lists, suggesting that the more proficient deaf readers had access to phonetic coding that interfered with their recall. Campbell and Wright (1988) in a British study of orally raised deaf adolescents and hearing controls found that deaf children performed poorly on a rhyme judgment task as a consequence of being susceptible to orthographic similarity. Moreover, in an effort to match the two groups on reading age (using the Neale reading test), the investigators found that the average chronological age of deaf subjects was almost twice that of their hearing counterparts (14.6 and 7.6, respectively).

In deaf users of sign language, Hanson and Fowler (1987) conducted a series of experiments employing a speeded lexical decision task in which college-aged deaf and hearing participants made decisions as to whether pairs of written items contained words or pseudowords. They found that phonological similarity between word pairs reduced the reading rate of both the hearing and the signing deaf participants, suggesting a similar phonetic coding strategy in the deaf and hearing participants. In another study, Hanson and McGarr (1989) found that signing deaf college students were able to demonstrate a certain level of PA in a rhyme generation task, but not as extensively as those expected of hearing peers, producing only 50% correct responses to written words. Because the participants were considered to be good readers, the authors speculated that PA abilities in these deaf adults may have developed as a consequence of reading experience and that in general, PA skills might not be expected to be present in young, developing readers. It should be noted that these studies by Hanson and colleagues did not identify whether deaf subjects were native users of ASL, making it difficult to infer possible relationships between deafness, signing experience, and PA skills.

In one of the few comparative studies investigating the phonological skills of children from oral, signing, and cueing backgrounds, Charlier and Leybaert (2000) conducted two experiments examining the rhyming abilities of deaf children in Belgium. In the first experiment, children were asked to make rhyme judgments in their native French based on picture stimuli. They found no differences between the hearing group and the group with extensive cued speech exposure (use of cued speech both at home and at school) and both of these groups outperformed all other deaf groups (including those who only used CS at school). In the second experiment, a different group of French deaf cuers and hearing children (mean age = 10.1) were asked to generate rhyming words for pictured and written target items. The results again indicated that the group of children who used cued speech at home and

school performed similarly to (although slightly lower than) the hearing control group. More recently, LaSasso and colleagues (LaSasso *et al.*, 2003) used a similar rhyme generation task as Hanson and McGarr (1989) to compare PA performance of college students matched on reading levels (using the Stanford Achievement Test-9, 1996). They compared three groups of skilled readers—hearing, deaf cuers, and deaf noncuers—and found that the deaf cuers had PA skills comparable to their hearing peers and superior to that of the deaf noncuers.

Taken together, these studies generally indicate lower performance on measures of PA in deaf compared to hearing students with evidence of strong PA skills among the more accomplished deaf readers, regardless of communication background. However, there is emerging evidence that the performance gap in measures of reading and PA between hearing and deaf students is considerably less in deaf students who have extensive exposure to cued speech.

Short-Term Memory and Deafness

In addition to PA, phonetic coding of linguistic items (digits, words, etc.) into short-term memory (STM) is also an important predictor of reading development in hearing children (Wagner & Torgeson, 1987). Hearing individuals have been shown to use a phonetic code during short-term recall of linguistic stimuli (Conrad, 1964, 1973, 1977; Healy, 1982); however, the encoding strategy employed by deaf individuals during STM tasks is less clear. An early STM study by Conrad (1970) claimed that deaf subjects, particularly those who are prelingually deaf, do not use this speech-based phonetic coding. However, other studies have noted some evidence of phonetic coding memory in deaf populations during short-term recall of linguistic items (Conrad, 1979; Hanson, 1982; Hanson, 1990), which is thought to be advantageous in their reading achievement (Hanson, Liberman, & Shankweiler, 1984; Lichtenstein, 1985; Lichtenstein, 1998). Specifically, Conrad (1979) tested deaf oral subjects on short-term recall of rhyming printed letters and found decreased performance with rhyming letters compared to unrhymed letters. Hanson (1982) found a similar effect in skilled deaf readers who were native users of ASL when their short-term recall of printed word items decreased with phonetically similar lists, but not orthographically similar lists. Later, Hanson (1990) examined deaf and hearing adults' temporal (and spatial) recall of letters following an articulatory interference task using letter sets that were designed to confuse subjects on the basis of phonetic, manual, and visual similarity. Both deaf and hearing groups were affected by phonetic similarity in the letters and showed no evidence of manual or visual coding during temporal recall.

Whereas the above studies examined the encoding strategies employed by deaf individuals, a number of studies have focused extensively on the amount of linguistic items that subjects recall. While Tractenberg (2002) found comparable digit recall performance between deaf signers and hearing nonsigning subjects, most other studies consistently indicate that deaf individuals recall fewer items than their hearing counterparts (Hanson, 1982; Hanson, 1990; Wallace & Corballis, 1973; Bellugi *et al.*, 1975; Conrad, 1970; Coryell, 2001; Boutla, Supalla, Newport, & Bavelier, 2004; Bavalier, Newport, Hall, Supalla, & Boutla, 2006). Using a computer for stimuli presentation, Coryell (2001) compared the digit span of deaf signers and deaf cuers to age-matched hearing controls and found that deaf signers recalled significantly fewer digit items than did hearing subjects, consistent with previous findings (Conrad, 1970; Wallace & Corballis, 1973; Bellugi *et al.*, 1975). Additional studies have shown that this lower capacity for recall in deaf signers compared to hearing subjects occurs even when rate of articulation and phonological similarity in item presentation is controlled for (Boutla *et al.*, 2004; Bavalier *et al.*, 2006). However, this discrepancy seems to be limited to serial recall, as deaf subjects exhibit recall performance comparable to that of hearing controls during free recall of linguistic items (Hanson, 1982; Boutla *et al.*, 2004).

Deaf cuers, on the other hand, showed comparable performance to hearing controls and significantly greater digit recall than deaf signers (Coryell, 2001). However, it should be noted that this study employed only the forward recall list of the test and that mental reordering skills, such as those required to perform the backward list, was not the focus of the study.

One criticism of these memory capacity studies described above is that differences in linguistic modality and the formational properties between ASL and spoken languages, rather than lack of audition, might account for the differences observed in STM capacities between hearing and deaf participants. More recent studies have addressed this issue with the inclusion of hearing native signers who share the same early ASL experience as deaf signers (Boutla *et al.*, 2004; Wilson & Emmorey, 1998; Bavalier *et al.*, 2006). These studies have found that hearing native signers of ASL recalled fewer items when stimuli were presented in ASL compared to English, suggesting that sign language, and not sensory experience, can negatively affect STM capacity. Considerable debate continues over whether the sequential nature of spoken languages is most advantageous for temporal-order STM tasks compared to the visuospatial nature of signed languages. Wilson and Emmorey (2006a, 2006b) have argued that memory capacity is not affected by language modality but is restricted by processing load and that items taking longer to produce, as in the case of signs, will result in a smaller capacity. In a study carefully controlling for intrinsic factors such as word length, articulation rate, and phonological similarity, hearing nonsigners and deaf signers demonstrated comparable STM span using letter stimuli presented in English and ASL respectively (Wilson & Emmorey, 2006a). In contrast, another study (Bavalier *et al.*, 2006) has asserted that the shorter span for ASL-presented items in deaf and hearing native users of ASL exists independently of such manipulations and is attributed to the differences between the auditory and visual modality during serial memory encoding. Their conclusions arose from their findings that deaf and hearing signers persist in showing decreased digit spans despite efforts to control for rate of stimulus presentation and phonological similarity across languages (Bavalier *et al.*, 2006). Taken together, the STM capacity of deaf individuals has largely been shown to be reduced, but the reason for this difference, whether it is attributed to language modality or cross-linguistic differences, is still poorly understood.

Present Study Questions

In short, the conclusions on the nature of PA and verbal STM in deaf populations remain unsettled. Importantly, these studies have been limited in their inclusion or description of the diverse communication backgrounds available to deaf people, thereby hindering a clear determination of whether any differences observed among hearing and deaf subjects in these two skills can be ascribed to the absence of audition or to their communication modality. While LaSasso and colleagues compared rhyme generation in deaf adult cuers with deaf noncuers (LaSasso *et al.*, 2003), the present study focuses on detection of phonemic units in lexical items and takes a step further by distinguishing deaf noncuers into two groups of oral and signing backgrounds. Likewise, even though the empirical literature is rife with STM studies of deaf oral users and ASL signers (Hanson, 1990; Hanson, 1982; Conrad, 1979; Boutla *et al.*, 2004; Bavalier *et al.*, 2006), the present study includes deaf cuers and extends the findings of Coryell (2001) to include backward digit-span recall (in addition to forward digit span) during verbal presentation of the stimuli in deaf groups of various communication backgrounds. American deaf adults from distinct language/communication backgrounds, ASL, oral English, and cued English were recruited and compared with one another as well as with two groups of hearing

subjects, hearing nonsigners, and hearing native signers. In order to specifically address the role of sensory and early language experience on phonemic knowledge and short-term memory, these groups were matched on their reading performance (measured by a test of word recognition) as well as performance IQ. The study of adults, as opposed to children, has the advantage of examining a population whose reading and reading-related skills have reached a mature stage and whose cognitive and linguistic abilities are reflective of lifelong experience with their auditory and communicative systems.

We made several predictions with regards to phonemic knowledge and short-term memory in skilled readers of distinct sensory and language backgrounds. First, because cued speech provides deaf users with unambiguous visual access to English phonology, we predicted that deaf cuers would do well in measures of phonological awareness. By comparison, orally raised deaf adults who without manual cues depend primarily on speech reading to access English and have incomplete visual access to English phonology, and they were predicted to be less proficient in phonemic awareness than cuers. Deaf native users of ASL were predicted to have the least access to English phonology and hence the lowest PA skills of the three deaf groups. Second, we predicted that the examination of STM capacity in the three aforementioned deaf groups compared to hearing subjects would provide valuable insight into potential differences in STM capacity between hearing and deaf proficient readers. Importantly, the present study allows us to examine the interplay of language modality and memory encoding skills. If deaf users of cued speech and oral users, whose visual communication system retains the sequential structure of spoken language, demonstrated comparable performance to that of hearing subjects, then Wilson and Emmorey's (2006a) claim of equal spans across language modalities (while taking language-specific differences into account) would be supported. In other words, as long as the individuals share the same native language (English), STM may be preserved even in the absence of audition. Such a finding could suggest that the lower digit-span scores seen in deaf signers might be attributed to articulatory differences between the two languages and not sensory differences *per se*. If, on the other hand, deaf cuers exhibited lower digit-span capacity than their hearing counterparts, this would support the claim made by Bavalier *et al.* (2006) that linguistic information presented in the visuo-gestural modality is not compatible with the temporal properties of STM in the auditory modality. To address these competing hypotheses, the present study employed two different versions of the digit span, verbal and visual, with the assumption that the visual version of the digit span negates any language-specific differences in stimulus item presentation, such as articulatory rate, duration, and mode of presentation. While it has already been established that digit-span capacity in deaf signers is significantly lower than that of hearing speakers for a number of possible reasons (Hanson, 1982; Wallace & Corballis, 1973; Bellugi *et al.*, 1975; Conrad, 1970), concerns about differences in articulatory rate and word length effect across languages (Wilson & Emmorey, 2006a; 2006b) are not at issue here because deaf cuers and oral users share English with hearing speakers as their native language.

Methods

Participants

A total of 51 subjects from five different categories of language and sensory backgrounds were recruited from the metropolitan Washington, DC area: deaf native users of American Sign Language (DA) ($n = 14$); deaf users of cued cpeech (DC) ($n = 9$); deaf oral users of English (DO) ($n = 8$); hearing native users of American Sign Language (HA) ($n = 10$); and hearing native speakers of English (H) ($n = 10$). Hearing controls were recruited from Georgetown University, and deaf and hearing native signers

were recruited via flyers posted at Gallaudet University (all participants were college educated with a minimum of 12 years of education). All deaf subjects were born deaf or became deaf before the age of 2 years, with >85 db hearing loss in the better ear. Subjects reported continuous use of their native languages and communication mode from before the age of 5 years until adolescence or beyond. All subjects were healthy with no reported history of reading, mental, or neurological disorders. All subjects were participants in a larger study involving functional brain imaging, and the tests given to subjects below were part of a larger battery of neuropsychological tests spanning two sessions of 3 hours each. For this analysis, subjects were chosen on the basis of their compatibility with regard to performance IQ and reading accuracy; to attain this goal four subjects with performance IQ standard scores of 127 or more were excluded from the analysis. IRB approval was obtained from Georgetown and Gallaudet Universities.

Neuropsychological and Behavioral Tests

All tests were administered to the subjects in their preferred language/communication mode by a hearing research assistant fluent in spoken English, ASL, and cued English, unless described otherwise.

Intelligence Quotient

Performance IQ (PIQ) was measured using the Wechsler Abbreviated Scale of Intelligence (WASI) test (Wechsler, 1999). This instrument contains four subtests, each measuring different aspects of intelligence and using items of increasing difficulty. The Performance IQ score was derived for each participant from the Block Design and the Matrix Reasoning subtest scores. A verbal IQ score was also obtained in four of the five groups using the WASI but will not be reported for the purpose of the current study as it was not obtained for the deaf ASL group.

Word Identification Fluency

The Test of Silent Word Reading Fluency (TSWRF) (Pro-Ed, Inc.) assesses word-identification fluency "as a valid estimate of general reading ability [which] can be used with confidence to identify poor readers" (Mather, Hammill, Allen, & Roberts, 2004). Subjects were presented with rows of words with no spaces between them and asked to draw lines between the boundaries of as many words as possible within 3 minutes. The TSWRF yielded raw scores for accuracy, which were then converted to standard scores through tables provided in the manual.

Reading Comprehension

The Passage Comprehension subtest of the Woodcock–Johnson III test measures silent reading comprehension without time constraints (Woodcock, McGrew, & Mather, 2001). The present reading achievement level of the subject dictates the starting point of the test and the level of difficulty of the test increases by increasing the level of vocabulary, the passage length, and the syntactic and semantic complexity of the items. The recommended starting point for an average adult requires the person to silently read a sentence or short paragraph and verbally supply the missing word that appropriately completes the sentence. This subtest yields raw scores and standard scores.

Phoneme Detection Test

Although rhyming tasks are often used as an indicator of phonological awareness, more direct measures of phonological awareness have been difficult to obtain in deaf populations in large part due to insensitive test administration protocols. Many current measures (e.g., Rosner Test of Auditory Analysis Skills, the Lindamood Auditory Conceptualization Test, or the Comprehensive Test of Phonological Processing) require stimulus items or the subject's responses to be spoken or verbalized, which can be problematic for deaf subjects who do not speech read or use speech to communicate. Here we introduce a computer-based phono-logical awareness measure, the Phoneme Detection Test (PDT), which addresses these administrative confounds. This test was developed to measure phonemic awareness via detection of the presence of a single phoneme in individual, visually presented words (computer generation of these stimuli was achieved with Presentation version 0.81; www.neurobs.com). The test includes 150 high-frequency words with multiple or opaque orthography-to-phonology correspondences (e.g., "c" maps to /s/ and /k/ phonemes such as "cent" and "call"), divided into five target-phoneme sets of 30 items each: /s/, /g/, /j/, and /k/ (/k/ repeated for "ch" and "c" sets). Half the items contained target phonemes appearing in initial, medial, or word-final positions and the other half served as orthographic foils in which an alternate grapheme-to-phoneme correspondence was used. Subjects were instructed to respond as quickly and accurately as possible with keyboard buttons indicating "Yes" or "No" if an item contained the target phoneme. Nonverbal stimuli and response modality remove undesirable confounds from subjects' different communication modes and allow between-group comparisons of accuracy and reaction time. Explicit instructions and examples were given at the beginning of the test to ensure that subjects understood that the task was not to detect orthographic units, but phonemic units. In addition, each set was preceded by a four-item practice session. The order of set presentation was counterbalanced across subjects.

Spatial Memory Span

The Spatial Span (SS) subtest from the Wechsler Memory Scale-III measures the ability to hold a visual-spatial sequence of events in working memory (Wechsler, 1997). A three-dimensional board of nine cubes positioned on a base is used to administer visual-spatial sequences, ranging in difficulty from two to nine movements, with two trials at each level. Subjects are instructed to manually respond by touching the blocks in correct sequences, either forwards or backwards for Spatial Span

Forward and Spatial Span Backward. Total raw score (from Forward and Backward trials) is converted to an age-referenced scaled score. This test was included to provide a spatial analogue to the verbal memory span.

Verbal Digit Span

The Wechsler Adult Intelligence Scale-III (WAIS-III) Digit Span subtest requires repetition of numbers in sequences of increasing length, from 2 to 9 numbers with two trials at each difficulty level (Wechsler, 1999). The subject is given two strings of each length, the length increasing with each pair. If the subject repeats both sequences correctly he or she receives a score of 2, if only one is correct a score of 1, and if neither is correct no points are earned. Hence it is these scores that are reflected in the raw score (not the longest correctly repeated sequence). The score from forward and backward lists were combined and converted to an age-reference scaled score. As is typical for this test, an experimenter administered the DST in English for hearing and deaf oral subjects. Prior to taking the test, deaf oral subjects were given opportunities to be familiarized with the experimenter's mouth movements. Deaf signers and deaf cuers viewed a prerecorded Quicktime video in which the experimenter presented the digits in their respective languages, ASL, and English (via cued speech). Subjects were given opportunity to respond in their preferred mode or language.

Visual Version of the Digit Span

Because of difficulties in interpreting between-group differences for the traditional version of the Digit Span described above and the existence of sensory and language differences during task presentation (Boutla *et al.*, 2004; Wilson & Emmorey, 1998; Wilson & Emmorey, 2006a, 2006b), we also administered a visual version of the Digit Span Test to our subjects. Written task instructions and practice sessions were presented on a computer screen at the beginning of the test to ensure subjects understood the task. Digits were pre-

sented centrally on the screen in large black font and at the same pace as the traditional verbal version of the Digit Span (Presentation version 0.81, www.neurobs.com). Immediately after the presentation of number strings, a red square flashed briefly on the screen to signal the end of the trial and begin recall. To visually simulate the falling intonation used when the last digit in a string is uttered in the Verbal Digit Span, the last digit in a string was presented using a different colored font (red),to prompt the subject that the sequence is about to end. Subjects responded using the number keypad and were given opportunity to delete their response if they made keyboard errors.

Data Analysis

We compared the five groups (deaf users of ASL, oral English, and cued English as well as hearing nonsigners and hearing native signers) on each behavioral measure using one-way ANOVAs with significance defined as alpha <0.05. Where main effect of group was observed, pairwise multiple comparisons were made among each of the five groups. To estimate inter-measure reliability, the traditional Verbal Digit Span and the experimental visual version of the Verbal Digit Span were entered into a correlation analysis (with forward and backward raw scores combined). In addition, to establish the relationship between measures of reading with measures of STM and PA, measures from the PDT and the Digit Span (both the traditional verbal version as well as for the experimental visual version) were entered into nonparametric correlation analyses with Passage Comprehension and Word Identification Fluency scores.

Results

Neuropsychological and Behavioral Tests

Table 1 shows the groups' demographics as well as their behavioral scores. As described

TABLE 1. Demographic, Neuropsychological, and Behavioral Measures Expressed as Mean Score (*SD*)

	Hearing	Hearing ASL	Deaf ASL	Deaf CS	Deaf Oral	Significance
N	8	9	13	9	8	
Demographics						
Age (years)	22.6 (3.1)	30.4 (5.8)	23.1 (3.6)	29.4 (3.6)	25.0 (3.5)	.000
Gender	4F	9F	7F	4F	2F	
Neuropsychological and Behavioral Scores						
Performance IQ	117.75 (6.7)	114.89 (10.5)	109.92 (10.0)	112.88 (8.8)	112.50 (8.7)	n.s.
Reading (accuracy)						
TSWRF (word identification)	115.62 (13.6)	108.56 (14.0)	105.15 (16.9)	122.55 (8.4)	113.87 (12.1)	n.s.
WJ-III Comprehension	119.5 (11.2)	112.67 (13.1)	100.15 (11.9)	106.0 (4.6)	102.5 (7.9)	.001
Short-term memory						
Spatial Span (SS)	109.37 (9.8)	106.67 (8.3)	108.85 (11.4)	97.77 (14.2)	101.87 (6.5)	n.s.
Digit Span Verbal (SS)	121.88 (16.2)	108.89 (14.5)	96.92 (13.9)	105.00 (10.3)	97.37 (10.0)	.002
Digit Span Verbal (raw)	23.75 (4.7)	19.78 (3.8)	16.46 (4.0)	18.22 (2.7)	16.75 (2.9)	.001
Visual version of Digit Span (raw)	22.33 (2.4)	21.44 (3.9)	15.81 (3.7)	15.87 (3.0)	11.86 (2.3)	.000
Phonemic awareness						
PDT accuracy (%)	93.7 (7.3)	93.4 (5.2)	65.2 (14.5)	86.4 (12.3)	87.6 (6.9)	0.000
PDT RT (ms)	1156 (335)	1854 (665)	2848 (1027)	1819 (777)	2577 (1332)	0.002

above, subjects were selected in such a way that they were matched for Performance IQ, $F(4, 42) = .985$, $P < 0.426$, and reading fluency as measured by TSWRF, $F(4, 42) = 2.461$, $P = 0.060$. However, despite their generally equivalent performance on word-recognition fluency, we found a main effect of group in the Passage Comprehension subtest, $F(4, 42) = 5.313$, $P < 0.001$. Post-hoc comparisons revealed that performance of the hearing nonsigning group was significantly higher on reading comprehension than the deaf signing (Tukey's HSD = 19.34, $P < 0.002$) and oral (Tukey's HSD = 17.00, $P < 0.018$) groups, but not the hearing signers or deaf cuers ($P > 0.05$). Hearing signers were not significantly different from any of the three deaf groups ($P > 0.05$), nor were there significant differences when comparing any of the three deaf groups with each other. Therefore the hearing nonsigning group was the only group at odds compared to the others with a significant advantage for reading comprehension.

Phoneme Detection Test

Computer difficulties resulted in data loss from six subjects for this test (H = 2, DC = 1, DO = 1, and DA = 2). Main effect of group was observed in the remaining PDT data on measures of performance accuracy, $F(4,36) = 12.26$, $P < 0.001$, and reaction time $F(4,36) = 4.33$, $P = 0.006$. Post-hoc comparisons revealed that the deaf signing group was significantly less accurate (Tamhane's T2, $P < 0.05$) on phoneme detection compared to the other four groups. However, deaf signers reported no significant difference in reaction times when compared to the other groups ($P > 0.05$) except for the hearing nonsigners, who were faster than the deaf signers (Tamhane's T2, $P = 0.002$). Accuracy and reaction times for the deaf cueing group was comparable to that of the hearing control group, hearing signers, and deaf oral users (Tamhane's T2, $P > 0.05$). The deaf oral group also demonstrated statistically indistinguishable accuracy and reaction times when compared to the hearing nonsigning group and hearing signing group (Tamhane's T2, $P > 0.05$).

Spatial Memory Span

WMS–Spatial Span revealed no significant group differences among the five groups, $F(4, 42) = 2.054$, $P = 0.104$.

Verbal Digit Span

The traditional verbal version of Digit Span test from the WAIS-III revealed significant group differences in raw scores, $F(4, 42) = 5.67$, $P < 0.001$. Post-hoc comparisons between the three deaf and two hearing groups showed that the hearing nonsigners performed significantly better (Tukey's HSD, $P < 0.05$) than all other groups except hearing signers (Tukey's HSD = 3.97, $P = 0.198$). The hearing ASL signers did not differ significantly from any of the deaf groups and no significant differences were found among the three deaf groups (Tukey's HSD, $P > 0.05$).

Visual Version of the Digit Span

Computer difficulties resulted in some data loss for the Visual Digit Span (H = 2, DA = 2, DC = 1, DO = 1). For the remaining data, significant between-group differences were observed in raw scores, $F(4, 36) = 12.63$, $P < 0.001$. Post-hoc comparisons indicated that all three deaf groups performed significantly lower than the two hearing groups in all pairwise contrasts (Tukey's HSD, $P < 0.01$). However, all deaf groups showed no significant differences with each other (Tukey's HSD, $P > 0.05$). Hearing nonsigners were not significantly different from hearing signers (Tukey's HSD = .889, $P = 0.986$).

Correlation Analyses

To assess the relationship between the standard verbal versions of the Digit Span and our experimental visual version of this test, we entered the data into a nonparametric correlation analyses and found that the two measures were significantly correlated to each other ($\tau = .602$, $P < 0.001$).

To estimate the relationship between phonemic awareness skills (as measured by the PDT) and reading ability, nonparametric correlation analysis (Kendall's tau) was performed between PDT accuracy scores and performance on the TSWRF as well as Passage Comprehension scores. Surprisingly, the first revealed no significant correlation between PDT accuracy and TSWRF. The second showed a positive correlation ($\tau = .305$, $P < 0.006$; two-tailed) between PA skills and reading comprehension. Reaction time from the PDT was negatively correlated to the above same measures (TSWRF: $\tau = -.291$, $P < 0.01$; two-tailed and Passage Comprehension: $\tau = -.248$; $P < 0.05$, two-tailed).

To estimate the relationship between STM memory and reading measures, both the traditional Verbal Digit Span and the experimental visually presented version of the Verbal Digit Span were entered into nonparametric correlation analyses and found to be significantly correlated with the Passage Comprehension (DS-Verbal: $\tau = .323$; DS-visual version of the verbal: $\tau = .409$, $P < 0.002$; two-tailed). However, neither version of the Digit Span was correlated to word identification fluency as measured by TSWRF (DS-Verbal: $\tau = .114$; DS-Visual: $\tau = .082$, $P > 0.05$).

Discussion

With a few exceptions (i.e., Charlier & Leybaert, 2000; LaSasso *et al.*, 2003), previous empirical studies examining the impact of deafness on skills that support reading have focused on deaf signers, making it difficult to dissociate the effect of deafness from early language experience. Inclusion of deaf individuals who acquired English natively via visual means (oral communication or cued speech) along with deaf users of ASL will help us disentangle the effect of deafness and language experience on phonological awareness and verbal short-term memory, two of the three core predictors of reading achievement (Wagner & Torgeson, 1987). The first aim of the present study was to explore the PA skills of deaf cuers (who have full, unambiguous access to the phonological structure of traditionally spoken languages) relative to other deaf and hearing groups. Then, by examining verbal working memory of deaf nonsigners as well as the more traditionally studied group of deaf signers, the second aim was to gain further insight into the role visual language plays in the capacity to retain lexical items in short-term memory.

Phonemic Awareness

Because commercially available measures of phonological awareness are not suitable for deaf populations (see Tractenberg, 2002), the PDT was developed to probe phonological coding skills in deaf participants using visual stimuli and nonverbal responses. As expected, deaf native signers of ASL did not perform well on phonemic detection of English words, reflecting their lack of experience with spoken English phonology. Specifically, the deaf signing group was significantly less accurate on the PDT than all other groups. Mean reaction time for the deaf signers was longer on the PDT, but this difference was significant only in comparison to the hearing nonsigning group. Only two deaf signers showed greater than 85% accuracy on the PDT, and deaf signers in general performed at or slightly above chance during the detection of phonemic units, despite being good readers.

On the other hand, deaf cuers and deaf oral users had accuracy scores that were statistically indistinguishable from those of either hearing groups. With an average accuracy above 85% on the PDT, both of the English-native deaf groups (cuers and oral users) clearly demonstrated robust awareness of the phonological structure of English lexical items, even when certain phonemes were not explicitly revealed in the orthography. To our surprise, deaf cuers and oral users were not different from each other during this phonological coding task (based on accuracy and reaction times). More direct access to the phonemic stream of English in deaf cuers would have predicted an advantage for this group over the oral group (cuers had shorter but not statistically different reaction times), but such a benefit was not observed on this test.

Correlation analyses revealed that although accuracy on the PDT was not correlated to performance on word identification fluency (measured by the TSWRF), it was correlated with Passage Comprehension; and reaction time on the PDT was correlated with both the TSWRF as well as reading comprehension, suggesting that a relationship does exist between reading and PA skills in the context of the speed by which subjects perform the PDT task. The absence of a correlation between accuracy in word-recognition fluency and PA is somewhat surprising, as studies of hearing populations frequently report that measures of phonemic coding skills correlate with word-reading accuracy. The reason for a lack of a correlation between the PA test and the TSWRF is most likely due to the fact that the TSWRF task relies more on sight word recognition than addressed phonology. Addressed phonology is probed more directly during tests of reading aloud, especially the reading of pseudowords.

In sum, PA skills are not well developed in deaf users of sign language, even though they have acquired proficient reading skills. This suggests that under some circumstances proficient reading can be attained in the absence of PA skills. Future studies will need to determine whether there are other skills, linguistic or otherwise, that are more strongly developed in deaf signers with good reading ability and how these facilitate their reading. We also found that deaf cuers performed more like hearing subjects and significantly better than deaf signers on the PA test. Their ability to detect phonemic units suggests they have been facilitated by lifelong use of manual cues to visually access English phonology. However, since our oral subjects performed equally well as the cuers, it seems that access to the phonological representation of English can also be obtained without the use of cues.

Short-Term Memory

There has been an ongoing debate as to whether retention spans in short-term verbal memory are lower in people who are deaf. Some have argued that studies in which differences have been observed in deaf population may be confounded by the delivery of the tests, that is, administration in sign language compared to English may introduce other variables that lead to shorter retention spans. Here we addressed this question using a two-pronged approach. First, the inclusion of deaf participants who use English to perform the task (instead of ASL) allows for a more comparable assessment between hearing and deaf groups. Second, we devised a visual version of the traditional Verbal Digit Span as a way to equalize the stimuli presentation and response mode between hearing and deaf groups. Together this allowed us to examine whether verbal STM is affected by sensory experience, language experience or modality of test presentation.

Our overall finding was that although all five groups were comparable on the Spatial Span tests, there were profound group differences on performance of the Verbal Digit Span. All three deaf groups showed shorter digit retention when compared to the nonsigning hearing group during the traditional version of the Digit Span and, further, all three deaf groups showed shorter digit retention when compared to both hearing groups in an experimental visual version of the Digit Span where subjects responded to visual stimuli using a keyboard.

Our first observation of lower performance on the Digit Span is consistent with recent findings (Boutla *et al.*, 2004; Bavalier *et al.*, 2006), that deaf signers exhibit shorter digit span for numbers presented in ASL compared to hearing nonsigners. When examining the longest correct digit length attained, our hearing subjects achieved spans of 7.2 (nonsigners) and 6.3 (signers) and our deaf subjects had spans of 4.9 (signers), 5.4 (cuers), and 5.0 (oral). These findings are largely consistent with the digit spans described by Bavalier *et al.* (2006) for signers. In addition to this observation, Boutla and colleagues also reported decreased serial item recall in hearing signers when they viewed the stimuli in ASL compared to when they heard the stimuli in English. Together these results suggest a detrimental effect of ASL on measures of verbal retention, but, perhaps somewhat surprisingly, our deaf cueing and oral groups also exhibited significantly lower digit spans than the hearing nonsigners. Since both the cueing and oral groups received the stimuli in their native English language and linguistic modality (cued or orally), the discrepancy in short-term recall of digits described in the literature cannot be solely attributed to signed languages. Our second test of verbal short-term verbal memory was given in the visual modality to all participants and resulted in all three deaf groups performing similarly to one another and significantly lower than the two hearing groups. Together these results suggest that even when language experience or modality of test presentation are taken into consideration, there are differences among hearing and deaf subjects in their ability to retain digits.

These findings suggest that the use of the visual-spatial modality (rather than the auditory modality used by hearing subjects) to receive and hold linguistic items in working memory presents a greater processing load, and results in lower item recall. This conclusion is consistent with the view put forward by Bavelier and colleagues, suggesting that visual modality is a limiting factor in working memory (Boutla *et al.*, 2004; Bavalier *et al.*, 2006). In this context it is also worth considering that deaf subjects did not only differ from the hearing subjects in their retention span and that all deaf groups performed similarly to one another, but also that the deaf signers did not show any improvements in performance on the experimental visual version of the digit span compared to the traditional verbal version. Specifically, our efforts to remove any linguistic or modality bias in stimuli presentation and recall responses had little positive effect on the performance of our deaf participants. This is consistent with findings where visually presented non-nameable items have reduced hearing subjects' capacity for serial item recall (Alvarez & Cavanagh, 2004; Cowan, 2001).

Finally, it is of interest to examine working memory spans in the context of our other measures. Deaf cuers performed similarly to the hearing subjects on word identification fluency, and phonemic awareness, but they had significantly lower digit-span performance. This suggests that good reading skill can be attained in the absence of strong working memory skills, and again suggests that skills traditionally thought of as predicting reading outcome in hearing subjects (Wagner & Torgeson, 1987) may not be suitable in gauging reading achievement in deaf students.

In sum, we found that deaf subjects regardless of communication or language background, had lower digit-span retention than hearing subjects, while spatial span was comparable amongst all groups. Further, we found no differences in performance among all three deaf groups even though their language background might have predicted differential ability on memory span. The findings suggest that longer digit recall in hearing compared to deaf subjects can be explained by the availability of the articulatory loop that is utilized for the sequential nature of the auditory channel in working memory.

Conclusion

The goal of the present study was to gain some insight into the cognitive and linguistic abilities of deaf people who are skilled readers yet have been raised with a variety of communication systems, namely ASL, cued speech, or the oral-aural method. We found deaf native signers of ASL did not do well on detection of hidden English phonology in visually presented words, while deaf cuers and deaf oral users had phonological performance comparable to those of hearing subjects. Second, we examined the digit span of deaf and hearing subjects and found that all three deaf groups performed similarly to one another and weaker than hearing subjects. Since deaf cuers and oral users receive the digit stimuli in the same language as hearing groups via a different visual medium, we conclude that the use of sign language does not have a detrimental effect on serial recall of linguistic items. Instead, it appears that linguistic information processing in the visual channel creates additional processing burden on short-term memory capacity and subsequent recall. This was confirmed by a second measure of the Digit Span that did not involve the use of manual languages in its administration. Taken together, the findings support the idea put forward by Bavalier *et al.* (2006) that the articulatory loop in working memory is most advantageous when speech articulation is used to encode linguistic items and that the visual nature of linguistic stimuli triggers a decrease in STM span. Finally, our results demonstrate that among deaf subjects skilled reading can be attained despite lower working memory abilities and, in the case of signers, despite lower STM and phonemic awareness skills. This strongly suggests that deaf subjects' reading skills are facilitated by abilities other than those traditionally considered to be important in hearing students.

Acknowledgments

This work was supported NICHD Grant HD40095, NIDCD Grant F32 DC007774, NSF Grant SBE 0541953, and by the General Clinical Research Center Program of the NCR-Resources (MO1-RR13297). We wish to thank Lynn Flowers, Eileen Napoliello, Jill Weisberg, and Alina Engelman for their help. We also thank our subjects for their participation.

Conflicts of Interest

The authors declare no conflicts of interest.

References

Adams, M. 1990. *Beginning to read: thinking and learning about print*. Cambridge, MA: MIT Press.

Allen, T. 1986. Patterns of academic achievement among hearing impaired students: 1974 and 1983. In A. Schildroth & M. Karchmer (Eds.), *Deaf children in America* (pp. 161–206). San Diego, CA: College-Hill.

Alvarez, G. A., & Cavanagh, P. 2004. The capacity of visual short-term memory is set both by visual information load and by number of objects. *Psychological Science* **15**: 106–111.

Bavalier, D., Newport, E. L., Hall, M., Supalla, T., & Boutla, M. 2006. Persistent difference in short-term memory span between sign and speech. *Psychological Science* **17**: 1090–1092.

Bellugi, U., Klima, E., & Siple, P. 1975. Remembering in signs. *Cognition* **3**: 93–125.

Bishop, D., & Adams, C. 1990. A prospective study of the relationship between specific language impairment, phonological disorders and reading retardation. *Journal of Child Psychology and Psychiatry and Allied Disciplines* **31**: 1027–1050.

Boutla, M., Supalla, T., Newport, E. L., & Bavelier, D. 2004. Short-term memory span: insights from sign language. *Nature Neuroscience* **7**: 997–1002.

Bradley, L., & Bryant, P. 1985. *Rhyme and reason in reading and spelling* (IARLD Monographs, No. 1). Ann Arbor: University of Michigan Press.

Campbell, R., & Wright, H. 1988. Deafness, spelling, and rhyme: how spelling supports written word and picture rhyming skills in deaf subjects. *Quarterly Journal of Experimental Psychology* **40A**(4): 771–788.

Charlier, B., & Leybaert, J. 2000. The rhyming skills of deaf children educated with phonetically augmented lipreading. *Quarterly Journal of Experimental Psychology* **53A**: 349–375.

Chincotta, D., & Underwood, G. 1996. Mother tongue, language of schooling, and bilingual digit span. *British Journal of Psychology* **87**(2): 193–208.

Clarke, B. R., & Ling, D. 1976. The effects of using Cued Speech: a follow-up study. *Volta Review* **78**: 23–34.

Conrad, R. 1964. Acoustic confusions in immediate memory. *British Journal of Psychology* **55**: 75–84.

Conrad, R. 1970. Short-term memory processes in the deaf. *British Journal of Psychology* **61**: 179–195.

Conrad, R. 1973. Some correlates of speech coding in the short-term memory of the deaf. *Journal of Speech and Hearing Research* **16**: 375–184.

Conrad, R. 1977. The reading ability of deaf school-leavers. *British Journal of Educational Psychology* **47**: 138–148.

Conrad, R. 1979. *The deaf school child*. London: Harper and Row.

Cornett, R. O. 1967. Cued speech. *American Annals of the Deaf* **112**: 3–13.

Coryell, H. 2001. *Verbal sequential processing skills and reading ability in deaf individuals using Cued Speech and signed communication*. Unpublished dissertation. Gallaudet University, Washington, DC.

Cowan, N. 2001. The magical number 4 in short-term memory: a reconsideration of mental storage capacity. *Behavioral Brain Science* **24**: 87–185.

Ehri, L., & Sweet, J. 1991. Fingerpoint-reading of memorized text: what enables beginners to process the print? *Reading Research Quarterly* **24**: 442–462.

Fleetwood, E., & Metzger, M. 1998. *Cued language structure: An analysis of Cued American English based on linguistic principles*. Silver Spring, MD: Calliope Press.

Furth, H. 1966. A comparison of reading test norms of deaf and hearing children. *American Annals of the Deaf* **111**: 461–462.

Gallaudet Research Institute. 2005. *Regional and national summary report of data from the 2004–2005 annual survey of deaf and hard of hearing children and youth*. Washington, DC: Gallaudet University.

Goodman, K. 1985. Unity in reading. In H. Singer & R. Ruddell (Eds.), *Theoretical models and processes of reading* (3rd ed.) (pp. 813–840). Newark, DE: International Reading Association.

Goswami, U., & Bryant, P. 1992. Rhyme, analogy, and children's reading. In P. B. Gough, L. C. Ehri, & R. Treiman (Eds.), *Reading acquisition* (pp. 49–64). Hillsdale, NJ: Erlbaum.

Hanson, V. 1982. Short-term recall by deaf signers of American Sign Language: Implication of encoding strategy for ordered recall. *Journal of Experimental Psychology* **8**: 572–583.

Hanson, V. 1989. Phonology and reading: evidence from profoundly deaf readers. In D. Shankweiler & E. Y. Liberman (Eds.), *Phonology and reading disability: Solving the reading puzzle* (pp. 67–89). Ann Arbor: University of Michigan Press.

Hanson, V. 1990. Recall of order information by deaf signers: phonetic coding in temporal order recall. *Memory & Cognition* **18**(6): 604–610.

Hanson, V., Liberman, I., & Shankweiler, D. 1984. Linguistic coding by deaf children in relation to beginning reading success. *Journal of Experimental Child Psychology* **37**: 378–393.

Hanson, V., & Fowler, C. 1987. Phonological coding in word reading: evidence from hearing and deaf readers. *Memory and Cognition* **15**: 199–207.

Hanson, V., & Lichtenstein, E. 1990. Short-term memory by deaf signers: the primary language coding hypothesis reconsidered. *Cognitive Psychology* **22**: 211–224.

Hanson, V., & McGarr, N. 1989. Rhyme generation in deaf adults. *Journal of Speech and Hearing Research* **32**: 2–11.

Healy, A. F. 1982. Short-term memory for order information. In G. H. Bower (Ed.), *The psychology of learning and motivation* Vol. 16 (pp. 191–238). New York: Academic Press.

Juel, C. 1988. Learning to read and write: a longitudinal study of 54 children from first through fourth grades. *Journal of Educational Psychology* **80:** 437–447.

Karchmer, M. A., Milone, M. N. Jr., & Wolk, S. 1979. Educational significance of hearing loss at three levels of severity. *American Annals of the Deaf* **124**(2): 97–109.

Klima, E., & Bellugi, U. 1979. *The signs of language*. Cambridge, MA: Harvard University Press.

LaSasso, C., Crain, K., & Leybaert, J. 2003. Rhyme generation in deaf students: the effect of exposure to cued speech. *Journal of Deaf Studies and Deaf Education* **8**(3): 250–270.

Lane, H., & Grosjean, F. (Eds.). 1980. *Recent perspectives on American Sign Language*. Hillsdale, NJ: Erlbaum.

Leybeart, J. 1993. Reading in the deaf: The roles of phonological codes. In M. Marcshark & M. Diane (Eds.), *Psychological perspectives on deafness* (pp. 269–309). Hillsdale, NJ: Erlbaum.

Lichtenstein, E. 1985. Deaf working memory processes and English language. In D. Martin (Ed.), *Cognition, education and deafness* (pp. 111–114). Washington, DC: Gallaudet College Press.

Lichtenstein, E. 1998. The relationship between reading processes and English skills of deaf college students. *Journal of Deaf Studies and Deaf Education* **3:** 80–134.

Lucas, C. (Ed.). 1990. *Sign language research*. Washington, DC: Gallaudet University Press.

Mather, N., Hammill, D., Allen, E., & Roberts, R. 2004. *Test of silent word reading fluency*. Austin, TX: Pro-Ed, Inc.

Nicholls, G., & Ling, D. 1982. Cued speech and the reception of spoken language. *Journal of Speech and Hearing Research* **25:** 262–269.

Olson, R., Forsberg, H., Wise, B., & Rack, J. 1994. Measurement of word recognition, orthographic, and phonological skills. In R. G. Lyon (Ed.), *Frames of reference from the assessment of learning disabilities* (pp. 243–277). Baltimore, MD: Brooks.

Perfetti, C. A., & Sandak, R. 2000. Reading optimally builds on spoken language. *Journal of Deaf Studies and Deaf Education* **5**(1): 32–50.

Quigley, S., & Paul, P. 1986. A perspective on academic achievement. In D. Luterman (Ed.), *Deafness in perspective* (pp. 55–86). San Diego: College-Hill.

Scarborough, H. 1989. Prediction of reading dysfunction from familial and individual differences. *Journal of Educational Psychology* **81:** 101–108.

Scarborough, H., & Brady, S. 2002. *Toward a common terminology for talking about speech and reading: a glossary of the "phon" words and some related terms*. Unpublished manuscript.

Shankweiler, D., Liberman, I. Y., Mark, L., Fowler, C., & Fischer, F. 1979. The speech code and learning to read. *Journal of Experimental Psychology: Human Learning and Memory* **5:** 531–545.

Snow, C., Burns, S., & Griffin, P. (Eds.). 1998. *Preventing reading difficulties in young children*. Washington, DC: National Academy Press.

Stokoe, W. C. Jr., Casterline, D., & Croneberg, C. 1965. *A dictionary of American Sign Language*. Washington, DC: Gallaudet College Press.

The Psychological Corporation. 1996. *The Stanford Achievement Test* (9th ed.), Houston, TX: Harcourt Educational Measurement.

Torgeson, J. K., Wagner, R. K., & Rashotte, C. A. 1994. Longitudinal studies of phonological processing and reading. *Journal of Learning Disabilities* **27**(5): 276–286.

Tractenberg, R. 2002. Exploring hypotheses about phonological awareness, memory, and reading achievement. *Journal of Learning Disabilities* **35**(5): 407–424.

Traxler, C. B. 2000. The Stanford Achievement Test, 9th edition: national norming and performance standards for deaf and hard-of-hearing students. *Journal of Deaf Studies and Deaf Education* **5**(4): 337–348.

Trybus, R., & Karchmer, M. 1977. School achievement scores of hearing impaired children: national data on achievement status and growth patterns. *American Annals of the Deaf Directory of Programs and Services* **122:** 62–69.

Wagner, R. K., & Torgeson, J. K. 1987. The nature of phonological processing and its causal role in the acquisition of reading skills. *Psychological Bulletin* **101**(2): 192–212.

Wallace, G., & Corballis, M. 1973. Short-term memory and coding strategy of the deaf. *Journal of Experimental Psychology* **99:** 334–348.

Wechsler, D. 1999. *Wechsler Abbreviated Scale of Intelligence*. San Antonio, TX: Harcourt Brace and Company.

Wechsler, D. 1997. *Wechsler Memory Scale–Third Edition (WMS-III) Spatial Span*. San Antonio, TX: Harcourt Brace and Company.

Wilbur, R. 1987. *American Sign Language: Linguistic and applied dimensions* (2nd ed.). Boston: Little, Brown.

Wilson, M., & Emmorey, K. 2006a. Comparing sign language and speech reveals a universal limit on short-term memory capacity. *Psychological Science* **17**(8): 682–683.

Wilson, M., & Emmorey, K. 2006b. No difference in short-term memory span between sign and speech. *Psychological Science* **17**(12): 1093–1094.

Wilson, M., & Emmorey, K. 1998. A "word length effect" for sign language: further evidence for the role of language in structuring working memory. *Memory and Cognition* **26**(3): 584–590.

Wilson, M., & Emmorey, K. 1997. A visuospatial "phonological loop" in working memory: evidence from American Sign Language. *Memory and Cognition* **25**: 313–320.

Woodcock, R. W., Mc Grew, K. S., & Mather, N. 2001. *Woodcock-Johnson III Tests of Achievement*. Itasca, IL: Riverside Publishing Company.

Signed Language and Human Action Processing

Evidence for Functional Constraints on the Human Mirror-Neuron System

David P. Corina and Heather Patterson Knapp

University of California, Davis, Davis, California, USA

In the quest to further understand the neural underpinning of human communication, researchers have turned to studies of naturally occurring signed languages used in Deaf communities. The comparison of the commonalities and differences between spoken and signed languages provides an opportunity to determine core neural systems responsible for linguistic communication independent of the modality in which a language is expressed. The present article examines such studies, and in addition asks what we can learn about human languages by contrasting formal visual-gestural linguistic systems (signed languages) with more general human action perception. To understand visual language perception, it is important to distinguish the demands of general human motion processing from the highly task-dependent demands associated with extracting linguistic meaning from arbitrary, conventionalized gestures. This endeavor is particularly important because theorists have suggested close homologies between perception and production of actions and functions of human language and social communication. We review recent behavioral, functional imaging, and neuropsychological studies that explore dissociations between the processing of human actions and signed languages. These data suggest incomplete overlap between the mirror-neuron systems proposed to mediate human action and language.

Key words: ASL; signed language; deaf; human action processing; mirror-neuron system; neurolinguistics

Introduction

The last forty years have seen a remarkable development of interest in the signed languages used within culturally Deaf communities around the world. Signed languages are structurally complex, naturally emerging communicative systems that display all of the linguistic, cognitive, and biological characteristics of spoken languages. They are produced by the hands and arms rather than the mouth and are perceived by the visual system rather than the auditory system. Linguistically allowable hand configurations, spatial locations, and movement trajectories are arbitrary, conventionalized, highly specified, and form a closed set that differs according to which of the world's many signed languages is being used. Their mere existence provides important insights into the remarkable diversity of human language, and to the flexibility of the cognitive and neurological systems that support language use. A fuller characterization of their properties is certain to help us better understand the perceptual, cognitive, and neurological processing of all visual representations of languages, including written language, visual speech and co-speech gestures, and of visual cognitions more generally.

Address for correspondence: David Corina, 267 Cousteau Place, Davis, CA 95618. Voice: 530-297-4421; fax: 530-297-4400. corina@ucdavis.edu

Historically, research into signed languages has been performed by comparing and contrasting them to spoken languages. For example, pioneering studies by Ursula Bellugi, Edward Klima, and colleages conducted in the 1970s and 1980s (e.g., Klima & Bellugi, 1979) compared the perception and production of American Sign Language (ASL) among deaf signers to that of spoken language use among hearing people. These comparisons, which took place along a number of perceptual and cognitive dimensions, laid the groundwork for decades of subsequent behavioral research that has been extraordinarily helpful in honing our understanding of the linguistic, psychological, and biological properties of human language.

Linguistic research has identified similarities in the formal patterning of grammatical properties across signed and spoken languages. For example, Lillo-Martin (1986, 1991) has shown how some aspects of pronoun use in ASL are similar to those of richly inflected languages like spoken Italian and Spanish. Sandler (1989, 1993) discusses how constructs such as the "syllable" may be useful for describing and predicting processes such as reduplication in both spoken and signed words.

Psycholinguistic research has examined how lexical properties such as frequency-of-occurrence and formational similarity can influence the rapid recognition of signs, as in speech (Carreiras, Gutirrez-Sigut, Baquero, & Corina, 2008; Dye & Shih, 2006; Emmorey, Norman, and O'Grady, 1991). Emmorey *et al.* (1991) show how processing of ASL sentences elicits patterns of selective grammatical reactivation that parallel spoken language processing, despite the sign language grammar's strong use of spatial mechanisms to signal pronominal reference.

Neurolinguistic studies have established that damage to regions in left hemisphere perisylvian areas disrupts language processing in remarkably similar ways for speakers and signers (Poizner, Klima, & Bellugi, 1987). These studies and hundreds others point to commonalities across sign and speech at structural, functional, and anatomical levels and have provided some of the strongest evidence to date for a core biological endowment of human language that can manifest with striking similarity in multiple modalities (see Emmorey, 2002, for a comprehensive review).

The present article examines signed languages from a different perspective. Here, we take the opportunity to ask what we can learn about human languages by contrasting formal visual-gestural linguistic systems (signed languages) with more general human action perception. To understand visual language perception (i.e., sign language), it is important to distinguish the tasks associated with perceiving human motion, generally, from the specialized operations that enable one to extract symbolic meaning from conventionalized linguistic human actions.

In this article we review data from recent behavioral studies that compare the perception of linguistic and nonlinguistic gestures in infants and adults, and signers and nonsigners. These data show that the perception of language expressed in the visual-manual modality is treated differently than other forms of complex visual-manual actions. We then turn to functional imaging studies and neuropsychological research, which also demonstrate that the brain honors a distinction between sign and nonlinguistic gesture processing. We discuss the importance of these findings in relation to understanding neural representation and processing of human languages. Finally, we discuss these results in light of recent proposals concerning neural systems underlying human action production and perception.

On the basis of these emerging data, we suggest that human sign languages require an integration of visual form and movement properties that are subserved by temporal-ventral and dorsal parietal-frontal neural systems in ways that differ from the perception of nonlinguistic gestures in deaf signers. These data suggest that the human action/perception system is highly malleable and adapts to the specialized demands of the input it receives.

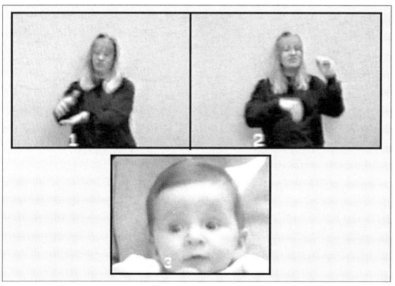

Figure 1. Split screen images of an infant monitoring sign language and pantomime (Adapted from Hildebrandt-Krentz & Corina, 2008).

Behavioral Studies of Linguistic and Nonlinguistic Gesture Perception

Recent behavioral studies have shown that for normally hearing infants, sign language may be treated qualitatively differently than pantomimic actions. In these studies, hearing 8-month-old babies who had not been previously exposed to sign language showed increased looking times to video displays that juxtapose sign language sentences and complex pantomimic "phrases" produced by the same actor (Hildebrandt-Krentz & Corina, 2008) (Fig. 1). This same pattern was not observed for 10-month-old hearing infants, who showed no preference. This study is important because it suggests that at a young age infants may be pre-equipped to be attuned to relevant differences between types of human action. Previous work has demonstrated the early sensitivity to linguistic versus nonlinguistic sounds (Vouloumanos & Werker, 2007), but this is the first study to show that these results may extend to the realm of manual-language processing. In the case of hearing infants, Hildebrant-Krentz and Corina (2008) proposed that viewing preferences diminish as visual linguistic stimuli cease to serve an ecological function (that is, the babies are being exposed to and are acquiring spoken languages in the home). Presumably, children who continue to receive sign language as a primary linguistic input continue to attune to human action processing in the service of linguistic communication, a hypothesis currently being tested.

In an attempt to delineate which aspects of signs and pantomime may drive the increased preference in the younger infants, this group was also shown point-light displays of the previously viewed actions (Hildebrandt-Krentz & Corina, 2008). In point-light displays, small white lights are attached to the arm and finger joints such that only the motion pattern (but not full-signal information) is conveyed to the person watching. Thus, point-light displays permitted the investigators to test whether movement qualities alone are sufficient to engage language-specific interests. Much to our surprise, and in contrast to the full signal displays, the point-light version did not differentially attract infants' attention as a function of movement type. This interesting finding suggested to us that movement properties alone were not fully responsible for the viewing preferences observed previously and that these infants might be seeking information from the full-signal human that was not available from arrays of lights. Post-hoc analysis of stimulus characteristics revealed that detailed qualities of handshape and facial movement in the full-signal videos may have contributed to observed differences between sign language and pantomime, further supporting this hypothesis.

Point-light displays preserve global properties of movement forms at the expense of local details of rigid body shape and form, and are believed to engage dorsal motion pathways that are specialized for analysis of optic flow information (Giese & Poggio, 2003). The present data suggest that local form information mediated by ventral perception pathways may differentially contribute to the infants' attraction to linguistic properties of human actions. It may be the case that young infants are highly attuned to local information conveyed in the faces and hands of those in their immediate environment. This attunement may have functional origins that extend beyond language per se: It is known that infants are close monitors of psychosocial content available from the eye, mouth, and head movements of adults (Meltzoff, 2007). Thus, infants' discrimination of linguistic from nonlinguistic motion in full-signal displays may be an even more sophisticated instantiation of their on-line attempts to learn whether or not the actions of the viewed adult have emotional-communicative relevance.

Using the point-light techniques with deaf adults signers and hearing nonsigners, we asked whether detection thresholds of signed versus pantomimic point-light movements embedded in a field of white noise dots were different for signers and nonsigners (Knapp, Cho, & Corina, 2008). These data indicated that for hearing subjects, sign movements were harder to detect than the pantomimic actions. Deaf subjects, however, showed equivalent abilities to detect sign and pantomimic movements under high noise conditions. These data are interesting for two reasons: Relative to nonsigners, the improved ability of signers to detect ASL movement patterns in noise suggests that familiarity with a particular motion class contributes to its absolute visual detectability. The equivalent detection of sign and nonsign point-light motion within this population, however, suggests that movement properties alone may not be sufficient to fully support a differential categorization of action classes. In other words, neither for infants nor for adults are movement patterns that have been divorced from other aspects of the signal sufficient to distinguish signs from nonlinguistic gestures. Thus, an important aspect of what we typically think of as human actions may encompass the integration of information about form and movement channels.

A recent series of behavioral experiments examined the effects of perceiving complex human action stimuli (signs and gestures) rotated in depth and in the picture plane. Deaf signers and hearing nonsigners were asked to quickly categorize viewed stimuli as either a sign or a gesture (Corina, Grosvald, & Lachaud, in preparation). The gestures used were intransitive self-directed actions (scratching one's neck, brushing back one's hair, etc.), similar to those used in our positron emission tomography (PET) study described below. On a small percentage of trials, identical stimuli were immediately repeated, permitting us to measure effects of repetition priming for these moving stimuli. Across the experiment the repeated items could consist of two identical upright video clips, or an upright clip followed by a depth rotated image (i.e., the same action video filmed from an approximately 45-degree angle) or the same image rotated in-plane 180 degree (i.e., upside down).

Not surprisingly, fluent signing deaf subjects were significantly quicker and more accurate at making the categorization judgments (deaf $\times =$ 768.5 msec, 81.2% correct; hearing $\times = 841$ msec, 75.9% correct; all *P*-values < .001). Both groups showed substantial repetition priming for both classes of stimuli. Here we focus on the comparison of the effects of repetition priming in cases in which the prime was presented

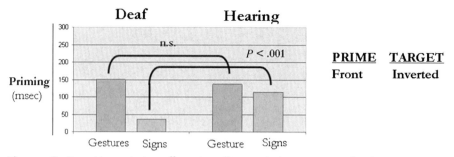

Figure 2. Repetition priming effects in milliseconds (reaction time for Prime categorization – reaction time for Target categorization) for Signs and Gestures in deaf signing ($n = 18$) and hearing ($n = 18$) nonsigning subjects. Robust priming for hearing subjects is found for both nonlinguistic gestures and signs. For deaf subjects, nonlinguistic gestures show robust priming, while repetition priming for signs is significantly reduced. These data indicate that sign and gesture are processed differently in deaf signers.

upright and the identical stimulus target was presented upside down.

For Upright$_{PRIME}$-Inverted$_{TARGET}$ pairs, all subjects showed a priming effect for nonlinguistic gestures. The nonsigners additionally showed a priming effect of similar magnitude for signs, indicating that they were processing gestures and signs in a similar fashion (see Figure 2). Critically, however, deaf signers' lexical decisions for upside-down ASL signs did not show a priming benefit from the prior upright presentation of signs. This suggests two things: *(a)* deaf signers process linguistic motion and nonlinguistic motion differently; and *(b)* inverted signs do not rapidly map to stored sign memory representations. These observations are intriguing because they suggest that during the time-course of motion perception, enough of the signal is perceived to allow for it to be recognized as belonging to a particular category of learned movement. If a movement pattern is obviously nonlinguistic in nature, it is processed in such a way as to allow for its subsequent recognition in a broader context (i.e., a different orientation). This "low bar" for pattern matching is raised for motion signals flagged as linguistic, however. For these higher-order patterns, it appears that a more rigorous standard of recognition is observed.

The constraints on the rapid perception of inverted signs are especially intriguing in light of our knowledge of face inversion effects. In-

verted faces are recognized far less accurately than other inverted objects, suggesting that upright faces are processed in a holistic manner in which both first- and second-order relational information is critical for recognition (Diamond & Carey, 1986; Bartett & Searcy, 1993; Murray, Yong, & Rhodes, 2000; Bertin & Bhatt, 2004). Inversion may make extraction and processing of second-order relational details (i.e., fine spatial information) more difficult. We speculate that in the context of this task, gestures and signs for nonsigners are processed in a similar fashion, one that places precedence on the global forms of the human actions. Computational models of biological movement processing have suggested that rotation-invariant aspects of biological movement processing may be subserved by dorsal-stream properties of the visual system (Giese & Poggio, 2003). The processing of the global properties is sufficient to engender a repetition priming effect despite the orientation changes.

In contrast, for deaf participants who are highly skilled signers, sign recognition may engage additional processing. This may include obligatory deconstruction of local properties (handshape, movement, facial information, etc.) and/or require integration of movement and form properties. In this case, the previous encounter with the identical upright stimuli provides little savings in the decomposition and integration of the novel inverted form. Visual linguistic information demands an integration of many different aspects of the signal, including fine spatial details that are not readily deduced under conditions of inversion.

Gestures, however, may not share this obligatory decomposition or demands for integration. These data suggest that local form properties subserved by ventral visual-stream networks may play a special role in the recognition of sign forms that differ from form processing in nonlinguistic gestures. Additional support for this claim comes from consideration of neuroimaging data discussed below.

The behavioral studies described above indicate differences in the processing of sign and human gestures—specifically, pantomimes and self-directed actions. Studies of infants suggest that this ability to distinguish forms of human movement, that is, language versus nonlinguistic pantomime, may be apparent at an early age. In cases in which local-form properties are masked (as in the case of point-light displays), deaf signers (and hearing babies) are not able to distinguish differences between sign and pantomimes based on movement properties alone. Studies of adult signers suggest that sign recognition in the context of a sign-gesture categorization task requires a decomposition of local-form properties of signs, but may differ from processes used to identify nonlinguistic gestures.

Neuroimaging Studies of Linguistic and Nonlinguistic Gesture Perception

Using functional brain imaging researchers have begun to explore dissociations of manual action perception and sign language processing (MacSweeney *et al.*, 2004; Corina *et al.*, 2007). MacSweeney *et al.* (2004) examined the contrast between the perception of British Sign Language (BSL) signs and a set of nonlinguistic gestures in Deaf and hearing signers and non-signers. This study was designed to provide a close comparison between a natural signed language (BSL) and a similar gesture display. The authors chose a highly constrained set of stylized, intransitive nonlinguistic gestures which are used in the United Kingdom as a signaling code by race-course bookmakers ("tic-tac"). These conventionalized stimuli (for example, two fists simultaneously brought together at the body's midline to indicate 10–1 betting odds) share many gestural and rhythmic qualities of natural signed languages such as BSL, but they do not constitute a linguistic system. A small set of tic-tac sequences were used in the nonlinguistic condition, and the stimuli were filmed with facial expressions so as to match the linguistic expressions used in BSL. Highly similar neural activation was seen for BSL and tic-tac sentence perception in all groups. Each contrast, set against a static low-level baseline, produced widespread bilateral posterior temporal-occipital, STS, and inferior temporal gyrus and inferior frontal lobe activation.

The direct comparison between the BSL condition relative to the tic-tac condition in the Deaf and hearing signing subjects did reveal a left-lateralized pattern of activation consistent with prototypical language effects. This activation included left perisylvian language regions, including temporal-ventral and inferior fusiform activations. In addition, these sign stimuli recruited dorsal parietal-frontal regions including the left SMG, which may reflect unique properties of sign language processing (Corina *et al.*, 1999).

In these signers, the comparison of tic-tac relative to BSL resulted in activation that was focused in a right hemisphere posterior temporal/occipital region anterior to the extrastriate body area (EBA) (Peelen, Wiggett, & Downing, 2006). The significance of this activation is discussed in more detail below. Given the authors' desire to match complexity of movement and form in these studies, the relatively sparse differences in activation between the BLS and tic-tac conditions suggest that signers may have treated tic-tac forms as linguistically possible but nonoccurring signs (analogous to phonotactcially possible nonwords such a "wug" or "fermp"). Numerous researchers have reported similarities in the neural activation during processing of possible but nonoccurring word forms compared to real words (Mechelli, Gorno-Tempini, & Price, 2003; Heim *et al.*, 2005).

A recent PET experiment furthers our understanding of differences between the neurological processing of signs and naturalistic human actions. This study sought to determine whether the focus and extent of neural activity during passive viewing of naturalistic human actions are modulated as a function of the type of action observed and the language experience of the viewer (Corina *et al.*, 2007). Hearing individuals unfamiliar with signed language and deaf signers observed three classes of actions: self-oriented, object-oriented, and communicative movements. The three classes of action were chosen to reflect increasing degrees of meaningfulness. Self-oriented actions, such as scratching one's head or rubbing one's eyes, are highly frequent but may not trigger conceptual elaboration. Impressionistically, in everyday interactions one tends to "look past" these gestures, perhaps because they are largely irrelevant for the viewer. Object-oriented actions (throwing a ball, folding a shirt, etc.) may be considered goal-directed actions that have clear, highly specific, and predictable functional consequences. Finally, linguistic gestures used in ASL are seen as clearly communicative in nature, even by individuals who are not users of signed languages. These stimulus forms were cast against a common complex baseline condition. The baseline, derived from the sign stimuli, served to control for stimulus luminance and low-level motion cues common to all human motions.

For hearing, sign language–naïve subjects, the passive viewing of these different classes of actions, relative to the common baseline, produced very similar patterns of neural activity despite the inherent differences in the content of these actions. Primary foci included regions previously identified as critical to a human ac-

tion recognition system: most notably, superior parietal (BA 40/7), ventral premotor (BA 6), and inferior regions of the middle frontal gyrus (BA 46).

Some between-task differences were also apparent. In the direct comparison between self-oriented and object-oriented actions, prominent bilateral activity was noted in visual association regions encompassing the left middle occipital gyrus and the right fusiform gyrus. The left middle occipital lobe is proximal to the extrastriate body area (EBA) described by Downing, Jiang, Shuman, and Kanwisher (2001). The right fusiform gyrus is a region that Decety *et al.* (1997) report as demonstrating greater activation to meaningless sequences of hand and arm actions compared to meaningful actions. This is interesting when one considers that viewing another person's self-oriented grooming actions is considerably less meaningful than viewing canonical actions performed with common, well-known objects.

The primarily lateral posterior occipital activations found when viewing self-oriented actions stands in contrast to medial posterior occipital regions more active in response to object-oriented actions. Medial visual areas are engaged when people speculate about attributes or actions of others. For example, lingual gyrus activations have been seen in cases in which subjects were required to make inferences about other human participants, including their personality traits (Kjaer, Nowak, & Lou, 2002) and motives governing unfair monetary offers from a human partner (Sanfey, Rilling, Aronson, Nystrom, & Cohen, 2003). Coupled with the activation of visual regions involved in the discernment of socially relevant cues was activation in bilateral medial frontal-orbital cortex (BA 11). Although highly speculative, the engagement of the medial posterior occipital and frontal orbital regions in response to object-oriented human actions is consistent with a more cognitive-evaluative assessment of the goal-directed properties of these movements.

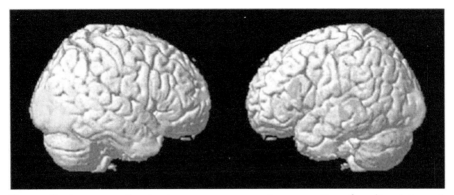

Figure 3. A contrast of activation patterns comparing perception of nonlinguistics actions (shown in green) and American Sign Language (red) (From Corina *et al.*, 2007 Reproduced by permission.)

For deaf signers, a different pattern was apparent. While the neural responses to self- and object-oriented actions showed a fair degree of similarity to one another, not unexpectedly, the neural responses to ASL were quite different. The direct contrast between data from ASL viewing relative to the combined responses of self-oriented and object-oriented actions provides a means of comparing linguistic and nonlinguistic human action perception in the deaf signers. As might be expected based on the concepts reviewed above, sign language viewing largely engendered neural activity in frontal and posterior superior temporal language areas, including left inferior frontal (BA 46/9) and superior temporal (BA 41) regions and the insula (BA 13) (shown in red in Figure 2). Thus, in this study, as in MacSweeney *et al.* (2004), the contrast between linguistic and nonlinguistic actions reveals the participation of left-hemisphere perisylvian and inferior frontal cortical regions in the perception of signed languages of the deaf.

When nonlinguistic actions are directly contrasted with ASL (shown in green in Fig. 3), prominent activity associated with their viewing was found bilaterally in middle occipital posterior visual association areas (BA 19/18) and ventral inferior temporal lobe (BA 20) and superior frontal (BA 10) regions. Prominent right hemisphere activity also included anterior regions of middle and superior temporal gyrus. We note that the right middle occipital posterior visual association activity found in this comparison is similar to that observed in the contrast between nonlinguistic and linguistic actions reported by MacSweeney *et al.* (2004).

The posterior middle occipital-temporal association areas are associated with specialized, high-level classes of visual stimulation. For example, regions of lateral posterior visual association cortex have been proposed to be selective for faces (Kanwisher, McDermott, & Chun, 1997; Kanwisher, 2000), images of bodies (Downing *et al.*, 2001), and biological movement (Grossman *et al.*, 2000; Grossman & Blake, 2001, 2002). A growing number of studies have begun further characterizing both the functional overlap and functional-anatomical specificities within these regions (Downing *et al.*, 2006; Morris, Pelphrey, & McCarthy, 2006; Peelen, Wiggett, & Downing, 2006). Our data show a clear focus of nonlinguistic human movement-generated activity in right hemisphere occipital-temporal association cortex. These regions correspond to the EBA and human MT (hMT) region described by Peelen, Wiggett, and Downing (2006). The differential processing of nonlinguistic and linguistic actions may reflect the gating of different classes of human motion in the deaf signers. Alternatively, deaf signers may show a greater reliance upon top-down processing in the recognition of highly familiar linguistically compositional human actions, thus leading to a more automatic and efficient early visual processing of highly familiar linguistic featural information. This is theoretically analogous to reports by Murray, Kersten, Olshausen, Schrater, and Woods (2002) that perceptually driven activity in primary visual cortex is reduced when higher visual areas group elements into coherent shapes, in line with predictive coding models of vision.

Taken together, these neuroimaging data suggest that human action processing in the deaf differentiates linguistic and nonlinguistic actions, especially in cases of naturalistic human actions. In direct comparisons of complex nonlinguistic human actions to linguistic signs, we observed increased activation in higher-order mid-temporal-occipital visual form-based regions. Nonlinguistic gesture detection may be driven by bottom-up processing, in which preliminary visual analysis is crucial to interpretation of the forms. In contrast, form-based processing of linguistic signs may be highly efficient and require less neural effort, providing a more direct mapping to meaning. The behavioral data discussed above are largely consistent. Reducing the availability of local form-based information for signs and gestures renders these signals largely indistinguishable for both infants and adults. However, potentially at odds with this interpretation are data from rotated sign and gestures. Recall that priming for signs suffered from effects of rotation, whereas nonlinguistic gestures continued to show priming even when rotated (for both deaf and hearing individuals). More work is required to better understand the temporal dynamics of these perceptual and cognitive processes.

Neuropsychological Studies

Data from neuropsychology also speak to the difference between the processing of linguistic and nonlinguistic actions. The reliance of signed language processing on left hemisphere regions is underscored by the unequivocal evidence for sign language aphasia occurring after left hemisphere lesions (Poizner *et al.*, 1987; Hickok, Bellugi, & Klima, 1997; Corina, 1998). Rare neuropsychological case studies of deaf signers have provided evidence for dissociations between the processing of sign language and human actions. Several reports have now documented cases in which, after damage to the left hemisphere, a deaf signer has completely or partially lost the ability to use sign language, but has retained an ability to use pantomime and nonlinguistic gesture (Poizner *et al.*, 1987; Corina *et al.*, 1992; Metz-Lutz *et al.*, 1999; Marshall, Atkinson, Smulovitch, Thacker, & Woll, 2004).

A sampling of this literature cuts a broad swath across patient age and primary language. For example, Metz-Lutz *et al.* (1999) report a case of a child with acquired temporal-lobe epileptic aphasia who was unable to acquire French Sign Language, but was unimpaired on ideomotor and visuospatial tasks and produced unencumbered nonlinguistic pantomime. Corina *et al.* (1992) reported that adult patient W.L. demonstrated marked ASL production and comprehension impairment after a lesion in left fronto-temporo-parietal regions, but retained intact pantomime comprehension and production, using gestures to convey symbolic information that he ordinarily would have imparted with sign language. Marshall *et al.* (2004) report an interesting case study patient, Charles, whose communicative behavior after a left-hemisphere stroke makes clear that sign and gesture production in BSL can be highly dissociated, even when the signs and gestures in question are physically quite similar. For example, when asked to produce the BSL sign for bicycle, he substituted a pantomimed bicycling motion. These cases emphasize that sign language impairments after left-hemisphere damage are not simply attributable to undifferentiated impairments in the motoric instantiation of symbolic representations, but in fact reflect disruptions to a manually expressed linguistic system that are not limited to any one language or stage of language development.

In summary, studies comparing differences in the processing of sign language and human actions in the deaf have shown frank disassociations in aphasic populations. Neuroimaging of deaf subjects shows further evidence of differentiation between perisylvian language systems and the engagement of bilateral ventral-lateral, and middle occipito-temporal regions and the right temporal lobe. The observation that sign activates left hemisphere perisylvian regions is not unexpected and is consistent with the growing literature showing that core aspects of human languages are mediated by left hemisphere structures regardless of language modality. What is new, and perhaps surprising, is that processing of nonlinguistic human actions in the deaf engages a system that might be attuned to cross-category properties of human body motion, and that this system differs from a frontal-parietal system commonly associated with human action recognition in hearing individuals.

Mirror-Neuron System and Human Action Understanding

Studies of human action perception have been influenced by neurophysiological data obtained from the macaque. Several studies report a unique neurophysiological response of a selective set of *mirror neurons:* cells which appear to couple the execution of goal-directed actions to the perception of similar goal-directed actions performed by another. These cells have been identified in a ventral premotor region (F5) (Gallese Fadiga, Fogassi, & Rizzolatti, 1996; Rizollatti, Fadiga, Gallese, & Fogassi, 1996) as well as in area 7b of parietal cortex (Fogassi, Gallese, Fadiga, & Rizzolatti, 1998; Gallese, Fogassi, Fadiga, & Rizzolatti, 2002). This F5–7b circuit in the macaque, often referred to as the mirror-neuron circuit, is speculated to be part of a larger mirror-neuron system (Rizzolatti & Craighero, 2004) forming the biological ba-

sis for understanding a wide range of human actions, including such complex behavioral constructs as imitation, social intent, empathy, and human language (e.g., Rizzolatti & Arbib, 1998; Iacoboni *et al.*, 1999; Rizzolatti, Fogassi, & Gallese, 2001; Ferrari, Gallese, Rizzolatti, & Fogassi, 2003; Rizzolatti & Craighero, 2004). Data from functional neuroimaging has been used to argue for a human homologue of a mirror-neuron system (Grezes & Decety, 2001; Grezes, Armony, Rowe, & Passingham, 2003; Aziz-Zadeh, Koski, Zaidel, Mazziotta, & Iacoboni, 2006). A growing consensus identifies this mirror-neuron system as a bilateral network involving superior temporal sulcus, intraparietal sulcus, the inferior parietal lobule, and the premotor cortex.

The account of the engagement of a bilateral frontal parietal human mirror-neuron system as a central component of human action understanding receives some support from the data reported above. When hearing subjects viewed self-directed and object-directed actions as well as unknown "tic-tac" gestures and signs, activation included bilateral inferior-parietal and frontal premotor regions. However, deviations from this network are readily apparent, such as the engagement of the frontal ventral-medial region indicative of social-evaluative judgments that was seen during the viewing of these goal-directed action sequences compared to self-directed actions. What is perhaps more difficult to incorporate within this general framework are the data from the deaf signers, who evidence a great deal of specialization of human action processing.

Sign language viewing engages classical language areas, which include perisylvian language regions, as well as inferior parietal regions such as the SMG and left frontal premotor and opercular regions. In contrast, the nonlinguistic gestures engage, to a greater extent, middle-temporal occipital regions known to participate in feature analysis of human form and movements. Behavioral and neuropsychological evidence indicate differential processing of signs and humans action in the deaf signers. Thus, it is unlikely that an undifferentiated mirror-neuron system underlies all aspects of human action perception (nonlinguistic or otherwise). Importantly, the accruing data suggest that the mirror-neuron system itself may be highly malleable. For example one may consider the well-attested left-hemispheric specialization for language (signed and spoken) as a case of specialization. In the case of deaf signers, the need for rapid differentiation of human gestures as language or nonlanguage may place processing demands on visual association regions not traditionally considered part of a mirror-neuron system.

Conclusions

The data presented here are important in that when brought together they provide another context for understanding language representation and processing. We suggest that unlike nonlinguistic gesture processing, neural systems subserving sign language in skilled signers benefit from efficient top-down processing, which may reduce the demands placed upon visual human form-recognition regions in lateral temporal-occipital cortex. Sign processing may require specialized form and movement integration to a degree not required for the recognition of nonlinguistic forms of movement. This efficiency and processing may come at a cost and may be selectively disrupted in cases of perisylvian lesions leading to sign aphasia. In contrast, nonlinguistic gesture processing may be more bottom-up and recruit large posterior and middle occipital regions during the dynamic processing of these less predicable forms of human action.

Taken together, these studies argue against a unitary human mirror-neuron system underlying human action perception, and force careful consideration of biological and functional factors which give rise to differentiated engagement of systems required for human communication and human action understanding.

References

Aziz-Zadeh, L., Koski, L., Zaidel, E., Mazziotta, J., & Iacoboni, M. 2006. Lateralization of the human mirror neuron system. *Journal of Neuroscience*, **26**(11): 2964–2970.

Bartlett, J. C., & Searcy, J. 1993. Inversion and configuration of faces. *Cognitive Psychology*, **25:** 281–316.

Bertin, E., & Bhatt, R. S. 2004. The Thatcher illusion and face processing in infancy. *Developmental Science*, **7**(4): 431–436.

Carreiras, M., Gutirrez-Sigut, E., Baquero, S., & Corina, D. 2008. Lexical processing in Spanish Sign Language (LSE). *Journal of Memory and Language*, **58**(1): 100–122.

Corina, D. P. 1998. Aphasia in atypical populations. In P. Coppens, Y. Lebrun, & A. Basso, (Eds.), *Aphasia in users of signed language*. London: Lawrence Erlbaum.

Corina, D. P., Chiu, Y., Knapp, H., Greenwald, R., San Jose-Robertson, L., & Braun, A. 2007. Neural correlates of human action observation in hearing and deaf subjects. *Brain Research*, **1152:** 111–129.

Corina, D. P., & Hildebrandt, U. 2002. Modality and structure in signed and spoken languages. In R. P. Meier, K. Cormier, & D. Quinto-Pozos (Eds.), *Psycholinguistic investigations of phonological structure in American Sign Language*. Cambridge: Cambridge University Press.

Corina, D. P., McBurney, S. L., Dodrill, C., Hinshaw, K., Brinkley, J., & Ojemann, G. 1999. Functional roles of Broca's area and Smg: evidence from cortical stimulation mapping in a deaf signer. *NeuroImage*, **10**(5): 570–581.

Corina, D. P., Poizner, H., Bellugi, U., Feinberg, T., Dowd, D., & O'Grady-Batch, L. 1992. Dissociation between linguistic and nonlinguistic gestural systems: a case for compositionality. *Brain and Language*, **43**(3): 414–447.

Corina, D., Grosvald, M., & Lachaud, C. (In preparation). *Repetition priming of signs and human actions in deaf and hearing subjects*.

Decety, J., Grezes, J., Costes, N., Perani, D., Jeannerod, M., Procyk, E., *et al.* 1997. Brain activity during observation of actions. Influence of action content and subject's strategy. *Brain*, **120:** 1763–1777.

Diamond, R., & Carey, S. 1986. Why faces are and are not special: an effect of expertise. *Journal of Experimental Psychology: General*, **115**(2): 107–117.

Downing, P. E., Chan, A. W., Peelen, M. V., Dodds, C. M., & Kanwisher, N. 2006. Domain specificity in visual cortex. *Cerebral Cortex*, **16**(10): 1453–1461.

Downing, P. E., Jiang, Y., Shuman, M., & Kanwisher, N. 2001. A cortical area selective for visual processing of the human body. *Science*, **293:** 2470–2473.

Dye, M. W. G., & Shih, S. 2006. Papers in Laboratory of Phonology 8. In L. M. Goldstein, D. H. Whalen, & C. T. Best (Eds.), *Phonological priming in British Sign Language*. Berlin: Mouton de Gruyter.

Emmorey, K. 2002. *Language, cognition, and the brain: Insights from sign language research*. Mahwah, NJ: Erlbaum.

Emmorey, K., Norman, F., & O'Grady, L. 1991. The activation of spatial antecedents from overt pronouns in American Sign Language. *Language and Cognitive Processes*, **6**(3): 207–228.

Ferrari, P. F., Gallese, V., Rizzolatti, G., & Fogassi, L. 2003. Mirror neurons responding to the observation of ingestive and communicative mouth actions in the monkey ventral premotor cortex. *European Journal of Neuroscience*, **17**(8): 1703–1174.

Fogassi, L., Gallese, V., Fadiga, L., & Rizzolatti, G. 1998. Neurons responding to the sight of goal directed hand/arm actions in the parietal area PF (7b) of the macaque monkey. *Society for Neuroscience Abstracts*, **24:** 257.5.

Gallese, V., Fadiga, L., Fogassi, L., & Rizzolatti, G. 1996. Action recognition in the premotor cortex. *Brain*, **119:** 593–609.

Gallese, V., Fogassi, L., Fadiga, L., & Rizzolatti, G. 2002. Attention and performance. In W. Prinz, B. Hommel (Eds.), *Action representation and the inferior parietal lobule*. New York: Oxford University Press.

Giese, M. A., & Poggio, T. 2003. Neural mechanisms for the recognition of biological movements. *Nature Neuroscience Reviews*, **4:** 179–192.

Grezes, J., Armony, J. L., Rowe, J., & Passingham, R. E. 2003. Activations related to "mirror" and "canonical" neurons in the human brain: An fMRI study. *NeuroImage*, **18:** 928–37.

Grezes, J., & Decety, J. 2001. Functional anatomy of execution, mental simulation, observation, and verb generation of actions: a meta-analysis. *Human Brain Mapping*, **12:** 1–19.

Grossman, E. D., & Blake, R. 2001. Brain activity evoked by inverted and imagined biological motion. *Vision Research*, **41:** 1475–1482.

Grossman, E. D., & Blake, R. 2002. Brain areas active during visual perception of biological motion. *Neuron*, **35**(6): 1167–1175.

Grossman, E., Donnelly, M., Price, R., Pickens, D., Morgan, V., Neighbor, G., *et al.* 2000. Brain areas active during visual perception of biological motion. *Journal of Cognitive Neuroscience*, **12:** 711–720.

Heim, S., Alter, K., Ischebeck, A. K., Amunts, K., Eickhoff, S. B., Mohlberg, H., *et al.* 2005. The role of the left Brodmann's areas 44 and 45 in reading words and pseudowords. *Brain Research. Cognitive Brain Research*, **25**(3): 982–993.

Hickok, G., Bellugi, U., & Klima, E. S. 1997. The basis of the neural organization for language: evidence from sign language aphasia. *Reviews in the Neurosciences*, **8**(3–4): 205–222.

Hildebrandt-Krentz, U., & Corina, D. 2008. Preference for language in early infancy: The human language bias is not speech specific. *Developmental Science*, **11**(1): 1–9.

Iacoboni, M., Woods, R. P., Brass, M., Bekkering, H., Mazziotta, J. C., & Rizzolatti, G. 1999. Cortical mechanisms of human imitation. *Science*, **286**(5449): 2526–2528.

Kanwisher, N. 2000. Domain specificity in face perception: review. *Nature Neuroscience*, **3**(8): 759–763.

Kanwisher, N., McDermott, J., & Chun, N. M. 1997. The fusiform face area: a module in human extrastriate cortex specialized for face perception. *Journal of Neuroscience*, **17**(11): 4302–4311.

Kjaer, T., Nowak, M., & Lou, H. 2002. Reflective self-awareness and conscious states: PET evidence for a common midline parietofrontal core. *NeuroImage*, **17**(2): 1080.

Knapp, H. P., Cho, H., & Corina, D. P. 2008. Perception of sign language and human actions. In M. R. de Quadros (Ed.), *TISLR 9: Theoretical Issues in Sign Language Research 9. 9 Congreso International de Aspectos Teóricos das Pesquisas nas Linguas de Sinais. December 6 to 9, 2006 Universidade Federal de Santa Catarina Florianópolis, SC Brasil*. Florianópolis: Lagoa Editora.

Lillo-Martin, D. 1986. Two kinds of null pronouns in American Sign Language. *Natural Language and Linguistic Theory*, **4:** 415–444.

Lillo-Martin, D. 1991. *Universal grammar and American Sign Language: Setting the null argument parameters. Studies in theoretical psycholinguistics*. Dordrecht: Kluwer.

MacSweeney, M., Campbell, R., Woll, B., Giampietro, V., David, A. S., McGuire, P. D., *et al.* 2004. Dissociating linguistic and nonlinguistic gestural communication in the brain. *NeuroImage*, **22**(4): 1605–1618.

Marshall, J., Atkinson, J., Smulovitch, E., Thacker, A., & Woll, B. 2004. Aphasia in a user of British Sign Language: dissociation between sign and gesture. *Cognitive Neuropsychology*, **21**(5): 537–554.

Mechelli, A., Gorno-Tempini, M. L., & Price, C. J. 2003. Neuroimaging studies of word and pseudoword reading: consistencies, inconsistencies, and limitations. *Journal of Cognitive Neuroscience*, **15**(2): 260–271.

Meltzoff, A. N. 2007. "Like me": a foundation for social cognition. *Developmental Science*, **10**(1): 126–134.

Metz-Lutz, M. N., de Saint Martin, A., Monpiou, S., Massa, R., Hirsch, E., & Marescaux, C. 1999. Early dissociation of verbal and nonverbal gestural ability in an epileptic deaf child. *Annals of Neurology*, **46**(6): 929–932.

Morris, J. P., Pelphrey, K. A., & McCarthy, G. 2006. Occipitotemporal activation evoked by the perception of human bodies is modulated by the presence or absence of the face. *Neuropsychologia*, **44**(10): 1919–1927.

Murray, J. E., Yong, E., & Rhodes, G. 2000. Revisiting the perception of upside-down faces. *Psychological Science*, **11:** 492–496.

Murray, S. O., Kersten, D., Olshausen, B. A., Schrater, P., & Woods, D. L. 2002. Shape perception reduces activity in human primary visual cortex. *Proceedings of the National Academy of Sciences of the United States of America*, **99:** 15164–15169.

Peelen, M. V., Wiggett, A. J., & Downing, P. E. 2006. Patterns of fMRI activity dissociate overlapping functional brain areas that respond to biological motion. *Neuron*, **49**(6): 815–822.

Poizner, H., Klima, E. S., & Bellugi, U. 1987. *What the hands reveal about the brain*. Cambridge: MIT Press.

Rizzolatti, G., & Arbib, M. A. 1998. Language within our grasp. *Trends in Neuroscience*, **21**(5): 188–194.

Rizzolatti, G., & Craighero, L. 2004. The mirror-neuron system. *Annual Review of Neuroscience*, **27:** 169–192.

Rizzolatti, G., Fadiga, L., Gallese, V., & Fogassi, L. 1996. Premotor cortex and the recognition of motor actions. *Brain Research. Cognitive Brain Research*, **3**(2): 131–141.

Rizzolatti, G., Fogassi, L., & Gallese, V. 2001. Neurophysiological mechanisms underlying the understanding and imitation of action. *Nature Reviews. Neuroscience*, **2**(9): 661–670.

Sandler, W. 1989. *Phonological representation of the sign: Linearity and non-linearity in American Sign Language*. Dordrecht: Foris.

Sandler, W. 1993. A sonority cycle in American Sign Language. *Phonology*, **10:** 243–279.

Sanfey, I. G., Rilling, J. K., Aronson, J. A., Nystrom, L. E., & Cohen, J. D. 2003. The neural basis of economic decision-making in the ultimatum game. *Science*, **300**(5626): 1755–1758.

Vouloumanos, A., & Werker, J. F. 2007. Listening to language at birth: evidence for a bias for speech in neonates. *Devopmental Science*, **10**(2): 159–164.

Neurocognitive Basis of Implicit Learning of Sequential Structure and Its Relation to Language Processing

Christopher M. Conway[a] and David B. Pisoni[a,b]

[a]*Speech Research Laboratory, Indiana University, Bloomington, Indiana, USA*

[b]*Devault Otologic Research Laboratory, Department of Otolaryngology–Head & Neck Surgery, Indiana University School of Medicine, Indianapolis, Indiana, USA*

The ability to learn and exploit environmental regularities is important for many aspects of skill learning, of which language may be a prime example. Much of such learning proceeds in an implicit fashion, that is, it occurs unintentionally and automatically and results in knowledge that is difficult to verbalize explicitly. An important research goal is to ascertain the underlying neurocognitive mechanisms of implicit learning abilities and understand its contribution to perception, language, and cognition more generally. In this article, we review recent work that investigates the extent to which implicit learning of sequential structure is mediated by stimulus-specific versus domain-general learning mechanisms. Although much of previous implicit learning research has emphasized its domain-general aspect, here we highlight behavioral work suggesting a modality-specific locus. Even so, our data also reveal that individual variability in implicit sequence learning skill correlates with performance on a task requiring sensitivity to the sequential context of spoken language, suggesting that implicit sequence learning to some extent is domain-general. Taking into consideration this behavioral work, in conjunction with recent imaging studies, we argue that implicit sequence learning and language processing are both complex, dynamic processes that partially share the same underlying neurocognitive mechanisms, specifically those that rely on the encoding and representation of phonological sequences.

Key words: implicit learning; sequence learning; language processing; modality-specificity; domain-generality; prefrontal cortex; basal ganglia

Introduction

An essential characteristic of skill learning is the necessity of encoding, representing, and/or producing structured sequences. Because the environment is characterized by the regular and coherent occurrence of sounds, objects, and events, any organism that can usefully encode and exploit such structure will have an adaptive advantage. Language and communication are excellent examples of structured sequential domains to which humans are sensitive. That is, spoken and written language units (letters, phonemes, syllables, words, etc.) each adhere to a semiregular, sequential structure that can be defined in terms of statistical or probabilistic relationships (Rubenstein, 1973). Sensitivity to such probabilistic information in the speech stream can improve the perception of spoken materials in noise; the more predictable a sentence is, the easier it is to perceive (Kalikow *et al.*, 1977; see also Miller & Selfridge, 1950). The presence of probabilistic, structured patterns is found in almost all aspects of our interaction with the world, whether it be in speaking, listening to music, learning a tennis swing, or perceiving complex scenes.

Address for correspondence: Christopher M. Conway, Department of Psychology, Saint Louis University, 3511 Laclede Ave., St. Louis, MO 63103. Voice: +314-977-2299; fax: +314-977-1014. cconway6@slu.edu.

Ann. N.Y. Acad. Sci. 1145: 113–131 (2008). © 2008 New York Academy of Sciences.
doi: 10.1196/annals.1416.009

How the mind, brain, and body encode and use structure that exists in time and space remains a formidable challenge for the cognitive and neural sciences (Port & Van Gelder, 1995). This issue has begun to be elucidated through the study of "implicit" learning (Cleeremans, Destrebecqz, & Boyer, 1998; Conway & Christiansen, 2006; Reber, 1993; Perruchet & Pacton, 2006). Implicit learning involves automatic learning mechanisms that are used to extract regularities and patterns distributed across a set of exemplars, typically without conscious awareness of the regularities being learned. Implicit learning is believed to be important for many aspects of skill learning, problem solving, and language processing.

One important research goal is to establish whether implicit learning is subserved by a single, domain-general mechanism that applies across a wide range of tasks, input, and domains, or instead consists of multiple task- or stimulus-specific subsystems. This is especially important if we are to usefully apply knowledge gained from laboratory studies of implicit learning to more real-world examples of language and skill learning. Two bodies of evidence have favored the former conclusion. First, many studies have demonstrated implicit learning across a wide range of stimulus domains and tasks, including but not limited to speech-like stimuli (Gomez & Gerken, 1999; Saffran, Aslin, & Newport, 1996), tone sequences (Saffran, Johnson, Aslin, & Newport, 1999), visual scenes and geometric shapes (Fiser & Aslin, 2001; Pothos & Bailey, 2000), colored light displays (Karpicke & Pisoni, 2004), and visuomotor sequences (Cleeremans & McClelland, 1991). Second, other studies using the artificial grammar learning (AGL) paradigm (Reber, 1967) have shown that participants can transfer their knowledge gained from one stimulus domain (e.g., visual symbols) to a different domain (e.g., nonsense syllables) if the underlying rule structure is the same (Altmann, Dienes, & Goode, 1995; Brooks & Vokey, 1991; Gomez & Gerken, 1999; Reber, 1969). Thus, implicit learning is argued to re-

sult in knowledge representations that are abstract or amodal in nature, independent of the physical qualities of the stimulus (Reber, 1993).

Despite this apparent evidence for a single, domain-general, and amodal implicit learning skill, there is reason to believe that implicit learning may be at least partly mediated by a number of separate specialized neurocognitive mechanisms. First, many views of the mind encompass to a greater or lesser extent the notion of functional specialization (Barrett & Kurzban, 2006; Fodor, 1983). As an example, working memory (Baddeley, 1986) consists in part of multiple, modality-specific processing components. Second, some of the transfer of knowledge data discussed above may suffer from methodological concerns (Redington & Chater, 1996); even if one disregards such concerns, it is not immediately clear that the results necessarily support the notion of amodal knowledge gained through implicit learning. Third, the fact that implicit learning has been demonstrated across numerous input types and tasks does not necessarily imply a single, domain-general system. It is just as possible logically that there may exist multiple implicit learning subsystems that all have similar computational principles, but that only some are engaged for specific task and input demands (Conway & Christiansen, 2005; Goschke, 1998; Seger, 1998). Finally, consistent with a multiple subsystems perspective, correlational analyses suggest that implicit learning is relatively task-specific (Feldman, Kerr, & Streissguth, 1995; Gebauer & Mackintosh, 2007).

In the first section below, we review recent behavioral work that examines the issues of domain-generality and modality-specificity in implicit learning. Our investigations explore the effect of sensory modality on implicit learning of sequential structures and the contribution of such abilities to language processing. Following the presentation of these studies, we review recent neural evidence that further illuminates the underlying neurocognitive basis of implicit sequence learning. Finally, we integrate the behavioral and imaging data and offer an account of the relation between implicit learning and language processing.

Cognitive Basis of Implicit Learning

Recent Behavioral Studies

The following three studies all use the artificial grammar learning (AGL) methodology (Reber, 1967). In a standard AGL task, a finite-state grammar is used to generate stimuli that conform to particular rules that determine the order in which each element of a sequence can occur (Fig. 1). Participants are exposed to the rule-governed stimuli under incidental and unsupervised learning conditions. Following exposure, participants' knowledge of the complex sequential structure is tested by giving them a test in which they must decide whether a set of novel stimuli follow the same rules or not. Generally, participants display adequate knowledge of the sequential structure despite having very little explicit awareness of what the underlying "rules" are; in fact, most participants report they were guessing during the test task. The similarities between implicit learning of artificial grammars and language acquisition are notable: both appear to involve the automatic extraction of sequential structure from a complex input domain that results in knowledge that is difficult to verbalize explicitly (Cleeremans *et al.*, 1998; Reber, 1967).

In the following sets of studies, we examine three important issues: the nature of modality constraints affecting implicit learning, the question of whether learning is mediated by multiple, independent learning mechanisms, and the extent to which implicit learning is a fundamental component of language-processing abilities.

Modality Constraints

To rigorously examine the effect of modality in implicit learning, we had three groups of participants engage in an AGL task, each assigned to a different sense modality: audition, vision, or touch (Conway & Christiansen, 2005). In

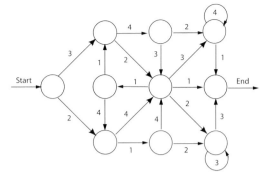

Figure 1. An example of an artificial grammar used to generate sequences in implicit learning experiments. To generate a sequence, the experimenter follows the paths of the grammar and notes the sequence of numbers that are encountered. For instance, the sequence 3-4-2-4-1 is grammatical with respect to this grammar, whereas the sequence 4-1-3-2-2 is not. The numbers 1–4 are then mapped onto stimulus elements needed for the experiment in question, allowing for the generation of a set of structured patterns occurring in virtually any stimulus modality or dimension as needed (tones, nonsense syllables, visual patterns, etc.).

these experiments, our strategy was to incorporate comparable experimental procedures and materials in the three sensory conditions in order to ensure a valid comparison of learning across modalities. These studies were also the first investigation of implicit learning in the tactile domain, a realm that had been previously ignored in earlier research.

Tactile stimulation was accomplished via vibrotactile pulses delivered to participants' five fingers of one hand (Fig. 2). The sequence pulses were generated from a finite-state grammar, where each element of the grammar corresponded to a pulse delivered to a particular finger. Each sequence generated from the grammar thus represented a series of vibration pulses delivered to the fingers, one finger at a time. For the visual group, visual sequences consisted of black squares appearing at different spatial locations, one at a time. Auditory sequences were composed of tone patterns. Like the vibrotactile sequences, the visual and auditory stimuli were nonlinguistic and thus participants could not easily rely on a verbal encoding strategy.

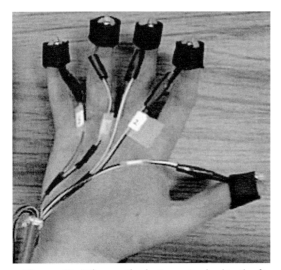

Figure 2. Vibrotactile devices attached to the fingers of a participant's hand. This setup was used by Conway and Christiansen (2005) to assess tactile implicit learning.

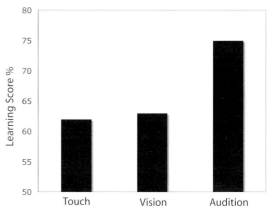

Figure 3. Implicit learning results for tactile, visual, and auditory sequences. (Adapted from Conway & Christiansen, 2005.)

The test results, which assess the ability to classify correctly novel sequences as being generated from the same grammar, revealed that visual learning performance was nearly identical to tactile learning (about 62%), whereas auditory learning was much higher than either tactile or visual learning (75% correct; Fig. 3). These data suggest a commonality among tactile, visual, and auditory implicit sequence learning: all three senses were able to mediate the encoding of the structured input. However, one striking difference among the senses was that the auditory performance was substantially (and significantly) greater than the other two modalities (75% vs. 62%). Thus, it appears that in this task, auditory implicit learning was more efficient than both tactile and visual learning. This is in accord with previous research emphasizing audition as being superior among the senses in regard to temporal processing tasks in general (e.g., Freides, 1974; Handel & Buffardi, 1969).

We were also interested in determining whether there were any other more subtle differences in learning across the senses. Additional analyses revealed that tactile learners were most sensitive to information at the beginning of a sequence, auditory learners were most sensitive to information at the end of a sequence, and visual learners displayed no biases toward either the beginning or the ending of the sequences. We determined this by comprehensively examining all training and test sequences in terms of their statistical structure. Learners in the tactile condition were more likely to make their classification judgments based on the extent to which a test sequence had statistical structure consistent with training items at the beginning of the sequence whereas auditory learners focused on structure at the endings of the sequences.

Taken together, the results from these experiments, confirmed and expanded in additional work (Conway & Christiansen, in press), suggest that not only does auditory implicit learning have a quantitative advantage over tactile and visual learning, but also that there may be qualitative differences in implicit learning among the three modalities. Specifically, tactile learning appears to be more sensitive to statistical structure at the beginnings of sequences, whereas auditory learning may be more sensitive to final-item structure. These biases suggest that each sensory system may apply slightly different computational strategies when processing sequential input. The auditory–recency bias is interesting because it mirrors findings on the modality effect in serial recall, in which a more pronounced recency effect (i.e., greater memory for items at the end of a list) is obtained with auditory lists as compared with visual lists (e.g., Crowder, 1986). This may indicate that similar constraints affect both explicit encoding of serial input and implicit learning of statistical structure. In both cases, learners appear to be more sensitive to auditory material at the end of a structured sequence or list of items.

Independent Stimulus-Specific Learning Mechanisms?

We recently attempted to determine whether implicit sequence learning consists of a single learning mechanism or multiple mechanisms that may operate simultaneously for different kinds of input or tasks (Conway & Christiansen, 2006). In order to distinguish between these two alternatives, we employed a dual-grammar, modified crossover AGL design. In a standard crossover design (see Redington & Chater, 1996), half of the participants are exposed to items from one grammar (e.g., grammar A) in the exposure phase, and then in the test phase must judge among items from both grammars A and B. The other half of participants receive grammar B at exposure but get the same test items as the first half of participants (from both grammars A and B). The novel modification we added is the inclusion of the second grammar during the acquisition phase. Thus, participants receive stimuli generated from both grammars A and B and are tested on novel stimuli also generated from both A and B. With this dual-grammar design, it is possible to assess to what extent learners can extract sequential structure from multiple input streams simultaneously; furthermore, we can test whether dual-grammar learning is easier or harder when both input streams are in the same sensory modality or same perceptual dimension.

In our study, participants viewed a subset of sequences from both grammars, arranged randomly. One grammar (A) was presented in the auditory modality as tone sequences. The other grammar (B) was presented as visual se-

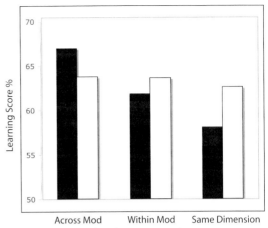

Figure 4. Implicit learning results comparing performance for dual-grammar (*black bars*) versus single-grammar (*white bars*) conditions. (Drawn from data presented in Conway & Christiansen, 2006.)

quences of colored patches in the center of the screen. After the acquisition phase, participants received novel sequences from both grammars, with some participants receiving visual sequences and others auditory. Like the standard AGL procedure, participants were told to classify each test sequence in terms of whether it followed the same underlying rules that generated the previous stimuli. This dual-grammar crossover design allowed us to assess to what extent learning two streams of sequential structure can occur simultaneously and independently of one another. In a second experiment, we varied the stimulus format of the two input streams, presenting both within the same sense modality but instantiated along two different perceptual dimensions (e.g., tones vs. nonwords or color sequences versus shape sequences). In a third experiment, both grammars were instantiated in the same perceptual dimension (e.g., two sets of nonword vocabularies or two sets of shape vocabularies).

The overall results are presented in Figure 4 for each of the three experimental dual-grammar conditions (black bars): across modality, within modality, and within the same perceptual dimension. We also compared performance levels with a different group of participants who received only one grammar at acquisition but were tested with the same stimulus materials that the dual-grammar participants received (white bars). This allowed us to assess to what extent learning two grammars proceeds as well as how learning one grammar proceeds for each of the three experimental input conditions. As Figure 4 shows, for the across-modality condition participants learned the two input structures, visual and auditory, quite well. In fact, the dual-grammar learning performance levels were actually higher than the performance of the single-grammar learners. These data suggest that participants learned the structural regularities from two artificial grammars in two different sense modalities just as well as if they had learned only one grammar alone, suggesting that the underlying learning systems operate simultaneously and independently of one another. For the other two input conditions, the results revealed that performance dropped slightly for the within-modal condition in which the two grammars were in the same sense modality, and performance broke down completely when the grammars were in the same perceptual dimension (Fig. 4).

Overall, the data revealed, quite remarkably, that participants were just as adept at learning structural regularities from two input streams as they were with one, as long as the two input types were in different sense modalities or perceptual dimensions. These findings suggest the operation of parallel, independent learning mechanisms that each handle a specific type of perceptual input, such as shapes, colors, tones, or word-like sounds (Goschke, Friederici, Kotz, & van Kampen, 2001; Keele, Ivry, Mayr, Hazeltine, & Heuer, 2003).

Contribution to Language Processing

Although it is commonly assumed that implicit learning is important for language processing, the evidence directly linking the two is equivocal. One approach is to assess language-impaired individuals on a putatively non-linguistic implicit learning task; if the group shows a deficit on the implicit learning task, this result is taken as support for a close link between the two cognitive processes. Using this approach, some researchers have found an implicit sequence learning deficit in dyslexics (Howard, Howard, Japikse, & Eden, 2006; Menghini, Hagberg, Caltagirone, Petrosini, & Vicari, 2006; Vicari, Marotta, Menghini, Molinari, & Petrosini, 2003), whereas others have found no connection between implicit learning, reading abilities, and dyslexia (Kelly, Griffiths, & Frith, 2002; Rüsseler, Gerth, & Münte, 2006; Waber *et al.*, 2003). At least with regard to reading and dyslexia, the role of implicit learning is not clear (though also see Bennett *et al.*, this volume, Folia *et al.*, this volume, and Stoodley *et al.*, this volume).

Given the data described previously, one complication with establishing an empirical link between implicit learning and language processing becomes apparent. If implicit learning involves multiple subsystems that each handle different types of input (e.g., Conway & Christiansen, 2006; Goschke *et al.*, 2001; Seger, 1998), then it is possible that some implicit learning systems (e.g., perhaps those handling phonological sequences) may be more closely involved with language acquisition and processing than others. To elucidate these issues, participants engaged in two AGL tasks, one using color patterns and the other using non-color spatial patterns, followed by a spoken sentence perception task (Conway, Karpicke, & Pisoni, 2007). For the AGL tasks, we used a procedure wherein participants observed a visual sequential pattern and then attempted to recall and reproduce the pattern by pressing appropriate buttons on a touch-screen monitor (Pisoni & Cleary, 2004). Implicit learning was assessed to the extent that serial recall for rule-governed sequences improves relative to non-structured sequences (Karpicke & Pisoni, 2004; Miller, 1958). This procedure has an advantage over traditional AGL performance scores because it provides a more valid assessment of implicit learning by relying on an indirect rather than direct measure of performance (Redington & Chater, 2002). Additionally, the use of the two types of visual sequences, colored patterns or noncolored spatial patterns, allowed us to examine possible differences for stimuli that differ in ease of verbal encoding.

The language-processing task involved participants listening to spoken sentences under degraded listening conditions and then identifying and writing down the final word in each sentence. Crucially, the sentences varied in the predictability of the final target word (see Kalikow *et al.*, 1977 and Clopper & Pisoni, 2006). Three types of sentences were used: high-predictability (HP), low-predictability (LP), and anomalous (AN). HP sentences had a final target word that is predictable given the semantic context of the sentence (e.g., "her entry should win first *prize*"); LP sentences had a target word that is not predictable given the semantic context of the sentence (e.g., "the man spoke about the *clue*"). AN sentences follow the same syntactic form as the HP and LP sentences, but the content words have been placed randomly to create semantically anomalous sentences (e.g., "the coat is talking about six *frogs*"). In this way, we were able to assess whether implicit sequence learning that is or is not phonologically mediated correlated with spoken language perception under degraded listening conditions for sentence materials that vary in their probabilistic structure. We first review the results for the color sequence learning task. The results revealed that performance on this task was significantly correlated with language-processing performance for the HP ($r = .48$) and LP ($r = .56$), but not for anomalous sentences (Fig. 5). Importantly, only participants' learning score on the sequencing task, not serial recall performance in general, correlated with the language task. That is, the contribution to language processing that we have demonstrated is not due merely to serial recall abilities, which has shown to be related to language development (Baddeley, 2003). It was only when we assessed how much memory span improved for grammatically consistent sequences did we find a significant correlation. Thus, what is important is the ability to im-

plicitly acquire knowledge about structured sequential patterns, not just the ability to encode and recall a sequence of items from memory.

Of interest, the sequence learning task that did not involve color sequences was not significantly correlated with performance on any of the sentence processing tasks (r's $< .38$). Whereas the sequences from the color learning task are very readily verbalized and coded into phonological forms (e.g., "red-blue-yellow-red"), those from the other task are not because they emphasize visual-spatial attributes. Thus, it is possible that implicit learning of phonological representations, not just spatiotemporal events more generally, contribute to success on the language-processing task. To examine this prediction further, we used a postexperiment debriefing on the noncolor learning task to divide participants into two groups: those who attempted to encode sequences using some kind of verbal code, such as labeling each of the four spatial positions with a digit (1–4; "phonological coders") and those who indicated they did not use a verbal code during the task ("nonphonological-coders"). We then assessed correlations between these two groups' learning scores and language perception measures and found that although none of the correlations quite reached statistical significance (presumably due to a lack of statistical power; N's $= 12$, 8), the difference in the correlations between the two groups was quite striking. The correlation results for the phonological coders and the noncoders are shown in Figures 6 and 7, respectively. Phonological coders' performance on the sequence task was positively correlated with their performance on the language task (r's $= .43, .28, .44$, for the HP, LP, and AN sentences, respectively), whereas the correlations for noncoders were much less or even negatively correlated with the language task (r's $= \pm.31, \pm.17, .14$, for the HP, LP, and AN sentences, respectively). This pattern of results further supports the conclusion that a crucial aspect of implicit sequence learning that contributes to spoken language processing is the learning of structured patterns from sequences

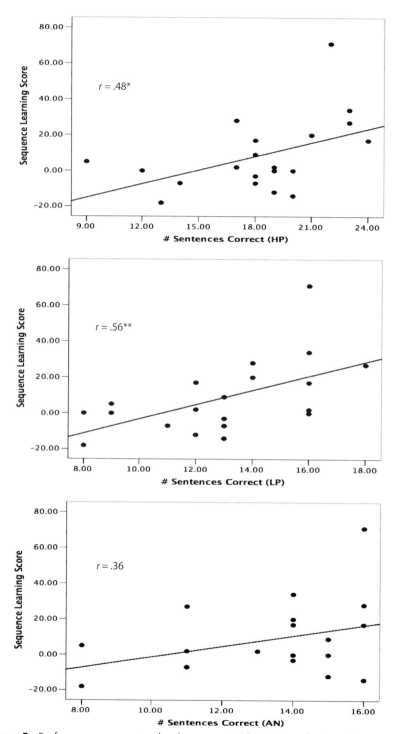

Figure 5. Performance on a visual color sequence learning task plotted against performance on a spoken language perception task under degraded listening conditions for high predictability (HP), low predictability (LP), and anomalous (AN) sentences. (Drawn from data presented in Conway & Christiansen, 2007.)

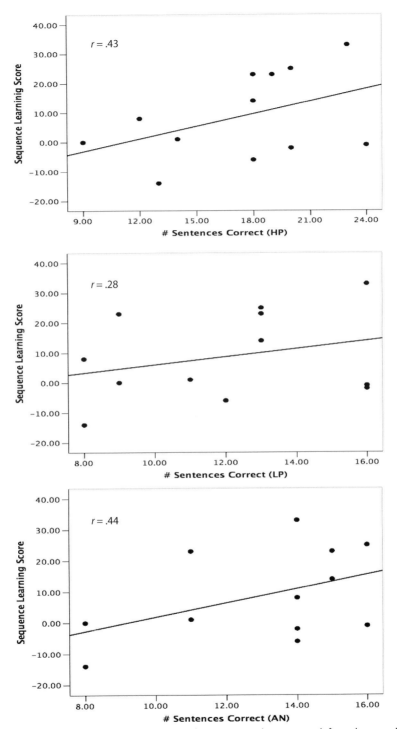

Figure 6. Performance on a visual noncolor sequence learning task for subjects who used a verbal coding strategy, plotted against performance on a spoken language perception task under degraded listening conditions for high predictability (HP), low predictability (LP), and anomalous (AN) sentences. (Drawn from data presented in Conway & Christiansen, 2007.)

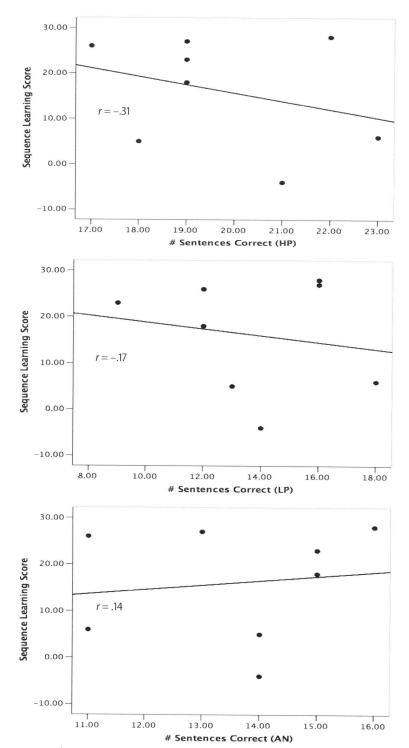

Figure 7. Performance on a visual noncolor sequence learning task for subjects who did not use a verbal coding strategy, plotted against performance on a spoken language perception task under degraded listening conditions for high predictability (HP), low predictability (LP), and anomalous (AN) sentences. (Drawn from data presented in Conway *et al.*, 2007.)

that can be easily represented using a verbal code.

These results provide the first empirical demonstration, to our knowledge, of individual variability in implicit learning performance correlating with language processing in typically developing subjects. We believe the evidence points to an important factor underlying spoken language processing: the ability to implicitly learn complex sequential patterns, especially those that can be represented phonologically.

Neural Basis of Implicit Sequential Learning

The behavioral data described above lead to two primary conclusions. First, implicit sequence learning involves multiple, modality-constrained mechanisms with each operating relatively independently of one another, and handling different kinds of input. Second, implicit learning for some kinds of stimuli, especially those that can be readily verbalized, has shared mechanisms with aspects of language processing. Considered together with data suggesting that implicit learning and sequence learning may also operate at more abstract levels of processing (e.g., Dominey, Ventre-Dominey, Broussolle, & Jeannerod, 1995; Tunney & Altmann, 2001), we should expect to find that there exists a combination of both modality-specific and more domain-general neural regions underlying implicit sequence learning. In fact, recent findings from neuroimaging studies support this general prediction. Although it is difficult to compare studies that rely on different methodologies, the general trends implicate both modality-specific and more abstract sequential processing brain areas. Below, we discuss neural evidence related to modality-specificity first and domain-generality second, followed by an integrative discussion to pinpoint the neurocognitive basis of implicit sequential learning and the relation to language processing.

Modality-Specificity

One of the central discoveries that has emerged out of the field of cognitive neuroscience is that cognition is grounded in sensorimotor function (Barsalou, Simmons, Barbey, & Wilson, 2003; Glenberg, 1997; Harris, Petersen, & Diamond, 2001). For instance, even conceptual knowledge, which has traditionally been proposed to be amodal or propositional in nature, appears to be based on perceptual representations (James & Gauthier, 2003). That is, neuroimaging studies have shown that concepts like "tools" or "animals" are represented by the same brain areas that are involved in perceiving or interacting with the actual physical items (e.g., visual and motor cortical areas, respectively; Pulvermüller, 2001). In a review of neural evidence from both humans and nonhumans, Harris *et al.* (2001) concluded that low-level sensory areas are involved not only in the online perception of information, but also in learning, memory, and storage of that information. These insights about the brain are paving a way for a new view of mind and behavior, one that focuses on sensorimotor constraints (Glenberg, 1997), brain–body–environment interactions (Clark, 1997), and the unity of perception, conception, and cognition (Goldstone & Barsalou, 1998).

Because of these insights, it may not be too surprising to discover that low-level, modality-specific brain regions also appear to underlie aspects of the temporal ordering and sequencing of stimuli. For instance, in both humans and rats, the auditory cortex mediates the learning and categorization of tone sequences (Gottselig, Brandeis, Hofer-Tinguely, Borbély, & Achermann, 2006; Kilgard & Merzenich, 2002; Ohl, Scheich, & Freeman, 2001). So too, visual areas such as IT in the monkey appear to be responsible for the learning of conditional associations among visual stimuli occurring in a sequential presentation format (Messinger, Squire, Zola, & Albright, 2001).

The best evidence, however, comes directly from neuroimaging studies of implicit sequence learning in humans. Although brain areas that may be considered to be domain-general are involved in implicit learning, there is also substantial evidence for a modality-specific component. Only a handful of neuroimaging studies have examined implicit learning using the AGL paradigm, but most of those reveal sensory-specific brain regions (e.g., occipital cortex) involved in the learning of rule-governed visual stimuli (e.g., Forkstam, Hagoort, Fernandez, Ingvar, & Petersson, 2006; Lieberman, Chang, Chiao, Bookheimer, & Knowlton, 2004; Petersson, Forkstam, & Ingvar, 2004; Seger, Prabhakaran, Poldrack, & Gabrieli, 2000; Skosnik *et al.*, 2002). For example, Lieberman *et al.* (2004) and Skosnik *et al.* (2002) observed increased medial occipital and superior occipital activation, respectively, when participants viewed grammatical test strings compared to ungrammatical test strings. Consistent with these data, the serial reaction time task (SRT; Nissen & Bullemer, 1987) has also revealed modality-specific brain regions responsible for learning sequential structure (e.g., Rauch *et al.*, 1995; 1997). On the basis of evidence such as this, Keele *et al.* (2003) recently presented a neurocognitive theory of implicit sequence learning and suggested the existence of multiple modality- or input-specific learning systems.

The modality-specificity revealed in these implicit learning tasks has a parallel in the implicit-memory literature. For example, repetition priming—that is, improvement in the ability to perceive or identify a stimulus on account of previous exposure to it—is known to involve modality-specific brain regions (see Schacter, Dobbins, & Schnyer, 2004). Reber, Stark, and Squire (1998) used an implicit memory task not unlike the AGL paradigm in which participants viewed complex dot patterns that were distortions of an underlying prototype pattern. Following exposure, participants attempted to classify novel dot patterns as either being similar to the prototype or not. The visual cortex showed different levels of activity for these new dot patterns, depending on whether they were similar to the prototype or not. Thus,

the similar nature of modality-specific brain regions involved in both implicit learning and implicit memory (e.g., priming) may implicate similar underlying computational processes involved in each. One likely possibility is that implicit sequence learning, like priming, at least partly is based on perceptual processing mechanisms that become tuned to particular stimuli based on previous experience (for similar proposals, see Chang & Knowlton, 2004; Kinder, Shanks, Cock, & Tunney, 2003).

In sum, consistent with the modality-constrained view outlined above, it is clear that brain regions traditionally thought to be modality-specific are active during implicit sequence learning tasks. However, it is possible that other brain networks are also involved in learning sequential structure including areas that process information in ways that may be considered to be more domain-general or abstract.

Domain-Generality

One of the most consistent findings from neuroimaging studies is that frontal cortical (prefrontal cortex, premotor cortex, supplementary motor areas, etc.) as well as subcortical areas (e.g., basal ganglia) play an essential role in sequence learning and representation (for general reviews, see Bapi, Pammi, Miyapuram, & Ahmed, 2005; Clegg, DiGirolamo, & Keele, 1998; Curran, 1998; Hikosaka *et al.*, 1999; Pascal-Leone, Grafman, & Hallett, 1995; Rhodes, Bullock, Verwey, Averbeck, & Page, 2004). For instance, the SRT task consistently activates premotor cortex (Berns, Cohen, & Mintun, 1997; Grafton, Hazeltine, & Ivry, 1995; Rauch *et al.*, 1995; Peigneux *et al.*, 2000), as well as parts of the basal ganglia, including the striatum (Berns *et al.*, 1997; Rauch *et al.*, 1995), the caudate (Peigneux *et al.*, 2000; Rauch *et al.*, 1995), and putamen (Grafton *et al.*, 1995). A recent meta-analysis shows that patients with Parkinson's disease are impaired on the SRT task (Siegert, Taylor, Weatherall, & Abernethy, 2006), highlighting the importance of the basal ganglia for this task. The AGL task also activates premotor (Opitz & Friederici, 2004) and prefrontal cortex (Fletcher, Büchel, Josephs, Friston, & Dolan, 1999; Skosnik *et al.*, 2002), often including Broca's area (Forkstam *et al.*, 2006; Petersson *et al.*, 2004; Seger *et al.*, 2000). The basal ganglia have also been implicated in some AGL studies (Forkstam *et al.*, 2006; Lieberman *et al.*, 2004), although unlike the SRT task, Parkinson's disease may not adversely affect AGL (Witt, Nühsman, & Deuschl, 2002). Other sequencing tasks besides SRT or AGL also show involvement of frontal lobe and basal ganglia (e.g., Bischoff-Grethe, Martin, Mao, & Berns, 2001; Carpenter, Georgopoulos, & Pellizzer, 1999; Huettel, Mack, & McCarthy, 2002).

The basal ganglia consist of a number of components, including the striatum, which itself is made up of the caudate and putamen (Nolte & Angevine, 1995). Although it has long been known that the basal ganglia are important for motor function, it is also becoming apparent that they are associated with other cognitive functions more generally, especially processes used for sequencing tasks (Middleton & Strick, 2000; Seger, 2006). The basal ganglia connect to multiple cortical sites including motor cortex, premotor cortex, and prefrontal cortex. The prefrontal cortex in turn is associated with executive function, cognitive control, and working memory (Miller & Cohen, 2001). More importantly, the prefrontal cortex is believed to play an essential role in learning, planning, and executing sequences of thoughts and actions (Fuster, 2001; 1995). The prefrontal cortex has many interconnections with various sensory, motor, and subcortical regions, making it an ideal candidate for more abstract, domain-general aspects of cognitive function (Miller & Cohen, 2001).

The corticostriatal loops connecting basal ganglia with cortex appear to be crucial for various forms of motor skill learning (e.g., Heindel, Butters, & Salmon, 1988) and non-motor cognitive processing (Seger, 2006). Interestingly, each of the parallel loops is believed to mediate a different aspect of cognitive processing, such

as "visual," "motor," or "executive" functions (Seger, 2006), thus constituting a form of specialization of function. The ways in which basal ganglia and prefrontal cortex interact appear to be complex and may partly depend on the nature of the task demands. In some cases, the prefrontal cortex appears necessary for learning new sequences, whereas the basal ganglia only become active once the sequences become well-practiced (Fuster, 2001). In other cases, learning appears to occur first in the basal ganglia, which then guide learning in prefrontal cortex (Pasupathy & Miller, 2005). A third possibility is that the basal ganglia contribute to reinforcement learning, while the cortex is specialized to handle unsupervised learning situations (Doya, 1999). Regardless of the actual ways in which these two brain structures interact, it appears likely that sequence learning relies heavily on the complex interaction of multiple corticostriatal loops, in a complex dynamic interplay that connect the basal ganglia to various cortical areas including circuits in the prefrontal cortex.

As is evident from this brief overview, implicit sequence learning appears to depend on a wide network of brain areas, including sensory, motor, frontal, and subcortical regions. Although we have focused here on frontal-striatal circuits, other brain regions including the parietal cortex (see Menghini *et al.*, this volume) and the cerebellum (Desmond & Fiez, 1998; Molinari, Filippini, & Leggio, 2002; Paquier & Mariën, 2005) have also been implicated in implicit learning. Implicit sequence learning likely involves multiple levels of learning, including learning simple stimulus-response associations as well as higher-order forms of learning that could be considered more abstract (Curran, 1998). Thus, the neural basis of implicit sequence learning not surprisingly involves a number of brain circuits that are active to a greater or lesser extent depending on the task's demands, learning situation, and nature of the input. The final question we address is to what extent neural mechanisms for implicit sequence learning are shared by those involved in language processing.

Sequential Learning and Language: A Synthesis

The traditional Broca–Wernicke model of language is now giving way to the recognition that language processing involves a much more distributed network of brain mechanisms including, interestingly enough, frontal/basal ganglia circuits (Friederici, Rüschemeyer, Hahne, & Fiebach, 2003; Lieberman, 2002; Ullman, 2004). For example, a recent fMRI study (Obleser, Wise, Dresner, & Scott, 2007) involving a speech perception task nearly identical to ours in which sentences varied on their semantic predictability (Conway *et al.*, 2007) showed that a network of frontal brain regions had increased activation for high predictability sentences. Thus, the frontal lobe and particularly the prefrontal cortex appear to be important for processing sequential context in spoken language. In addition, the two classic language dysfunctions, Broca's and Wernicke's aphasia, are now known to be driven just as much if not more from damage to subcortical basal ganglia structures as from cortical lesions (Lieberman, 2002). Even so, Broca's area and other frontal lobe structures still certainly play an important role in linguistic tasks, but they do not appear to be language-specific. For example, several theories ascribe Broca's area to be a "supramodal" sequence or structural processor, especially for complex hierarchical sequences be they linguistic or not (Conway & Christiansen, 2001; Forkstam *et al.*, 2006; Friederici, 2004; Greenfield, 1991; Tettamanti *et al.*, 2002). Thus, the frontal lobe, basal ganglia, and corticostriatal circuits appear to be active for both implicit sequence learning and several aspects of language processing.

However, the behavioral data reviewed above indicate that not all aspects of implicit sequence learning will necessarily recruit the same neurocognitive mechanisms as language processing. Performance on an implicit learning task only correlated with spoken language processing when the sequences were composed of verbal items. Thus, we ought to expect to find that certain brain regions are involved specifically in verbal sequencing, and these may be the regions that underlie both the implicit sequence learning and the spoken language tasks. There are two likely candidates for a verbal-specific sequencing brain system. One possibility is that there may be corticostriatal circuits that are specifically devoted to sequencing of verbal-mediated material. This possibility is consistent with suggestions that different corticostriatal loops perform analogous computations (i.e., sequencing), but handle different input domains (Ullman, 2004. A second likely possibility is that regions of Broca's area specifically handle phonological sequences. This idea is supported by data showing that Broca's aphasics can perform a spatiomotor implicit sequence learning task, but not one involving phonological sequences (Goschke *et al.*, 2001).

In sum, there appear to be both domain-general and modality-specific neurocognitive mechanisms that underlie both language and implicit sequence learning. The extent to which these neural mechanisms will be shared across linguistic and nonlinguistic tasks will depend on several factors, one being related to the perceptual dimension of the input (visual, auditory, verbal, etc.). For instance, we predict that the neural mechanisms that are devoted to sequence processing more generally (frontal/basal ganglia circuits) will interact with modality-specific (e.g., visual and auditory unimodal and association areas) brain regions when the task requires it. Furthermore, there may be phonological-specific processing areas (e.g., specific components of the frontal lobe, such as Broca's region) that will be preferentially recruited when the task involves phonological sequencing, whether the input itself is visual or auditory. This complex dynamic of domain-general and modality-specific neural mechanisms has been recently demonstrated in a neuroimaging study examining the effect of input modality and linguistic complexity during spoken and written language processing tasks (Jobard, Vigneau, Mazoyer, & Tzourio-Mazoyer, 2007). Both reading and listening tasks involved a common phonological or supramodal network of brain regions, including the inferior frontal area, whereas visual and auditory unimodal and association areas were preferentially active during reading and listening tasks, respectively.

Conclusions

We have reviewed evidence that implicit sequential learning is mediated by a combination of modality-specific and domain-general neurocognitive learning mechanisms that likely contribute to the successful acquisition and processing of linguistic input. Sequence learning and language are both complex, dynamic processes that involve a wide network of brain areas acting in concert. The behavioral work suggests some of the ways in which the underlying neurocognitive mechanisms are both constrained by input modality and how they rely on neural mechanisms shared with language processing that are of a more abstract or supramodal nature. We suggest that a full understanding of language acquisition and processing—whether it be for written or spoken material—will likely benefit from increased exploration into the understanding of the neurocognitive basis of implicit sequence learning.

Acknowledgments

Preparation of this manuscript was supported by NIH Grant DC00012.

Conflicts of Interest

The authors declare no conflicts of interest.

References

Altmann, G. T. M., Dienes, Z., & Goode, A. 1995. Modality independence of implicitly learned grammatical knowledge. *Journal of Experimental Psychology: Learning, Memory, & Cognition*, **21:** 899–912.

Baddeley, A. D. 2003. Working memory and language: an overview. *Journal of Communication Disorders*, **36:** 189–208.

Baddeley, A. D. 1986. *Working memory.* Oxford, UK: Oxford University Press.

Bapi, R. S., Pammi, V. S. C. Miyapuram, K. P., & Ahmed. 2005. Investigation of sequence processing: a cognitive and computational neuroscience perspective. *Current Science*, **89:** 1690–1698.

Barrett, H. C., & Kurzban, R. 2006. Modularity in cognition: framing the debate. *Psychological Review*, **113:** 628–647.

Barsalou, L. W., Simmons, W. K., Barbey, A. K., & Wilson, C. D. 2003. Grounding conceptual knowledge in modality-specific systems. *Trends in Cognitive Sciences*, **7:** 84–91.

Berns, G. S., Cohen, J. D., & Mintun, M. A. 1997. Brain regions responsive to novelty in the absence of awareness. *Science*, **276:** 1272–1275.

Bischoff-Grethe, A., Martin, M., Mao, H., & Berns, G. S. 2001. The context of uncertainty modulates the subcortical response to predictability. *Journal of Cognitive Neuroscience*, **13:** 986–993.

Brooks, L. R., & Vokey, J. R. 1991. Abstract analogies and abstracted grammars: comments on Reber (1989) and Mathews *et al.* (1989). *Journal of Experimental Psychology: General*, **120:** 316–323.

Carpenter, A. F., Georgopoulos, A. P., & Pellizzer, G. 1999. Motor cortical encoding of serial order in a context-recall task. *Science*, **283:** 1752–1757.

Chang, G. Y., & Knowlton, B. G. 2004. Visual feature learning in artificial grammar classification. *Journal of Experimental Psychology: Learning, Memory, & Cognition*, **30:** 714–722.

Clark, A. 1997. *Being there: Putting brain, body, and world back together again.* Cambridge, MA: MIT Press.

Cleeremans, A., Destrebecqz, A., & Boyer, M. 1998. Implicit learning: news from the front. *Trends in Cognitive Sciences*, **2:** 406–416.

Cleeremans, A. & McClelland, J. L. 1991. Learning the structure of event sequences. *Journal of Experimental Psychology: General*, **120:** 235–253.

Clegg, B. A., DiGirolamo, G. J., & Keele, S. W. 1998. Sequence learning. *Trends in Cognitive Sciences*, **2:** 275–281.

Clopper, C. G. & Pisoni, D. B. 2006. The Nationwide Speech Project: a new corpus of American English dialects. *Speech Communication*, **48:** 633–644.

Conway, C. M. & Christiansen, M. H. 2001. Sequential learning in non-human primates. *Trends in Cognitive Sciences*, **5:** 529–546.

Conway, C. M. & Christiansen, M. H. 2005. Modality-constrained statistical learning of tactile, visual, and auditory sequences. *Journal of Experimental Psychology*, **31:** 24–39.

Conway, C. M., & Christiansen, M. H. 2006. Statistical learning within and between modalities: pitting abstract against stimulus-specific representations. *Psychological Science*, **17:** 905–912.

Conway, C. M., & Christiansen, M. H. in Press. Seeing and hearing in space and time: effects of modality and presentation rate on implicit statistical learning. *European Journal of Cognitive Psychology*.

Conway, C. M., Karpicke, J., & Pisoni, D. B. 2007. Contribution of implicit sequence learning to spoken language processing: some preliminary findings from normal-hearing adults. *Journal of Deaf Studies and Deaf Education*, **12:** 317–334.

Crowder, R. G. 1986. Auditory and temporal factors in the modality effect. *Journal of Experimental Psychology: Learning, Memory, and Cognition*, **2:** 268–278.

Curran, T. 1998. Implicit sequence learning from a cognitive neuroscience perspective: what, how, and where? In M. A. Stadler & P. A. Frensch (Eds.), *Handbook of implicit learning* (pp. 365–400). London: Sage Publications.

Desmond, J. E., & Fiez, J. A. 1998. Neuroimaging studies of the cerebellum: language, learning, and memory. *Trends in Cognitive Sciences*, **2:** 355–361.

Dominey, P. F., Ventre-Dominey, J., Broussolle, E., & Jeannerod, M. 1995. Analogical transfer in sequence learning. In J. Grafman, K. J. Holyoak, & F. Boller (Eds.), *Structure and functions of the human prefrontal cortex* (pp. 173–181). New York: New York Academy of Sciences.

Doya, K. 1999. What are the computations of the cerebellum, the basal ganglia and the cerebral cortex? *Neural Networks*, **12:** 961–974.

Feldman, J., Kerr, B., & Streissguth, A. P. 1995. Correlational analyses of procedural and declarative learning performance. *Intelligence*, **20:** 87–114.

Fiser, J., & Aslin, R. N. 2001. Unsupervised statistical learning of higher-order spatial structures from visual scenes. *Psychological Science*, **12:** 499–504.

Fletcher, P., Büchel, C., Josephs, O., Friston, K., & Dolan, R. 1999. Learning-related neuronal responses in prefrontal cortex studied with functional neuroimaging. *Cerebral Cortex*, **9:** 168–178.

Fodor, J. A. 1983. *The modularity of mind: an essay on faculty psychology.* Cambridge, MA: Bradford Books, MIT Press.

Forkstam, C., Hagoort, P., Fernandez, G., Ingvar, M., & Petersson, K. M. 2006. Neural correlates of artificial syntactic structure classification. *NeuroImage*, **32:** 956–967.

Freides, D. 1974. Human information processing and sensory modality: cross-modal functions, information complexity, memory, and deficit. *Psychological Bulletin*, **81:** 284–310.

Friederici, A. D. 2004. Processing local transitions versus long-distance syntactic hierarchies. *Trends in Cognitive Sciences*, **8:** 245–247.

Friederici, A. D., Rüschemeyer, S.-A., Hahne, A., & Fiebach, C. J. 2003. The role of left inferior frontal and superior temporal cortex in sentence comprehension: Localizing syntactic and semantic processes. *Cerebral Cortex*, **13:** 170–177.

Fuster, J. 2001. The prefrontal cortex—an update: time is of the essence. *Neuron*, **30:** 319–333.

Fuster, J. 1995. Temporal processing. In J. Grafman, K. J. Holyoak, & F. Boller (Eds.), *Structure and functions of the human prefrontal cortex* (pp. 173–181). New York: New York Academy of Sciences.

Gebauer, G. F., & Mackintosh, N. J. 2007. Psychometric intelligence dissociates implicit and explicit learning. *Journal of Experimental Psychology: Learning, Memory, & Cognition*, **33:** 34–54.

Glenberg, A. M. 1997. What memory is for. *Behavioral and Brain Sciences*, **20:** 1–55.

Goldstone, R. L., & Barsalou, L. W. 1998. Reuniting perception and conception. *Cognition*, **65:** 231–262.

Gomez, R. L., & Gerken, L. 1999. Artificial grammar learning by 1-year-olds leads to specific and abstract knowledge. *Cognition*, **70:** 109–135.

Goschke, T. 1998. Implicit learning of perceptual and motor sequences: evidence for independent learning systems. In M. A. Stadler & P. A. Frensch (Eds.), *Handbook of implicit learning* (pp. 410–444). London: Sage Publications.

Goschke, T., Friederici, A. D., Kotz, S. A., & van Kampen, A. 2001. Procedural learning in Broca's aphasia: dissociation between the implicit acquisition of spatio-motor and phoneme sequences. *Journal of Cognitive Neuroscience*, **13:** 370–388.

Gottselig, J. M., Brandeis, D., Hofer-Tinguely, G., Borbély, A. A., & Achermann, P. 2006. Human central auditory plasticity associated with tone sequence learning. *Learning & Memory*, **11:** 162–171.

Grafton, S. T., Hazeltine, E., & Ivry, R. 1995. Functional mapping of sequence learning in normal humans. *Journal of Cognitive Neuroscience*, **7:** 497–510.

Greenfield, P. M. 1991. Language, tools and brain: the ontogeny and phylogeny of hierarchically organized sequential behavior. *Behavioral and Brain Sciences*, **14:** 531–595.

Handel, S., & Buffardi, L. 1969. Using several modalities to perceive one temporal pattern. *Quarterly Journal of Experimental Psychology*, **21:** 256–266.

Harris, J. A., Petersen, R. S., & Diamond, M. E. 2001. The cortical distribution of sensory memories. *Neuron*, **30:** 315–318.

Heindel, W. C., Butters, N., & Salmon, D. P. 1988. Impaired learning of a motor skill in patients with Huntington's disease. *Behavioral Neuroscience*, **102:** 141–147.

Hikosaka, O., Nakahara, H., Rand, M. K., Sakai, K., Lu, X., Nakamura, K., *et al*. 1999. Parallel neural networks for learning sequential procedures. *Trends in Neurosciences*, **22:** 464–471.

Howard, J. H., Jr., Howard, D. V., Japikse, K. C., & Eden, G. F. 2006. Dyslexics are impaired on implicit higher-order sequence learning, but not on implicit spatial context learning. *Neuropsychologia*, **44:** 1131–1144.

Huettel, S. A., Mack, P. B., & McCarthy, G. 2002. Perceiving patterns in random series: dynamic processing of sequence in prefrontal cortex. *Nature Neuroscience*, **5:** 485–490.

James, T. W., & Gauthier, I. 2003. Auditory and action semantic features activate sensory-specific perceptual brain regions. *Current Biology*, **13:** 1792–1796.

Jobard, G., Vigneau, M., Mazoyer, B., & Tzourio-Mazoyer, N. 2007. Impact of modality and linguistic complexity during reading and listening tasks. *NeuroImage*, **34:** 784–800.

Kalikow, D. N., Stevens, K. N., & Elliott, L. L. 1977. Development of a test of speech intelligibility in noise using sentence materials with controlled word predictability. *Journal of the Acoustical Society of America*, **61:** 1337–1351.

Karpicke, J. D., & Pisoni, D. B. 2004. Using immediate memory span to measure implicit learning. *Memory & Cognition*, **32:** 956–964.

Keele, S. W., Ivry, R., Mayr, U., Hazeltine, E., & Heuer, H. 2003. The cognitive and neural architecture of sequence representation. *Psychological Review*, **110:** 316–339.

Kelly, S. W., Griffiths, S., & Frith, U. 2002. Evidence for implicit sequence learning in dyslexia. *Dyslexia*, **8:** 43–52.

Kilgard, M. P., & Merzenich, M. M. 2002. Order-sensitive plasticity in adult primary auditory cortex. *Proceedings of the National Academy of Sciences*, **99:** 3205–3209.

Kinder, A., Shanks, D. R., Cock, J., & Tunney, R. J. 2003. Recollection, fluency, and the explicit/implicit distinction in artificial grammar learning. *Journal of Experimental Psychology: General*, **132:** 551–565.

Lieberman, M. D., Chang, G. Y., Chiao, J., Bookheimer, S. Y., & Knowlton, B. J. 2004. An event-related fMRI study of artificial grammar learning in a balanced chunk strength design. *Journal of Cognitive Neuroscience*, **16:** 427–438.

Lieberman, P. 2002. On the nature and evolution of the neural bases of human language. *Yearbook of Physical Anthropology*, **45:** 36–62.

Menghini, D., Hagberg, G. E., Caltagirone, C., Petrosini, L., & Vicari, S. 2006. Implicit learning deficits in dyslexic adults: An fMRI study. *NeuroImage*, **33:** 1218–1226.

Messinger, A., Squire, L. R., Zola, S. M., & Albright, T. D. 2001. Neuronal representations of stimulus associations develop in the temporal lobe during learning. *Proceedings of the National Academy of Sciences of the United States of America*, **98:** 12239–12244.

Middleton, F. A., & Strick, P. L. 2000. Basal ganglia output and cognition: evidence from anatomical, behavioral, and clinical studies. *Brain and Cognition*, **42:** 183–200.

Miller, E. K., & Cohen, J. D. 2001. An integrative theory of prefrontal cortex function. *Annual Review of Neuroscience*, **24:** 167–202.

Miller, G. A. 1958. Free recall of redundant strings of letters. *Journal of Experimental Psychology*, **56:** 485–491.

Miller, G. A., & Selfridge, J. A. 1950. Verbal context and the recall of meaningful material. *American Journal of Psychology*, **63:** 176–185.

Molinari, M., Filippini, V., & Leggio, M. G. 2002. Neuronal plasticity of interrelated cerebellar and cortical networks. *Neuroscience*, **111:** 863–870.

Nissen, M. J., & Bullemer, P. 1987. Attentional requirements of learning: evidence from performance measures. *Cognitive Psychology*, **19:** 1–32.

Nolte, J. N., & Angevine, J. B. 1995. *The human brain in photographs and diagrams*. New York: Mosby.

Obleser, J., Wise, R. J. S., Dresner, M. A., & Scott, S. K. 2007. Functional integration across brain regions improves speech perception under adverse listening conditions. *The Journal of Neuroscience*, **27:** 2283–2289.

Ohl, F. W., Scheich, H., & Freeman, W. J. 2001. Change in pattern of ongoing cortical activity with auditory category learning. *Nature*, **412:** 733–736.

Opitz, B., & Friederici, A. D. 2004. Brain correlates of language learning: The neuronal dissociation of rule-based versus similarity-based learning. *The Journal of Neuroscience*, **24:** 8436–8440.

Paquier, P. F., & Mariën, P. 2005. A synthesis of the role of the cerebellum in cognition. *Aphasiology*, **19:** 3–19.

Pascal-Leone, A., Grafman, J., & Hallett, M. 1995. Procedural learning and prefrontal cortex. In J. Grafman, K. J. Holyoak, & F. Bollers (Eds.), *Structure and functions of the human prefrontal cortex* (pp. 61–70). New York: New York Academy of Sciences.

Pasupathy, A., & Miller, E. K. 2005. Different time courses of learning-related activity in the prefrontal cortex and striatum. *Nature*, **433:** 873–876.

Peigneux, P., Maquet, P., Meulemans, T., Destrebecqz, A., Laureys, S., Degueldre, C., *et al*. 2000. Striatum forever, despite sequence learning variability: a random effect analysis of PET data. *Human Brain Mapping*, **10:** 179–194.

Perruchet, P., & Pacton, S. 2006. Implicit learning and statistical learning: two approaches, one phenomenon. *Trends in Cognitive Sciences*, **10:** 233–238.

Petersson, K. M., Forkstam, C., & Ingvar, M. 2004. Artificial syntactic violations activate Broca's region. *Cognitive Science*, **28:** 383–407.

Pisoni, D. B., & Cleary, M. 2004. Learning, memory, and cognitive processes in deaf children following cochlear implantation. In F.-G. Zeng, A. N. Popper, & R. R. Fay (Eds.), *Springer handbook of auditory research Vol. 20. Cochlear implants: Auditory protheses and electric hearing* (pp. 377–426). New York: Springer-Verlag.

Port, R. F., & Van Gelder, T. 1995. *Mind as motion: Explorations in the dynamics of cognition.* Cambridge, MA: MIT Press.

Pothos, E. M., & Bailey, T. M. 2000. The role of similarity in artificial grammar learning. *Journal of Experimental Psychology: Learning, Memory, & Cognition*, **26:** 847–862.

Pulvermüller, F. 2001. Brain reflections of words and their meaning. *Trends in Cognitive Sciences*, **5:** 517–524.

Rauch, S. L., Savage, C. R., Brown, H. D., Curran, T., Alpert, N. M., Kendrick, A., *et al*. 1995. A PET investigation of implicit and explicit sequence learning. *Human Brain Mapping*, **3:** 271–286.

Rauch, S. L., Whalen, P. J., Savage, C. R., Curran, T., Kendrick, A., Brown, H. D., *et al*. 1997. Striatal recruitment during an implicit sequence learning task as measured by functional magnetic resonance imaging. *Human Brain Mapping*, **5:** 124–132.

Reber, A. S. 1967. Implicit learning of artificial grammars. *Journal of Verbal Learning and Verbal Behavior*, **6:** 855–863.

Reber, A. S. 1969. Transfer of syntactic structure in synthetic languages. *Journal of Experimental Psychology*, **81:** 115–119.

Reber, A. S. 1993. *Implicit learning and tacit knowledge: An essay on the cognitive unconscious.* Oxford, England: Oxford University Press.

Reber, P. J., Stark, C. E. L., & Squire, L. R. 1998. Cortical areas supporting category learning identified using functional MRI. *Proceedings of the National Academy of Sciences of the United States of America*, **95:** 747–750.

Redington, M., & Chater, N. 2002. Knowledge representation and transfer in artificial grammar learning (AGL). In R. M. French & A. Cleeremans (Eds.), *Implicit learning and consciousness: An empirical, philosophical, and computational consensus in the making* (pp. 121–143). Hove, East Sussex: Psychology Press.

Redington, M., & Chater, N. 1996. Transfer in artificial grammar learning: a reevaluation. *Journal of Experimental Psychology: General*, **125:** 123–138.

Rhodes, B. J., Bullock, D., Verwey, W. B., Averbeck, B. B., & Page, M. P. A. 2004. Learning and production of movement sequences: behavioral, neurophysiological, and modeling perspectives. *Human Movement Science*, **23:** 699–746.

Rubenstein, H. 1973. Language and probability. In G. A. Miller (Ed.), *Communication, language, and meaning: Psychological perspectives* (pp. 185–195). New York: Basic Books, Inc.

Rüsseler, J., Gerth, I., & Münte, T. F. 2006. Implicit learning is intact in developmental dyslexic readers: Evidence from the serial reaction time task and artificial grammar learning. *Journal of Clinical and Experimental Neuropsychology*, **28:** 808–827.

Saffran, J. R., Aslin, R. N., & Newport, E. L. 1996. Statistical learning by 8-month-old infants. *Science*, **274:** 1926–1928.

Saffran, J. R., Johnson, E. K., Aslin, R. N., & Newport, E. L. 1999. Statistical learning of tone sequences by human infants and adults. *Cognition*, **70:** 27–52.

Schacter, D. L., Dobbins, I. G., & Schnyer, D. M. 2004. Specificity of priming: a cognitive neuroscience perspective. *Nature Reviews Neuroscience*, **5:** 853–862.

Seger, C. A. 2006. The basal ganglia in human learning. *The Neuroscientist*, **12:** 285–290.

Seger, C. A. 1998. Multiple forms of implicit learning. In M. A. Stadler & P. A. Frensch (Eds.), *Handbook of implicit learning* (pp. 295–320). London: Sage Publications.

Seger, C. A., Prabhakaran, V., Poldrack, R. A., & Gabrieli, J. D. E. 2000. Neural activity differs between explicit and implicit learning of artificial grammar strings: an fMRI study. *Psychobiology*, **28:** 283–292.

Siegert, R. J., Taylor, K. D., Weatherall, M., & Abernethy, D. A. 2006. Is implicit sequence learning impaired in Parkinson's disease? A meta-analysis. *Neuropsychology*, **20:** 490–495.

Skosnik, P. D., Mirza, F., Gitelman, D. R., Parrish, T. B., Mesulam, M-M., & Reber, P. J. 2002. Neural correlates of artificial grammar learning. *NeuroImage*, **17:** 1306–1314.

Tettamanti, M., Alkadhi, H., Moro, A., Perani, D., Kollias, S., Weniger, D. 2002. Neural correlates for the acquisition of natural language syntax. *NeuroImage*, **17:** 700–709.

Tunney, R. J., & Altmann, G. T. M. 2001. Two modes of transfer in artificial grammar learning. *Journal of Experimental Psychology: Learning, Memory, & Cognition*, **27:** 614–639.

Ullman, M. T. 2004. Contributions of memory circuits to language: the declarative/procedural model. *Cognition*, **92:** 231–270.

Vicari, S., Marotta, L., Menghini, D., Molinari, M., & Petrosini, L. 2003. Implicit learning deficit in children with developmental dyslexia. *Neuropsychologia*, **41:** 108–114.

Waber, D. P., Marcus, D. J., Forbes, P. W., Bellinger, D. C., Weiler, M. D., Sorensen, L. G., *et al*. 2003.

Motor sequence learning and reading ability: Is poor reading associated with sequencing deficits? *Journal of Experimental Child Psychology*, **84:** 338–354.

Witt, K., Nühsman, A., & Deuschl, G. 2002. Intact artificial grammar learning in patients with cerebellar degeneration and advanced Parkinson's disease. *Neuropsychologia*, **40:** 1534–1540.

Implicit Learning and Dyslexia

Vasiliki Folia,[a,b,c] Julia Uddén,[a,b,c] Christian Forkstam,[a,b,c] Martin Ingvar,[b,d] Peter Hagoort,[a,c] and Karl Magnus Petersson[a,b,c,d]

[a]Max Planck Institute for Psycholinguistics, Nijmegen, the Netherlands

[b]Cognitive Neurophysiology Research Group, Stockholm Brain Institute, Karolinska Institute, Stockholm, Sweden

[c]F. C. Donders Centre for Cognitive Neuroimaging, Radboud University, Nijmegen, the Netherlands

[d]Cognitive Neuroscience Research Group, Universidade do Algarve, Faro, Portugal

Several studies have reported an association between dyslexia and implicit learning deficits. It has been suggested that the weakness in implicit learning observed in dyslexic individuals may be related to sequential processing and implicit sequence learning. In the present article, we review the current literature on implicit learning and dyslexia. We describe a novel, forced-choice structural "mere exposure" artificial grammar learning paradigm and characterize this paradigm in normal readers in relation to the standard grammaticality classification paradigm. We argue that preference classification is a more optimal measure of the outcome of implicit acquisition since in the preference version participants are kept completely unaware of the underlying generative mechanism, while in the grammaticality version, the subjects have, at least in principle, been informed about the existence of an underlying complex set of rules at the point of classification (but not during acquisition). On the basis of the "mere exposure effect," we tested the prediction that the development of preference will correlate with the grammaticality status of the classification items. In addition, we examined the effects of grammaticality (grammatical/nongrammatical) and associative chunk strength (ACS; high/low) on the classification tasks (preference/grammaticality). Using a balanced ACS design in which the factors of grammaticality (grammatical/nongrammatical) and ACS (high/low) were independently controlled in a 2 × 2 factorial design, we confirmed our predictions. We discuss the suitability of this task for further investigation of the implicit learning characteristics in dyslexia.

Key words: artificial grammar learning; structural mere-exposure effect; dyslexia; inferior frontal cortex; basal ganglia

Introduction

During the acquisition of reading and writing skills, children develop the ability to represent aspects of the phonological component of language by an orthographic representation and relate this to a visuographic input-output code. This is typically achieved by means of a supervised learning process (i.e., teaching), in contrast to natural language acquisition, which is largely a spontaneous, non-supervised, and self-organized acquisition process (Petersson, 2005a; Petersson, Ingvar, & Reis, 2009). Aspects of language can also be an object of metalinguistic awareness: the intentional and explicit control over aspects of phonology, syntax, semantics,

Address for correspondence: Karl Magnus Petersson, Max Planck Institute for Psycholinguistics, P.O. Box 310, 6500 AH Nijmegen, the Netherlands. Voice: +0031-2436-10984; fax: +0031-2436-10652. karl.magnus.petersson@fcdonders.ru.nl and discourse, as well as pragmatics. Children gradually create explicit representations and acquire processing mechanisms that allow for reflecting and analyzing different aspects of language use (Karmiloff-Smith, Grant, Sims, Jones, & Cuckle, 1996). When children subsequently learn to read, this has repercussions on the phonological representations of spoken language (Morais, 1993; Petersson, Reis, Askelöf, Castro-Caldas, & Ingvar, 2000; Petersson, Reis, & Ingvar, 2001; Ziegler & Goswami, 2005; see Goswami, this volume). Learning to read involves both explicit as well as implicit processes; typically children initially learn grapheme–phoneme mappings explicitly, after which they apply and continue to learn how phonology is mapped onto its written representation implicitly (Gombert, 2003; Petersson & Reis, 2006; Ziegler & Goswami, 2005). Karmiloff-Smith (1992) proposed that cognitive development relies on implicit/procedural learning mechanisms to initiate the setup of a new stage of representational development. A deficit in implicit acquisition mechanisms might therefore have a negative impact on the acquisition of reading and writing skills and therefore affect literacy acquisition. Dyslexia is rarely studied within the framework of learning, and a deficit in implicit learning might contribute to difficulties associated with dyslexia (Howard, Howard, Japikse, & Eden, 2006; see also Bennet *et al.*, this volume; Menghini *et al.*, this volume; Stoodley *et al.*, this volume). Recently, Howard *et al.* (2006) provided evidence suggesting that the weakness in implicit learning observed in dyslexic individuals might be narrowed down to paradigms that involve sequential processing and they argued that the implicit sequence learning deficit in dyslexia is associated with selective deficits in the fronto-striatal-cerebellar circuits that underlie implicit sequence learning. It has been shown that fronto-striatal circuits are involved in sequence processing after implicit grammar acquisition (Forkstam, Hagoort, Fernandez, Ingvar, & Petersson, 2006; Petersson, Forkstam, & Ingvar, 2004).

Implicit Learning

Humans are equipped with acquisition mechanisms that extract structural regularities implicitly from experience without the induction of an explicit model (Reber, 1967, 1993; Stadler & Frensch, 1998). This capacity was explored in the seminal work of Reber (1967), showing that humans can successfully classify strings generated from an implicitly acquired artificial grammar and proposed that this process is intrinsic to natural language acquisition. Following this suggestion, it has been argued that artificial grammar learning (AGL) is a relevant model for investigating aspects of language learning in infants (Gomez & Gerken, 2000), exploring differences between human and animal learning relevant to the narrow faculty of language (Hauser, Chomsky, & Fitch, 2002), and language learning in adults (Friederici, Steinhauer, & Pfeifer, 2002; Petersson *et al.*, 2004). We suggest that it can serve as a device for investigating the implicit aspects of structure learning related to reading and writing acquisition as well. Reber (1967) suggested that humans can acquire implicit knowledge of the underlying structure of grammar through a statistical learning process and that the acquired knowledge is put to use during grammaticality classification. Reber (1967; but see Reber, 1993) argued that implicit learning mechanisms abstracted "rule-based" knowledge, and more recent studies seem to suggest that dual mechanisms might be engaged (Forkstam *et al.*, 2006; Knowlton & Squire, 1996; Meulemans & Van der Linden, 1997). Following Reber (1967) and Seger (1994), Forkstam & Petersson (2005) adapted four proposed defining characteristics of implicit learning: *(a)* explicit access is limited to the knowledge acquired—subjects typically cannot provide a sufficient explicit account of what they have learned; *(b)* the nature of the knowledge acquired is more complex than simple associations or simple exemplar-specific frequency counts; *(c)* implicit learning does not involve explicit hypothesis testing, but is an automatic (incidental) consequence of the type and amount of processing performed on the stimuli; and *(d)* implicit learning does not rely on declarative memory mechanisms that engage the medial temporal lobe memory system.

Dyslexia: An Implicit Learning Deficit?

Developmental dyslexia is commonly defined as a reading disability, a deficit in learning to spell and write, occurring in children despite normal intelligence, no sensory or neurological impairment, and conventional instruction and socioeconomic opportunity (Dilling, Mombour, & Schmidt, 1991; Habib, 2000; Shaywitz, 1998). However, dyslexia is rarely studied in the framework of the contemporary learning literature (Howard *et al.*, 2006). Learning to read involves both explicit as well as implicit processes; children initially learn the grapheme–phoneme correspondence explicitly, typically in a supervised manner, after which they apply and continue to learn them implicitly in an unsupervised manner (Gombert, 2003). A deficit in implicit learning might contribute to difficulties associated with dyslexia, but the literature on implicit learning and dyslexia has yielded mixed results (Howard *et al.*, 2006). Most studies of implicit learning in dyslexics have investigated serial reaction time (SRT) types of tasks and there are, to our knowledge, only two studies that investigate artificial grammar learning (AGL). For a recent review of these experimental task, see Forkstam and Petersson (2005).

An important weakness of all studies of implicit learning in dyslexics to date is that they lack a developmental design (Goswami, 2003). Another weakness of some of the studies is that they report null findings. These null findings are difficult to interpret in the context of small study samples and experimental designs that are not always carefully controlled. Therefore, it is likely that the absence of significant results reflects a lack of statistical power as well as the presence of confounding factors. On the other hand, the conflicting literature on im-

plicit learning and dyslexia might suggest that it is not enough to investigate simple implicit acquisition tasks or just to contrast implicit and explicit learning. In this brief but comprehensive review, we will give priority to those studies which find an implicit learning deficit in dyslexics, but we will also comment on those which report null findings, beginning with those studies that have investigated SRT-type tests and subsequently turning our attention to the AGL studies.

Vicari *et al.* (2003) reported deficient implicit learning in dyslexic children on visuomotor SRT-type tasks that used sequences of colors. They also included a test of declarative (explicit) memory capacities. Their main finding suggests that individuals with developmental dyslexia are impaired in the acquisition of implicit sequence knowledge, while there was no significant difference between the dyslexic and control groups in terms of explicit sequence learning. Some studies have reported null-findings on similar SRT-type tasks (Kelly, Griffiths, & Frith, 2002; Waber *et al.*, 2003), and Rüsseler *et al.* (2006) questioned the implicit learning deficit in dyslexia based on these and their own null findings. However, Waber *et al.* (2003) investigated a sample of children with "heterogeneous learning problems," which makes their findings difficult to interpret in the context of dyslexia, and although there was no significant learning difference between the dyslexic and normal readers in Rüsseler *et al.* (2006), the dyslexic subjects showed consistently longer response times (RTs) on the SRT task compared to the normal controls. This was also the case in Kelly *et al.* (2002). Of inportance, in a follow-up study, Vicari *et al.* (2005) used the classical SRT task as well as an implicit mirror drawing test, and showed that the children with developmental dyslexia were impaired on both tasks. Their SRT results suggest a deficit in sequential learning and that the deficit does not depend on the material being learned (with or without motor sequence of response action), but only on the implicit character of the task. These behavioral findings were further replicated in an fMRI study of adult dyslexics (Menghini, Hagberg, Caltagirone, Petrosini, & Vicari, 2006). Consistent with this perspective, both Stoodley *et al.* (2006) and Howard *et al.* (2006) provided further evidence that the implicit learning deficits observed in dyslexic individuals can be narrowed down to paradigms that involve sequential processing. Stoodley *et al.* (2006) found significant differences in implicit learning between good and poor readers on the SRT task. In addition, the dyslexic group showed less of an RT decrease on the repeated sequence, while the RTs were similar to that of the control group on the random trials. Recently, Sperling *et al.* (2004) argued that poor implicit learning could hinder the establishment of good phonological processing as well as learning orthographic–phonological representations, whereas Gombert (2003) proposed that children with dyslexia have a phonological deficit that prevents normal implicit learning of linguistic regularities and hence interferes with reading development. Howard *et al.* (2006) showed that adult dyslexics are impaired on implicit acquisition in an alternating (higher-order) SRT task in which sequential dependences exist across nonadjacent elements. They compared the performance on the alternating SRT task with the performance on a simple spatial context learning task in which the global configuration of a display cues the location of a search target. Their results suggest that college students with a history of dyslexia are impaired in implicit higher-order sequence learning, but unimpaired in spatial context learning. They also argue that evidence from functional neuroimaging, and transcranial magnetic stimulation investigations in patients suggest that sequence learning depends on fronto-striatal-cerebellar circuitry and that the acquisition of nonadjacent, higher-order, sequential regularities calls on fronto-striatal-cerebellar circuitry, whereas spatial contextual learning depends on medial temporal lobe structures (Chun & Phelps, 1999; Howard *et al.*, 2006; Packard & Knowlton, 2002a). The fMRI results of Menghini *et al.* (2006) suggest that an implicit learning deficit in dyslexia is associated with a level of activation in higher cerebellar and parietal regions (see also the morphometric results reported by Menghini *et al.* in this volume). These investigators speculate that automatization is required to achieve reading fluency and that the cerebellum might be important for the development of automaticity. However, it is important to note that the development of automaticity does not necessarily overlap with implicit learning. Automaticity can also arise from repetitive application of explicit, conscious procedures, over and over again, until adequate performance is achieved (Cohen, Dunbar, & McClelland, 1990; Cohen, Servan-Schreiber, & McClelland, 1992; Logan, 1988; MacLeod & Dunbar, 1988; Petersson, Elfgren, & Ingvar, 1997, 1999; Petersson, Sandblom, Gisselgård, & Ingvar, 2001). Howard *et al.* (2006) also reported significant positive correlations between measures of reading ability and accuracy-based implicit acquisition measures. Notably, they were able to rule out several nonspecific explanations for their results, including a general cognitive or attention deficit, task difficulty, or age, and established that deficits in implicit sequence learning occur even when explicit learning can be ruled out. They emphasize that dyslexics do not suffer from a general implicit learning deficit, but that this deficit is specific to sequential processing, highlighting the importance of sequence complexity (i.e., the level of structure present in the sequences), consistent with the findings of Vicari *et al.* (2003, 2005).

Much less is known about the implicit acquisition of artificial grammars in dyslexics. To date, only two studies on dyslexia have been conducted using this paradigm. Rüsseler *et al.* (2006) used a short acquisition session and reported null findings only in terms of correct responses on the grammaticality classification task; no baseline classification was included in the experiment, and they did not control for local substring regularities (i.e., ACS-type information, cf. below). Although there was no significant difference between the dyslexic and normal readers, the dyslexic subjects performed at a lower level (mean number of correct responses) on the classification task. In an interesting study by Pothos and Kirk (2004), the artificial grammar of Knowlton and Squire (1996) was used in two AGL tasks of equal formal complexity, but with different stimulus format in a between-subject design: in one of the tasks (the geometric-shapes-embedded AGL task), the stimuli were created so as to encourage whole stimulus perception, deemphasizing the constituent elements, while in the other task (geometric-shapes-sequential AGL task) the constituent elements were emphasized by presenting them serially. Pothos and Kirk (2004) controlled for local substring regularities (i.e., ACS), but did not manipulate this dimension experimentally. The dyslexic group performed equally well on the "grammaticality" classification in both tasks, and the nondyslexic group performed as well as the dyslexic group on the visual-embedded, but less well on the visual-sequential task. These findings were interpreted as indicating that the dyslexic participants were less able to process the individual stimulus elements, suggesting that dyslexic individuals are sometimes prevented from adopting an explicit strategy, which would have interfered with the implicit acquisition mechanisms supporting geometric-sequential AGL. This is consistent with recent work associating dyslexia with problems in focused attention and attention shifting. Thus, Pothos and Kirk (2004) proposed that competent real-world learning is achieved via an interaction of implicit and explicit learning processes.

In summary, there is a cumulating series of investigations of implicit learning in dyslexia, and taken as a whole, these studies suggest that there are aspects of implicit learning that might operate at subnormal levels in dyslexic individuals. The lack of a developmental design in these studies (Goswami, 2003) prevents us from making any conclusions concerning the causal role of an implicit acquisition deficit in dyslexia. It might be an outcome of dyslexia rather than

a cause, similar in character to the many parallel findings between the dyslexic and illiterate brain (Petersson *et al.*, 2009; Petersson & Reis, 2006; Petersson, Reis, *et al.*, 2001). A few tentative conclusions are warranted, however: *(a)* dyslexia does not seem to be associated with a general implicit learning deficit; *(b)* the implicit learning deficit observed does not seem to be related to nonspecific factors such as general cognitive or attention deficit, task difficulty, or age; *(c)* the implicit acquisition deficit seems to be related to sequence processing, which is likely related to sequence complexity (i.e., the level of structure present in the sequences; for a short review see Petersson, 2005b) and for a comprehensive review see Davis *et al.*, 1994); and *(d)* the implicit learning deficit in dyslexia can be observed when explicit learning is intact.

Implicit Artificial Grammar Acquisition

The artificial grammar used by Reber (1967), here and subsequently referred to as the Reber grammar, is an example of a right-linear phrase structure grammar which generates a rational language (Perrin & Pin, 2004). This type of grammar represents the simplest formal model that captures the idea of the "infinite use of finite means" (Petersson, 2005b; Petersson, Grenholm, & Forkstam, 2005). The Reber grammar, like any right-linear phrase structure grammar, can be implemented in a finite-state architecture (see Fig. 1; from Petersson, 2005). We used this grammar in the present study as a generator of the stimulus material. The finite-state machine can be viewed as an explicit generating mechanism and as a recognition device for a formal language (e.g., Davis *et al.*, 1994). In general, a formal (artificial) grammar serves as an intentional definition (Chomsky, 1986) of a language, and represents a formal specification of the mechanism that generates structural regularities in the output. Here, it should be noted that the term *language* in formal language is technical and does not entail anything beyond what is outlined above and that a formal (or

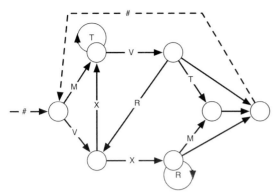

Figure 1. The transition graph representation of the Reber grammar, which was used to generate the grammatical strings in the present study (Petersson, 2005).

artificial) grammar represents a specification of a mechanism that generates (or recognizes) certain types of sequential structural regularities (Petersson *et al.*, 2004). It is also important to note that the finite-state architecture is not limited to capturing local substring dependencies, but that this architecture can also incorporate long-distance dependencies (as long as there is a fixed finite upper bound for these dependencies; cf. Petersson, 2005b; Petersson *et al.*, 2005).

The typical artificial grammar learning (AGL) experiment includes an acquisition phase followed by a grammaticality classification. During the acquisition phase, participants are engaged in a short-term memory task using an acquisition sample of symbol sequences generated from an artificial grammar. Subsequent to the acquisition phase, subjects are informed that the symbol sequences were generated according to a complex system of rules and they are asked to classify new items as grammatical or not based on their immediate impression (guessing based on "gut feeling"). The subjects typically perform reliably above chance (Forkstam *et al.*, 2006; Petersson *et al.*, 2004), and it can be concluded that participants have acquired knowledge about aspects of the underlying generative structure. It is assumed that the classification performance is based on implicit acquisition mechanisms because subjects

are typically unable to provide sufficient reasons to motivate their classification decisions (Forkstam *et al.*, 2006; Forkstam & Petersson, 2005; Stadler & Frensch, 1998). An alternative way of assessing the implicit acquisition of an artificial grammar is the structural mere-exposure version of AGL. This version is based on the "mere exposure" effect, which refers to the finding that repeated exposure to a stimulus induces an increased preference for that stimulus compared to novel stimuli (Zajonc, 1968). The mere-exposure version might be a more sensitive measure of implicitly acquired knowledge because the participants are never made aware of the existence of an underlying generative mechanism.

Goals of the Current Study

In the present study we characterize a new forced-choice structural mere-exposure AGL paradigm in normal readers based on preference classification. We compare this preference classification paradigm with the standard grammaticality classification paradigm. We predict, on the basis of the mere-exposure effect (Zajonc, 1968), that the development of preference will start to correlate with grammaticality. In order to achieve these objectives, we used a balanced associative chunk strength (ACS) design (Forkstam *et al.*, 2006; Meulemans & Van der Linden, 1997). In the balanced ACS design, the factors grammaticality status (grammatical/nongrammatical) and ACS (high/low) are independently controlled in a 2×2 factorial design. It has been argued that sensitivity to the level of ACS is a reflection of a statistical fragment-based learning mechanism, whereas sensitivity to the grammaticality status of the items, independent of ACS, is related to an implicit structure-based acquisition mechanism. Moreover, it is not implausible that learning based on ACS reflects an explicit declarative memory mechanism involving the medial temporal lobe (Forkstam *et al.*, 2006; Lieberman, Chang, Chiao, Bookheimer, & Knowlton, 2004), while implicit learning of grammaticality status independent of ACS reflects a procedural learning mechanism involving the basal ganglia and the prefrontal cortex (Forkstam *et al.*, 2006). In this study, the subjects participated in one implicit acquisition session per day for 5 days; symbol strings were presented visually one letter at a time, which requires temporal integration of information. Before the first acquisition session on the first day, subjects participated in a baseline preference classification task. Finally, after the last acquisition session on the 5th day, subjects performed a preference classification and then the standard grammaticality classification task.

In summary, the objectives of the present study were to investigate the behavioral equivalence of the forced-choice preference classification to the standard grammaticality classification task and to explore the effects of the factors *(a)* grammaticality status (grammatical/nongrammatical) and *(b)* ACS (high/low) on the classification task (preference/grammaticality). In the Discussion section, we argue that these AGL paradigms are suitable for further investigation of the implicit learning characteristics in dyslexia.

Methods

Participants

Thirty-two right-handed (16 females and 16 males; mean age $\pm$ SD = 22 $\pm$ 3 years; mean years of education $\pm$ SD = 16 $\pm$ 2), healthy Dutch university students volunteered to participate in the study (part of a larger fMRI project; data not shown). They were all prescreened, and none of the subjects used any medication, had a history of drug abuse, head trauma, neurological or psychiatric illness, or a family history of neurological or psychiatric illness. All subjects had normal or corrected-to-normal vision. Written informed consent was obtained from all participants according to the protocol of the Declaration of Helsinki, and the local medical ethics committee approved the study.

Stimulus Material

We generated 569 grammatical (G) strings from the Reber grammar (5–12 consonants from the alphabet [M, S, V, R, X]; see Fig. 1). For each item we calculated frequency distribution of 2- and 3-letter chunks for both terminal and complete string positions in order to derive the associative chunk strength (ACS) for each item (cf. Knowlton & Squire, 1996; Meulemans & Van der Linden, 1997). Then, iteratively, we randomly selected 100 strings, generating an acquisition set that was comparable in terms of 2- and 3-letter chunks to the complete string set. Subsequently we generated the nongrammatical string, derived from each remaining grammatical string by a switch of letters in two nonterminal positions, and these were selected to match the grammatical strings in terms of both terminal and complete string ACS (i.e., collapsed over order information within strings). Finally, in an iterative procedure, we randomly selected three sets of 60 strings each from the remaining grammatical strings, in order to generate the three classification sets consisting of 50% grammatical and nongrammatical strings, as well as 50% high and low ACS strings relative to ACS information in the acquisition set and independent of grammaticality status. Thus the stimulus material included an acquisition set and two classification sets (all sets were disjoint). The classification sets were used for the 2 × 2 factorial design of the classification task. Thus each classification set consisted of 30 strings of each string type: high ACS grammatical (HG), low ACS grammatical (LG), high ACS nongrammatical (HNG), and low ACS nongrammatical (LNG).

Experimental Procedures

The subjects were informed on the first day that they were to participate in a short-term memory experiment. The complete experiment was conducted over 5 days with an acquisition session each day. An initial preference classification test (PC) was performed before the first acquisition session on the first day (AGL1). A second preference test was performed after the last session on the 5th day (AGL2). After the AGL2, the grammaticality instruction was introduced (AGL3). During both acquisition and classification sessions, each string was centrally presented letter-by-letter on a computer screen (2.7–6.9 s corresponding to 5–12 letters; 300 ms letter-presentation duration, 300 ms inter-letter interval) using the Presentation software (http://nbs.neuro-bs.com).

Implicit Acquisition Task

During each acquisition session, all subjects were presented with the 100 acquisition strings (acquisition set) on a computer screen (presentation order randomized for each acquisition session). When the last letter in a string disappeared, the subject was instructed to immediately reconstruct the string from memory by typing on a keyboard in a self-paced fashion. No performance feedback was given and only positive examples (i.e., grammatical strings) were presented during acquisition. The acquisition phase lasted approximately 20–40 min.

Classification Tasks

The classification task consisted of a yes/no forced-choice procedure, and the subjects were instructed to make their choice based on their immediate impression ("gut feeling"). On the first day, the subjects were given the preference classification instruction (AGL1); they were instructed to classify novel strings as preferable or not (likeable/pleasant or not) and told that there was no right or wrong response. The subjects were given the same preference instruction on the last day (AGL2). After the AGL2, participants were informed about the grammatical nature of the grammar and were instructed to classify new strings as grammatical or not (AGL3). During classification on days 1 and 5, the participants were presented with novel letter strings from the classification set in the same way as during acquisition. During a classification session 30 strings were presented one at a time on a computer screen. After a 1-s prestimulus period, the strings were presented for 3 s, followed by a 1-s motor preparation delay period. The subject then had 2.5 s to make his or her classification decision and push the corresponding key with the left or right index finger, based on the preference. The classification sets and string presentation order were balanced over subjects. Each classification session was split in two in order to balance response finger within subject, each lasting approximately 20 min. The stimuli were presented via an LCD projector, projecting the computer display onto a semitransparent screen that the subject comfortably viewed through a mirror device. At the end of the experimental procedure on day 5, participants were presented with a generation task and then a 31-item fragment-completion task. In the generation task, participants were instructed to generate 10 letter strings that they regarded as grammatical; in the fragment-completion task they were instructed to complete each item with the letter they thought would render the string grammatical.

Data Analysis

Repeated-measures ANOVAs were used for the analysis of the data, unless otherwise stated (statistical software package SPSS). A significance level of $P < 0.05$ was used. Scores were based on hit and endorsement rates. The hit rate is defined as the sum of all hits (accepted grammatical strings) and correct rejections (rejected nongrammatical strings). The endorsement rate is defined as the number of all strings classified as grammatical, independent of the actual grammaticality status (cf. Forkstam *et al.*, 2006; Meulemans & Van der Linden, 1997).

Results

On the baseline preference classification (AGL1; that is, before any exposure to the

TABLE 1. Endorsement Rates over Grammaticality and ACS levels[a]

	AGL1		AGL2		AGL3	
	High ACS	Low ACS	High ACS	Low ACS	High ACS	Low ACS
G	53 (15)%	45 (18)%	73 (16)%	62 (20)%	82 (20)%	71 (21)%
NG	51 (21)%	48 (13)%	41 (22)%	34 (17)%	32 (22)%	27 (21)%

[a]Percentage of items endorsed (i.e., item classified as grammatical independent of actual grammaticality status) by condition (grammatical/nongrammatical × high/low associative chunk strength (ACS) status; mean performance level and standard deviation). G = grammatical; NG = nongrammatical; ACS = associative chunk strength.

grammar) subjects classified at the expected chance level [50 ± 7% correct, $T(31) = 0.42$, $P = 0.67$]. Consistent with previous findings (Forkstam *et al.*, 2006; Petersson *et al.*, 2004) the overall correct classification performance was clearly above chance on preference [AGL2; 65 ± 14% correct, $T(31) = 5.7$, $P < 0.0001$] and grammaticality classification [AGL3; 73 ± 16% correct, $T(31) = 7.7$, $P < 0.0001$]. Thus, subjects classified items reliably above chance on both the preference classification (AGL2) and the grammaticality classification (AGL3) tasks. The classification performance improved after the grammaticality instruction was provided [$F(1, 31) = 8.8$, $P = 0.006$].

Classification Performance: Hit Rates

The analysis of hit rate (classification performance) showed that the subjects were sensitive to the grammaticality status of the items [$F(2, 62) = 26$, $P < 0.0001$]. In particular, the participants classified the grammatical strings correctly more often (AGL2 > AGL1), and the hit increased further on the AGL3 task compared to both AGL1 and AGL2. Specific contrast comparisons revealed that the group improved its classification performance for LG strings [$F(2, 62) = 15.6$, $P < 0.0001$] and LNG strings [$F(2, 62) = 17.8$, $P < 0.0001$] after the grammaticality instruction (AGL3) in comparison to both the AGL2 and AGL1 tasks, whereas the classification performance for HNG strings improved in comparison only to the AGL1 task [$F(2, 62) = 10.8$, $P < 0.0001$].

Classification Performance: Endorsement Rates

We then analyzed the performance data in terms of endorsement rate (i.e., item classified as grammatical independent of actual grammaticality status). Both grammaticality and ACS status influenced the endorsement rate (Table 1, Figs. 2 and 3). A repeated-measures ANOVA with task (AGL1/2/3), grammaticality (G/NG), and ACS (H/L) as within-factors showed significant main effects of grammaticality [$F(1, 31) = 47$, $P < 0.0001$] and ACS [$F(1, 31) = 18$, $P < 0.0001$], whereas the main effect of task type was nonsignificant [$F(2, 62) = 1.4$, $P = 0.25$]. In addition, there was a significant interaction between task and grammaticality [$F(2, 62) = 37$, $P < 0.0001$], while the interaction between task and ACS was nonsignificant [$F(2, 62) = 0.48$, $P = 0.57$]. This shows that grammaticality is the main contributor to the increased classification performance between the baseline and the two classification tasks after implicit acquisition of the grammar. These results suggest that subjects implicitly acquired knowledge about the underlying grammar after only 5 days of acquisition. Moreover, there was a significant interaction between grammaticality and ACS [$F(1, 31) = 8.9$, $P < 0.05$]. Post-hoc analysis revealed that this interaction was due to the overall difference in classification performance of AGL2/3 compared to the baseline performance (AGL1), as well as the comparison between AGL2 and AGL3. No other interactions reached significance ($P > 0.9$).

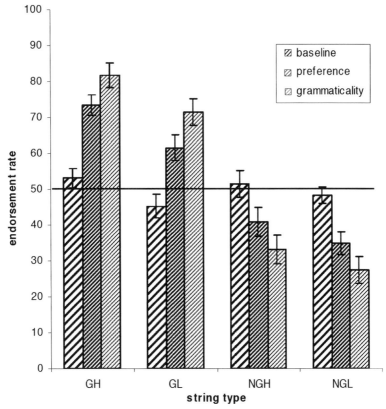

Figure 2. Endorsement rates over grammaticality and ACS levels. The endorsement rates (i.e., item classified as grammatical independent of actual grammaticality status) as a function of grammaticality status as well as associative chunk strength (GH: grammatical high ACS strings, GL: grammatical low ACS strings, NGH: nongrammatical high ACS strings, NGL: nongrammatical low ACS strings). The endorsement rate of grammatical versus nongrammatical items increases as a function of repeated acquisition for both high and low ACS strings. Error bars correspond to standard error of the mean.

Specifically, preference classification (AGL2) was significantly affected by grammaticality status [$F(1, 31) = 31.7, P < 0.0001$] and ACS status [$F(1, 31) = 15.4, P < 0.0001$]. These effects were also observed in grammaticality classification [AGL3; grammaticality status, $F(1, 31) = 61.6, P < 0.0001$; ACS status, $F(1, 31) = 13.6, P < 0.001$], while the interaction between grammaticality and ACS was not significant on either task [AGL2: $F(1, 31) = 3.8, P = 0.059$; AGL3: $F(1, 31) = 2.6, P = 0.11$].

We further investigated the effects of grammaticality, following Chang and Knowlton (2004), who argued that ACS might not be a useful cue for the low ACS items, but that correct performance on these items has to be based on knowledge of structural regularities rather than local substring familiarity. Similarly to Lieberman *et al.* (2004), we found no effects of grammaticality status for both high and low ACS strings on the baseline test [AGL1; HG vs. HNG: $F(1, 31) = 0.42, P = 0.52$; LG vs. LNG: $F(1, 31) = 0.65, P = 0.43$], while we observed significant effects for preference classification [AGL2; HG vs. HNG: $F(1, 31) = 34, P < 0.0001$; LG vs. LNG: $F(1, 31) = 24, P < 0.0001$] and grammaticality classification [AGL3; HG vs. HNG: $F(1, 31) = 59, P < 0.0001$; LG vs. LNG: $F(1, 31) = 55, P < 0.0001$]. We also observed a significant effect of ACS for both grammatical and nongrammatical strings during preference classification

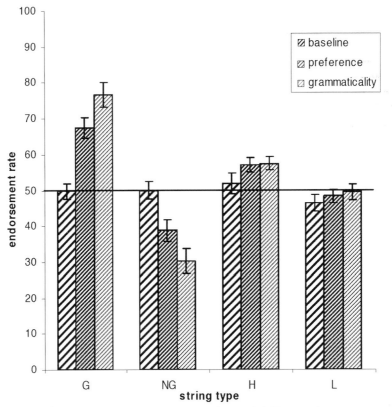

Figure 3. Endorsement rates over grammaticality and ACS main factor categories. The endorsement rates (i.e., item classified as grammatical independent of actual grammaticality status) as a function of grammaticality status (G = grammatical strings, NG = nongrammatical strings) as well as associative chunk strength (H = high ACS strings, L = low ACS strings). The endorsement rate for grammatical versus nongrammatical items, but not for high versus low ACS items, increases as a function of repeated acquisition sessions. Error bars correspond to standard error of the mean.

[AGL2; HG vs. LG: $F(1, 31) = 22$, $P < 0.0001$; HNG vs. LNG: $F(1, 31) = 4.04$, $P = 0.05$]. However, for grammaticality classification, ACS only had an effect on the grammatical strings [AGL3; HG vs. LG: $F(1, 31) = 21$, $P < 0.0001$], but not on the nongrammatical strings (HNG vs. LNG: $F(1, 31) = 2.9$, $P = 0.09$].

In addition, we compared LG versus HNG based on the argument that this maximally contrasts structural versus substring knowledge; if grammaticality status is used for classification, the acceptance of an LG item would crucially depend on the grammaticality status of the item, whereas if substring knowledge is used, the low ACS status would pro-

mote a rejection decision. On the other hand, if substring knowledge is used for classification, the acceptance of HNG items would depend on the high ACS status, while if grammatical status is used, the grammaticality status would indicate a rejection decision. As predicted, we found a significant advantage for LG over HNG strings in both preference classification [AGL2; LG > HNG: $T(31) = 3.28$, $P = 0.003$] and grammaticality classification [AGL3; LG > HNG; $T(31) = 5.82$, $P < 0.0001$]. Taken together, these results show that grammaticality status independent of ACS is used for structural generalization in classifying novel strings and provide support for the notion that grammatical structure other than substring or fragment features is used for successful classification.

Signal Detection and Bias: Analysis of the d-Prime and Beta Values

The subjects showed a stable d-prime effect in discriminating between grammatical (G) and nongrammatical (NG) strings [except in the baseline AGL1 test; mean d-prime values: AGL1 = 0.006, AGL2 = 0.94; AGL3 = 1.53; AGL2 > AGL1: $T(31) = -4.91$, $P = 0.0001$; AGL3 > AGL2: $T(31) = -2.95$, $P = 0.006$, AGL3 > AGL1: $T(31) = -7.63$, $P = 0.0001$]. No significant response bias was found (mean beta-values: AGL1 = 1.02; AGL2 = 1.01; AGL3 = 1.17; all $P > 0.6$). However, participants showed no d-prime effect in discriminating between high and low ACS strings (mean d-prime values: AGL1 = 0.15, AGL2 = 0.22; AGL3 = 0.21; all $P > 0.66$). In other words, no difference in the ability to discriminate better high than low chunks was found. In addition, no significant response bias was observed (mean beta-values: AGL1 = 0.99; AGL2 = 0.98; AGL3 = 1.00; all $P > 0.8$). We also investigated the behavioral data for training effects on day 5 by dividing each classification task (preference/grammaticality) into four separate blocks for each task. The statistical analysis yielded no differences in the performance between the four blocks within each classification task.

Subjective Reports

During each classification session (AGL1/2/3), each subject was asked to rate his or her level of attention, distraction, engagement, boredom, and perceived difficulty ("VAS" ratings four times evenly distributed over each session). There was no significant difference on these measures except for a small increase in the level of attention [AGL1: 7.9 ± 1.1; AGL2: 7.9 ± 1.1; AGL3: 8.3 ± 1.0; $F(2, 58) = 9.2$, $P = 0.0001$] and the participants also rated grammaticality classification as more difficult than preference classification [AGL1: 3.4 ± 2.3; AGL2: 3.2 ± 2.3; AGL3: 4.8 ± 2.8; $F(2, 62) = 8.96$, $P = 0.001$]. Most participants reported that the stimuli presented in the classification tasks were similar to what they saw during the acquisition sessions, and they noticed some regularity in the stimulus during the acquisition task (typically, that the strings would start with M or V). All but one participant reported only vague criteria for his or her preference and grammaticality decisions (which would apply equally to all item types).

Fragment Completion and Generation Performance

A fragment completion and a generation task were administered after the last grammaticality classification AGL3. In the fragment completion task, the participants had to fill in a missing letter in 31 strings that they had never encountered before. All participants scored significantly above chance levels (20%; mean correct completions = 74 ± 16%). Statistically significant correlation between the number of correct completions and the percentage of correct responses on both classification tasks (AGL2/3) was found (AGL2: $P = 0.025$; AGL3: $P = 0.013$). In the generation task, the participants were asked to generate ten grammatically correct strings; 27 participants could generate grammatically correct strings (mean = 5.3 ± 3.7). The generated strings were categorized as new (correct grammatical strings that were never presented to the participants), exact copies (correct grammatical strings that were not new, but already presented during the acquisition sessions), and copies with more or less repeated trigrams. In the latter case, correct grammatical strings were not "new," because if a repeated substring was deleted then they would also have been presented already. For example, if a participant were to write MSVRXVRXVRXVS, and if some but not all of the VRXs are deleted, then the string was part of stimuli of the acquisition sessions. According to this classification, participants generated on average 2.3 new grammatical strings and 2.3 exact copies. A significant correlation was found between the generation of grammatical items and the percentage of correct responses on AGL3 ($P = 0.0001$), but not on AGL2. The rating of perceived performance did not correlate with the percentage of correct responses on AGL3 (participants were asked to rate this only after AGL3).

Discussion

The artificial grammar learning paradigm has been used as a model of several aspects of language acquisition and implicit learning. In this experiment we modified the original version of the paradigm by investigating both grammaticality and preference classification. It can be argued that preference classification might be more optimal in characterizing the outcome of implicit acquisition since in the preference version participants are kept completely unaware of the underlying generative mechanism, whereas in the grammaticality version, the subjects have at least, in principle, been informed about the existence of an underlying complex set of rules at classification (but not during acquisition). The results of the present study showed that the participants implicitly acquired knowledge about the underlying artificial grammar, since participants performed well above chance levels on both preference (AGL2) and grammaticality classification (AGL3) in comparison to baseline classification (AGL1). Participants improved their performance in AGL3 compared to AGL2. Thus the instruction type did influence the final classification proficiency. However, this difference is quantitative rather than qualitative in nature since all effects significant in grammaticality classification (AGL3) were already significant in preference classification (AGL2), as well as the reverse; only the pattern of results was strengthened in AGL3 compared to AGL2. We found that being informed about the existence of an underlying generative mechanism during

the utilization of ACS did not increase in grammaticality classification and the significant effect of LG versus HNG was already present in preference classification (AGL2; LG > HNG). These results suggest that grammaticality status independent of ACS is used for structural generalization in classifying novel strings and provides support for the notion that grammatical structure other than local substring regularities is to a large extent used for classification. Thus, the abstraction of grammatical structure takes place during implicit artificial grammar acquisition. This can be seen especially in the quantitative performances between the two classification tasks that take place without an increase in the use of ACS-type information. Furthermore, the use of a preference classification baseline ensures that the effects observed in the classification task are actually attributable to information learned during the acquisition phase. Subjective reports also suggested that the participants did not utilize an explicit rule-searching strategy, but that their classification decisions were reached by guessing based on "gut feeling." In addition, the subjective ratings of perceived performance did not correlate with the actual classification performance. These results show that preference and grammaticality classification are equivalent in terms of behavioral effects and strongly support the notion that humans can implicitly acquire knowledge about a complex system of interacting rules by mere exposure to the acquisition material that can also be effectively put to use (Reber, 1967). In other words, preference starts to correlate with the grammaticality status of the classification items without any explicit awareness of the underlying generative mechanisms as predicted by the mere exposure effect (Zajonc, 1968).

Dual Mechanisms in Implicit Artificial Grammar Acquisition

Additional support for the implicit character of AGL comes from lesion studies on amnesic patients. Knowlton and Squire (1996) investigated amnesic patients and normal controls on the original AGL task as well as a transfer version of the task. The patients and their normal controls performed similarly on both AGL versions, while the amnesic patients could not explicitly retrieve complete strings or any substring information. Knowlton and Squire (1996) argued that AGL depends on implicit acquisition of both abstract (i.e., rule-based) and exemplar-specific information, the latter indicated by the acquisition of distributional information of local substring regularities (i.e., ACS-type information). The acquisition of long-distance dependencies, as opposed to local substring dependencies, has been demonstrated both in visuomotor sequence learning and in AGL (Poletiek, 2002). Moreover, it is known that infants can rapidly acquire and generalize over local sequential regularities, and several studies have shown rapid (on the order of 2–10 min) "rule abstraction" (Marcus, Vijayan, Bandi Rao, & Vishton, 1999), AGL (Gomez & Gerken, 1999), and transition probability acquisition in artificial syllable sequences (Saffran, Aslin, & Newport, 1996) capacities in 8-month-old infants. It is also clear from these studies that distributional information of local sequential regularities are acquired and used for grammaticality classification in addition to implicit abstraction of grammatical structure (Forkstam *et al.*, 2006; Meulemans & Van der Linden, 1997).

Artificial Grammar Learning and Functional Neuroimaging

A number of functional magnetic resonance imaging (fMRI) studies have investigated implicit (e.g., Forkstam *et al.*, 2006; Lieberman *et al.*, 2004; Petersson *et al.*, 2004; Seger, Prabhakaran, Poldrack, & Gabrieli, 2000) and explicit learning of material generated from artificial grammars (e.g., Fletcher, Buchel, Josephs, Friston, & Dolan, 1999; Strange, Henson, Friston, & Dolan, 2001) and artificial languages (e.g., Opitz & Friederici, 2003). In the explicit learning studies (e.g., Fletcher *et al.*, 1999; Opitz & Friederici, 2003; Strange *et al.*, 2001), the

experimental task can be characterized as explicit problem solving with performance feedback (Petersson *et al.*, 2004). In this setup, the participants are explicitly instructed to try to extract the underlying rules based on feedback (trial-and-error search). To overcome the explicit nature of the acquisition task in these experiments, we have, as in this study, investigated grammaticality classification task after implicit acquisition without performance feedback in which the participants only are exposed to positive examples (i.e., well-formed strings, Forkstam *et al.*, 2006; Petersson *et al.*, 2004). The latter two studies showed that artificial syntactic violations activated Broca's region (left Brodmann's area (BA) 44/45; Fig. 4). In Forkstam *et al.* (2006), the activated frontal regions were more extensive and also included right homotopic regions. Importantly, the left inferior frontal region (BA 45) was the only frontal region that was selectively sensitive to grammaticality, but not to the level of associative chunk strength (ACS). This lends support for the suggestion that the left inferior frontal cortex (BA 45) has a specific role in processing structural regularities (Petersson *et al.*, 2004). This is also consistent with recent results showing that the left prefrontal cortex subserves structured sequence processing (Fig. 4; Bookheimer, 2002; Hagoort, 2005).

A recent study by Lieberman *et al.* (2004) using an AGL paradigm similar to that of Forkstam *et al.* (2006) also reported that the caudate nucleus was sensitive to grammaticality (Fig. 4). These findings are in line with a difference between the processing mechanisms that retrieve linguistic structures and the procedural processing mechanisms that apply syntactic "rules" (see, e.g., Ullman, 2004). Here the basal ganglia support the procedural aspects of processing. In this context, it is of interest to note that the basal ganglia learning system (Packard & Knowlton, 2002b) and the medial temporal lobe memory system (Squire & Zola-Morgan, 1991) might interact in complex ways, competitively (Poldrack *et al.*, 2001) as well as cooperatively (Voermans *et al.*, 2004).

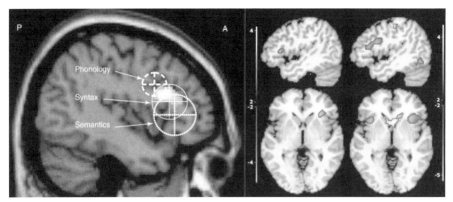

Figure 4. Regions related to phonological, syntactic, and semantic processing (cf. Bookheimer, 2002, and Hagoort, 2005). *Left:* Activation related to artificial syntactic violations (Petersson *et al.*, 2004). *Right:* Regions active in artificial grammatical versus nongrammatical items in red and nongrammatical versus grammatical in blue (Forkstam *et al.*, 2006). (In color in *Annals* online.)

Neural systems supporting procedural learning, and important for online governing of the parsing process, are thought to depend on recurrent networks implemented in corticostriatal loops (see, for example, Luciana, 2003; Nelson & Webb, 2003). Classifications of G items correlated with the activation of the caudate nucleus when contrasted with NG items. Moreover, the opposite contrast of comparing classifications of NG versus G items correlated with activation of the left inferior frontal region. In terms of laterality of the corticostriatal circuits, both the caudate and the inferior frontal region were active bilaterally during processing of grammaticality. The observed selective sensitivity to grammaticality, as opposed to ACS, in the left inferior frontal BA 45 suggests a left-lateral bias in the use of corticostriatal circuits for processing sequence structure.

Artificial Grammar Learning and Dyslexia

As noted in the introduction, very little is known about the AGL in dyslexic subjects. On the basis of the tentative conclusions outlined in the Introduction, we would like to suggest that the AGL paradigm is a suitable device for further investigation into the implicit learning characteristics in dyslexia. In particular,

since the implicit acquisition deficit observed in dyslexia seems to be related to sequence processing and to sequence complexity (i.e., the level of structure present in the sequences), the use of the artificial (formal) language framework for defining and precisely quantifying sequence complexity seems highly relevant (Cutland, 1980; Davis *et al.*, 1994; Hopcroft, Motwani, & Ullman, 2000). Structural complexity can be systematically varied in artificial grammars, thus making it possible to experimentally manipulate the level of structure available in the stimulus material in a precise and quantitative manner (Petersson, 2005b; Petersson *et al.*, 2005). The AGL paradigm is modality- and material-independent, which allows for experimental investigation into the role of material, sensory modality, and cross-modality transfer effects: for example, results on pure tone- and syllable sequences suggest that performance is higher for syllables compared to pure tone sequences $(P = 0.01)$, and while grammaticality classification was significant for both types of sequences on day 5 $(P < 0.001)$, implicit acquisition effects for preference classification on day 5 were only observed for the syllable group $(P = 0.01)$ (cf. Faísca, Bramão, Forkstam, Reis, & Petersson, 2007). As previously illustrated, issues related to temporal- and spatial integration can be investigated as well (e.g., Forkstam *et al.*, 2006; Petersson *et al.*, 2004; Pothos & Kirk, 2004). It is possible to separate the effects related to local substring regularities from those of structure abstraction in a precise manner. Finally, sequence processing after implicit artificial grammar acquisition is known to involve fronto-striatal loops as well as the cerebellum (Forkstam *et al.*, 2006; Lieberman *et al.*, 2004; Petersson *et al.*, 2004), which is relevant given the proposed fronto-striatal-cerebellar circuit deficit in dyslexics (Howard *et al.*, 2006).

Ziegler and Goswami (2005) argue that atypical development of reading skills can arise from variations in the initial conditions or constraints on learning, or from variations in the training environment, or from an interaction between the two. They suggest that explicit access to phonemes is not readily available prior to reading and that all major theories of reading acquisition argue that gaining access to phoneme-size units is a crucial step for the beginning reader of an alphabetic language (Ziegler & Goswami, 2005). A major cause of the early difficulty of reading acquisition is that phonology and orthography initially favor different grain sizes and that structural regularities present in the lexicon of spoken word forms may form the basis of incidental/implicit learning about phonology (Ziegler and Goswami, 2005). Building on an implicit foundation of phonological knowledge, learning to read involves explicit as well as implicit processes; typically children initially learn grapheme–phoneme mappings explicitly, after which they apply and continue to learn how phonology is mapped onto its written representation implicitly (Gombert, 2003; Petersson & Reis, 2006; Ziegler & Goswami, 2005). Ziegler and Goswami (2005) suggest that it is these explicit processes and their potential interactions with the more implicit aspects of lexical processing that are missing from the models. The relationship between reading ability and phoneme awareness is necessarily reciprocal (Petersson *et al.*, 2009; Ziegler & Goswami, 2005). Awareness of sounds at the smallest grain size (phonemes) does not develop automatically

as children get older and the discovery of the phoneme as a psycholinguistic unit depends largely on direct instruction in reading and spelling (Ziegler & Goswami, 2005). Therefore, in order to fully understand nonoptimal reading and writing development it might be necessary to investigate not only implicit acquisition or explicit learning mechanisms, but their interaction as well.

Conclusions

In this article we reviewed the literature on implicit learning and dyslexia and tentatively concluded that: *(a)* dyslexia does not seem to be associated with a general implicit learning deficit; *(b)* the implicit learning deficit observed in dyslexia does not seem to be related to nonspecific factors like general cognitive or attention deficit, task difficulty, or age; *(c)* the implicit acquisition deficit seems to be related to sequence processing, which is likely related to sequence complexity; and *(d)* the implicit learning deficit in dyslexia can be observed when explicit learning is intact. We also characterized a novel forced-choice structural mere-exposure artificial grammar learning paradigm in normal readers in relation to the standard grammaticality classification paradigm. We explored the outcome of an acquisition mechanism capable of extracting structural regularities from experience in an implicit fashion from positive examples alone and without any external supervision or feedback. The results showed that preference and grammaticality classification are equivalent in terms of behavioral effects and strongly support the notion that humans can implicitly acquire knowledge about a complex system of interacting rules by mere exposure to the acquisition material that also can be effectively put to use.

Acknowledgments

This work was supported by the Max Planck Institute for Psycholinguistics, the F. C.

Donders Centre for Cognitive Neuroimaging, Vetenskapsrådet (8276), Hedlunds Stiftelse, and Stockholm County Council (ALF, FoUU).

Conflicts of Interest

The authors declare no conflicts of interest.

References

Bookheimer, S. 2002. Functional MRI of language: new approaches to understanding the cortical organization of semantic processing. *Annual Review of Neuroscience*, **25:** 151–188.

Chang, G. Y., & Knowlton, B. J. 2004. Visual feature learning in artificial grammar classification. *Journal of Experimental Psychology: Learning, Memory, and Cognition*, **30:** 714–722.

Chomsky, N. 1986. *Knowledge of language*. New York: Praeger.

Chun, M. M., & Phelps, E. A. 1999. Memory deficits for implicit contextual information in amnesic subjects with hippocampal damage. *Nature Neuroscience*, **2:** 844–847.

Cohen, J. D., Dunbar, K., & McClelland, J. L. 1990. On the control of automatic processes: a parallel distributed processing model of the Stroop effect. *Psychological Review*, **99:** 45–77.

Cohen, J. D., Servan-Schreiber, D., & McClelland, J. L. 1992. A parallel distributed processing approach to automaticity. *American Journal of Psychology*, **105:** 239–269.

Cutland, N. J. 1980. *Computability: An introduction to recursive function theory*. Cambridge, UK: Cambridge University Press.

Davis, M. D., Sigal, R., & Weyuker, E. J. 1994. *Computability, complexity, and languages: Fundamentals of theoretical computer science* (2nd ed.). San Diego, CA: Academic Press.

Dilling, H., Mombour, W., & Schmidt, M. H. 1991. *International classification of mental diseases: ICD-10*. Bern: Huber.

Faísca, L., Bramão, I., Forkstam, C., Reis, A., & Petersson, K. M. 2007. *Implicit learning of structured auditory sequences: An advantage for verbal stimulus*. Presented at the Annual Mid-Year Meeting of the International Neuropsychological Society. Bilbao, Spain.

Fletcher, P., Buchel, C., Josephs, O., Friston, K., & Dolan, R. 1999. Learning-related neuronal responses in prefrontal cortex studied with functional neuroimaging. *Cerebral Cortex*, **9:** 168–178.

Forkstam, C., Hagoort, P., Fernandez, G., Ingvar, M., & Petersson, K. M. 2006. Neural correlates of artificial syntactic structure classification. *NeuroImage*, **32:** 956–967.

Forkstam, C., & Petersson, K. M. 2005. Towards an explicit account of implicit learning. *Current Opinion in Neurology*, **18:** 435–441.

Friederici, A. D., Steinhauer, K., & Pfeifer, E. 2002. Brain signatures of artificial language processing: Evidence challenging the critical period hypothesis. *Proceedings of the National Academy of Sciences of the United States of America*, **99:** 529–534.

Gombert, J. E. 2003. Implicit and explicit learning to read: implication as for subtypes of dyslexia. *Current Psychology Letters: Behavior, Brain and Cognition* **10**(1):

Gomez, R. L., & Gerken, L. 1999. Artificial grammar learning by 1-year-olds leads to specific and abstract knowledge. *Cognition*, **70:** 109–135.

Gomez, R. L., & Gerken, L. 2000. Infant artificial language learning and language acquisition. *Trends in Cognitive Sciences*, **4:** 178–186.

Goswami, U. 2003. Why theories about developmental dyslexia require developmental designs. *Trends in Cognitive Sciences*, **7:** 534–540.

Habib, M. 2000. The neurological basis of developmental dyslexia: an overview and working hypothesis. *Brain*, **123:** 2373–2399.

Hagoort, P. 2005. On Broca, brain and binding: a new framework. *Trends in Cognitive Sciences*, **9:** 416–423.

Hauser, M. D., Chomsky, N., & Fitch, W. T. 2002. The faculty of language: what is it, who has it, and how did it evolve? *Science*, **298:** 1569–1579.

Hopcroft, J. E., Motwani, R., & Ullman, J. D. 2000. *Introduction to automata theory, languages, and computation* (2nd ed.). Reading, MA: Addison-Wesley.

Howard, J. H., Howard, D. V., Japikse, K. C., & Eden, G. F. 2006. Dyslexics are impaired on implicit higher-order sequence learning, but not on implicit spatial context learning. *Neuropsychologia*, **44:** 1131–1144.

Karmiloff-Smith, A. 1992. *Beyond modularity: a developmental perspective on cognitive science*. Cambridge, MA: MIT Press.

Karmiloff-Smith, A., Grant, J., Sims, K., Jones, M. C., & Cuckle, P. 1996. Rethinking metalinguistic awareness: representing and accessing knowledge about what counts as a word. *Cognition*, **58:** 197–219.

Kelly, S. W., Griffiths, S., & Frith, U. 2002. Evidence for implicit sequence learning in dyslexia. *Dyslexia*, **8:** 43–52.

Knowlton, B. J., & Squire, L. R. 1996. Artificial grammar learning depends on implicit acquisition of both abstract and exemplar-specific information. *Journal of Experimental Psychology: Learning, Memory, and Cognition*, **22:** 169–181.

Lieberman, M. D., Chang, G. Y., Chiao, J., Bookheimer, S. Y., & Knowlton, B. J. 2004. An event-related fMRI study of artificial grammar learning in a balanced chunk strength design. *Journal of Cognitive Neuroscience*, **16:** 427–438.

Logan, G. D. 1988. Toward an instance theory of automatization. *Psychological Review*, **95:** 492–527.

Luciana, M. 2003. The neural and functional development of human prefrontal cortex. In M. de Haan & M. H. Johnson (Eds.), *The cognitive neuroscience of development* (pp. 157–179). New York: Psychology Press.

MacLeod, C. M., & Dunbar, K. 1988. Training and Stroop-like interference: evidence for a continuum of automaticity. *Journal of Experimental Psychology: Learning, Memory, and Cognition*, **14:** 126–135.

Marcus, G. F., Vijayan, S., Bandi Rao, S., & Vishton, P. M. 1999. Rule learning by seven-month-old infants. *Science*, **283:** 77–80.

Menghini, D., Hagberg, G. E., Caltagirone, C., Petrosini, L., & Vicari, S. 2006. Implicit learning deficits in dyslexic adults: an fMRI study. *NeuroImage*, **33:** 1218–1226.

Meulemans, T., & Van Der Linden, M. 1997. Associative chunk strength in artificial grammar learning. *Journal of Experimental Psychology: Learning, Memory, and Cognition*, **23**(4): 1007–1028.

Morais, J. 1993. Phonemic awareness, language and literacy. In R. M. Joshi & C. K. Leong (Eds.), *Reading disabilities: diagnosis and component processes* (pp. 175–184). Dordrecht, the Netherlands: Kluwer Academic Publishers.

Nelson, C. A., & Webb, S. J. 2003. A cognitive neuroscience perspective on early memory development. In M. de Haan & M. H. Johnson (Eds.), *The cognitive neuroscience of development* (pp. 99–125). New York: Psychology Press.

Opitz, B., & Friederici, A. D. 2003. Interactions of the hippocampal system and the prefrontal cortex in learning language-like rules. *NeuroImage*, **19**(4): 1630–1737.

Packard, M. G., & Knowlton, B. J. 2002a. Learning and memory functions of the basal ganglia. *Annual Review of Neuroscience*, **25:** 563–593.

Packard, M. G., & Knowlton, B. J. 2002b. Learning and memory functions of the basal ganglia. *Annual Review of Neuroscience*, **25:** 563–593.

Perrin, D., & Pin, J.-E. 2004. *Infinite words: Automata, semigroups, logic, and games*. Amsterdam, the Netherlands: Elsevier.

Petersson, K. M. 2005a. *Learning and memory in the human brain*. Stockholm: Karolinska University Press.

Petersson, K. M. 2005b. On the relevence of the neurobiological analogue of the finite state architecture. *Neurocomputing*, **65–66:** 825–832.

Petersson, K. M., Elfgren, C., & Ingvar, M. 1997. A dynamic role of the medial temporal lobe during retrieval of declarative memory in man. *NeuroImage*, **6:** 1–11.

Petersson, K. M., Elfgren, C., & Ingvar, M. 1999. Learning-related effects and functional neuroimaging. *Human Brain Mapping*, **7**(4): 234–243.

Petersson, K. M., Forkstam, C., & Ingvar, M. 2004. Artificial syntactic violations activate Broca's region. *Cognitive Science*, **28:** 383–407.

Petersson, K. M., Grenholm, P., & Forkstam, C. 2005. Artificial grammar learning and neural networks. Proceedings of the Cognitive Science Society, 1726–1731.

Petersson, K. M., Ingvar, M., & Reis, A. 2009. Language and literacy from a cognitive neuroscience perspective. In D. Olson & N. Torrance (Eds.), *Cambridge handbook of literacy* (pp. 152–181). Cambridge, UK: Cambridge University Press.

Petersson, K. M., & Reis, A. 2006. Characteristics of illiterate and literate cognitive processing: Implications for brain-behavior co-constructivism. In P. B. Baltes & F. Rösler & P. A. Reuter-Lorenz (Eds.), *Lifespan development and the brain: The perspective of biocultural co-constructivism* (pp. 279–305). New York: Cambridge University Press.

Petersson, K. M., Reis, A., Askelöf, S., Castro-Caldas, A., & Ingvar, M. 2000. Language processing modulated by literacy: a network-analysis of verbal repetition in literate and illiterate subjects. *Journal of Cognitive Neuroscience*, **12:** 364–382.

Petersson, K. M., Reis, A., & Ingvar, M. 2001. Cognitive processing in literate and illiterate subjects: a review of some recent behavioral and functional data. *Scandinavian Journal of Psychology*, **42:** 251–167.

Petersson, K. M., Sandblom, J., Gisselgård, J., & Ingvar, M. 2001. Learning related modulation of functional retrieval networks in man. *Scandinavian Journal of Psychology*, **42:** 197–216.

Poldrack, R. A., Clark, J., Pare-Blagoev, E. J., Shohamy, D., Creso Moyano, J., Myers, C., *et al.* 2001. Interactive memory systems in the human brain. *Nature*, **414:** 546–550.

Poletiek, F. H. 2002. Implicit learning of a recursive rule in an artificial grammar. *Acta Psychologica*, **111:** 323–335.

Pothos, E. M., & Kirk, J. 2004. Investigating learning deficits associated with dyslexia. *Dyslexia*, **10:** 61–76.

Reber, A. S. 1967. Implicit learning of artificial grammars. *Journal of Verbal Learning and Verbal Behavior*, **5:** 855–863.

Reber, A. S. 1993. *Implicit learning and tacit knowledge: An essay on the cognitive unconscious*. New York: Oxford University Press.

Rüsseler, J., Gerth, I., & Münte, T. F. 2006. Implicit learning is intact in adult developmental dyslexic readers: evidence from the serial reaction time task and artificial grammar learning implicit learning in dyslexia.

Journal of Clinical and Experimental Neuropsychology, **28:** 808–827.

Saffran, J. R., Aslin, R. N., & Newport, E. L. 1996. Statistical learning by 8-month-old infants. *Science*, **274:** 1926–1928.

Seger, C. A. 1994. Implicit learning. *Psychological Bulletin*, **115:** 163–196.

Seger, C. A., Prabhakaran, V., Poldrack, R. A., & Gabrieli, J. D. 2000. Neural activity differs between explicit and implicit learning of artificial grammar strings: an fMRI study. *Psychobiology*, **28:** 283–292.

Shaywitz, S. E. 1998. Dyslexia. *New England Journal of Medicine*, **338:** 307–312.

Sperling, A. J., Lu, Z. L., & Manis, F. R. 2004. Slower implicit categorical learning in adult poor readers. *Annals of Dyslexia*, **54:** 281–303.

Squire, L. R., & Zola-Morgan, S. 1991. The medial temporal lobe memory system. *Science*, **253:** 1380–1386.

Stadler, M. A., & Frensch, P. A. (Eds.). 1998. *Handbook of implicit learning*. Thousand Oaks, CA: Sage.

Stoodley, C. J., Harrison, E. P., & Stein, J. F. 2006. Implicit motor learning deficits in dyslexic adults. *Neurosychologia*, **44:** 795–798.

Strange, B. A., Henson, R. N. A., Friston, K. J., & Dolan, R. J. 2001. Anterior prefrontal cortex mediates rule learning in humans. *Cerebral Cortex*, **11:** 1040–1046.

Ullman, M. T. 2004. Contributions of memory circuits to language: the declarative/procedural model. *Cognition*, **92:** 231–270.

Vicari, S., Finzi, A., Menghini, D., Marotta, L., Baldi, S., & Petrosini, L. 2005. Do children with developmental dyslexia have an implicit? *Journal of Neurology, Neurosurgery, and Psychiatry*, **76:** 1392–1397.

Vicari, S., Marotta, L., Menghini, D., Molinari, M., & Petrosini, L. 2003. Implicit learning deficit in children with developmental dyslexia. *Neuropsychologia*, **41:** 108–114.

Voermans, N. C., Petersson, K. M., Daudey, L., Weber, B., van Spaendonck, K. P., Kremer, H. P. H., *et al.* 2004. Interaction between the human hippocampus and caudate nucleus during route recognition. *Neuron*, **43:** 427–435.

Waber, D. P., Marcus, D. J., Forbes, P. W., Bellinger, D. C., Weiler, M. D., Sorensen, L. G., *et al.* 2003. Motor sequence learning and reading ability: Is poor reading associated with sequencing deficits? *Journal of Experimental Child Psychology*, **84:** 338–354.

Zajonc, R. B. 1968. Attitudinal effects of mere exposure. *Journal of Personality and Social Psychology Monograph Supplement*, **9**(2): Part 2.

Ziegler, J. C., & Goswami, U. 2005. Reading acquisition, developmental dyslexia, and skilled reading across languages: a psycholinguistic grain size theory. *Psychological Bulletin*, **131:** 3–29.

Motor Sequence Learning and Developmental Dyslexia

Pierre Orban,[a,b] Ovidiu Lungu,[a] and Julien Doyon[a]

[a] Functional Neuroimaging Unit, Geriatric Institute and Psychology Department,
University of Montréal, Montréal, Québec, Canada

[b] Cyclotron Research Center, University of Liège, Liège, Belgium

Beyond the reading-related deficits typical of developmental dyslexia (DD), recent evidence suggests that individuals afflicted with this condition also show difficulties in motor sequence learning. To date, however, little is known with respect to the characteristics of the learning impairments, nor to the neural correlates associated with this type of procedural deficit in DD patients. Here, we first summarize the results of the few behavioral and brain imaging studies that have investigated the effects of DD on motor sequence learning. To help guide research in this field, we then discuss relevant psychophysical and neuroimaging work conducted in healthy volunteers in relation to three different conceptual perspectives: *when*, *how*, and *what*. More specifically, we examine the cognitive boundaries that affect performance across the different stages of learning (i.e., "when"), the different cognitive processes (i.e., "how") under which learning occurs, and the mental representations (i.e., "what") that are elicited when acquiring this type of skilled behavior. It is hoped that this conceptual framework will be useful to researchers interested in further studying the nature of the motor learning impairment reported in DD.

Key words: motor sequence learning; developmental dyslexia; functional brain imaging; adults; children; explicit learning; implicit learning; motor representations; learning stages

Introduction

From early childhood, an impressive variety of skills are gradually acquired, ranging from simple motor and perceptual skills to more complex cognitive ones like reading. Throughout life, such procedural abilities are learned so that they eventually come to be performed automatically and implicitly, meaning that the learned material can be retrieved without consciousness. In developmental dyslexia (DD), children classically exhibit a core literacy deficit and fail to master efficient reading despite normal intelligence and adequate conventional

education. More recently, however, accumulating evidence has led to the view that this developmental disorder may also be characterized by a wider disorder in skill acquisition and automatization. According to this viewpoint, literacy deficits would thus represent but one facet of a more general impairment in procedural learning.

Several new studies have demonstrated that DD patients show signs of a marked impairment in implicit motor sequence learning (Howard, Howard, Japikse, & Eden, 2006; Menghini, Hagberg, Caltagirone, Petrosini, & Vicari, 2006; Stoodley, Harrison, & Stein, 2006; Stoodley, Ray, Jack & Stein, 2008, this volume; Vicari *et al.*, 2005; Vicari, Marotta, Menghini, Molinari, & Petrosini, 2003; but see Kelly, Griffiths, & Frith, 2002; Russeler, Gerth, & Munte, 2006 for contradictory results), as

Address for correspondence: Julien Doyon, Functional Neuroimaging Unit, Research Center of the Geriatric Institute, University of Montreal, 4565, Queen Mary, Montréal, Québec H3W 1W5, Canada. julien.doyon@umontreal.ca

Ann. N.Y. Acad. Sci. 1145: 151–172 (2008). © 2008 New York Academy of Sciences.
doi: 10.1196/annals.1416.016

revealed through variants of the serial reaction time task (SRT) (Nissen & Bullemer, 1987). In this paradigm, subjects are required to respond to stimuli which, unbeknownst to them, follow an 8–12-elements sequential pattern. Learning is evidenced by decreases in reaction time and number of errors in response to the sequential pattern as compared to random stimulus presentation. Using such a paradigm, researchers have generally found that dyslexic individuals are as able as controls to produce appropriate motor responses when confronted with stimuli presented at random, but are impaired at detecting the occurrence of a sequential configuration of successive stimulus–motor response associations, as reflected by the lack of a progressive reduction in reaction time and errors. Such a pattern of results has been obtained in children and adolescents (Vicari *et al.*, 2005; Vicari *et al.*, 2003; Stoodley *et al.*, 2008, this volume) as well as in young adults (Howard *et al.*, 2006; Menghini *et al.*, 2006; Stoodley *et al.*, 2006), using either the classical deterministic version (Menghini *et al.*, 2006; Stoodley *et al.*, 2006; Vicari *et al.*, 2005; Vicari *et al.*, 2003) or an alternative form of the SRT paradigm (Howard *et al.*, 2006; Stoodley *et al.*, 2008, this volume). Altered performance on this task has been thought to depend mainly on implicit learning processes, as explicit knowledge of the sequence is usually not demonstrated when participants are asked to generate it at the end of the training session. Moreover, DD children have been shown to perform as well as controls when the ordering of stimuli is explicitly memorized and verbalized prior to the training period, hence further supporting the claim that the learning deficit seen in this condition is mostly implicit in nature (Vicari *et al.*, 2003).

Although the functional and structural brain differences associated with the reading-related deficits observed in DD are relatively well documented (Hoeft *et al.*, 2006; Shaywitz, Lyon, & Shaywitz, 2006; Temple, 2002), little is known with regard to these functional differences coupled with the motor sequence learning impair-

ment seen in this syndrome. Only two studies have focused on this issue, and the results so far have been inconsistent. Nicolson and colleagues (1999) were the first to report on the existence of an altered level of cerebellar functioning during a trial-and-error motor sequence task in DD using positron emission tomography (PET). These authors found an abnormal, decreased level of activation in the ipsilateral anterior cerebellum of DD subjects during both the acquisition of a novel motor sequence and the execution of a pre-learned sequence of movements. More recently, however, Menghini and colleagues (2006) used functional magnetic resonance imaging (fMRI) to look at differences in brain activations between DD and control adults as they practiced a deterministic version of the SRT task. Contrary to Nicolson and coworkers (1999), the latter investigators revealed that the cerebellum was more active in DD subjects than in control subjects, particularly in the late learning phase. Although discrepancies between these two experiments may be due to differences in the type of motor sequence learning tasks used, as they differed in terms of the amount of awareness involved, both groups of researchers did underscore the fact that DD groups presented levels of activity in the cerebellar cortex that differed from those of the matched control groups. On the basis of such findings, investigators in this field have proposed the "cerebellar deficit hypothesis," which postulates that a dysfunction within the cerebellum is responsible for the entire array of symptoms observed in DD (Nicolson, Fawcett, & Dean, 2001; see Zeffiro & Eden, 2001, for discussion). Yet the cerebellum is but one component of the brain network known to support motor sequence learning in healthy subjects. As discussed below, numerous other cerebral regions are engaged during this type of motor learning, notably the striatum and motor-related cortical regions, which play a key role in the encoding and retention of a motor sequence. Consequently, it is possible that the motor learning deficits seen in DD may be related to a concurrent dysfunction in brain structures other than the cerebellum.

With the recent increase of interest in exploring the specificity of the motor sequence learning deficit in DD using brain imaging techniques, we believe that further integration between this field of research and the vast knowledge base already acquired through psychophysical and neuroimaging work in typically reading subjects will be necessary to pinpoint the real nature of this memory impairment in DD subjects. In the present article, we will thus describe the work done so far in reading disability but will mainly focus on the cognitive boundaries and neuroanatomic underpinnings known to mediate motor sequence learning in typical individuals. At the outset, it is important to note that, unlike the majority of DD studies, those in the area of motor sequence learning in normal control subjects have mostly been conducted in adults, but rarely in children. Therefore, most of the conceptual issues discussed in this review will be based upon results from studies carried out in human adults, but findings from developmental research will also be included when possible. Motor sequence learning will be discussed in relation to three different conceptual perspectives: *when*, *how*, and *what*. The first looks at the cognitive boundaries that affect performance across the different stages of learning during practice over short or long periods of time. The second addresses the question of how subjects learn new sequences of movements, and especially the role of both implicit and explicit memory processes. Finally, the third considers the type of mental representation that is elicited during the acquisition of this procedural ability. Although each of these issues will be discussed separately, it should also be noted that this taxonomic separation serves only a didactic purpose, as any motor sequence learning task is likely to involve a unique combination of these three factors (Fig. 1). Methodological considerations will also be emphasized in order to guide future investigators in their use of optimal experimental designs for investigating further the

effects of DD on both behavioral performance and brain changes.

Cognitive Boundaries of Motor Sequence Learning

Compared to the vast literature available on motor sequence learning in typical subjects, only a few studies have looked at the effects of DD on this type of motor learning, and thus several conceptual and methodological issues remain to be addressed. For instance, it is commonly agreed that motor learning follows at least two distinct stages: an early, fast learning stage that is accompanied by dramatic improvements in performance within the first training session, and a slow learning stage, in which further improvements in performance occur over multiple sessions and longer periods of time (Karni *et al.*, 1998). Motor learning studies with DD subjects have focused exclusively on the fast learning stage. Consequently, it is unclear whether individuals with DD have a deficit in encoding motor sequences at all, or whether they are simply slower to learn, hence necessitating longer and greater number of training sessions than control subjects. Similarly, most studies investigating sequence learning among DD subjects have claimed that the motor learning deficit observed in this population is specifically related to impaired implicit learning processes. Because researchers have not yet manipulated this learning process to check directly its effects on the subjects' performance, however, a thorough examination is needed to determine whether the motor learning deficit seen in DD is really due to impaired difficulties in implicit or explicit memory processes. Finally, the issue pertaining to the representational changes occurring during learning have not been directly addressed in studies employing DD participants. Thus, it is still unknown whether the motor sequence learning deficit in dyslexia is perceptual or motoric in nature, or whether it is related to the acquisition and retrieval of

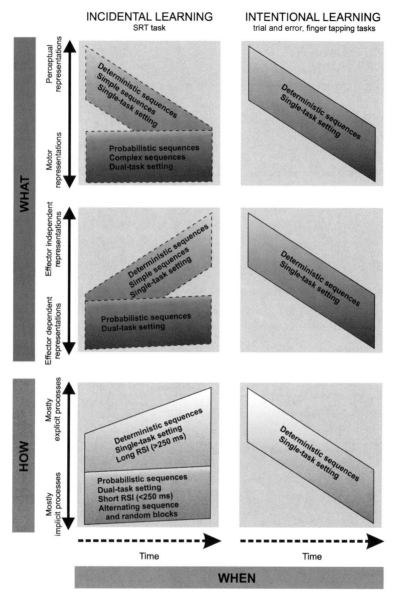

Figure 1. Conceptual framework describing the methodological factors influencing incidental and intentional motor sequence learning in its early phase. This figure shows the changes over time (WHEN) that occur in the type of learning processes (HOW) and mental representations (WHAT) during the fast, early stage of motor sequence learning. The *left* and *right panels* contrast these changes for incidental and intentional learning paradigms, respectively. The polygonal shapes within each panel illustrate the extent to which a particular type of process (implicit versus explicit) or representation (perceptual versus motor and effector-dependent versus effector-independent) dominates at a particular point in time during the fast acquisition phase. The presence of *continuous lines* defining the polygons indicates that there is direct experimental evidence for the temporal changes described by them. In contrast, the *dashed lines* indicate that the evidence is limited or indirect, as it is deduced from studies that looked at particular time points during motor learning, but not at the actual changes over time. The experimental factors known to induce these temporal changes are reported within each polygon.

effector-specific or effector-independent representations of the motor sequence (however, see Bennett, Romano, Howard & Howard, 2008, this volume).

When: Stages of Learning

Learning, be it motor or not, comprises dynamic processes through which information is manipulated and transformed over time. From the start, the field of motor learning has been dominated by studies in adult subjects that explored the behavioral changes occurring in the fast learning stage until they reach asymptotic performance. These behavioral changes usually happen within one or across several training sessions and take place over a short period of time lasting no longer than a few hours of practice. However, in recent years, there has been growing interest in uncovering the learning processes that span over longer time frames, as there is evidence that changes in performance can occur over multiple sessions encompassing days, weeks, or even months of practice (Doyon & Benali, 2005; Doyon & Ungerleider, 2002). This longer temporal perspective is particularly suited for motor learning, given that most motor skills are known to evolve slowly, requiring a considerable amount of practice before they can be performed automatically and recalled without any drop in performance.

In addition to investigating the effects of practice on performance at different stages of learning a new skill, greater attention has recently been paid to the offline changes that occur in the consolidation phase, defined as the process during which a newly learned motor trace goes from a labile representation into a more robust trace. In the motor domain, this process has been operationally defined in two different ways: first, by showing that the memory trace is susceptible to permanent disruption (i.e., interference) after the administration of a competing task within a time window of 6–8 hours (Walker, Brakefield, Hobson, & Stickgold, 2003); and second, by demonstrating the existence of delayed gains in performance

after a sleep-dependent consolidation process (Korman, Raz, Flash, & Karni, 2003; Walker *et al.*, 2003). Altogether, a plethora of studies thus suggests that motor learning follows different stages and that the cognitive processes and representations subserving learning in the early stages are most likely different from those supporting automatic performance and long-term retention after extended periods of time. Indeed, with extended training, the new skill is thought to become resistant to interference after consolidation and to the effects of time such that it can be readily retrieved despite long periods without practice.

Interestingly, a few studies have recently shown that motor sequence learning in children follows similar phases. Researchers have reported that the latter are as effective as adults in retaining a motor trace in long-term memory (as revealed through the presence of spontaneous gains in performance after long periods of time including sleep) using both the SRT task (Meulemans, Van der Linden, & Perruchet, 1998), as well as a self-initiated sequential finger-to-thumb opposition task (Dorfberger, Adi-Japha, & Karni, 2007). However, the role of sleep on motor memory consolidation among children still remains unclear. For example, in a study using a probabilistic variant of the SRT task, Fischer, Wilhelm, & Born (2007) revealed that compared to that of adults, the children's performance worsens after sleep, but not after a similar amount of daytime during wakefulness. Although conjectural, these inconsistencies may be due to differences in the type of tasks and experimental conditions, which lead to the development of distinct representations during motor learning. Such issues will be addressed in the subsequent sections of this review.

How: Learning Processes

Explicit learning is characterized by awareness of the material being learned, whereas implicit learning refers to the acquisition of a skill without awareness. In the motor sequence learning domain, ample evidence exists to conclude that the structure of the sequence, the timing of the stimulus presentation, and the experimental instructions given to the subjects prior to training all constitute important methodological factors in determining which of these two types of processes will be recruited during learning. For example, motor sequences may be probabilistic (where transitions from one element to the next are variable and occur with a given probability) or deterministic in nature (where transitions are perfectly predictable and occur according to a fixed rule). Previous behavioral studies performed among adult subjects have shown that implicit processes tend to predominate in the case of probabilistic sequences, while explicit processes are likely to develop in parallel when sequences are deterministic (Jimenez, Vaquero, & Lupianez, 2006). Similarly, it has been demonstrated that learning is mostly explicit when the sequence of movements is acquired intentionally, memorized in advanced, or discovered by trial and error, while it is mostly implicit when, unbeknownst to subjects, the sequence of movements is acquired incidentally through repetition of seemingly random executed movements. In the following paragraphs, we will analyze the methodological factors that may lead to the use of explicit or implicit processes during motor sequence learning, with a strong emphasis on the SRT task and its variants, as most of the research in DD has used this paradigm. It is important to note, however, that the distinction between implicit and explicit processes serves only a practical purpose as no task is process-pure (Destrebecqz et al., 2003, 2005; Jacoby, 1991). Most likely, in any given motor learning task, the two types of processes always coexist in various degrees.

The SRT task is the most widely used paradigm to study motor sequence learning among healthy and clinical populations (Nissen & Bullemer, 1987). In a typical setting, a stimulus is presented on the screen at one of four locations, and subjects are required to press the button corresponding to that location using one of four fingers of their hand. As mentioned in the introduction, unbeknownst to subjects, a sequence of 8–12-elements long is usually repeated 8–10 times in a given block of practice trials. With repetition, subjects come to perform sequences of movements more efficiently, leading to decreases in reaction time (RT) and in the number of errors. Scores in this condition are then compared to those in which stimuli are presented at random, and the difference in performance is then used to show that procedural motor learning has taken place. Even though the SRT task was originally designed to tap into implicit processes, a number of studies have shown that motor sequence learning tested with this paradigm can be implicit, explicit, or based on a combination of both processes, depending on various methodological conditions (Destrebecqz et al., 2003, 2005). Here are some factors that can determine whether explicit or implicit processes are recruited during motor sequence learning:

The first and most important aspect affecting how learning will take place is the subject's awareness of the learned material. On the one hand, the level of awareness of the motor sequence can be manipulated at the beginning of the task through specific experimental instructions given to subjects. In this situation, the participants are told beforehand that a motor sequence exists and that it has to be learned (i.e., intentional learning), or that they are only required to respond to stimuli as quickly as possible while making as few errors as possible (i.e., incidental learning). On the other hand, the subjects' awareness about the sequence may also develop naturally during incidental learning, and may then be assessed at the end of the allocated period of practice through various tests. In the majority of studies using the SRT task, learning has been incidental, and awareness about the sequence has been probed at the end of the experiment using both recognition and generation tests (Destrebecqz et al., 2003, 2005; Willingham & Goedert-Eschmann, 1999). In a typical recognition task, subjects are presented with parts of the sequence and asked to decide whether the items correspond or not to the stimuli (sequence) presented during training. In the generation tests, however, subjects are informed that there was a sequence during practice and are asked to retrieve and reproduce as many elements as possible without any help from external cues.

Of interest, several studies of children have observed the same differences in performance under conditions of incidental and intentional motor sequence learning. Some researchers have employed only one of these approaches and showed that children are as able as adults to learn a sequence either incidentally (Meulemans *et al.*, 1998) or intentionally (Dorfberger *et al.*, 2007). Others have compared the two conditions and showed that adults and children show a similar performance during incidental learning, whereas adults outperform children and older children far better than younger ones during intentional learning. (Karatekin, Marcus, & White, 2007; Thomas & Nelson, 2001).

During incidental learning, implicit processes are more likely to dominate at the beginning of the acquisition process, whereas with more and more practice, explicit processes may then develop in parallel (Willingham & Goedert-Eschmann, 1999). Given this mixture of implicit and explicit processes by the end of the practice session, it then becomes particularly important to be able to dissociate their influence on motor performance. Unfortunately, to date, there is no perfect technique permitting the evaluation of implicit and explicit processes online while subjects are performing the task. Consequently, researchers have relied on the administration of the "process dissociation procedure" (Destrebecqz *et al.*, 2003, 2005; Jacoby, 1991) at the end of the practice period to assess the effects of these means of learning the sequence. This technique is based on the idea that automatic and controlled behaviors are associated with unconscious and conscious processes, respectively. Subjects are then given two types of tests, where these approaches can act together (inclusion tests) or in opposition to each other (exclusion tests). For example, typical retrieval and recognition tasks are thought to refer to inclusion tests as their performance is based on both types of processes. In contrast, asking subjects to reproduce a sequence that bears no resemblance to the original one (i.e., avoiding reproduction of the learned material) is thought to represent an exclusion test. The difference between the inclusion and exclusion scores is then believed to express the influence of the conscious processes alone. Yet it is important to point out that the presence of awareness at the beginning of a task (intentional learning) as compared to its occurrence later in the practice period (incidental learning) may have different effects on motor performance. Although it is generally agreed that subjects who develop explicit knowledge during incidental learning are responding to the sequence faster than those relying on implicit processes, presumably on account of the anticipation of the next stimulus (Marcus, Karatekin, & Markiewicz, 2006), there is also evidence that the intention to learn the sequence explicitly may actually hinder motor performance (Fletcher *et al.*, 2005).

Second, another important variable that may influence whether learning will be implicit or explicit is the structure of the sequence. Two distinct aspects of the sequence structure may affect how it is acquired: the overall nature of the sequence (e.g., deterministic versus probabilistic) and the type of element-to-element transitions (e.g., first- versus second-order transitions) required in a particular sequence. Thus, as we have already mentioned, the learning of deterministic sequences is considered to depend upon both implicit and explicit learning (Willingham & Goedert-Eschmann, 1999), whereas the acquisition of probabilistic sequences is believed to be mostly implicit (Peigneux *et al.*, 2000). In addition, the presence of second-order transitions in a deterministic sequence (i.e., when a combination of two elements preceding the trial perfectly predicts the appearance of the next stimulus) will typically lead to implicit sequence learning, while the presence of first-order transitions will usually facilitate the emergence of explicit learning.

Third, the way stimuli are administered may also determine whether implicit or explicit processes will be recruited during motor sequence learning. For instance, the presentation of sequence blocks interleaved with random ones, as opposed to the successive and repeated administration of blocks of practice with a sequence, ensures that subjects will not learn the sequence explicitly (Bischoff-Grethe, Goedert, Willingham, & Grafton, 2004; Thomas *et al.*, 2004). By the same token, there is also evidence that the response-to-stimulus interval (the time between subject's response to a stimulus and the presentation of the subsequent one) impairs explicit learning when it is very short (fewer than 250 ms), while leaving implicit learning intact (Destrebecqz *et al.*, 2003, 2005).

Finally, the use of a dual-task paradigm, in which the motor sequence learning condition (i.e., the primary task) is performed at the same time as that of a distracting task (e.g., counting tones = secondary task) may have two distinct effects on learning. The first consequence is that such experimental designs prevent the development of an explicit learning process, because it requires additional attentional resources. These resources are thought to be recruited by the distracting task, thus enhancing the implicit nature of the main motor task. The second effect is that the distracter task may suppress the expression of motor performance (e.g., the usual decrease in RT) during the learning phase. The magnitude of this effect depends on the complexity of the sequence and on the dimensional overlap (i.e., share common characteristics in terms of stimuli or responses) between the two tasks, and it may be used to control for behavioral changes during the learning stage (Seidler *et al.*, 2002, 2005).

Apart from the SRT task and its variants, other paradigms have also been used to investigate motor sequence learning in humans. For instance, one paradigm uses a trial-and-error approach (Jenkins, Brooks, Nixon, Frackowiak, & Passingham, 1994; Jueptner & Weiller, 1998; Toni, Krams, Turner, & Passingham, 1998), in which subjects have to initiate motor responses by themselves in the proper order (sequence) using auditory or visual feedback. In this paradigm, when subjects make a mistake by choosing the wrong subsequent element in the sequence, they are required to start again from the beginning, until they perform the sequence of movements correctly. In this case, subjects are aware that there is a sequence right from the beginning of the experiment, and thus explicit processes dominate at the beginning of the learning session. Another approach employs tasks that require subjects to explicitly memorize the sequence prior to the onset of the training, and then asks them to execute movements (Doyon *et al.*, 2002; Karni *et al.*, 1995; Lehéricy *et al.*, 2005). In this situation, subjects usually employ an explicit verbal code (made up of numbers or letters) to learn the sequence before initiating any movement. Thus, similar to the intentional SRT task or the learning by trial and error, explicit processes are expected to be prevalent in the early stages of the task, with the implicit ones developing later with automatization.

What: Content of Learning

It is difficult to focus on the processes subserving motor sequence learning while ignoring the content itself, that is, *what* people are learning and how the information about the sequence is represented. These are obviously key issues that need to be addressed (Bapi, Doya, & Harner, 2000; Bird & Heyes, 2005) as their exploration can lead to a better understanding of several behavioral phenomena that have already been reported. These include the transfer and generalization of motor sequence knowledge from one effector to another and from one modality to another, the consolidation of procedural memories over time, as well as the interference and facilitation effects seen when several motor skills are being learned at once.

The SRT paradigm not only requires that subjects physically respond to stimuli, but also involves the visual presentation of sequentially displayed stimuli. Hence, one real concern when using this paradigm is whether subjects are learning a sequence of motor responses or a sequence of visual stimuli with little bearing on the motor aspect of the sequence. Furthermore, if subjects acquire both perceptual and motor knowledge about the sequence, one can then ask whether these two types of representations are independent of each other or not. On way to address this issue has been to test two groups of subjects, one performing the task in the usual way (motor condition) and the other observing the sequence of stimuli (perceptual condition). At the end of the training session, both groups of subjects are then tested in a generation task (explicit condition) or in a motor task (implicit condition). A series of studies used this approach (Bird & Heyes, 2005; Bird, Osman, Saggerson, & Heyes, 2005; Osman, Bird, & Heyes, 2005), but their goal was to assess whether perceptual sequence learning is implicit or explicit and whether it is effector-dependent or -independent. Another way to investigate this issue has been to employ a series of distinct stimuli (e.g., colors, shapes) that are located at the center of the screen, and to require subjects to perform spatially distinct motor responses (e.g., with four fingers of their hand). At the testing phase, the colors or shapes are spatially separated such that either the original sequence of responses (motor condition) or the original sequence of stimuli is preserved (perceptual condition). Studies employing these kinds of design have found mixed results. Some researchers (Witt & Willingham, 2006) have reported that subjects develop both perceptual and motor knowledge, but that those representations are independent of each other. While some have shown that subjects can only form a perceptual or motor representation, others re-

vealed that these two types of representations are dependent on each other. Such discrepancies in the pattern of results may be explained by various methodological differences among studies, for example, whether subjects were given instructions to intentionally learn the motor sequence or whether they were aware of the sequence, the structure of the sequence, or the tests used to assess the representation of the sequential knowledge. Regardless of these differences, however, these findings suggest that motor sequence learning is supported by multiple types of representations that may also change over time. In line with this conclusion are the results of two well-controlled studies employing a trial-and-error, bidimensional sequence learning task (Bapi *et al.*, 2000; Bapi, Miyapuram, Graydon, & Doya, 2006), where the orientation of the display (perceptual dimension) or of the response keypad (motor dimension) was manipulated. The authors found that the perceptual representation of the motor sequence dominated early, whereas the motor representation formed more slowly and was more prevalent later within the learning session. The study by Bapi *et al.*, (2000) is particularly important as it shows that the types of sequence representations are not stationary but change over time.

Given the fact that the information regarding motor sequences can be coded using multiple modalities (auditory, visual, tactile,) and that it can be expressed using different output systems (motor, verbal), another issue concerns whether or not a transfer and generalization of knowledge occurs within and between modalities. Is learning of the sequence effector-dependent or effector-independent? Does one code the sequence using allocentric or egocentric frames of reference? Do we use single or multiple codes to store the sequence? Although still a matter of debate, a large body of studies points to the fact that subjects form both effector-dependent and effector-independent representations of the sequential knowledge (Bapi *et al.*, 2000; Bapi *et al.*, 2006; Deroost, Zeeuws, & Soetens, 2006; Grafton, Hazeltine, & Ivry,

1998). There is also evidence that the sequence may be coded with egocentric and allocentric frames of reference (Liu, Lungu, Waechter, Willingham, & Ashe, 2007; Witt & Willingham, 2006). However, a brief review of these studies suggests that the two types of representations seem to depend on the way in which learning takes place. Thus, effector-dependent and egocentric representations are thought to be used during both implicit and explicit learning, whereas effector-independent representations and allocentric coding of the sequence appear specific to explicit learning (Liu *et al.*, 2007).

Conceptual Framework

As mentioned earlier, motor sequence learning is very dynamic, involving changes in a variety of memory processes and representations with repeated practice of a newly learned skilled behavior. Figure 1 illustrates how different methodological factors may affect the temporal evolution of these changes as they occur during a single training session for both incidental and intentional types of motor learning tasks. For example, taking such a conceptual framework into account, one can see that the use of deterministic sequences in a single-task paradigm will have different effects on the temporal distribution of implicit and explicit processes (the HOW panel), depending on the type of motor skill task that is administered. Thus, during incidental learning (HOW, left side), implicit processes are believed to dominate at the beginning of the learning process, while explicit processes may also develop later, in parallel, with more practice. By contrast, during intentional learning (HOW, right side) of deterministic sequences in a single-task setting, the acquisition is thought to be explicit at the beginning and then to become more and more implicit as the sequence is learned. Apart from the temporal evolution of the learning processes (HOW) or of the representations about the sequence (WHAT), one can also observe that these two dimensions correlate. For instance, during

incidental learning (left panels), the temporal change in the type of representations (from perceptual to motor or from effector-independent to effector-dependent) is associated with parallel transitions from explicit to implicit processes. Given the interaction between the processes involved (HOW) and the content (WHAT) of learning, the interpretation of behavioral or neuroimaging results from a single point of view must thus be made with caution.

Brain Correlates of Motor Sequence Learning

The neural underpinnings of the cognitive boundaries associated with motor sequence learning have been explored *in vivo* in groups of healthy volunteers using functional brain imaging techniques like PET and fMRI. By using various experimental designs and by manipulating different task parameters, a clearer picture of how cortical and subcortical structures contribute to the learning and production of a motor sequence has recently emerged (Ashe, Lungu, Basford, & Lu, 2006; Doyon & Benali, 2005; Doyon & Ungerleider, 2002). In fact, a plethora of studies demonstrate that both the striatum, cerebellum and motor-related cortical areas play a major role in this type of motor memory, and that plasticity within and between these cortico-subcortical systems occur during the different phases of learning a sequence of movements. Up to now, however, only two brain imaging reports using either PET during a trial-and-error task (Nicolson *et al.*, 1999) or fMRI during a deterministic SRT task (Menghini *et al.*, 2006) have been conducted in DD patients. Overall, these investigators' results suggest that the procedural learning deficit seen in dyslexia is related to abnormal cerebellar functioning. Yet this hypothesis still remains conjectural. First, given that a large set of brain areas, not just the cerebellum, are recruited during motor sequence learning in healthy subjects, it is possible that a dysfunction within structures other than the cerebellum may also explain the motor learning deficit seen in DD. Second, because these studies have only looked at the early learning phase, it is unknown whether differences in behavior and in the underlying plastic neural changes occur beyond this time window (e.g., during the consolidation and/or slow acquisition phases). Third, it is unclear how the differences in functional anatomy associated with this motor learning deficit relate to the type of processes (implicit versus explicit) called into play and to the mode of memory representations (perceptual versus motor, effector-dependent versus effector-independent) that are formed during motor learning. To gain some insights into these issues, we present below a brief review of the studies conducted in cohorts of healthy human subjects that illustrate how brain activity is modulated during motor sequence learning. More specifically, this section focuses, respectively, on the effects of the amount of practice (*when*), the level of awareness (*how*), and the type of memory representation (*what*) that is acquired.

When: Stages of Learning

There is now ample evidence demonstrating that the improvement in performance typically observed after practice on a motor sequence memory task is associated with plastic neuronal changes within a large set of cerebral structures (Ashe *et al.*, 2006; Doyon & Benali, 2005; Doyon & Ungerleider, 2002). To study the learning-dependent functional reorganization of such a motor memory trace, several experimental designs have been employed. Among them, a first approach has been to compare the intensity of activation in specific brain regions while subjects are scanned over successive sessions of practice of a single motor sequence. An alternative option has been to look at differences in brain activation between the execution of a new motor sequence and that of a previously learned sequence. Finally, more complex parametric analyses have also been employed to provide a more detailed description of the changes in brain activity mea-

sured as performance on the motor sequence task improves. In most neuroimaging studies, these approaches have been implemented to study the effect of practice in the early phase of the learning process, that is, during training or scanning periods lasting no more than a few hours. These studies will first be discussed and findings from experiments demonstrating practice effects on brain activity beyond that time window will then be described. Because practice effects on brain activity are likely to be different depending on whether learning is incidental or intentional, studies that used such paradigms will also be considered separately.

Incidental motor sequence learning has essentially been explored using a deterministic version of the SRT task. Functional imaging studies using this experimental approach have revealed a partial dissociation in brain networks subtending the production of a motor sequence, depending on whether subjects were still improving their performance or had already reached an asymptotic level of performance at the end of the training session. For example, in a PET study, Doyon, Owen, Petrides, Sziklas, and Evans (1996) reported that, compared to a motor control (random) condition, the execution of a well-learned sequence of limb movements produces significant activations in the cerebellum, striatum, anterior cingulated, and posterior parietal cortices, while practice of a different and newly learned motor sequence does not. In another PET study, Grafton, Hazeltine, and Ivry (1995) scanned a group of young participants while they were performing a SRT task under single- or dual-task conditions. With learning, monotonic increases in brain activity were observed in the premotor cortex and the prefrontal and parietal areas as well as in the putamen, but not in the cerebellum. In a more recent fMRI study using a version of the SRT task, Seidler *et al.* (2002, 2005) have reported that the primary motor cortex and the putamen were respectively engaged in both initial and later phases of learning. By contrast, the cerebellum was not recruited at any step of the learning process. The authors explained the lack of cerebellar activation by the fact that the performance changes were fully prevented on account of the concurrent practice of the secondary task (an argument that will be discussed below). Altogether, results of the SRT studies looking at the early learning phase suggest that the striatum is engaged from the onset of the acquisition of a motor memory trace, and that it remains a key structure once asymptotic performance level is reached. By contrast, the involvement of the cerebellar cortex is less crucial once the motor sequence can be performed more efficiently.

Looking at intentional learning, several experimental tasks have been employed in order to unravel the brain correlates associated with practice of a new sequence. In an fMRI study (Doyon *et al.*, 2002), subjects were trained on a deterministic SRT task in which the sequence had previously been memorized, hence making learning intentional in nature. Learning-dependent brain plasticity was explored by looking at three separate scanning sessions interspersed with periods of practice over a day. The involvement of the striatum increased during the entire course of training. A transient shift in neuronal activity from the cerebellar cortex to the deep nuclei was also detected in the first two training sessions, while the cerebellum was no longer activated by the end of training (i.e., the third training session). A functional reorganization also developed at the cortical level, notably in prefrontal, premotor, and parietal cortices, thus suggesting that the cortico-striatal system is important for maintaining the learned representation of a motor sequence. In a study using a trial-and-error task to assess intentional motor sequence learning (Jenkins *et al.*, 1994), the authors revealed that the cerebellum, the prefrontal cortex, and the premotor areas are more importantly recruited during the initial learning of a new sequence of movements than during the production of a well-practiced sequence. By contrast, the supplementary motor area (SMA) appeared to subtend specifically the execution of a prelearned

sequence. Additional findings regarding the cerebral correlates associated with practice on a trial-and-error task were later reported (Jueptner & Weiller, 1998). Of particular interest was the observation that a learning-dependent shift in brain activity developed from the anterior to the posterior striato-thalamo-cortical loops, at both the cortical and subcortical levels. A shift of activity from the prefrontal cortex to the SMA was paralleled by increases and decreases of activity in the caudal and rostral areas of the putamen, respectively. These results have recently been extended through an experiment conducted by Lehéricy *et al.* (2005), in which volunteers were scanned over three sessions administered over a few hours as they executed an explicitly known sequence of movements at a particular pace under auditory guidance. A similar neural plasticity within the subterritories of the putamen was reported: the activity of the associative area decreased with practice, whereas that of the sensorimotor area increased. Finally, although studies regarding the cerebral plasticity that develops over successive sessions of practice are very informative, they do not give much insight into the dynamic physiological changes occurring within training sessions. To investigate this issue, Toni and colleagues (1998) employed a parametric approach to characterize linear and nonlinear changes of neural activity developing on a single practice session of a trial-and-error task. These authors showed that the pattern of activations in the cerebellum, the striatum, and multiple cortical areas followed complex dynamics that could not be captured solely by the average level of activity within the session. In conclusion, in accord with findings from the incidental learning paradigms, tasks that look at intentional learning point again to a crucial role for the striatum in supporting the execution of a relatively well-mastered motor sequence. More specifically, the storage of a motor sequence memory trace appears to be localized in the sensorimotor putamen and related structures of the entire striato-thalamo-cortical loop. Although the cerebellum does play a role in the very early acquisition of a new motor sequence, it is less crucial once the sequence can be executed at an asymptotic level of performance by the end of the early learning phase.

As pointed out above, there is a large consensus that brain plasticity continues to develop well beyond a time window of one day as practice goes on, hence shaping and reorganizing the motor engram until complete automatization after days or weeks of training. In the study by Lehéricy and colleagues (2005), the early shift in the motor representation of the sequence in the sensorimotor territory of the putamen was maintained even when scanning was carried out after 28 days of training. Parallel to this shift, the neural responses during production of auditorily paced sequential movements decreased in the cerebellar cortex and deep nuclei with long-term practice. The long-term practice of timed motor sequences, requiring subjects to produce button pushes of different temporal lengths across the sequence, was also investigated with PET (Penhune & Doyon, 2002). Differences in activation were observed between early training and recall after 5 days of practice. Extensive activation of the cerebellum was detected on day 1, whereas decreased cerebellar activity and increased involvement of the striatum were observed on day 5. Recall of the sequence 1 month later without additional practice was characterized by increased activity in the primary cortex, in line with the seminal demonstration that extensive training over weeks leads to the recruitment of a larger primary motor cortical map during automatic production of a motor sequence (Karni *et al.*, 1995). Finally, in addition to the long-term changes seen with online practice, it is important to note that the offline consolidation process of a motor memory trace has also been shown to produce functional brain reorganization, especially when a night of sleep has intervened before the retest session (Fischer, Nitschke, Melchert, Erdmann & Born, 2005; Peigneux *et al.*, 2003; Walker, Stickgold, Alsop, Gaab & Schlaug, 2005).

In a recent model, Doyon and coworkers (Doyon & Benali, 2005; Doyon & Ungerleider, 2002) attempted to integrate the results obtained in brain imaging studies of motor sequence learning. They postulated that, as for motor adaptation, the acquisition of new motor sequences involves interactions between the cortico-striatal and cortico-cerebellar systems in the early phase of the learning process. Once sequential movements have been consolidated and overlearned so that they can be executed automatically after extended practice, however, the cerebellum is no longer called into play. By contrast, the striatum and its motor-related cortical regions are implicated, not only in the encoding, but in long-term retention of the sequence, thus constituting a possible repository site of the motor memory trace. In particular, the sensorimotor subterritory of the striatum, but not the associative territory, is believed to subserve the automatic production of a motor sequence. Interestingly, the studies described above also indicate that a similar functional reorganization along the rostro-caudal axis of the (pre)motor cortex develops at the cortical level with extended practice. In the prefrontal cortex, neural activity has been found to evolve differently depending on the task employed during the early acquisition phase, as increases were observed during incidental learning, while decreases were reported in intentional learning. After extensive practice, however, once the execution of the motor sequence has become automatic, the prefrontal cortex would no longer be engaged.

How: Learning Processes

When investigating the functional anatomy associated with motor sequence learning, one needs to be careful before attributing the changes in brain activity that occur with training to a pure practice effect. In fact, depending on the nature of the motor task administered, the successive phases of the acquisition process may preferentially engage implicit or explicit processes, thus producing a major confound with respect to the underlying cerebral plasticity. As mentioned earlier, task performance during incidental learning is known to rely on implicit and then explicit processes, whereas performance during intentional learning first involves explicit processes early in training, but then tends to be supported later by implicit processes. Below, we will review some studies that explored the extent to which implicit and explicit processes recruit segregated or overlapping brain circuitries, and how these brain networks may interact with one another during practice of a motor sequence.

In early PET studies, some researchers used a secondary distracter task to manipulate the subject's level of awareness of a reoccurring sequential pattern of stimuli in a SRT paradigm (Grafton *et al.*, 1995; Hazeltine, Grafton, & Ivry, 1997). In such studies, subjects were first asked to practice the SRT task (with spatially coded or color-coded stimuli) concurrently with a counting task in the first training session, and then to produce the motor sequence without any distractor in a second session. Because subjects did not report any awareness during the first dual-task session, the authors concluded that the increased activity in the motor cortex, the SMA, and the putamen reflect the recruitment of implicit processes. When subjects could focus all their attentional resources on the SRT task in the second session, however, explicit knowledge emerged in a majority of participants and activated a somewhat distinct brain network composed of the dorsolateral prefrontal and premotor cortices as well as of the putamen. In another study, using fMRI this time, subjects were trained on two SRT tasks that are known to elicit preferentially either implicit or explicit processes, respectively (Schendan, Searl, Melrose, & Stern, 2003). In the implicit condition, subjects were naive with respect to the repeating pattern. Implicit learning was also promoted by varying the first sequence element at the beginning of the blocks of practice rather than by using a dual-distractor task. By contrast, participants in the explicit condition were instructed to memorize

the locations of a repeating series of stimuli and were then asked to chunk together elements of the sequence. Their results revealed the existence of largely overlapping brain networks in both conditions. The common cerebral network included the striatum, premotor cortex, and the prefrontal region. The medial temporal lobe was also significantly activated, thus suggesting that part of the limbic system contributes to the development of sequential motor routines.

One important limitation of the experimental designs used in the studies described above relates to order effects that cannot be excluded as the explicit condition always followed the implicit one. To overcome this potential confounding effect, variants of the SRT task have been employed to ensure that participants acquire both explicit and implicit sequential knowledge in parallel, assuming that concurrent learning of both types of knowledge does not interfere with one another. In the first study, the simultaneous acquisition of sequential movements under both explicit and implicit conditions was promoted by manipulating the subjects' instructions (Willingham, Salidis, & Gabrieli, 2002). Subjects were aware that a repeating pattern was present when red stimuli were displayed on the screen, therefore promoting the use of explicit processes. By contrast, when black stimuli were used to elicit motor responses, the subjects were told that no repeating pattern was present. However, unbeknownst to them, either the sequence practiced in the explicit (red) condition or a novel sequence was displayed in the black condition, thus promoting the use of implicit processes in what was called an explicit-covert and a more conventional implicit condition. In this task, a common network of brain areas, notably composed of the putamen and the prefrontal cortex, was found to mediate both explicit and implicit acquisition processes of sequential motor responses. In another study favoring concurrent learning, Aizenstein and colleagues (2004) tested subjects on a variant of the probabilistic SRT task under dual-task type of constraints. The participants had to respond to colors (implicit learning component of the task) while paying attention to the motor sequence based on the shape of the stimulus (explicit component). A significant overlap in the brain circuitry was reported for both explicit and implicit motor sequence learning: concurrent learning notably elicited activation in striatal and prefrontal areas.

The studies described above suggest that a set of common cerebral structures mediate both the implicit and explicit acquisition of a motor sequence. However, one cannot entirely rule out the possibility that both implicit and explicit processes were present to some degree in each experimental condition, meaning that a so-called assumption of exclusiveness can hardly be postulated. To better tease apart the respective brain networks recruited by implicit and explicit processes, the process dissociation procedure described in the previous section was used in two PET studies by Destrebecqz *et al.* (2003, 2005). The response-to-stimulus interval (RSI) was also manipulated during practice to promote the use of explicit (long RSI) or implicit (minimal RSI) learning mechanisms. Subjects were not scanned during the actual learning phase, but rather while they were performing a posttraining, sequence-generation task that allowed them to better dissociate the contribution of both conscious and nonconscious processes to the production of the learned sequence. Using such an approach, the authors demonstrated that the striatum supports implicit retrieval while the prefrontal cortex is mainly engaged in the explicit recollection of sequential knowledge. A similar role of the striatum to the implicit sequence learning process has also been seen in a study by Peigneux *et al.* (2000), who used a probabilistic sequence defined by an artificial grammar, a procedure manipulating the sequence complexity known to foster the engagement of implicit processes.

Given that some brain areas preferentially support either implicit or explicit processes, the possibility that interactive mechanisms between neural systems may act during learning has also been investigated. In the study by Destrebecqz *et al.* (2005), a functional connectivity analysis revealed that activity within the striatum was inhibited by that of the prefrontal cortex, an interaction effect indicating that explicit learning negatively affects the implicit acquisition process of a motor sequence. Fletcher *et al.* (2005) also addressed this issue by manipulating the instructions given to subjects (to search for a sequence or simply to respond to stimuli) as well as the difficulty of the sequence (classical SRT or alternating SRT). The results showed that the prefrontal cortex was more active when subjects had explicit intentions to learn a difficult (alternating) motor sequence than when they simply responded or searched for the simpler sequence. The functional connectivity analysis showed that the activity within the prefrontal cortical area was positively correlated with bilateral activity in the thalamus (a relay in cortico-striatal circuits) when learning was intentional, whereas an opposite pattern was apparent when learning was essentially incidental. These findings indicate that brain networks interact with one another depending on the nature of the learning process involved.

The results from this set of studies suggest that a number of brain structures are commonly involved in motor sequence learning, irrespective of whether performance on the task is implicit or explicit in nature. However, it also appears that some nodes of this cerebral circuit are preferentially engaged in one of these memory processes. The implicit component of task performance is mediated by the striatum, a finding that is consistent with the observation that this structure is particularly important for the execution of a well-practiced sequence of movements when performance is automatic and implicitly produced. By contrast, the explicit component of motor learning is mostly dependent upon activity of the prefrontal cortex, a finding that explains the different practice effects on brain activity observed in incidental and intentional motor sequence learning tasks.

What: Content of Learning

Unlike the case in behavioral studies where the representation (*what*) aspect of a motor sequence has been studied in some detail, little attention has been given to this issue using brain imaging techniques. Only a few studies have tried to pinpoint the neural substrate underlying perceptual and motor representations of a sequence while controlling in various ways for the type of learning process. For instance, in a study in which analysis was restricted to subjects who learned a motor sequence implicitly, Bischoff-Grethe *et al.* (2004) found that both mesial motor and premotor areas supported the motoric representation of the sequence. Similarly, in a study using an explicit learning design, other researchers (Bapi *et al.*, 2006) examined the neural changes associated with the perceptual versus motor representation of a motor sequence early in its learning process. The authors found neural shifts of activation at both cortical (e.g., from parietal to premotor) and subcortical levels (e.g., from anterior to posterior putamen). In addition, the results showed that the activation of the anterior cerebellum was more related to the visual than to the motor representation of the sequence.

The brain regions underlying effector-dependent and -independent representations of the motor sequence have also been described in a PET study (Grafton *et al.*, 1998), where subjects first practiced a version of the SRT task using the four fingers of their dominant hand and were then tested using arm movements. From the practice to the test period, a shift of activity was observed in the somatosensory cortex, indicating that this region subserves effector-dependent representations of the sequence. At the same time, significant activation was also seen in the inferior parietal cortex, suggesting that this region mediates the effector-independent representations of the motor sequence.

Given the relationship that exists between the types of representations of sequential knowledge and the way in which the latter is acquired (implicitly versus explicitly), it is difficult to dissociate between the neural substrates that underlie the memory process from those mediating the content of motor sequence learning. For instance, it has been shown that the hippocampus not only supports the explicit learning processes involved in motor sequence learning, but the use of allocentric codes or effector-independent representations of sequences as well (Bapi *et al.*, 2006; Schendan *et al.*, 2003). Similarly, changes in representation of the motor sequence that occur over time, as the skill becomes consolidated and automatized, are also reflected by neural shifts of activation. For example, sleep-based consolidation of a motor sequence has been associated with a reduction of activity in prefrontal, premotor, and primary motor areas as well as with an increase of activity in parietal cortices (Fischer *et al.*, 2005). Therefore, it is necessary to control or to account for the type of processes that are likely to be elicited during motor learning and their changes over time in order to isolate the neural substrate specific to a given type of mental representation.

Methodological Issues

As detailed above, the nature of the motor sequence task (incidental versus intentional), the stage of learning (early versus late), the type of processes (implicit versus explicit), and the modality used to express the extent of learning are all conditions that contribute to the variability seen in reported cerebral networks. In addition to these conceptual aspects, however, a number of methodological factors may also influence the pattern of results that one obtains in brain imaging studies of motor sequence learning (Doyon & Ungerleider, 2002). Indeed, the choice of an appropriate baseline condition to control for nonspecific contributions to task-related activations is also of particular importance. While some studies compared signals related to practice of the motor sequence using an SRT task with a simple rest condition, others have used perceptual or active motor conditions. Another source of variability also comes from the method employed during data analyses. While the classical subtraction approach allows researchers to compare the effects of different experimental conditions or of changes across practice sessions, a parametric analysis can provide a more accurate description of how brain activity is modulated by the level of improvement in performance within a single session. Whether reflected through a subtraction or a parametric analysis, however, changes in brain activity are sometimes attributed erroneously to the learning process per se, because they may actually depend on how learning is expressed.

Here are two reasons that support such a statement: The first is that internally and externally triggered movements are not entirely subtended by overlapping brain networks. Indeed, compared to movements executed in response to external cues, movements produced in a self-initiated manner are characterized by distinct brain responses in the SMA and basal ganglia (Cunnington, Windischberger, Deecke, & Moser, 2002; Jenkins, Jahanshahi, Jueptner, Passingham, & Brooks, 2000). In the SRT as well as in other externally cue-driven tasks, movements are first initiated solely in response to the appearance of visual or auditory stimuli. With practice, however, an internal rhythm is more likely to play a role in movement generation, and consequently the resulting brain plasticity may be biased because of this confounding "movement initiation" effect. A second reason comes from the fact that learning may hardly be dissociated from changes in performance (Ashe *et al.*, 2006). Although improvements in performance (as reflected by a reduction in reaction time on the SRT task) usually constitute the grounds for inferring that learning occurred, they may also modulate brain activity irrespective of any learning per se. Indeed, it is well known that the rate of simple finger movements covaries with the amplitude of neural activity in a variety of cortical and subcortical structures (Riecker, Wildgruber, Mathiak, Grodd, & Ackermann, 2003; Turner, Grafton, Votaw, Delong, & Hoffman, 1998). To address this issue, Seidler *et al.* (2002) used a different experimental manipulation, which consisted in introducing a secondary distracter task concurrent with practice on the classical SRT, such that learning of the sequential pattern, but not its behavioral expression, could develop. Using such an approach in the framework of an fMRI study, these authors found that the cerebellum was not activated during the encoding phase of a motor sequence for as long as performance changes were suppressed by concurrent practice of the visual distracter task (Seidler *et al.*, 2002). Because the cerebellum, and lobule VI in particular, was activated only when the secondary task was no longer present, the authors concluded that the cerebellum does not mediate learning per se, but rather is involved in its unspecific expression. These findings are intriguing and raise important concerns as numerous other imaging studies of motor sequence learning have consistently reported that the same lobule of the neocerebellum is subserving motor sequence learning (see Desmond & Fiez, 1998, for a review). However, one should be aware that the prevention of performance changes strongly modifies the learning context, therefore modifying the very nature of the task.

Conclusions

Overall, the results of numerous studies in typical subjects indicate that motor sequence learning is a dynamic memory process. The studies reviewed here demonstrate that, depending on the experimental conditions and the material to be learned, this type of learning may (1) be modulated over time, both within a single training session (fast learning phase) as well as through longer time frames (slow learning phase); (2) be more or less implicit or explicit; and (3) involve a mixture of perceptual and motoric representations of the sequence.

In comparison, evidence for a deficit in motor sequence learning in DD is much more limited, as it relies mostly on studies that have investigated incidental learning in the fast acquisition phase using the SRT task. In fact, the nature of the procedural deficit reported for DD is still a matter of debate (see Bennett *et al.*, 2008, this volume).

Motor sequence learning studies in DD subjects have been carried out using the assumption that SRT tasks capture mostly implicit processes. Therefore, the deficit has been interpreted as owing to impairment in the implicit, but not the explicit memory system. In this review, we have shown that there is a mixture of implicit and explicit processes during motor sequence learning on the SRT and that the involvement of these processes changes over time, depending on various conceptual and methodological factors (Fig. 1). Future studies will have to address this issue vis-à-vis dyslexia. Indeed, to support the hypothesis that the learning deficit is mostly implicit, it will be critical to manipulate experimental factors that favor the use of such processes, for example, using probabilistic sequences in an SRT task. In addition it will also be important to determine whether a presumably intact explicit system would help individuals with DD in intentional learning of motor sequences, in which case explicit processes play a role at the onset of learning. Thus, subsequent experiments will need to test whether this motor impairment is observed by means of other experimental paradigms like the trial-and-error and sequential finger-tapping tasks. Finally, tests such as the process dissociation procedure could help in revealing to what extent the deficit is implicit in nature or involves both implicit and explicit processes.

To date, all studies in DD showed a motor sequence learning impairment in the early learning phase; hence it appeared that there is no reason to investigate this issue beyond this learning stage. However, it would be interesting to assess whether individuals with DD also present deficits during the consolidation, slow learning, and automatization phases of a motor sequence. In order to attain this goal, one will have to ensure that the subjects with dyslexia overcome their shortcomings during the early learning phase. Two experimental strategies could then be employed: one would be to extend the number of training sessions during the early learning phase, while the other would be to rely on experimental factors that enhance the role of explicit processes at the onset of learning, as described above. By means of such an approach, DD subjects would be helped in their initial acquisition of the motor skill, and it could then be possible to investigate whether or not they are impaired at later stages of the whole learning process. Given that consolidation of the motor skill, taking place during wakefulness or sleep depends on functional reorganization of the brain, this might provide additional cues on the dysfunctional brain circuitry seen in DD.

With respect to the brain changes associated with DD, some researchers have postulated that the motor sequence learning deficit in this population results primarily from a dysfunction within the cerebellum (Nicolson *et al.*, 2001). There are two aspects that need to be further addressed in relation to this hypothesis. First, the mechanism of this dysfunction is unknown; based only on the results reported so far, it is unclear whether the differential involvement of the cerebellum in DD relates to the processes (explicit or implicit) or to the content (e.g., representation or coding of the sequence) of the newly learned motor skilled behavior. Second, an important question that remains to be addressed is whether the cerebellum is the only dysfunctional region that explains motor sequence learning deficits in DD. Research in typical volunteers clearly indicates that the striatum, along with other motor-related areas, is particularly important for the creation and automatic execution of a motor memory trace.

In conclusion, the present review identified a series of experimental factors that are known to affect the way learning processes and mental representation unfold in time during the fast early phase of motor sequence learning (Fig. 1). These are known to be an important source of variability in the patterns of activation observed in brain imaging studies of motor learning. Therefore, we believe that future brain imaging research in DD aimed at characterizing the neural substrate of this deficit will need to take these aspects into account. Moreover, the motoric confounding effect of performance is also particularly relevant here as controls consistently perform better than DD patients, even when these latter demonstrate some improvement in performance. It is thus critical to control for or, at least, to account for these between-group differences. Finally, the overwhelming majority of studies investigating motor sequence learning among healthy subjects have been carried out in adult subjects. Because dyslexia is a developmental disorder, it will be important to consider behavioral and neurological differences that appear between children and adults. Indeed, one imaging study that compared typically developing children and adults showed dissimilarities in areas considered essential for the initial acquisition and automatization of the sequence, notably in the striatum (Thomas *et al.*, 2004). Thus, one will have to dissociate the normal developmental effects observed in motor sequence learning from those arising from the etiology of developmental dyslexia.

The presence of motor learning deficits among people with DD is puzzling, and, at the moment, it is unclear how these deficits relate to the literacy deficits typical of DD and their neural correlates. It is hoped that the conceptual framework presented here regarding the stages, processes, and content of motor sequence learning, based on evidence from studies with typically reading subjects, will help DD researchers to address these issues and to place the motor deficits within the clinical, functional, and neurologic tableau of developmental dyslexia.

Acknowledgments

This work was supported by Grants CIHR (MOP-66990) and NSERC (42909-04) to J.D. P.O. is a research fellow at the Belgian National Funds for Scientific Research (FNRS) and O.V. is supported by a grant from the Multidisciplinary Team in Locomotion Rehabilitation at the University of Montreal. We are grateful to Dr. Philippe Peigneux for his comments on a previous draft of this manuscript.

Conflicts of Interest

The authors declare no conflicts of interest.

References

Aizenstein, H. J., V. A. Stenger, J. Cochran, K. Clark, M. Johnson, R. D. Nebes, *et al.* 2004. Regional brain activation during concurrent implicit and explicit sequence learning. *Cerebral Cortex* **14**(2): 199–208.

Ashe, J., O. V. Lungu, A. T. Basford & X. Lu. 2006. Cortical control of motor sequences. *Current Opinion in Neurobiology* **16**(2): 213–221.

Bapi, R. S., K. Doya & A. M. Harner. 2000. Evidence for effector independent and dependent representations and their differential time course of acquisition during motor sequence learning. *Experimental Brain Research* **132**(2): 149–162.

Bapi, R. S., K. P. Miyapuram, F. X. Graydon & K. Doya. 2006. fMRI investigation of cortical and subcortical networks in the learning of abstract and effector-specific representations of motor sequences. *NeuroImage* **32**(2): 714–727.

Bennett, I. J., C. J. Romano, J. H. Howard, Jr. & D. V. Howard. 2008. Two forms of implicit learning in young adults with dyslexia. *Annals of the New York Academy of Sciences*, this volume.

Bird, G. & C. Heyes. 2005. Effector-dependent learning by observation of a finger movement sequence. *Journal of Experimental Psychology: Human Perception and Performance* **31**(2): 262–275.

Bird, G., M. Osman, A. Saggerson & C. Heyes. 2005. Sequence learning by action, observation and action observation. *British Journal of Psychology* **96**(Pt 3): 371–388.

Bischoff-Grethe, A., K. M. Goedert, D. T. Willingham & S. T. Grafton. 2004. Neural substrates of response-based sequence learning using fMRI. *Journal of Cognitive Neuroscience* **16**(1): 127–138.

Cunnington, R., C. Windischberger, L. Deecke & E. Moser. 2002. The preparation and execution of self-initiated and externally-triggered movement: a study of event-related fMRI. *NeuroImage* **15**(2): 373–385.

Deroost, N., I. Zeeuws & E. Soetens. 2006. Effector-dependent and response location learning of probabilistic sequences in serial reaction time tasks. *Experimental Brain Research* **171**(4): 469–480.

Desmond, J. E. & J. A. Fiez. 1998. Neuroimaging studies of the cerebellum: language, learning and memory. *Trends in Cognitive Sciences* **2**(2): 355–362.

Destrebecqz, A., P. Peigneux, S. Laureys, C. Degueldre, G. Del Fiore, J. Aerts, *et al.* 2003. Cerebral correlates of explicit sequence learning. *Brain Research : Cognitive Brain Research* **16**(3): 391–398.

Destrebecqz, A., P. Peigneux, S. Laureys, C. Degueldre, G. Del Fiore, J. Aerts, *et al.* 2005. The neural correlates of implicit and explicit sequence learning: interacting networks revealed by the process dissociation procedure. *Learning & Memory* **12**(5): 480–490.

Dorfberger, S., E. Adi-Japha & A. Karni. 2007. Reduced susceptibility to interference in the consolidation of motor memory before adolescence. *PLoS ONE* **2**: e240.

Doyon, J. & H. Benali. 2005. Reorganization and plasticity in the adult brain during learning of motor skills. *Current Opinion in Neurobiology* **15**(2): 161–167.

Doyon, J., A. M. Owen, M. Petrides, V. Sziklas & A. C. Evans. 1996. Functional anatomy of visuomotor skill learning in human subjects examined with positron emission tomography. *European Journal of Neuroscience* **8**(4): 637–648.

Doyon, J., A. W. Song, A. Karni, F. Lalonde, M. M. Adams & L. G. Ungerleider. 2002. Experience-dependent changes in cerebellar contributions to motor sequence learning. *Proceedings of the National Academy of Sciences USA* **99**(2): 1017–1022.

Doyon, J. & L. G. Ungerleider. 2002. Functional anatomy of motor skill learning. In L. R. Squire & D. L. Schacter (Eds.), *Neuropsychology of memory* (pp. 225–238). New York: Guilford Press.

Fischer, S., M. F. Nitschke, U. H. Melchert, C. Erdmann & J. Born. 2005. Motor memory consolidation in sleep shapes more effective neuronal representations. *Journal of Neuroscience* **25**(49): 11248–11255.

Fischer, S., I. Wilhelm & J. Born. 2007. Developmental differences in sleep's role for implicit off-line learning: comparing children with adults. *Journal of Cognitive Neuroscience* **19**(2): 214–227.

Fletcher, P. C., O. Zafiris, C. D. Frith, R. A. Honey, P. R. Corlett, K. Zilles, *et al.* 2005. On the benefits of not trying: brain activity and connectivity reflecting the interactions of explicit and implicit sequence learning. *Cerebral Cortex* **15**(7): 1002–1015.

Grafton, S. T., E. Hazeltine & R. Ivry. 1995. Functional mapping of sequence learning in normal humans. *Journal of Cognitive Neuroscience* **7**(4): 497–510.

Grafton, S. T., E. Hazeltine & R. B. Ivry. 1998. Abstract and effector-specific representations of motor sequences identified with PET. *Journal of Neuroscience* **18**(22): 9420–9428.

Hazeltine, E., S. T. Grafton & R. Ivry. 1997. Attention and stimulus characteristics determine the locus of motor-sequence encoding: a PET study. *Brain* **120**(Pt 1): 123–140.

Hoeft, F., A. Hernandez, G. McMillon, H. Taylor-Hill, J. L. Martindale, A. Meyler, *et al.* 2006. Neural basis of dyslexia: a comparison between dyslexic and nondyslexic children equated for reading ability. *Journal of Neuroscience* **26**(42): 10700–10708.

Howard, J. H. Jr., D. V. Howard, K. C. Japikse & G. F. Eden. 2006. Dyslexics are impaired on implicit higher-order sequence learning, but not on implicit spatial context learning. *Neuropsychologia* **44**(7): 1131–1144.

Jacoby, L. 1991. A process dissociation framework: separating automatic from intentional uses of memory. *Memory and Language* **30**: 513–541.

Jenkins, I. H., D. J. Brooks, P. D. Nixon, R. S. Frackowiak & R. E. Passingham. 1994. Motor sequence learning: a study with positron emission tomography. *Journal of Neuroscience* **14**(6): 3775–3790.

Jenkins, I. H., M. Jahanshahi, M. Jueptner, R. E. Passingham & D. J. Brooks. 2000. Self-initiated versus externally triggered movements. II. The effect of movement predictability on regional cerebral blood flow. *Brain* **123**(Pt 6): 1216–1228.

Jimenez, L., J. M. Vaquero & J. Lupianez. 2006. Qualitative differences between implicit and explicit sequence learning. *Journal of Experimental Psychology: Learning, Memory, and Cognition* **32**(3): 475–490.

Jueptner, M. & C. Weiller. 1998. A review of differences between basal ganglia and cerebellar control of movements as revealed by functional imaging studies. *Brain* **121**(Pt 8): 1437–1449.

Karatekin, C., D. J. Marcus & T. White. 2007. Oculomotor and manual indexes of incidental and intentional spatial sequence learning during middle childhood and adolescence. *Journal of Experimental Child Psychology* **96**(2): 107–130.

Karni, A., G. Meyer, P. Jezzard, M. M. Adams, R. Turner & L. G. Ungerleider. 1995. Functional MRI evidence for adult motor cortex plasticity during motor skill learning. *Nature* **377**(6545): 155–158.

Karni, A., G. Meyer, C. Rey-Hipolito, P. Jezzard, M. M. Adams, R. Turner, *et al.* 1998. The acquisition of skilled motor performance: fast and slow experience-driven changes in primary motor cortex. *Proceedings of the National Academy of Sciences USA* **95**(3): 861–868.

Kelly, S. W., S. Griffiths & U. Frith. 2002. Evidence for implicit sequence learning in dyslexia. *Dyslexia* **8**(1): 43–52.

Korman, M., N. Raz, T. Flash & A. Karni. 2003. Multiple shifts in the representation of a motor sequence during the acquisition of skilled performance. *Proceedings of the National Academy of Sciences USA* **100**(21): 12492–12497.

Lehéricy, S., H. Benali, P. F. Van de Moortele, M. Pelegrini-Issac, T. Waechter, K. Ugurbil, *et al*. 2005. Distinct basal ganglia territories are engaged in early and advanced motor sequence learning. *Proceedings of the National Academy of Sciences USA* **102**(35): 12566–12571.

Liu, T., O. V. Lungu, T. Waechter, D. T. Willingham & J. Ashe. 2007. Frames of reference during implicit and explicit learning. *Experimental Brain Research.* **180**(2): 273–280.

Marcus, D. J., C. Karatekin & S. Markiewicz. 2006. Oculomotor evidence of sequence learning on the serial reaction time task. *Memory & Cognition* **34**(2): 420–432.

Menghini, D., G. E. Hagberg, C. Caltagirone, L. Petrosini & S. Vicari. 2006. Implicit learning deficits in dyslexic adults: an fMRI study. *NeuroImage* **33**(4): 1218–1226.

Meulemans, T., M. Van Der Linden & P. Perruchet. 1998. Implicit sequence learning in children. *Journal of Experimental Child Psychology* **69**(3): 199–221.

Nicolson, R. I., A. J. Fawcett, E. L. Berry, I. H. Jenkins, P. Dean & D. J. Brooks. 1999. Association of abnormal cerebellar activation with motor learning difficulties in dyslexic adults. *Lancet* **353**(9165): 1662–1667.

Nicolson, R. I., A. J. Fawcett & P. Dean. 2001. Developmental dyslexia: the cerebellar deficit hypothesis. *Trends in Neuroscience* **24**(9): 508–511.

Nissen, M. J. & P. Bullemer. 1987. Attentional requirements of learning: evidence from performance measures. *Cognitive Psychology* **19:** 1–32.

Osman, M., G. Bird & C. Heyes. 2005 Action observation supports effector-dependent learning of finger movement sequences. *Experimental Brain Research* **165**(1): 19–27.

Peigneux, P., S. Laureys, S. Fuchs, A. Destrebecqz, F. Collette, X. Delbeuck, *et al*. 2003. Learned material content and acquisition level modulate cerebral reactivation during posttraining rapid-eye-movements sleep. *NeuroImage* **20**(1): 125–134.

Peigneux, P., P. Maquet, T. Meulemans, A. Destrebecqz, S. Laureys, C. Degueldre, *et al*. 2000. Striatum forever, despite sequence learning variability: a random

effect analysis of PET data. *Human Brain Mapping* **10**(4): 179–194.

Penhune, V. B. & J. Doyon. 2002. Dynamic cortical and subcortical networks in learning and delayed recall of timed motor sequences. *Journal of Neuroscience* **22**(4): 1397–1406.

Riecker, A., D. Wildgruber, K. Mathiak, W. Grodd & H. Ackermann. 2003. Parametric analysis of rate-dependent hemodynamic response functions of cortical and subcortical brain structures during auditorily cued finger tapping: a fMRI study. *NeuroImage* **18**(3): 731–739.

Russeler, J., I. Gerth & T. F. Munte. 2006. Implicit learning is intact in adult developmental dyslexic readers: evidence from the serial reaction time task and artificial grammar learning. *Journal of Clinical and Experimntal Neuropsychology* **28**(5): 808–827.

Schendan, H. E., M. M. Searl, R. J. Melrose & C. E. Stern. 2003. An FMRI study of the role of the medial temporal lobe in implicit and explicit sequence learning. *Neuron* **37**(6): 1013–1025.

Seidler, R. D., A. Purushotham, S. G. Kim, K. Ugurbil, D. Willingham & J. Ashe. 2002. Cerebellum activation associated with performance change but not motor learning. *Science* **296**(5575): 2043–2046.

Seidler, R. D., A. Purushotham, S. G. Kim, K. Ugurbil, D. Willingham & J. Ashe. 2005. Neural correlates of encoding and expression in implicit sequence learning. *Experimental Brain Research* **165**(1): 114–124.

Shaywitz, B. A., G. R. Lyon & R. E. Shaywitz. 2006. The role of functional magnetic resonance imaging in understanding reading and dyslexia. *Developmental Neuropsychology* **30**(1): 613–632.

Stoodley, C. J., E. P. Harrison & J. F. Stein. 2006. Implicit motor learning deficits in dyslexic adults. *Neuropsychologia* **44**(5): 795–798.

Stoodley, C. J., N. J. Ray, A. Jack & J. F. Stein. 2008. Implicit learning in control, dyslexic, and garden-variety poor readers. *Annals of the New York Academy of Sciences*, this volume.

Temple, E. 2002. Brain mechanisms in normal and dyslexic readers. *Current Opinion in Neurobiology* **12**(2): 178–183.

Thomas, K. M., R. H. Hunt, N. Vizueta, T. Sommer, S. Durston, Y. Yang, *et al*. 2004. Evidence of developmental differences in implicit sequence learning: an fMRI study of children and adults. *Journal of Cognitive Neuroscience* **16**(8): 1339–1351.

Thomas, K. M. & C. A. Nelson. 2001. Serial reaction time learning in preschool- and school-age children. *Journal of Experimental Child Psychology* **79**(4): 364–387.

Toni, I., M. Krams, R. Turner & R. E. Passingham. 1998. The time course of changes during motor sequence learning: a whole-brain fMRI study. *NeuroImage* **8**(1): 50–61.

Turner, R. S., S. T. Grafton, J. R. Votaw, M. R. Delong & J. M. Hoffman. 1998. Motor subcircuits mediating the control of movement velocity: a PET study. *Journal of Neurophysiology* **80**(4): 2162–2176.

Vicari, S., A. Finzi, D. Menghini, L. Marotta, S. Baldi & L. Petrosini. 2005. Do children with developmental dyslexia have an implicit learning deficit? *Journal of Neurology, Neurosurgery, and Psychiatry* **76**(10): 1392–1397.

Vicari, S., L. Marotta, D. Menghini, M. Molinari & L. Petrosini. 2003. Implicit learning deficit in children with developmental dyslexia. *Neuropsychologia* **41**(1): 108–114.

Walker, M. P., T. Brakefield, J. A. Hobson & R. Stickgold. 2003. Dissociable stages of human memory consolidation and reconsolidation. *Nature* **425**(6958): 616–620.

Walker, M. P., R. Stickgold, D. Alsop, N. Gaab & G. Schlaug. 2005. Sleep-dependent motor memory plasticity in the human brain. *Neuroscience* **133**(4): 911–917.

Willingham, D. & K. Goedert-Eschmann. 1999. The relation between implicit and explicit learning: evidence for parallel development. *Psychological Science* **10:** 531–534.

Willingham, D. B., J. Salidis & J. D. Gabrieli. 2002. Direct comparison of neural systems mediating conscious and unconscious skill learning. *Journal of Neurophysiology* **88**(3): 1451–1460.

Witt, J. K. & D. T. Willingham. 2006. Evidence for separate representations for action and location in implicit motor sequencing. *Psychonomic Bulletin & Review* **13**(5): 902–907.

Zeffiro, T. & G. Eden. 2001. The cerebellum and dyslexia: perpetrator or innocent bystander? *Trends in Neuroscience* **24**(9): 512–513.

Implicit Learning in Control, Dyslexic, and Garden-Variety Poor Readers

Catherine J. Stoodley, Nicola J. Ray, Anthea Jack, and John F. Stein

Department of Physiology, Anatomy and Genetics, University of Oxford, Oxford, United Kingdom

Developmental dyslexia is diagnosed when children fail to acquire literacy skills despite adequate education and intellectual ability. There is evidence of impaired implicit learning in dyslexia, and it is possible that poor implicit learning in dyslexic children affects their acquisition of complex skills such as reading. To assess whether children with dyslexia show evidence of poor implicit motor learning, 45 dyslexic children completed a serial reaction time task (SRTT). Age-matched controls ($n = 44$) and nondyslexic poor readers ("garden-variety" poor readers, $n = 20$) were used as comparison groups. The inclusion of the garden-variety poor-reader group allows us to address the specificity of implicit learning deficits to dyslexics, as opposed to poor readers who do not have a discrepancy between their intellectual and literacy skills. There were no significant differences between the three groups in performance accuracy. However, whereas the controls and garden-variety poor readers showed good implicit learning (measured by a significant reduction in response times from a block of random to a block of sequenced trials), the dyslexic group did not. These data suggest that implicit motor learning deficits may underlie the laborious learning seen in developmental dyslexia. Because garden-variety poor readers were as able as control children to use the sequence cues to achieve better task performance, there may be differences in how garden-variety poor readers and dyslexic children acquire knowledge. This has important implications for remediation programs that are specific to children with dyslexia and for distinguishing among varieties of poor readers.

Key words: developmental dyslexia; implicit learning; serial reaction time task; cerebellum

Introduction

Developmental dyslexia is characterized by difficulty acquiring literacy skills despite normal to above-normal cognitive ability and education. While the most obvious deficit in dyslexia is in phonological processing (Snowling, 2000), evidence of a range of other difficulties has been found in sensorimotor domains (for review, see Stein, 2001; see also

Ramus, 2003). In recent years, dyslexic children's difficulty with learning—and in particular, automatizing information and skills—has gained attention, leading Nicolson and Fawcett to propose the cerebellar deficit hypothesis of dyslexia (Nicolson & Fawcett, 1990; Nicolson, Fawcett, & Dean, 2001).

The cerebellum ("little brain") is a subcortical structure that contains more than half the neurons in the brain, conferring upon it a considerable computational capacity (Ito, 1984). The cerebellum has reciprocal connections to regions of the cerebral cortex and spinal cord, and these connections are thought to enable the modification of cortical activities, thereby optimizing motor

Address for correspondence: Dr. Catherine Stoodley, Cognitive/Behavioral Neurology Group, Massachusetts General Hospital/Harvard Medical School, 175 Cambridge Street, Suite 340, Boston, MA 02114, USA. Voice: +617-726-3669; fax: +617-724-7836. cstoodley@partners.org

Ann. N.Y. Acad. Sci. 1145: 173–183 (2008). © 2008 New York Academy of Sciences.
doi: 10.1196/annals.1416.003

programs (Ito, 2005). More recently, it has been suggested that the lateral regions of the cerebellum, which receive information from and project to prefrontal cortical areas (Allen *et al.*, 2005; Schmahmann & Pandya, 1997), are involved in cognitive processing. Studies of patients with cerebellar damage have uncovered evidence of a range of cognitive difficulties, including problems with language and reading (Gasparini *et al.*, 1999; Gottwald, Wilde, Mihajlovic, & Mehdorn, 2004; Greve, Stanford, Sutton, & Foundas, 1999; Moretti, Bava, Torre, Antonello, & Cazzato, 2002; Silveri, Leggio, & Molinari, 1994), visual spatial deficits (Levisohn, Cronin-Golomb, & Schmahmann, 2000; Riva & Giorgi, 2000; Schmahmann & Sherman, 1998), and behavioral symptoms, including changes in affect, impulsivity, and a general dysregulation of emotion (Baillieux *et al.*, 2006; Schmahmann & Sherman, 1998; Schmahmann, Weilburg, & Sherman, 2007). Furthermore, alterations in cerebellar anatomy have been found in several developmental disorders, including dyslexia (Eckert *et al.*, 2003; Rae *et al.*, 2002), autism (Courchesne, Redcay, Morgan, & Kennedy, 2005; Penn, 2006), and attention deficit disorder (Castellanos *et al.*, 2002; Seidman, Valera, & Makris, 2005).

Both lesion and imaging studies suggest that the cerebellum is involved in implicit motor learning, by which a participant shows practice-dependent improvement on a task without conscious awareness of learning the task. Patients with cerebellar lesions are impaired on implicit motor learning (Beldarrain, Grafman, Pascual-Leone, & Garcia-Monco, 1999; Gomez-Beldarrain, Garcia-Monco, Rubio, & Pascual-Leone, 1998; Molinari *et al.*, 1997; Quintero-Gallego, Gomez, Casares, Marquez, & Perez-Santamaria, 2006), and several neuroimaging studies have shown that the cerebellum is active during motor sequence learning (Toni, Krams, Turner, & Passingham, 1998; Ungerleider, Doyon, & Karni, 2002). Implicit motor learning is often assessed using serial reaction time tasks (SRTTs) (Nissen & Bullemer,

1987; Reber & Squire, 1994, 1998; Robertson, 2007). In these tasks, participants are told that they are to perform a reaction time task by pressing buttons as quickly as possible when the appropriate stimuli are presented. First, stimuli are presented in a random order. These are followed by a set of stimuli presented in a sequence that is repeated several times. Finally, a set of randomly ordered stimuli conclude the task. Typically participants improve their performance during the sequence blocks (i.e., response times drop as the sequence is repeated), but not during the random blocks. This discrepancy between the reaction times for processing sequential versus random stimuli is used to assess implicit learning.

Using a variety of tasks, several studies have investigated implicit learning in dyslexia, and these have reported mixed results. Vicari and colleagues have conducted two studies investigating implicit learning in children using a SRTT; both studies found that dyslexic participants did not improve on the implicit task, in contrast with their normal performance on an explicit learning task (Vicari, Finzi, Menghini, Marotta, Baldi, & Petrosini, 2005; Vicari, Marotta, Menghini, Molinari, & Petrosini, 2003). In adult dyslexics, there is also evidence that implicit learning is impaired (Howard, Howard, Japikse, & Eden, 2006; Sperling, Lu, & Manis, 2004; Stoodley, Harrison, & Stein, 2006), although some studies have found that adult dyslexics show intact learning (Howard *et al.*, 2006; Kelly, Griffiths, & Frith, 2002; Rüsseler, Gerth, & Münte, 2006). These studies employed different tasks, which may account for some of the disagreement. For example, Rüsseler and colleagues (2006) found that dyslexic adults were not impaired on either a traditional SRTT or an implicit artificial grammar task. Kelly *et al.* (2002) used learning of both a spatial and nonspatial sequence and again did not find a deficit in adult dyslexics. Howard *et al.* (2006) found that dyslexic college students were impaired in sequence learning, but not in a context-learning task, both of which were implicit in nature.

Because the above-cited studies do not allow for an unequivocal conclusion to be made, further studies are needed. In addition, the specificity of an implicit learning deficit in dyslexia still remains to be investigated. One of the major questions emerging in the literature on reading disorders is whether dyslexic children differ from garden-variety poor readers on certain tasks. Unlike developmental dyslexics, garden-variety poor readers have no discrepancy between their cognitive ability and literacy scores; rather, they perform equally low on both. The demonstration of a deficit in dyslexic, but not garden-variety poor readers, speaks to the specificity of the impairment to dyslexia, as opposed to a general weakness that accompanies all forms of poor reading. This study aimed (1) to confirm the existence of an implicit motor sequence learning deficit in dyslexic children using a task with no alpha-numeric confounds in order to discourage verbal rehearsal, and (2) to investigate whether such an implicit learning deficit in dyslexic children extends to all children who are poor readers regardless of their general intelligence. To this end, control, dyslexic, and garden-variety poor readers were compared on the degree of implicit learning achieved during a SRTT.

Methods

Participants

Participants were 109 children (age range, 7:0 to 15:8 years:months). Informed parental consent was obtained for all participants. Cognitive ability was measured by the Similarities and Matrices subtests of the British Abilities Scales-II (BAS-II; Elliot, Smith, & McCulloch, 1996) and literacy skills were measured using the Reading and Spelling subtests of the BAS-II. The children were divided into groups based on the following criteria: control children had both mean literacy and mean cognitive scores in the normal range (i.e., scores no more than 1 SD below average, such that the

mean of the Similarities and Matrices T scores was 40+ and the mean of the Reading and Spelling standard scores was 85+), and had no discrepancy between their cognitive and literacy scores. Dyslexic children had a greater than 1 SD discrepancy between their cognitive ability and their literacy skills. Garden-variety poor readers had no discrepancy between their cognitive and literacy scores, but both were more than 1 SD below the age-referenced norms. On the basis of these criteria, there were 44 control children, 45 dyslexic children, and 20 garden-variety poor readers.

Four of the garden-variety readers had mean cognitive scores between -2.5 and 2 SD below normal (Similarities and Matrices mean T scores of 25–30); one dyslexic child had a mean cognitive z-score of -1.3 on account of a low score on the Matrices, but a normal score on the Similarities subtest. So we conducted analyses both including and excluding these children, and no difference in the pattern of results was found. All the children understood the task and were able to complete the task. Therefore, in the analyses reported here, these cases were included.

The groups were matched for age (one-way ANOVA, $P = 0.32$). All children were right-handed. There were 18 boys and 26 girls in the control group; 34 boys and 11 girls in the dyslexic group; and 11 boys and 9 girls in the garden-variety poor-reader group.

Cognitive and Literacy Measures

Cognitive ability was assessed using the BAS-II Similarities (verbal), Matrices (nonverbal), and Digit Span (short-term verbal memory) subtests. These scores are expressed as T scores, with a mean of 50 and a standard deviation of 10. All participants also completed the single-word Reading and Spelling subtests of the BAS-II. These scores are given as standard scores, with a mean of 100 and SD of 15. Children's raw scores were converted into age-referenced normed standard scores. In order to calculate the discrepancy between the Cognitive and

You will see one of four animals on the screen.

 When you see the FISH, press the GREEN button

When you see the BIRD, press the BLUE button

 When you see the PIG or CAT, don't press any buttons!

Please go as quickly as you can without making silly mistakes!

Do you have any questions?

Press any button to begin!

Figure 1. Instructions and stimuli for the SRTT.

Literacy scores, all scores were converted into z-scores.

Serial Reaction Time Task

The SRTT was based on that designed by Nissen and Bullemer (1987), but adapted for use with children. Because a task of 300 trials proved too difficult for children in pilot studies, who became bored and would pause at unpredictable points late in the task, we used two types of cues (color and object) to shorten the time required for implicit learning to occur (Robertson & Pascual-Leone, 2001).

The SRTT was programmed in SuperLab Pro (version 2.0; Cedrus, San Pedro, CA, USA). The stimuli were animals, including a fish, bird, cat, and pig (Fig. 1). The animals were different colors (green, blue, yellow and pink, respectively) to further cue the responses. The children responded using a button box, which had a blue button and a green button. Participants were instructed to press the blue button when they saw the blue bird, and the green button when they saw the green fish. They were not to press any buttons when they saw the cat or the pig. The bird and fish stimuli appeared and

remained on the screen until the correct response was entered. The pig and cat remained on the screen for 1000 msec before disappearing. The interstimulus interval was 400 msec for the stimuli that did not require a button press; when a button press was required, the next stimulus would appear 400 msec after the button was pressed. Children were instructed that they were to respond as quickly as possible with the correct button when the animals appeared.

The task was divided into three sections: a block of 40 randomly ordered trials, followed directly by a sequence block consisting of 14 repetitions of a six-item sequence (cat-fish-cat-bird-fish-pig), which was followed by a final random block of 30 trials. All sections were run together in one 154-trial experiment. Accuracy and response times (RTs) were recorded and analyzed offline. To assess explicit learning, after the task the child was asked "Did you notice anything about the task?" "Did you notice anything different during the middle of the task?" and their verbal responses (if any) were written down.

For data analysis, trials were grouped into 11 blocks: first two random blocks; then seven sequence blocks (each block contained two

TABLE 1. Cognitive and Literacy Scores

Task	Controls $n = 44$	Dyslexics $n = 45$	Garden-variety $n = 20$	ANOVA P-value	C vs. Dys P-value	Dys vs. G-V P-value	C vs. G-V P-value
Age	9.4 ± 2.0 (7.0–15.8)	10.1 ± 1.9 (7.25–14.6)	9.6 ± 1.8 (7.6–14.9)	n.s.	n.s.	n.s.	n.s.
Matrices	53.0 ± 8.4 (37–68)	55.1 ± 10.4 (29–86)	39.3 ± 10.3 (20–54)	<0.001	n.s.	<0.001	<0.001
Similarities	52.1 ± 8.8 (37–72)	55.3 ± 11.8 (20–77)	36.4 ± 9.2 (20–50)	<0.001	n.s.	<0.001	<0.001
Digit span	48.0 ± 10.0 (20–68)	43.0 ± 7.2 (18–68)	42.4 ± 8.1 (30–59)	0.018	0.015	n.s.	0.03
Read	105.4 ± 14.1 (82–142)	80.9 ± 12.9 (55–108)	76.9 ± 6.2 (65–88)	<0.001	<0.001	n.s.	<0.001
Spell	102.9 ± 13.2 (79–130)	80.6 ± 11.6 (55–107)	80.5 ± 6.5 (66–89)	<0.001	<0.001	n.s.	<0.001
Discrep.	−0.02 ± 0.65 (−2.1 – 0.9)	1.80 ± 0.62 (1.0–3.5)	0.20 ± 0.49 (−1.0–0.7)	<0.001	<0.001	<0.001	n.s.

Key: Scores given as mean ± SD; ranges are given in parentheses. Age is given in years. Matrices, similarities, and digit span scores are T-scores (mean 50, SD 10); reading and spelling are standard scores (mean 100, SD 15). All measures are from the BAS-II. C = controls; Dys = dyslexics; G-V = garden-variety poor readers. Read = single word reading; spell = spelling; discrep. = (Sim and Mat mean Z score) – (Read and Spell mean Z score). C vs. Dys, Dys vs. G-V, and C vs. G-V columns give P-values based on independent samples t-test. n.s. = $P > 0.05$.

repeats of the sequence); and two final random blocks. For individual participants, the median RT values for each block were used for analysis. To assess the degree of implicit learning, the following measures were calculated: accuracy (percent correct); RTs; and the percent decrease in RTs during the sequence condition compared to the first random condition. Data analyses were performed using SPSS version 13.0.

Results

Cognitive and Literacy Scores

Table 1 gives the cognitive and literacy scores for the three participant groups. There was no significant difference between the control and dyslexic groups on mean cognitive ability (mean of the Similarities and Matrices scores). The control group had significantly higher scores than the dyslexic and garden-variety readers on the Digit Span, Reading, and Spelling subtests of the BAS-II. Both the control and dyslexic groups had higher cognitive scores than the garden-variety poor readers, but the dyslexics' literacy scores were on a par with the garden-variety poor-reader group.

Serial Reaction-Time Task

Table 2 and Figure 2 show the results from the SRTT. Because the RT scores were not normally distributed, the nonparametric Kruskall–Wallis test was used to compare the three groups, and Mann–Whitney tests were used to compare the dyslexic and control, control and garden-variety, and garden-variety and dyslexic groups. The accuracy scores and the raw RTs did not differ between the groups, with the exception of the dyslexic group, which was faster than the control and garden-variety readers during the first block. This difference was due to the presence of five very slow control participants (with average RTs of >1 sec during the random RT block) as opposed to a generally faster group of dyslexic participants. When the analyses were repeated, removing these five

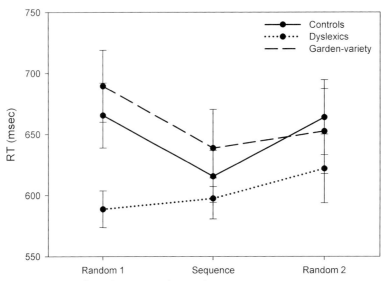

Figure 2. Patterns of RTs by group during the SRTT. RT = response time in msec. *Dots* represent group mean RTs; error bars = Standard Error Mean (SEM).

TABLE 2. SRTT Task Results

Task	Controls $n = 44$	Dyslexics $n = 45$	Garden-variety $n = 20$	Group comparison P-value	C vs. Dys P-value	Dys vs. G-V P-value	C vs. G-V P-value
Accuracy	93.8 ± 3.6 (84.4–100.0)	92.2 ± 4.5 (80.5–98.7)	93.7 ± 3.7 (84.4–100.0)	n.s.	n.s.	n.s.	n.s.
Ran1–4	665.5 ± 176.5 (472.5–1210.0)	588.7 ± 101.0 (401.7–855.7)	689.5 ± 131.7 (453.5–954.0)	0.013	n.s.	0.004	n.s.
Seq1–14	615.5 ± 141.3 (420.5–1030.2)	597.4 ± 112.5 (416.4–950.7)	638.8 ± 141.3 (398.6–1025.0)	n.s.	n.s.	n.s.	n.s.
Ran5–7	663.9 ± 204.0 (451.8–1361.0)	621.9 ± 189.0 (434.0–1392.9)	652.5 ± 155.7 (411.5–1043.0)	n.s.	n.s.	n.s.	n.s.
% RT decrease	6.0 ± 12.7 (−16.0–45.5)	−1.7 ± 9.7 (−30.8–24.5)	7.4 ± 9.3 (−21.3–19.6)	0.001	0.002	0.001	n.s.

Key: Scores given as mean ± SD (range). Accuracy = % correct. Other values are in msec. Accuracy and % RT decrease scores were normally distributed; parametric tests (ANOVA and independent samples t-tests) were used to compare the groups. The RT scores were not normally distributed (one-sample Kolmogorov–Smirnov test, $P < 0.05$), and therefore non-parametric Kruskal–Wallis tests were used to compare groups, and Mann–Whitney tests were used to compare control vs. dyslexic groups. C = controls; Dys = dyslexics; G-V = garden-variety poor readers. n.s. = $P > 0.05$.

control participants, the pattern of the results described below remained the same, despite the fact that the groups' RTs no longer differed on the first random block.

The non-normal response time data were log-transformed before conducting repeated-measures analysis and paired sample *t*-tests. In the repeated-measures analysis, there was a sig-

nificant effect of block type (sequence versus random; $P < 0.001$) and a significant block by group interaction ($P = 0.001$). The difference between the RTs during the random and sequence conditions was significant in the control ($P = 0.002$) group, indicating that the control group showed successful learning on the SRTT. The garden-variety poor readers

($P = 0.001$) also showed a significant difference between the RTs during the first random condition and the sequence condition, but the dyslexic group showed no evidence of sequence learning ($P = 0.38$). When the degree of learning was examined using the percent decrease in RTs during the sequence condition, this measure was significantly smaller in the dyslexic group as compared with the other two groups (ANOVA, $P = 0.001$; control versus dyslexic group, $P = 0.002$; garden-variety versus dyslexic group, $P = 0.001$), indicating a reduced degree of implicit learning in the dyslexic group (in fact, on average the dyslexic group's RTs *increased* by 2% during the sequence block).

Correlation Analyses

The RT scores were log-transformed for Pearson's correlation and partial correlation analyses in the whole group. Accuracy on the task mildly correlated with literacy scores ($r = 0.22$, $P = 0.02$), such that more accurate children tended to have higher literacy scores. The degree of learning on the task (indicated by the % decrease in RTs between the first random and the sequence blocks) significantly correlated with the size of the cognitive-literacy discrepancy in the whole group ($r = -0.25$, $P = 0.008$); thus, the children with a large discrepancy showed the least motor learning on the SRTT.

Partial correlations controlling for age and cognitive ability (mean of the Similarities and Matrices subtests of the BAS-II) showed significant relationships between certain measures of SRTT performance and literacy scores (mean of the Reading and Spelling subtests of the BAS-II). Mean literacy scores significantly correlated with SRTT accuracy ($r = 0.25$, $P = 0.009$) and the % reduction in RT between the first random and the sequence blocks ($r = 0.23$, $P = 0.01$).

If we use a cutoff point of a 10% reduction in RTs in the sequence condition compared to the first random block to indicate that

a participant "learned" during the task, 32% of controls, and 50% of garden-variety poor readers, but only 11% of dyslexics, showed evidence of implicit learning. With a less stringent criterion of a 5% reduction in RTs, 54% of the control group learned compared with 22% of the dyslexic group and 70% of the garden-variety poor readers. Therefore, a much smaller percentage of the dyslexic group showed motor learning on the SRTT compared to the other two reader groups, including the garden-variety group, even though the garden-variety readers had significantly lower cognitive scores than the dyslexic group.

Discussion

On our measure of implicit motor learning, both control children and garden-variety poor readers showed evidence of learning on the SRTT, whereas the dyslexic children did not. Furthermore, the size of the discrepancy between cognitive and literacy scores correlated with the degree of learning on the SRTT, suggesting that a weakness in implicit learning is observed in children whose reading is discrepant from their IQ, rather than in all poor readers.

These results are consistent with a previous report using a numeric SRTT in adult dyslexic and control participants (Stoodley *et al.*, 2006). They are also similar to those of Vicari and colleagues (2003, 2005), who found that dyslexic children performed significantly worse than control children on implicit-learning SRTT tasks. However, not all studies have shown such a deficit in poor readers. Using a longer version of the SRTT with 50 repeats of a six-item sequence (compared to the present study, in which the sequence was repeated only 14 times), Waber *et al.* (2003) found that good and poor readers showed similar learning patterns during the SRTT; they also found that children of higher cognitive ability were faster and more accurate when performing the SRTT. Crucially, Waber and colleagues

(2003) did not differentiate between discrepant and garden-variety poor readers, which—given that we found that garden-variety poor readers showed normal learning—may explain the difference in results. It is also possible that, had we lengthened the task to include more repeats of the sequence, the dyslexic group would have eventually achieved the same degree of learning as the control and garden-variety poor readers. However, the tasks employed by Vicari and colleagues were much longer than the task used in this study (60 repeats of a five-item sequence in the 2003 study, and 24 repeats of a nine-item sequence in the 2005 study), suggesting that even had we increased the number of trials, the dyslexic group might still show a deficit in implicit learning.

We kept the length of the task short for four main reasons: first, the children lost interest during an earlier version of the task with 300 trials; second, the task was included as part of a larger battery in clinic and school settings, and therefore time was at a premium; third, we did not want some of the children acquiring explicit knowledge of the sequence; and finally, we were interested in whether such a quick task (<3 minutes) would be able to discriminate the groups in terms of sequence learning. We found that the task was well tolerated by the children and did show differences in learning between the groups.

A recent study showed that implicit learning deficits in dyslexia, when found, may extend outside the motor domain: Boada and Pennington (2006) have shown that dyslexic children have poorer implicit phonological representations than both chronological and reading age-matched controls. If a child has a lack of implicit learning that extends across different domains, it may be useful to adapt a different educational approach with that child. The present study has shown that the children with poorer implicit learning also tended to have larger discrepancies between their cognitive and literacy skills. This pattern was also shown in a high-functioning adult dyslexic sample (Stoodley *et al.*, 2006), in which dyslexic university stu-

dents who did not show implicit learning on an SRTT were less likely to have compensated for their reading difficulties, as evidenced by an ongoing discrepancy between their cognitive and literacy scores. Thus it is possible that the children who cannot benefit from implicit learning may have greater difficulty compensating for their literacy problems.

How does this implicit learning deficit arise? Implicit motor learning is believed to involve cerebellar processing, and the cerebellum is also implicated in the automatization of learned movements (for recent examples, see Floyer-Lea & Matthews, 2004; Lang & Bastian, 2002). It is likely that implicit learning is mediated by the long-term depression of parallel fiber–Purkinje cell synapses in the cerebellum (Ito, 1984) to build up the neural models of sensorimotor relations that allow already learned movements to be automatically performed. The lack of automaticity under dual-task conditions in some dyslexic children was what led Nicolson and Fawcett to propose the cerebellar theory of dyslexia (Nicolson & Fawcett, 1990; Nicolson, Fawcett, & Dean, 2001); the implicit learning deficits found in dyslexic children further implicate cerebellar dysfunction in dyslexia. However, there are alternative explanations for a "cerebellar" implicit learning deficit in dyslexia. For example, the magnocellular system of large neurons feeds heavily from the parietal lobes to the cerebellum for the visual guidance of movement (Stein, 2001; Stein & Glickstein, 1992; Stein & Walsh, 1997). Hence, a more global explanation could be that the cerebellar deficit represents just one component of the neural systems that are disrupted in dyslexia. Finally, learning in general requires consistent, millisecond-level timing of neural circuits. If there is any jitter or noise in dyslexics' brains due to abnormalities in the development or migration of neurons comprising larger circuits, implicit learning would potentially be disrupted. Inconsistency in the timing and patterns of information reaching the cerebellum could disrupt the cerebellum's ability to automatize a series of movements, as is required to show learning on the SRTT. Thus, an implicit learning deficit in dyslexia could be due to a variety of disruptions in neural processing—and it is difficult to distinguish whether the cerebellum is not functioning properly (as per the cerebellar theory) or whether its input is impaired (magnocellular theory). Alternatively, the overall level of "noise" in multiple neural systems could be responsible for a disruption in the timing required for implicit sequence learning. A recent imaging study of dyslexic and control adults performing a SRTT found that dyslexic adults had differing activation in the supplementary motor area (involved in motor planning), the inferior parietal areas, and the cerebellum (Menghini, Hagberg, Caltagirone, Petrosini, & Vicari, 2006), again suggesting that the cerebellum is part of a larger network of regions that may be functioning differently in dyslexia.

A second important outcome of this study shows a difference in learning patterns between dyslexic and garden-variety poor readers, which suggests that these two groups, who show similar literacy profiles, may have deficits in different mechanisms underlying literacy acquisition. The garden-variety poor readers showed a pattern similar to that of the control group, whereas the dyslexic readers showed a flat learning curve. Vicari *et al.* (2003) and Sperling *et al.* (2004) show that dyslexics have intact declarative, but impaired implicit, learning. Perhaps garden-variety poor readers have more difficulty with conscious, explicit, learning, which affects their acquisition of cognitive and literacy skills. Future studies are needed to examine this possibility.

If these results can be generalized to other forms of learning, and related to classroom learning, there will be important implications for both research and practice. In terms of research, perhaps not all poor readers should be considered together because the problems of discrepant readers may have different causes from those of garden-variety poor readers. In terms of educational practice, if it is known that a child may not be implicitly picking up on cues

from the environment and benefiting from exposure to print in the way that his or her peers may, the child could be taught strategies to consciously acquire the necessary skills that he or she cannot acquire implicitly. Indeed, many remediation programs train dyslexic children to use such explicit strategies (for an example, see Lovett, Lacerenza, & Borden, 2000).

In conclusion, the findings of this study are two-fold: First, we confirmed that some dyslexic children do not show implicit motor sequence learning; second, we found that not all poor readers have this deficit—garden-variety poor readers, who have impaired reading and low cognitive ability, performed as well as controls on the implicit learning task. These results should be considered with respect to teaching dyslexic readers as well as in the classification of participants in future research.

Acknowledgments

We would like to thank the schools and children who participated in this study, and members of the Dyslexia Research Trust clinic for aiding in data acquisition. C.J. Stoodley was funded by a Goodger/Schorstein Research Fellowship from the University of Oxford and by the Garfield Weston and Dyslexia Research Trusts.

Conflicts of Interest

The authors declare no conflicts of interest.

References

Allen, G., R. McColl, H. Barnard, W. Ringe, J. Fleckenstein & C. Cullum. 2005. Magnetic resonance imaging of cerebellar-prefrontal and cerebellar parietal functional connectivity. *NeuroImage* **28:** 39–48.

Baillieux, H., H. D. Smet, G. Lesage, P. Paquier, P. D. Deyn & P. Marien. 2006. Neurobehavioral alterations in an adolescent following posterior fossa tumor resection. *Cerebellum* **5:** 289–295.

Beldarrain, M. G., J. Grafman, A. Pascual-Leone & J. C. Garcia-Monco. 1999. Procedural learning is impaired in patients with prefrontal lesions. *Neurology* **52:** 1853–1860.

Boada, R. & B. Pennington. 2006. Deficient implicit phonological representations in children with dyslexia. *Journal of Experimental Child Psychology* **95:** 153–193.

Castellanos, F., P. Lee, W. Sharp, N. Jeffries, D. Greenstein, L. Clasen, *et al.* 2002. Developmental trajectories of brain volume abnormalities in children and adolescents with attention-deficit/hyperactivity disorder. *Journal of the American Medical Association* **288:** 1740–1748.

Courchesne, E., E. Redcay, J. Morgan & D. Kennedy. 2005. Autism at the beginning: microstructural and growth abnormalities underlying the cognitive and behavioral phenotype of autism. *Developmental Psychopathology* **17:** 577–597.

Eckert, M., C. Leonard, T. Richards, E. Aylward, J. Thomson & V. Berninger. 2003. Anatomical correlates of dyslexia: frontal and cerebellar findings. *Brain* **126:** 482–494.

Elliot, C., P. Smith & K. McCulloch. 1996. *British abilities scales – II*. Windsor: NFER-Nelson.

Floyer-Lea, A. & P. Matthews. 2004. Changing brain networks for visuomotor control with increased movement automaticity. *Journal of Neurophysiology* **92:** 2405–2412.

Gasparini, M., V. DiPiero, O. Ciccarelli, M. M. Cacioppo, P. Pantano & G. L. Lenzi. 1999. Linguistic impairment after right cerebellar stroke: a case report. *European Journal of Neurology* **6:** 353–356.

Gomez-Beldarrain, M., J. Garcia-Monco, B. Rubio & A. Pascual-Leone. 1998. Effect of focal cerebellar lesions on procedural learning in the serial reaction time task. *Experimental Brain Research* **120:** 25–30.

Gottwald, B., B. Wilde, Z. Mihajlovic & H. Mehdorn. 2004. Evidence for distinct cognitive deficits after focal cerebellar lesions. *Journal of Neurology, Neurosurgery and Psychiatry* **75:** 1124–1131.

Greve, K., M. Stanford, C. Sutton & A. Foundas. 1999. Cognitive and emotional sequelae of cerebellar infarct: a case report. *Archives of Clinical Neuropsychology* **14:** 455–469.

Howard, J. H., Jr., D. V. Howard, K. C. Japikse & G. F. Eden. 2006. Dyslexics are impaired on implicit higher-order sequence learning, but not on implicit spatial context learning. *Neuropsychologia* **44:** 1131–1144.

Ito, M. 1984. *The cerebellum and neural control*. New York: Raven Press.

Ito, M. 2005. Bases and implications of learning in the cerebellum: adaptive control and internal model mechanism. *Progress in Brain Research* **148:** 95–109.

Kelly, S., S. Griffiths & U. Frith. 2002. Evidence for implicit sequence learning in dyslexia. *Dyslexia* **8:** 43–52.

Lang, C. E. & A. J. Bastian. 2002. Cerebellar damage impairs automaticity of a recently practiced movement. *Journal of Neurophysiology* **87:** 1336–1347.

Levisohn, L., A. Cronin-Golomb & J. Schmahmann. 2000. Neuropsychological consequences of cerebellar tumour resection in children: cerebellar cognitive affective syndrome in a paediatric population. *Brain* **123:** 1041–1050.

Lovett, M., L. Lacerenza & S. Borden. 2000. Putting struggling readers on the PHAST track: a program to integrate phonological and strategy-based remedial reading instruction and maximise outcomes. *Journal of Learning Disabilities* **33:** 458–476.

Menghini, D., G. Hagberg, C. Caltagirone, L. Petrosini & S. Vicari. 2006. Implicit learning deficits in dyslexic adults: an fMRI study. *NeuroImage* **33:** 1218–1226.

Molinari, M., M. Leggio, A. Solida, R. Ciorra, S. Misciagna, M. Silveri, *et al.* 1997. Cerebellum and procedural learning: evidence from focal cerebellar lesions. *Brain* **120:** 1753–1762.

Moretti, R., A. Bava, P. Torre, R. Antonello & G. Cazzato. 2002. Reading errors in patients with cerebellar vermis lesions. *Journal of Neurology* **249:** 461–468.

Nicolson, R., A. Fawcett & P. Dean. 2001. Developmental dyslexia: the cerebellar deficit hypothesis. *Trends in Neuroscience* **24:** 508–511.

Nicolson, R. I. & A. J. Fawcett. 1990. Automaticity: a new framework for dyslexia research? *Cognition* **35:** 159–182.

Nissen, M. & P. Bullemer. 1987. Attentional requirements of learning: evidence from performance measures. *Cognitive Psychology* **19:** 1–32.

Penn, H. 2006. Neurobiological correlates of autism: a review of recent research. *Child Neuropsychology* **12:** 57–79.

Quintero-Gallego, E. A., C. M. Gomez, E. V. Casares, J. Marquez & F. J. Perez-Santamaria. 2006. Declarative and procedural learning in children and adolescents with posterior fossa tumours. *Behavioral and Brain Functions* **2:** 9.

Rae, C., J. Harasty, T. Dzendrowskyj, J. Talcott, J. Simpson, A. Blamire, *et al.* 2002. Cerebellar morphology in developmental dyslexia. *Neuropsychologia* **40:** 1285–1292.

Ramus, F. 2003. Developmental dyslexia: specific phonological deficit or general sensorimotor dysfunction? *Current Opinion in Neurobiology* **13:** 212–218.

Reber, P. J. & L. R. Squire. 1994. Parallel brain systems for learning with and without awareness. *Learning and Memory* **1:** 217–229.

Reber, P. J. & L. R. Squire. 1998. Encapsulation of implicit and explicit memory in sequence learning. *Journal of Cognitive Neuroscience* **10:** 248–263.

Riva, D. & C. Giorgi. 2000. The cerebellum contributes to higher functions during development: evidence from a series of children surgically treated for posterior fossa tumours. *Brain* **123:** 1051–1061.

Robertson, E. 2007. The serial reaction time task: implicit motor skill learning? *Journal of Neuroscience* **27:** 10073–10075.

Robertson, E. & A. Pascual-Leone. 2001. Aspects of sensory guidance in sequence learning. *Experimental Brain Research* **137:** 336–345.

Rüsseler, J., I. Gerth & T. F. Münte. 2006. Implicit learning is intact in adult developmental dyslexic readers: evidence from the serial reaction time task and artificial grammar learning. *Journal of Clinical and Experimental Neuropsychology* **28:** 808–827.

Schmahmann, J. & D. Pandya. 1997. The cerebrocerebellar system. In J. Schmahmann (Ed.), *The cerebellum and cognition* (pp. 31–60). San Diego: Academic Press.

Schmahmann, J. & J. Sherman. 1998. The cerebellar cognitive affective syndrome. *Brain* **121:** 561–579.

Schmahmann, J. D., J. B. Weilburg & J. C. Sherman. 2007. The neuropsychiatry of the cerebellum: Insights from the clinic. *Cerebellum* **6:** 254–267.

Seidman, L., E. Valera & N. Makris. 2005. Structural brain imaging of attention-deficit/hyperactivity disorder. *Biological Psychiatry* **57:** 1263–1272.

Silveri, M., M. Leggio & M. Molinari. 1994. The cerebellum contributes to linguistic production: a case of agrammatic speech following a right cerebellar lesion. *Neurology* **44:** 2047–2050.

Snowling, M. 2000. *Dyslexia*. Oxford: Blackwell.

Sperling, A., Z.-L. Lu & F. Manis. 2004. Slower implicit categorical learning in adult poor readers. *Annals of Dyslexia* **54:** 281–303.

Stein, J. 2001. The sensory basis of reading problems. *Developmental Neuropsychology* **20:** 509–534.

Stein, J. & M. Glickstein. 1992. Role of the cerebellum in visual guidance of movement. *Physiological Review* **72:** 967–1017.

Stein, J. & V. Walsh. 1997. To see but not to read: the magnocellular theory of dyslexia. *Trends in Neurosciences* **20:** 147–152.

Stoodley, C. J., E. P. D. Harrison & J. F. Stein. 2006. Implicit motor learning deficits in dyslexic adults. *Neuropsychologia* **44/54:** 795–798.

Toni, I., M. Krams, R. Turner & R. Passingham. 1998. The time course of changes during motor sequence learning: a whole-brain fMRI study. *NeuroImage* **8:** 50–61.

Ungerleider, L. G., J. Doyon & A. Karni. 2002. Imaging brain plasticity during motor skill learning. *Neurobiology of Learning Memory* **78:** 553–564.

Vicari, S., A. Finzi, D. Menghini, L. Marotta, S. Baldi & L. Petrosini. 2005. Do children with developmental dyslexia have an implicit learning deficit? *Journal of Neurology, Neurosurgery and Psychiatry* **76:** 1392–1397.

Vicari, S., L. Marotta, D. Menghini, M. Molinari & L. Petrosini. 2003. Implicit learning deficit in children with developmental dyslexia. *Neuropsychologia* **41:** 108–114.

Waber, D., D. Marcus, P. Forbes, D. Bellinger, M. Weiler, L. Sorenson, *et al*. 2003. Motor sequence learning and reading ability: Is poor reading associated with sequencing deficits? *Journal of Experimental Child Psychology* **84:** 338–354.

Two Forms of Implicit Learning in Young Adults with Dyslexia

Ilana J. Bennett,[a] Jennifer C. Romano,[b] James H. Howard, Jr.,[b,c] and Darlene V. Howard[a]

[a]Department of Psychology, Georgetown University, Washington, DC, USA

[b]Department of Psychology, Catholic University of America, Washington, DC, USA

[c]Department of Neurology, Georgetown University, Washington, DC, USA

Implicit learning is thought to underlie the acquisition of many skills including reading. Previous research has shown that some forms of implicit learning are reduced in individuals with dyslexia (e.g., sequence learning), whereas other forms are spared (e.g., spatial context learning). However, it has been proposed that dyslexia-related motor dysfunction may have contributed to the implicit sequence learning deficits reported earlier. To assess implicit sequence learning in the absence of a motor sequence, 16 young adults diagnosed with dyslexia (20.6 ± 1.5 years) and 18 healthy controls (20.8 ± 2.0 years) completed a triplet frequency learning task (TRIP) that involved learning a sequential regularity in which the location of certain events followed a repeating pattern, but motor responses did not. Participants also completed the spatial contextual cueing task (SCCT), which involved learning a spatial regularity in which the location of distractors in some visual arrays predicted the target location. In addition, neuropsychological tests of real-word and pseudo-word reading were administered. TRIP task analyses revealed no between-group differences in pattern learning, but a positive correlation between individual learning scores and reading ability indicated that poor readers learned less well than did good readers. Thus, earlier reports of reduced implicit sequence learning in dyslexics cannot be entirely accounted for by motor sequencing deficits. No significant correlations or group differences in learning were found for SCCT. These findings offer additional evidence for a link between poor reading and impaired implicit sequence learning.

Key words: implicit learning; sequence learning; spatial context learning; dyslexia; reading ability

Introduction

Developmental dyslexia is characterized by low reading achievement despite normal intelligence and ample education or learning opportunity (American Psychiatric Association [APA], 2000). The reading weakness is typically attributed to phonological processing deficits whereby individuals with dyslexia have diffi-

culty learning associations between how words appear in print (graphemes) and how they sound (phonemes) (Bradley & Bryant, 1983; Ramus *et al.*, 2003; Snowling, 2001). However, this explanation does not account for the wide range of sensory, cognitive, and motor deficits also observed in dyslexia (Habib, 2000; Ramus *et al.*, 2003).

An alternative theory is that deficits associated with dyslexia are due to underlying impairments in skill learning (e.g., Nicolson & Fawcett, 1990; Rudel, 1985). This view is in line with dyslexia technically being classified as a learning disorder (APA, 2000). Skills

Address for correspondence: Ilana J. Bennett, Georgetown University, Department of Psychology, 301 N White Gravenor Hall, Washington, DC 20057. Voice: +202-687-4099; fax: +202-687-6050. ijb5@georgetown.edu

Ann. N.Y. Acad. Sci. 1145: 184–198 (2008). © 2008 New York Academy of Sciences.
doi: 10.1196/annals.1416.006

such as reading can be acquired through both explicit and implicit processes. For example, grapheme–phoneme associations are initially learned through explicit memorization, but implicit rule-based decoding skill evolves through repeated exposures to regularly formed words (Gombert, 2003; Uhry & Clark, 2005). Research has shown that explicit, effortful forms of skill learning are spared in poor readers and dyslexics (Sperling, Lu, & Manis, 2004; Vicari, Marotta, Menghini, Molinari, & Petrosini, 2003, Exp. 2), whereas studies of implicit learning have revealed a mixed pattern of spared (Howard, Howard, Japikse, & Eden, 2006; Kelly, Griffiths, & Frith, 2002; Russeler, Gerth, & Munte, 2006) and impaired (Howard *et al.*, 2006; Sperling *et al.*, 2004; Vicari *et al.*, 2005) learning.

Implicit learning occurs in a wide range of tasks that reveal nonconscious, unintentional sensitivity to regularities among stimuli (Seger, 1994). Studies have shown that these tasks differ not only in the nature of the regularity present, but also in the underlying neural systems they engage (Forkstam & Petersson, 2005; Stadler & Frensch, 1997). For example, implicit sequence learning tasks examine the learning of sequential regularities. In the serial reaction time task (SRTT) (Nissen & Bullemer, 1987), participants respond faster and more accurately to visual stimuli that follow a repeating sequence of locations versus stimuli that occur at randomly determined locations. On the other hand, implicit spatial context learning tasks investigate how spatial regularities are learned. In the spatial contextual cueing task (SCCT) (Chun & Jiang, 1998), search performance is better for visual arrays in which the configuration of distractors predicts the location of a target compared to nonpredictive arrays. Sequence learning tasks such as the SRTT have been shown to rely on a frontal-striatal-cerebellar network, whereas spatial context learning in the SCCT is mediated by medial temporal lobe structures, specifically the hippocampus and/or parahippocampal cortex (Chun & Phelps, 1999; Greene, Gross, Elsinger, & Rao, 2007; Prull, Gabrieli, & Bunge, 2000).

One study by Howard and colleagues (2006) found a dissociation between these two forms of implicit learning in the same group of young adults with dyslexia. Sequence learning was measured with a modified version of the SRTT, the alternating serial reaction time task (ASRT) (Howard & Howard, 1997), in which stimuli that follow a repeating sequence of locations (pattern) alternate with randomly determined stimuli (random). Analyses showed that the dyslexic group learned significantly less than age-matched controls on the ASRT task as determined by faster and more accurate responses to pattern versus random stimuli. But on the SCCT, there was no group difference in spatial context learning. In addition, correlations between reading ability and implicit learning revealed that poor reading ability was associated with reduced sequence learning, but preserved spatial context learning. These outcomes are consistent with data indicating that differences in brain function associated with dyslexia overlap with the neural systems involved in implicit sequence learning, but not with those involved in implicit spatial context learning. That is, compared to controls, individuals with dyslexia show reduced activation in inferior frontal and left temporal-parietal areas during language-based tasks (Collins & Rourke, 2003; Habib, 2000). Other imaging studies find that dyslexics have abnormal structure and function of the cerebellum (Eckert *et al.*, 2003; Finch, Nicolson, & Fawcett, 2002; Menghini, Hagberg, Caltagirone, Petrosini, & Vicari, 2006; Nicolson *et al.*, 1999; Rae *et al.*, 2002) and striatum (Brown *et al.*, 2001). Together these results suggest that frontal-striatal-cerebellar regions are affected in dyslexia. In contrast, abnormalities in medial temporal lobe structures are not known to be characteristic of dyslexia.

Implicit sequence learning deficits, like those observed by Howard and colleagues in 2006, have been reported in multiple studies of children and young adults with dyslexia (Menghini *et al.*, 2006; cf. Russeler *et al.*, 2006; Stoodley, Harrison, & Stein, 2006; Vicari *et al.*, 2005; Waber *et al.*, 2003). However, all of these studies used tasks in which a motor sequence was present. This is potentially important because there is evidence that dyslexic individuals have problems executing sequential motor movements. For example, deficient planning and timing of the sequential motor plans involved in speech production have been proposed to underlie dyslexia-related difficulties in repeating series of syllables and reading complex phrases (Catts, 1989; Wolff, Cohen, & Drake, 1984; Wolff, Michel, & Ovrut, 1990a). Nonlinguistic tasks also reveal motor sequencing problems in dyslexia. For instance, poor readers perform worse on finger-tapping tasks when they require alternating movements between hands versus repeating them with a single finger (Wolff, Michel, Ovrut, & Drake, 1990b), and dyslexic children demonstrate inferior coordination of movements during copying tasks (Denckla, 1985). Therefore, the question arises as to whether such motor sequencing deficits may have been the sole source of impairment reported in the earlier implicit sequence learning studies.

The present study was designed to assess implicit sequence learning in the absence of motor sequencing in young adults with and without dyslexia using a variation of the ASRT that contained no motor sequence (Howard, Howard, Dennis, & Kelly, 2008; Howard *et al.*, 2004). The same individuals completed the SCCT, which also does not require participants to use motor sequencing. In addition to examining group differences, correlation analyses were performed using measures of the two types of implicit learning and reading ability because previous studies have indicated that continuous measures of reading skill may be more sensitive than the dichotomous group variable (Conlon, Sanders, & Zapart, 2004; Howard *et al.*, 2006; Shaywitz, Escobar, Shaywitz, Fletcher, & Makuch, 1992). It was expected that if earlier reports of reduced implicit sequence learning in poor readers and individuals with dyslexia were solely due to motor sequencing deficits, then there should be no group differences on the nonmotor sequence

learning task and no relationship between nonmotor sequence learning and reading ability. However, if the deficits were due at least in part to a more general sequencing deficit, then the dyslexic group should learn less than the nondyslexic group in the present task, and poor reading should be associated with less learning. For spatial context learning, it was expected that there would be no group differences in learning and no relationship between measures of learning and reading ability, indicating preserved spatial context learning in young adult poor readers.

Methods

Participants

Participants were 16 individuals with dyslexia and 18 nondyslexic controls. Inclusion criteria for all participants were being an undergraduate student at the Catholic University of America between the ages of 18 and 25 years. Participants in the dyslexic group met criteria for a diagnosis of dyslexia according to the Catholic University Disability Support Services Office, which was based on current and comprehensive neuropsychological evaluations and interviews with qualified professionals. Individuals were excluded from the dyslexic group if they also met criteria for dysgraphia, or had an unspecified learning disorder. Participants in the control group had no history of learning disability. Table 1 presents demographic and neuropsychological characterizations for each group. Participants received either payment or course credit and gave informed consent for experimental procedures approved by the Catholic University of America Institutional Review Board.

General Procedure

Participants completed 1-hour testing sessions on each of three separate days. On the first day, they signed an informed consent form and then completed the triplet task (TRIP). The

TABLE 1. Demographics and Neuropsychological Test Results

	Dyslexic ($n = 16$)	Control ($n = 18$)	t
Demographics			
Age	20.6 ± 1.5	20.8 ± 2.0	n.s.
Male/female	4/12	5/13	
Neuropsychological tests			
WASI Two-Subtest IQ SS	109.8 ± 10.5	115.6 ± 9.1	n.s.
WJ-III Word Identification SS	92.0 ± 8.2	103.5 ± 6.8	4.1**
WJ-III Word Attack SS	87.1 ± 10.0	98.8 ± 10.7	3.6*
WJ-III Spelling SS	93.4 ± 10.4	110.2 ± 7.4	5.4**
RAN average speed	28.3 ± 3.7	23.9 ± 3.9	-3.4*
RAN average errors	1.8 ± 4.1	0.9 ± 0.7	n.s.
WAIS-III Digit Symbol coding	69.4 ± 16.0	85.1 ± 23.3	2.3*
WAIS-III Digit Symbol pairing	14.8 ± 2.8	14.8 ± 3.2	n.s.
WAIS-III Digit Symbol recall	7.7 ± 1.4	7.8 ± 1.1	n.s.
WAIS-III Digit Span forward	9.8 ± 2.1	11.7 ± 2.1	2.7*
WAIS-III Digit Span backward	6.6 ± 2.5	8.1 ± 2.1	n.s.
Auditory Consonant Trigrams	5.4 ± 2.9	8.1 ± 1.8	3.2**

Notes. All scores are given as mean $\pm$ SD based on raw data, except where standard scores are noted. Independent sample *t*-tests show group effects (*$P < .05$, **$P < .001$, n.s. = not significant). WASI = Wechsler Abbreviated Scale of Intelligence; WJ-III = Woodcock-Johnson, 3rd edition; SS = age-adjusted standard score with a mean of 100 and standard deviation of 15; RAN = Rapid Automatized Naming; and WAIS-III = Wechsler Adult Intelligence Scale, 3rd edition.

spatial contextual cueing task (SCCT) was completed on the second day. Neuropsychological tests were administered on the third day. The three testing sessions were completed within a 1-week period for all participants, except for one dyslexic subject whose testing spanned 12 weeks.

Triplet Frequency Learning Task (TRIP)

For the TRIP task, participants viewed four black outlined open circles presented in a horizontal row on a 15 in. (38 cm) Apple iMac computer monitor. For purposes of description below, the four stimulus locations are referred to as 1, 2, 3, and 4, where 1 is the leftmost position and 4 is the rightmost position. However, numbers never appeared on the screen. Each trial, referred to as a triplet, comprised three discrete events, in which two red circles appear, one after the other, followed by a green circle. Participants were instructed to respond to the location of the green event using the middle and index fingers of each hand to press the corresponding buttons ("z", "x", "/" and

"." on the keyboard). Each of the three events was presented for 120 ms with a 150 ms inter-stimulus interval. The green event remained on the screen until the correct response was made, and 650 ms later the next trial began. Participants completed thirty 50-trial blocks. They were encouraged to take short breaks after each block.

Like the ASRT (Howard *et al.*, 2006), the TRIP task contained a second-order sequential structure, in which the location of every other stimulus follows a repeating pattern. As a result of this sequential regularity in the ASRT task, stimulus location on trial n predicts the location of trial $n + 2$. For example, in the sequence 1r2r3r4r, numbers represent the predictable, alternating trials that follow the repeating pattern, with 1 through 4 denoting the location of the filled-in circle, and the letter "r" referring to trials where the stimulus could occur at any of the four locations. The same sequential regularity occurred in the TRIP task, with the location of the first event within a triplet predicting the location of the third event. For example, in the triplet 1r2, where 1 and "r" refer to red events and 2 refers to the green event, the first red circle at location 1 predicts that the green circle will occur at location 2, with the location of the second red event being randomly determined. Thus, the triplet 1r2 is consistent with the repeating pattern 1r2r3r4r. In the ASRT, runs of three consecutive trials (i.e., triplets) that were consistent with the pattern (high-frequency triplets) occurred 75% of the time, and pattern-inconsistent triplets (low-frequency triplets) occurred 25% of the time. However, in this TRIP task, high-frequency and low-frequency triplets occurred 90% and 10% of the time, respectively.

Participants received feedback at the end of each block that was designed to direct responding to 92% accuracy. The feedback consisted of mean reaction time and mean accuracy for a given block, plus a statement prompting them to "focus more on accuracy" if their mean accuracy was below 90% or to "focus more on speed" if their mean accuracy was above 94%.

A recognition task and an interview were used to assess explicit knowledge of the sequential regularity. In a 24-trial recognition task (Howard *et al.*, 2004), all possible combinations of triplet events were presented with the black circles, not red and green circles. For each triplet, participants were instructed to indicate whether that combination of events occurred "frequently" or "infrequently" during the task by pressing one of two buttons. A postexperiment interview was also administered. Questions ranged from general inquiries about strategies used to improve performance and the frequency of events occurring at each location to more specific questions about the relationships between the red and green events, asking participants to describe the regularity if they noticed one.

Spatial Contextual Cueing Task

Stimuli and procedures for the SCCT used here are identical to those described previously (Howard *et al.*, 2006). Participants viewed visual arrays on a 15 in. (38 cm) Apple iMac com-

puter monitor. Arrays were made up of 11 distractors (the letter *L* rotated by 0, 90, 180, or 270 degrees) and one target (horizontal letter T) that were white against a gray background. Distractors were made more similar to the target by offsetting the L legs by 3 pixels (Chun & Phelps, 1999, Exp. 2). On each trial, a fixation dot appeared for one second, followed by an array. Participants were instructed to search the array for the target and respond as quickly and accurately as possible by pressing "z" if the tail of the horizontal T was pointing left or "/" if it was pointing right, using their left and right index fingers, respectively. Auditory feedback after each response indicated correct (short beep) and incorrect (long tone) responses. If responses did not occur within 6 seconds, the trial ended with a long tone indicating an incorrect response, and the next trial began. Participants completed one practice block of 24 novel arrays, and then thirty 24-trial test blocks. They were encouraged to take short breaks after each block.

Twelve arrays repeated across all test blocks. In these familiar arrays, the locations of the distractors predicted the location of the target but not its orientation. Therefore, this regularity could not be used to predict the correct response. The remaining 12 arrays for each block were novel across the experiment. Within each block, presentation of familiar and novel arrays was randomized.

A recognition task and an interview were used to assess explicit knowledge of the spatial regularity. In a 24-trial recognition task (Chun & Jiang, 2003) the screen was divided into four quadrants by short lines placed at the midpoints of each side of the screen. The 12 familiar arrays from the test blocks and 12 novel arrays were presented with a distractor in place of the target location. For each array, participants were instructed to indicate which quadrant the target would most likely have occurred in by pressing one of four buttons on the keyboard. A postexperiment interview was also administered, with questions ranging from general inquiries about the task and material to more specific questions asking participants whether they noticed that certain displays repeated across trials.

Neuropsychological Testing

A battery of neuropsychological tests was administered to characterize the cognitive profiles of each group. Some tests were later correlated with measures of implicit learning. An intelligence quotient (IQ) was calculated using two subtests of the Wechsler Abbreviated Scale of Intelligence (WASI) (Wechsler, 1999): the Vocabulary subtest that involved defining orally presented words, and the Matrix Reasoning subtest that entailed identifying the missing piece of an abstract visual display. Real-word and pseudo-word reading were assessed with the Woodcock–Johnson (WJ-III) (Woodcock, McGrew, & Mather, 2001) Word Identification and Word Attack subtests, respectively, in which participants read aloud lists of English words or pronounceable nonsense words. The WJ-III Spelling subtest measured participants' ability to write orally presented words. Rapid Automatized Naming (RAN) (Denckla & Rudel, 1974) assessed the speed of naming separate series of colors, objects, letters, and numbers. The Wechsler Adult Intelligence Scale (WAIS-III) (Wechsler, 1997) Digit Symbol Coding subtest measured hand–eye coordination and processing speed by giving participants 2 minutes to fill in the symbols that corresponded to a series of digits. Cued recall of the digit–symbol pairs and free recall of the symbols were assessed with the WAIS-III Digit Symbol Pairing and Recall subtests, respectively. Working memory was measured with WAIS-III Digit Span Forward and Backward, and Consonant Trigrams (Peterson & Peterson, 1959). The digit span task involved repeating progressively longer strings of numbers in the same (forward) or reverse (backward) order they were presented, and Consonant Trigrams required that participants recall three consonants after short intervals during which they performed a distracting counting task.

Results

Demographics and Neuropsychological Data

Demographic information and neuropsychological test results are presented in Table 1. The dyslexic and control groups were matched on age and gender. Neuropsychological tests revealed a pattern characteristic of dyslexia in that both groups were of normal intelligence, but the dyslexic group performed significantly worse than the control group on measures of real-word and pseudo-word reading (WJ-III Word Identification and Word Attack subtests, respectively), spelling (WJ-III Spelling), naming speed (RAN average speed of the four stimulus sets), hand–eye coordination and processing speed (WAIS-III Digit Symbol Coding), and working memory (WAIS-III Digit Span Forward and Consonant Trigrams).

Implicit Learning Data: Group Analyses

Implicit learning was examined in each task using separate repeated-measures ANOVAs for reaction time and accuracy measures. For each block, median reaction times on correct trials and mean accuracy scores were calculated for high-frequency and low-frequency triplets in the TRIP task and for familiar and novel arrays in the SCCT. A variable of epoch was then created by taking the mean of these scores across groups of five blocks.

Implicit Sequence Learning (TRIP)

To assess potential group differences in implicit sequence learning, group (dyslexic, control) × triplet type (high-frequency, low-frequency) × epoch (1–6) mixed-design ANOVAs were conducted separately for reaction time and accuracy measures (Fig. 1).

For reaction time, the dyslexic group (423.4 ± 51.8 ms) responded significantly slower than the control group (390.1 ± 54.6 ms), $F(1, 32) = 5.9$, $P < .03$. A main effect of epoch, $F(5, 160) = 67.7$, $P < .001$, and a

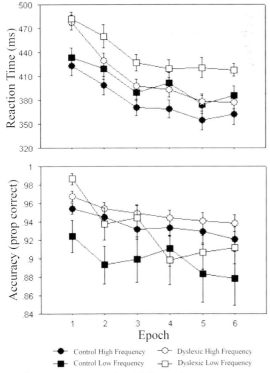

Figure 1. For the TRIP task, responses to high-frequency (*circles*) and low-frequency (*squares*) triplets for the control (*solid symbols*) and dyslexic (*open symbols*) groups on mean of median reaction time (ms) and mean accuracy (proportion correct) measures.

group × epoch interaction, $F(5, 160) = 2.5$, $P < .04$, showed that overall speed increased more across epochs for the dyslexic group compared to controls. Sequence learning was revealed by significant effects of triplet type, $F(1, 32) = 112.9$, $P < .001$, and triplet type × epoch, $F(5, 160) = 4.4$, $P < .001$, with faster responses to high-frequency (393.4 ± 54.0 ms) versus low-frequency (418.1 ± 54.8 ms) triplets, a difference that increased across epochs. Group × triplet type and group × triplet type × epoch interactions were not significant, P's $> .10$, indicating that we did not detect group differences in sequence learning.

For accuracy, the dyslexic group ($94.0 \pm 5.9\%$) did not differ from the control group ($91.7 \pm 8.0\%$), $P > .15$, showing that, as intended, the feedback provided after every block successfully matched the groups on overall ac-

curacy. A significant main effect of epoch, $F(5, 160) = 7.2$, $P < .001$, showed that accuracy decreased across epochs, which is typical in sequence learning tasks as participants make increasingly more errors on pattern-inconsistent trials as they learn the regularity. Sequence learning was seen as a main effect of triplet type, $F(1, 32) = 13.6$, $P < .001$, with more accurate responses to high-frequency ($94.2 \pm 4.0\%$) versus low-frequency ($91.4 \pm 9.2\%$) triplets. In line with the reaction time results, group differences in sequence learning were not observed in either the group × triplet type or group × triplet type × epoch interactions, P's $> .21$.

Implicit Spatial Context Learning (SCCT)

To assess implicit spatial context learning, group (dyslexic, control) × array type (familiar, novel) × epoch (1–6) mixed-design ANOVAs were conducted for both behavioral measures (Fig. 2). One control participant was not included in this analysis because the data were lost because of a computer error.

For reaction time, responses were significantly slower in the dyslexic group (2.1 ± 0.4 sec) compared to the control group (1.8 ± 0.5 sec), $F(1, 31) = 4.8$, $P < .04$. There was a significant main effect of epoch, $F(5, 155) = 64.8$, $P < .001$, with responses speeding up across epochs. Spatial context learning was revealed by faster responses to familiar arrays (1.9 ± 0.5 sec) compared to novel arrays (2.0 ± 0.4 sec), $F(1, 31) = 4.3$, $P < .05$. There were no significant group differences in learning (group × array type, $P > .68$; group × array type × epoch, $P > .06$). However, the marginal three-way interaction was followed up with separate array type × epoch ANOVAs for each group, which revealed significant learning in the control group (array type, $F(1, 16) = 5.1$, $P < .04$; array type × epoch, $F(5, 80) = 2.9$, $P < .03$), but not in the dyslexic group (P's $> .34$).

For accuracy, the dyslexic group ($92.9 \pm 6.2\%$) made significantly more errors than the control group ($96.0 \pm 3.5\%$), $F(1, 31) = 6.9$, $P < .02$. A main effect of epoch, $F(5,$

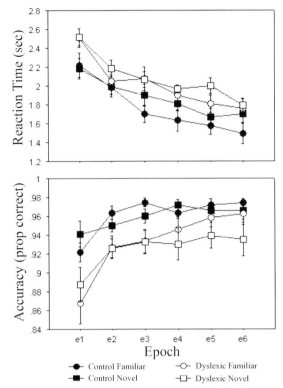

Figure 2. For the SCCT, responses to familiar (*circle*) and novel (*square*) arrays for the control (*solid symbols*) and dyslexic (*open symbols*) groups on mean of median reaction time (sec) and mean accuracy (proportion correct) measures.

$155) = 22.1$, $P < .001$, showed that accuracy increased across epochs. The array type effect did not attain significance, $P > .19$, but spatial context learning was seen with a significant array–type $\times$ epoch interaction, $F(5, 155) = 3.3$, $P < .01$. Group $\times$ array type and group $\times$ array type $\times$ epoch interactions were not significant, P's $> .29$, indicating that there were no group differences in learning.

Correlations between Implicit Learning and Reading Ability

As indicated earlier, it is important to conduct correlations between individual measures of reading ability and implicit learning because these analyses may better capture relationships with reading skill, especially when there is a broad range of reading ability within both groups, and an overlap between the groups. Learning scores for each behavioral measure were calculated for each participant by taking the difference, in the final epoch, between high-frequency versus low-frequency triplets for the TRIP task and familiar versus novel arrays for the SCCT. Real-word and pseudo-word reading were measured for each participant, using age-adjusted standard scores from the WJ-III Word Identification and Word Attack subtests.

A significant positive correlation was observed for the TRIP accuracy learning score and pseudo-word reading, $r = +.38$, $P < .03$. Thus, although there were no group differences in sequence learning, this correlation shows that poor reading is associated with reduced sequence learning. There was also a nonsignificant trend, $r = +.31$, $P < .09$, for poor pseudo-word reading to be associated with lower SCCT reaction time learning scores, which is in line with the group analyses that revealed spatial context learning on the reaction time measure in the control group, but not the dyslexic group. Scatter plots for these correlations are presented in Figure 3. Correlations between implicit learning scores and real-word reading were in the same direction as above, but they did not attain significance, P's $> .40$.

Correlations between Implicit Learning and Rapid Naming

Because of the similarities between sequential processing in implicit sequence learning and rapid naming (e.g., sequential eye movements, processing sequentially presented stimuli, and executing sequential motor responses), correlations were also conducted between TRIP learning scores and measures of average speed and average errors from the four stimulus sets of the RAN. In line with previous studies that show that poor reading is associated with worse performance on the RAN (Denckla & Rudel, 1976; Wolf, Bowers, & Biddle, 2000), a significant negative correlation was seen between pseudo-word reading and average RAN

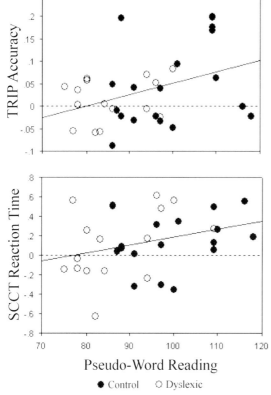

Figure 3. Scatter plots separately comparing learning scores for the TRIP task (accuracy) and SCCT (reaction time) to the measure of pseudo-word reading (age-scaled score) for the control (*solid circle*) and dyslexic (*open circle*) groups.

speed, $r = -.44$, $P < .01$. More importantly, results revealed a significant negative correlation between RAN speed and the TRIP accuracy learning score, $r = -.39$, $P < .03$, indicating that individuals who performed more slowly on the rapid naming task also learned less on the TRIP task.

Measures of Implicitness

After the TRIP task, participants completed a recognition task in which they judged the frequency of all combinations of triplet events. Mean recognition ratings were calculated for each participant as the proportion of times high-frequency and low-frequency triplets were reported as having occurred "frequently" during the task. A group (dyslexic, control) × triplet

type (high-frequency, low-frequency) mixed-design ANOVA showed no significant effects (P's $> .14$), indicating that high-frequency ($.42 \pm .14$) and low-frequency ($.45 \pm .08$) triplets were rated as occurring equally often in both the dyslexic and control groups. Similarly, analyses of the postexperiment interview did not reveal any explicit awareness. Three dyslexic and six control participants indicated that they noticed a relationship between either of the two red events and the third green event, but no individual accurately described the nature of the regularity.

After the SCCT, participants completed a recognition task that involved viewing arrays in which the targets were replaced by distractors and indicated in which quadrant the target would most likely have occurred. Mean accuracy scores were calculated for each participant for familiar and novel arrays. A group (dyslexic, control) × array type (familiar, novel) mixed-design ANOVA revealed no significant effects (P's $> .08$). That is, target quadrants were recognized equally often for familiar and novel arrays for both groups. Thus, as for the TRIP task, analyses of the postexperiment interviews did not reveal any explicit awareness of the spatial regularity. Eight dyslexic and five control participants indicated that they noticed certain displays repeated across trials. However, none of them reported explicitly trying to memorize the displays to facilitate performance.

Taken together, recognition tests and postexperiment interviews for both the TRIP and SCCT indicated that no participant had explicit awareness of either regularity even though they responded faster and/or more accurately to high-frequency versus low-frequency triplets and familiar versus novel arrays.

Discussion

This study examined the relationship between two forms of implicit learning (sequence learning and spatial context learning) and reading ability in young adults with and without dyslexia. Implicit sequence learning was assessed in the absence of motor sequencing using the TRIP task to determine whether motor sequencing deficits could be the sole source of sequence learning impairment previously seen in poor readers and individuals with dyslexia (Howard *et al.*, 2006; Menghini *et al.*, 2006; Stoodley *et al.*, 2006; Vicari *et al.*, 2005). In contrast to previous studies that used motor sequence learning tasks, between-group analyses revealed no group differences in learning. However, in line with those studies, pseudo-word reading was positively correlated with the TRIP accuracy learning score, indicating that poor readers had sequence learning deficits even when there was no motor sequence to be learned. Implicit spatial context learning, measured with the SCCT task, revealed no group differences in learning as previously reported (Howard *et al.*, 2006), and there were no significant correlations between spatial context learning and reading ability. Unlike some previous studies that could not rule out explicit learning, results observed here must be due to implicit learning because there was no evidence of explicit awareness in either the TRIP or SCCT task, as assessed via recognition tests and verbal reports. The findings are discussed in more detail below.

Implicit Sequence Learning

A significant positive correlation between pseudo-word reading and TRIP learning on the accuracy measure was found in the current study. The analogous correlation was also observed in a study by Howard and colleagues (2006), using the ASRT learning task. This suggests that poor (pseudo-word) readers are relatively worse at sequence learning whether or not a motor sequence is present, because the ASRT task contained a sequence of motor responses but the TRIP task does not. Thus, earlier reports of sequence learning deficits (Howard *et al.*, 2006; Menghini *et al.*, 2006; Stoodley *et al.*, 2006; Vicari *et al.*, 2005) cannot be explained by motor sequencing

deficits alone. Instead, implicit sequence learning deficits in poor readers are likely due, at least in part, to difficulty learning other forms of sequential information that are present in both the TRIP and ASRT tasks, such as the perceptual sequence of stimuli and/or the sequence of eye movements to fixate the target stimuli (Goschke, 1998; Mayr, 1996; Seger, 1997).

In fact, there is existing evidence that poor readers have perceptual sequence learning deficits. For example, one study found significantly less learning in dyslexics versus controls using a task that contained a perceptual sequence, but not motor response or eye movement sequences (Vicari *et al.*, 2003). Perceptual sequence learning deficits are predicted by the temporal processing theory, which states that individuals with dyslexia are poorer at integrating sequential sensory information, especially when stimuli are presented rapidly (Habib, 2000). This theory developed from work showing that children and young adults with dyslexia have difficulty on tasks that involve processing rapid sequences of auditory (Helenius, Uutela, & Hari, 1999; Tallal, 1980) and visual (Conlon *et al.*, 2004; Eden, Stein, Wood, & Wood, 1995) stimuli. Other explanations have been proposed for the perceptual sequencing deficits in dyslexia, including deficient sensory processing in the magnocellular pathway (Stein, 2001), delayed attention shifting (Hari & Renvall, 2001), and limited perceptual memory (Ben-Yehudah, Sackett, Malchi-Ginzberg, & Ahissar, 2001). According to the latter explanation, individuals with dyslexia have a limited capacity to retain perceptual traces and compare them across short intervals. In the TRIP task, learning involves retaining perceptual traces across the three events within a trial, binding these events into a triplet, and then comparing triplets across trials. Thus, an inability to retain and compare perceptual traces could manifest as implicit sequence learning deficits in poor readers.

It could also be argued that difficulty learning the sequence of eye movements to fixate the targets contributes to sequence learning deficits in poor readers. However, support for this view is hard to establish because there are conflicting results from examinations of oculomotor control in poor readers. Some studies report that individuals with dyslexia make more eye movements and have difficulty maintaining fixation compared to controls (Biscaldi, Gezeck, & Stuhr, 1998; Eden, Stein, Wood, & Wood, 1994; Pavlidis, 1981), whereas others find no group differences (Black, Collins, De Roach, & Zubrick, 1984; Olson, Kliegl, & Davidson, 1983; Stanley, Smith, & Howell, 1983). If present, abnormal eye movements in poor readers would affect their ability to fixate the targets during sequence learning tasks, which may influence their perception of the sequential stimuli, and ultimately affect their sequence learning performance. In either case, the TRIP task does not allow us to separate perceptual and eye movement sequencing deficits in poor readers

Sequencing deficits in poor readers have also been observed in analyses of the rapid automatized naming task (RAN). Although the RAN is usually thought of as a measure of phonological retrieval (Wagner & Torgesen, 1987) or processing speed (Wolf & Bowers, 1999), the nature of the task suggests that sequential processing is also involved. Stimuli for the RAN include separate cards that display series of colored squares, objects, letters, and numbers. Participants are instructed to name the items on each card out loud as fast as possible. Thus, successful completion of the task involves making sequential eye movements to fixate the items, processing the perceptual sequence of stimuli, and then executing the speech-related sequence of motor movements. Results from both group analyses and correlations between pseudo-word reading and RAN average speed replicated previous findings of reduced rapid naming ability in poor readers (Denckla & Rudel, 1976; Wolf et al., 2000). Interestingly, slow naming was significantly associated with less learning on the TRIP accuracy learning score, supporting the notion that both RAN

and TRIP tasks reflect a sequencing deficit in poor readers.

The relationship between implicit sequence learning, reading ability, and speech production makes sense from an evolutionary perspective. According to this view, language skills such as speech and reading may have evolved from similar but more basic processes like sequence learning. Speech production involves sequential motor movements and is therefore thought to have been adapted from neural networks involved in motor sequencing (Lieberman, 2002). Similarly, reading, an even more recent sequential skill than speech, may have evolved from more primitive sequencing functions (Dehaene, 2004). This perspective is strengthened by the fact that these three processes rely on similar neural structures including frontal regions, cortical motor areas, the striatum, and the cerebellum (Bohland & Guenther, 2006; Fiez & Petersen, 1998; Lieberman, 2002; Riecker et al., 2005; Wildgruber, Ackerman, & Grodd, 2001).

When dyslexic and control groups were combined, both the present TRIP study and a previous study that employed the ASRT (Howard et al., 2006) found positive correlations between reading ability (pseudo-word reading) and implicit sequence learning. However, unlike the previous study, the current study did not find significant group differences in learning. Interpreting the between-group effects is complicated because, in addition to differences in the presence (ASRT) or absence (TRIP) of motor sequencing, the TRIP and ASRT tasks differ in ways that do not allow for direct comparison across tasks. For example, although both tasks had the same structural complexity (i.e., event n + 2 is predicted by event n), the ratio of high-frequency triplets to low-frequency triplets was higher in the TRIP task (9:1) compared to the ASRT task (3:1), perhaps making the TRIP task easier to learn. The TRIP task also isolated the triplets from the sequence by presenting each triplet as a discrete trial, whereas triplets in the ASRT task occur in a continuous overlapping stream. Nonetheless, because correlation analyses revealed similar effects for reading ability across studies, it suggests that, as previously indicated by others (Conlon *et al.*, 2004; Howard *et al.*, 2006; Shaywitz et al., 1992), our understanding of this heterogeneous disorder might be clarified if future research includes correlation analyses that treat reading ability as a continuous variable in addition to group analyses that treat reading skill as a dichotomous variable based on diagnoses of dyslexia.

Implicit Spatial Context Learning

Results for implicit spatial context learning in this study were only partially consistent with our predictions based on an earlier examination of spatial context learning in young adults with dyslexia (Howard *et al.*, 2006). As expected, there were no significant group differences in learning on the SCCT. However, there was a trend for a positive correlation between pseudo-word reading and SCCT learning on the reaction time measure, whereas a negative correlation had been reported previously (Howard *et al.*, 2006). Direct comparisons of the results from these two studies are complicated because in the present study, but not in the earlier study, the dyslexic group was significantly less accurate than the control group. In addition, none of the group comparisons or correlations between reading ability and SCCT learning in the present study is significant, revealing only marginal trends. Thus, results from both studies suggest that implicit spatial context learning is preserved in poor readers.

Future Considerations

Additional research is necessary to clarify the impaired and spared implicit learning abilities in poor readers and individuals diagnosed with dyslexia. Deficits have been reported for sequence learning (Howard *et al.*, 2006; Menghini *et al.*, 2006; Stoodley *et al.*, 2006; Vicari *et al.*, 2005), mirror drawing (Vicari *et al.*, 2005), and categorical learning (Sperling *et al.*, 2004).

However, other forms of implicit learning, such as spatial context learning (Howard *et al.*, 2006) and some types of artificial grammar learning (Pothos & Kirk, 2004; Russeler *et al.*, 2006), appear to be relatively spared. This information may be relevant to training programs that could improve reading fluency in dyslexia by either targeting underlying deficits in implicit learning or by capitalizing on intact implicit learning processes.

Acknowledgments

This research was funded by Grant R37 AG15450 from the National Institute on Aging/National Institutes of Health. We want to thank Carly Shoupe, Elizabeth Bonner, Tara Kraft, Richard Garlipp, and Lauren Mays for their help with data collection. Preliminary findings from this project were presented at the 25th Rodin Remediation Academy Conference in Washington, DC in October 2006.

Conflicts of Interest

The authors declare no conflicts of interest.

References

American Psychiatric Association. 2000. *Diagnostic and statistical manual of mental disorders,* (4th ed, text revision). Washington, DC: Author.

Ben-Yehudah, G., E. Sackett, L. Malchi-Ginzberg & M. Ahissar. 2001. Impaired temporal contrast sensitivity in dyslexics is specific to retain-and-compare paradigms. *Brain* **124:** 1381–1395.

Biscaldi, M., S. Gezeck & V. Stuhr. 1998. Poor saccadic control correlates with dyslexia. *Neuropsychologia* **36**(11): 1189–1202.

Black, J. L., D. W. Collins, J. N. De Roach & S. Zubrick. 1984. A detailed study of sequential saccadic eye movements for normal- and poor-reading children. *Perceptual and Motor Skills* **59**(2): 423–434.

Bohland, J. W. & F. H. Guenther. 2006. An fMRI investigation of syllable sequence production. *NeuroImage* **32**(2): 821–841.

Bradley, L. & P. E. Bryant. 1983. Categorizing sounds and learning to read: a causal connection. *Nature* **301:** 419–421.

Brown, W. E., S. Eliez, V. Menon, J. M. Rumsey, C. D. White & A. L. Reiss. 2001. Preliminary evidence of widespread morphological variations in the brain in dyslexics. *Neurology* **56**(6): 781–783.

Catts, H. W. 1989. Speech production deficits in developmental dyslexia. *Journal of Speech and Hearing Disorders* **54**(3): 422–428.

Chun, M. M. & Y. Jiang. 1998. Contextual cueing: implicit learning and memory of visual context guides spatial attention. *Cognitive Psychology* **36**: 28–71.

Chun, M. M. & Y. Jiang. 2003. Implicit, long-term spatial contextual memory. *Journal of Experimental Psychology: Learning, Memory, & Cognition* **29**(2): 224–234.

Chun, M. M. & E. A. Phelps. 1999. Memory deficits for implicit contextual information in amnestic subjects with hippocampal damage. *Nature Neuroscience* **2**(9): 844–847.

Collins, D. W. & B. P. Rourke. 2003. Learning-disabled brains: a review of the literature. *Journal of Clinical and Experimental Neuropsychology* **25**(7): 1011–1034.

Conlon, E., M. Sanders & S. Zapart. 2004. Temporal processing in poor adult readers. *Neuropsychologia* **42**: 142–157.

Dehaene, S. 2004. Evolution of human cortical circuits for reading and arithmetic: the "neuronal recycling" hypothesis. In S. Dehaene, J. R. Duhamel, M. Hauser & G. Rizzolatti (Eds.), *From monkey brain to human brain* (pp. 133–158). Cambridge, MA: MIT Press.

Denckla, M. B. 1985. Motor coordination in dyslexic children: theoretical and clinical implications. In F. H. Duffy & N. Geschwind (Eds.), *Dyslexia: A neuroscientific approach to clinical evaluation* (pp. 187–195). Boston, MA: Little, Brown and Company.

Denckla, M. B. & R. D. Rudel. 1976. Rapid automatized naming (R.A.N.): dyslexia differentiated from other learning disabilities. *Neuropsychologia* **14**: 471–479.

Denckla, M. B. & R. G. Rudel. 1974. Rapid "automatized" naming of pictured objects, colors, letters, and numbers by normal children. *Cortex* **10**: 186–202.

Eckert, M. A., C. M. Leonard, T. L. Richards, E. H. Aylward, J. Thomson & V. W. Berninger. 2003. Anatomical correlates of dyslexia: frontal and cerebellar findings. *Brain* **126**(2): 482–494.

Eden, G. F., J. F. Stein, H. M. Wood & F. B. Wood. 1994. Differences in eye movements and reading problems in dyslexic and normal children. *Vision Research* **34**(10): 1345–1358.

Eden, G. F., J. F. Stein, H. M. Wood & F. B. Wood. 1995. Temporal and spatial processing in reading disabled and normal children. *Cortex* **31**: 451–468.

Fiez, J. A. & S. E. Petersen. 1998. Neuroimaging studies of word reading. *Proceedings of the National Academy of Sciences USA* **95**(3): 914–921.

Finch, A. J., R. I. Nicolson & A. J. Fawcett. 2002. Evidence for a neuroanatomical difference within the olivo-cerebellar pathway of adults with dyslexia. *Cortex* **38**(4): 529–539.

Forkstam, C. & K. M. Petersson. 2005. Towards an explicit account of implicit learning. *Current Opinions in Neurology* **18**: 435–441.

Gombert, J. E. 2003. Implicit and explicit learning to read: implication as for subtypes of dyslexia. *Current Psychology Letters: Behavior, Brain & Cognition* **10**(1): 25–40.

Goschke, T. 1998. Implicit learning of perceptual and motor sequences. In M. A. Stadler & P. A. Frensch (Eds.), *Handbook of implicit learning* (pp. 401–444). Thousand Oaks, CA: Sage Publications, Inc.

Greene, A. J., W. L. Gross, C. L. Elsinger & S. M. Rao. 2007. Hippocampal differentiation without recognition: an fMRI analysis of the contextual cueing task. *Learning and Memory* **14**(8): 548–554.

Habib, M. 2000. The neurological basis of developmental dyslexia. An overview and working hypothesis. *Brain* **123**: 2373–2399.

Hari, R. & H. Renvall. 2001. Impaired processing of rapid stimulus sequences in dyslexia. *Trends in Cognitive Sciences* **5**(12): 525–532.

Helenius, P., K. Uutela & R. Hari. 1999. Auditory stream segregation in dyslexic adults. *Brain* **122**(5): 907–913.

Howard, J. H. Jr. & D. V. Howard. 1997. Age differences in implicit learning of higher order dependencies in serial patterns. *Psychology and Aging* **12**: 634–656.

Howard, J. H. Jr., D. V. Howard, N. A. Dennis & A. J. Kelly. 2008. Implicit learning of predictive relationships in three element visual sequences by young and old adults. *Journal of Experimental Psychology: Learning, Memory and Cognition* **34**: 1139–1157.

Howard, J. H. Jr., D. V. Howard, K. C. Japikse & G. F. Eden. 2006. Dyslexics are impaired on implicit higher-order sequence learning but not on implicit spatial context learning. *Neuropsychologia* **44**(7): 1131–1144.

Howard, J. H. Jr., A. J. Kelly, N. A. Dennis, C. J. Vaidya, R. F. Barr & D. V. Howard. 2004. *Age-related deficits in implicit learning of higher-order sequential structure in the absence of motor sequencing.* Paper presented at the Ninth Cognitive Aging Conference, Atlanta, GA.

Kelly, S. W., S. Griffiths & U. Frith. 2002. Evidence for implicit sequence learning in dyslexia. *Dyslexia* **8**(1): 43–52.

Lieberman, P. 2002. On the nature and evolution of the neural bases of human language. *American Journal of Physical Anthropology* **119**(S35): 36–62.

Mayr, U. 1996. Spatial attention and implicit sequence learning: evidence for independent learning of spatial and nonspatial sequences. *Journal of Experimental Psychology: Learning, Memory, & Cognition* **22**: 350–364.

Menghini, D., G. E. Hagberg, C. Caltagirone, L. Petrosini & S. Vicari. 2006. Implicit learning deficits in dyslexic adults: an fMRI study. *NeuroImage* **33:** 1218–1226.

Nicolson, R. I. & A. J. Fawcett. 1990. Automaticity: a new framework for dyslexia research? *Cognition* **30:** 159–182.

Nicolson, R. I., A. J. Fawcett, E. L. Berry, I. H. Jenkins, P. Dean & D. J. Brooks. 1999. Association of abnormal cerebellar activation with motor learning difficulties in dyslexic adults. *Lancet* **15**(353): 1662–1667.

Nissen, M. J. & P. Bullemer. 1987. Attentional requirements of learning: evidence from performance measures. *Cognitive Psychology* **19:** 1–32.

Olson, R. K., R. Kliegl & B. J. Davidson. 1983. Dyslexic and normal readers' eye movements. *Journal of Experimental Psychology: Human Perception and Performance* **9**(5): 816–825.

Pavlidis, G. T. 1981. Do eye movements hold the key to dyslexia? *Neuropsychologia* **19**(1): 58–64.

Peterson, L. R. & M. J. Peterson. 1959. Short-term retention of individual verbal items. *Journal of Experimental Psychology* **58:** 193–198.

Pothos, E. M. & J. Kirk. 2004. Investigating learning deficits associated with dyslexia. *Dyslexia* **10:** 61–76.

Prull, M. W., J. D. Gabrieli & S. A. Bunge. 2000. Age-related changes in memory: a cognitive neuroscience perspective. In F. I. Craik & T. A. Salthouse (Eds.), *The handbook of aging and cognition* (pp. 91–153). Mahwah, NJ: Lawrence Erlbaum.

Rae, C., J. A. Harasty, T. E. Dzendrowskyj, J. B. Talcott, J. M. Simpson, A. M. Blamire, *et al.* 2002. Cerebellar morphology in developmental dyslexia. *Neuropsychologia* **40**(8): 1285–1292.

Ramus, F., S. Rosen, S. C. Dakin, B. L. Day, J. M. Castellote, S. White, *et al.* 2003. Theories of developmental dyslexia: insights from a multiple case study of dyslexic adults. *Brain* **126:** 841–865.

Riecker, A., K. Mathiak, D. Wildgruber, M. Erb, I. Hertrich, W. Grodd, *et al.* 2005. Fmri reveals two distinct cerebral networks subserving speech motor control. *Neurology* **644:** 700–706.

Rudel, R. D. 1985. The definition of dyslexia: language and motor deficits. In F. H. Duffy & N. Geschwind (Eds.), *Dyslexia: A neuroscientific approach to clinical evaluation* (pp. 33–53). Boston, MA: Little, Brown.

Russeler, J., I. Gerth & T. F. Munte. 2006. Implicit learning is intact in adult developmental dyslexic readers: evidence from the serial reaction time task and artificial grammar learning. *Journal of Clinical and Experimental Neuropsychology* **28**(5): 808–827.

Seger, C. A. 1994. Implicit learning. *Psychological Bulletin* **115**(2): 163–196.

Seger, C. A. 1997. Two forms of sequential implicit learning. *Consciousness and Cognition* **6**(1): 108–131.

Shaywitz, S. E., M. D. Escobar, B. A. Shaywitz, J. M. Fletcher & R. Makuch. 1992. Evidence that dyslexia may represent the lower tail of a normal distribution of reading ability. *New England Journal of Medicine* **326:** 145–150.

Snowling, M. J. 2001. From language to reading and dyslexia. *Dyslexia* **7:** 37–46.

Sperling, A. J., Z. L. Lu & F. R. Manis. 2004. Slower implicit categorical learning in adult poor readers. *Annals of Dyslexia* **54**(2): 281–303.

Stadler, M. A. & P. A. Frensch (Eds.). 1997. *Handbook of implicit learning*. Thousand Oaks, CA: Sage Publications, Inc.

Stanley, G., G. A. Smith & E. A. Howell. 1983. Eye movements and sequential tracking in dyslexic and control children. *British Journal of Psychology* **74:** 181–187.

Stein, J. 2001. The magnocellular theory of developmental dyslexia. *Dyslexia* **7**(1): 12–36.

Stoodley, C. J., E. P. Harrison & J. F. Stein. 2006. Implicit motor learning deficits in dyslexic adults. *Neuropsychologia* **44**(5): 795–798.

Tallal, P. 1980. Auditory temporal perception, phonics, and reading disabilities in children. *Brain and Language* **9:** 182–198.

Uhry, J. K. & D. B. Clark. 2005. *Dyslexia theory and practice of instruction* (3rd ed.). Baltimore, MD: York Press.

Vicari, S., A. Finzi, D. Menghini, L. Marotta, S. Baldi & L. Petrosini. 2005. Do children with developmental dyslexia have an implicit learning deficit? *Journal of Neurology, Neurosurgery, and Psychiatry* **76:** 1392–1397.

Vicari, S., L. Marotta, D. Menghini, M. Molinari & L. Petrosini. 2003. Implicit learning deficit in children with developmental dyslexia. *Neuropsychologia* **41:** 108–114.

Waber, D. P., D. J. Marcus, P. W. Forbes, D. C. Bellinger, M. D. Weiler, L. G. Sorensen, *et al.* 2003. Motor sequence learning and reading ability: Is poor reading associated with sequencing deficits? *Journal of Experimental Child Psychology* **84**(4): 338–354.

Wagner, R. K. & J. K. Torgesen. 1987. The nature of phonological processing and its causal role in the acquisition of reading skill. *Psychological Bulletin* **101**(2): 192–212.

Wechsler, D. 1997. *Wechsler adult intelligence scale* (3rd ed.). San Antonio, TX: The Psychological Corporation.

Wechsler, D. 1999. *Wechsler abbreviated scale of intelligence*. San Antonio, TX: The Psychological Corporation.

Wildgruber, D., H. Ackerman & W. Grodd. 2001. Differential contributions of motor cortex, basal ganglia, and cerebellum to speech motor control: effect of syllable repetition rate evaluated by fMRI. *NeuroImage* **13**(1): 101–109.

Wolf, M. & P. G. Bowers. 1999. The double-deficit hypothesis for the developmental dyslexias. *Journal of Educational Psychology* **91**: 415–438.

Wolf, M., P. G. Bowers & K. Biddle. 2000. Naming-speed processes, timing, and reading: a conceptual review. *Journal of Learning Disabilities* **33**(4): 387–407.

Wolff, P. H., C. Cohen & C. Drake. 1984. Impaired motor timing control in specific reading retardation. *Neuropsychologia* **22**(5): 587–600.

Wolff, P. H., G. F. Michel & M. Ovrut. 1990a. The timing of syllable repetitions in developmental dyslexia. *Journal of Speech and Hearing Research* **33**: 281–289.

Wolff, P. H., G. F. Michel, M. Ovrut & C. Drake. 1990b. Rate and timing precision of motor coordination in developmental dyslexia. *Developmental Psychology* **26**(3): 349–359.

Woodcock, R. W., K. S. McGrew & N. Mather. 2001. *Woodcock-Johnson III tests of achievement*. Itasca, IL: Riverside Publishing.

Impaired Serial Visual Search in Children with Developmental Dyslexia

Ruxandra Sireteanu,[a,b,c,*] **Claudia Goebel,**[a] **Ralf Goertz,**[a,b]
Ingeborg Werner,[a] **Magdalena Nalewajko,**[a] **and Aylin Thiel,**[a,b]

[a]*Department of Neurophysiology, Max-Planck-Institute for Brain Research, Frankfurt, Germany*

[b]*Department of Biological Psychology, Institute for Psychology, Johann Wolfgang Goethe-University, Frankfurt, Germany*

[c]*Department of Biomedical Engineering, College of Engineering, Boston University, Boston, Massachusetts, USA*

In order to test the hypothesis of attentional deficits in dyslexia, we investigated the performance of children with developmental dyslexia on a number of visual search tasks. When tested with conjunction tasks for orientation and form using complex, letter-like material, dyslexic children showed an increased number of errors accompanied by faster reaction times in comparison to control children matched to the dyslexics on age, gender, and intelligence. On conjunction tasks for orientation and color, dyslexic children were also less accurate, but showed slower reaction times than the age-matched control children. These differences between the two groups decreased with increasing age. In contrast to these differences, the performance of dyslexic children in feature search tasks was similar to that of control children. These results suggest that children with developmental dyslexia present selective deficits in complex serial visual search tasks, implying impairment in goal-directed, sustained visual attention.

Key words: developmental dyslexia; serial visual search; sustained attention

Introduction

Developmental dyslexia is a neurological condition affecting about 5–10% of the school-age population and characterized by a marked deficit in reading and writing abilities without impairments in general intelligence. Children with developmental dyslexia present deficits in phonological processing—the awareness of the sound structure of words. In spite of cultural diversity, dyslexia appears to have a unified underlying biological cause in alphabetic languages (Paulesu *et al.*, 2001). Both juvenile and adult dyslexics show reduced cortical activity in areas located in the temporo-parietal lobe on the left side of the brain when tested by tasks involving phonological processing (for review, see Eden & Zeffiro, 1999).

In addition to the phonological impairment, it has been argued by some that dyslexic subjects show deficits in the processing of rapidly changing auditory information, implying that the phonological impairment might result from this more fundamental deficit (Temple *et al.*, 2003). The auditory deficit is correlated with a severe disturbance in the left inferior prefrontal cortex (Temple *et al.*, 2003), divisions of which are reported to be specialized for semantic and phonological processing.

Contrast sensitivity has been reported to be impaired in dyslexic subjects, but the impairment depends on the type of dyslexia and the investigation performed (cf.

*We dedicate this paper to the memory of Ruxandra Sireteanu (year of birth–2008)

Address for correspondence: Ruxandra Sireteanu, Ph.D., Department of Neurophysiology, Max-Planck-Institute for Brain Research, Deutschordenstrasse 46, 60528 Frankfurt, Germany. sireteanu@mpih-frankfurt.mpg.de

Cornelissen, Richardson, Mason, Fowler, & Stein, 1995; Gross-Glenn *et al.*, 1995; Williams, Stuart, Castles, & McAnally, 2003). Recently, dyslexic adults were reported to show selective impairments on sequential tasks, both auditory and visual. Ben-Yehudah and Ahissar (2004) suggested that dyslexia might involve a deficit in "retain and compare" types of tasks, which are reported to involve the parietal cortex.

Deficits in higher-order, global visual tasks like motion coherence sensitivity, visual contour integration, and visual change detection have been reported in developmental dyslexia, suggesting an involvement of higher-order cortical areas and/or abnormal cooperative associations between distant cortical loci (Simmers & Bex, 2001; Rutkowski, Crewther, & Crewther, 2003). These tasks are thought to be based on activity of the posterior parietal cortex of the right hemisphere of the brain. Recent corroborating evidence for a possible deficiency in the right posterior parietal cortex comes from the reports of left visual field inattention and right field overdistractability in visual flanker and reaction time tasks in developmental dyslexics (Facoetti & Molteni, 2001; Facoetti & Turatto, 2000; Hansen, Stein, Orde, Winter, & Talcott, 2001).

Various attentional deficits have been reported in developmental dyslexics. These include prolonged attentional dwell time (Hari, Valta, & Uutela, 1999), a tendency not to focus visual attention as much as normal readers do (Facoetti, Paganoni, & Lorusso, 2000; Facoetti, Paganoni, Turatto, Marzola, & Mascetti, 2000), and a general attentional deficit across visual and auditory modalities, related to "sluggish attentional shifts" (Hari & Renvall, 2001). Other reported deficits of attention have been related to the syntactic deficits of poor readers (Deutsch & Bentin, 1996), to their contrast sensitivity deficits (Stuart, McAnally, & Castles, 2001), to their impaired visual search (Casco & Prunetti, 1996; Vidyasagar & Pammer, 1999; Vidyasagar, 2001), and to their left neglect (Eden, Stein, & Wood, 1996).

In previous studies, we suggested that developmental dyslexia might reflect a weakness in a number of cortical areas, including the parietal and the frontal cortex on both sides of the brain (Sireteanu, Goebel, Goertz, & Wandert, 2006; Sireteanu, Goertz, Bachert, & Wandert, 2005). To probe the involvement of the right hemisphere, we investigated the performance on a visual line bisection task. Dyslexic children did not show the overestimation of the left visual field (pseudoneglect) characteristic of normal adult vision. Instead, they showed a consistent "mini neglect" (overestimation of the right visual field), suggesting that developmental dyslexia might be associated with selective deficits in visual attention, probably involving neural structures located in the right posterior parietal cortex (Sireteanu *et al.*, 2005).

The present study involves three independent experiments in which we tested whether developmental dyslexics might present selective deficits in different types of visual search tasks. Previous studies have yielded conflicting results: some studies found increased reaction times in dyslexic subjects (Casco & Prunetti, 1996; Vidyasagar & Pammer, 1999), whereas others showed decreased latencies in highly demanding conjunction search tasks (Sireteanu *et al.*, 2006). In a visual search task, subjects are asked to search for an odd item among a number of distracting items. If the time needed to complete the search is independent of the number of distractors, the search is said to be parallel; if the time needed to detect the odd item increases with the number of distractors, the search is said to be serial. For another type of task, a search for conjunctions task, the subjects are required to locate the item in the display that differs from the surrounding items by a combination of features (for example, orientation and color). The time needed to complete the search for a conjunction of features usually increases linearly with the number of distractors, indicating serial search, while the time needed to locate the target in a feature search task is independent of the number of distractors

(Treisman & Gelade, 1980; Treisman & Gormican, 1988). Studies employing brain imaging technology have shown that visual conjunction search tasks rely on a cortical network that includes the right parietal lobe, thought to be activated by successive shifts of attention (Corbetta, Shulman, Miezin, & Petersen, 1995), and the right superior prefrontal region, thought to be involved in spatial working memory (Goebel *et al.*, 1997; Leonards, Sunaert, Van Hecke, & Orban, 2000).

Our first experiment employed several highly demanding, complex feature tasks for orientation and form, as well as a conjunction task for orientation and form. The distracting items were identical in the two types of tasks. A second experiment involved two feature search tasks (search for items differing from the distractors by color or orientation), as well as a conjunction search task, in which the target item differed from the distractors by color and orientation. Previous studies have shown that in normal observers, both feature search tasks for orientation and for color elicit parallel search, while for the conjunction task, search time increases with the number of distractors, indicating serial search (cf. Sireteanu, & Rettenbach, 2000; Treisman & Gormican, 1988). In the third experiment, dyslexic and control children were tested with a number of basic visual feature search tasks in which target and distractors differed by a specific visual attribute (a circle with a gap among complete circles, a circle with an added line amid complete circles, pairs of convergent lines amid parallel lines, a tilted line amid vertical lines). These tasks have been shown to elicit a parallel visual search (Rettenbach, Diller & Sireteanu, 1999; Sireteanu & Rettenbach, 1995; Treisman & Gelade, 1980). We hypothesize that dyslexic children would show impairments in the conjunction, but not in the feature search tasks. In addition, our expectation was that more pronounced impairments would be seen in dyslexic children for the complex tasks involving letter-like material than for the tasks involving geometric items.

Methods

Subject Recruitment and Inclusion Criteria

All subjects were recruited by leaflets distributed to schools in the Frankfurt area and by word of mouth. Dyslexia was defined by a difference of at least two grades as assessed by a number of psychometric tests. To be included in the study, the subjects had to satisfy the following criteria: to have no known neurologic or psychiatric abnormalities; no ophthalmologic disorders; no medication; and fully corrected refraction. Dyslexic and control children were matched by age, gender and, as far as possible, general intelligence and socioeconomic level. Only right-handed subjects were included in the study. Both dyslexic and control children were recruited from the same schools and lived in the same geographic area.

Testing Procedures

Prior to the experiments, the subjects were given a complete orthoptic and psychometric examination. Orthoptic examination consisted in the measurement of eye alignment, using a cover–uncover test; stereopsis, assessed with the Titmus, Randot, and TNO tests; objective refraction; Snellen corrected visus for single and crowded optotypes; color vision, assessed with the Ishihara test; and contrast sensitivity, tested for near and far with the VisTech Contrast Sensitivity Charts. The results of the orthoptic tests showed no deficits in basic visual functions in dyslexic children. These children did not show an increased incidence of refraction errors or of errors in eye alignment. Their visual acuities and contrast sensitivities were in the normal range (for examples, see Figures 1 and 2).

Psychometric examination of the subjects consisted of intelligence tests; vocabulary and arithmetic tests; tests for writing proficiency, reading proficiency, sustained attention, short-term memory, and phonological awareness (syllable sequences; for details, see Sireteanu

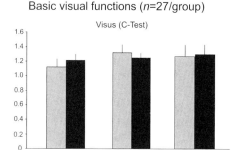

Figure 1. Visual acuity for single and crowded optotypes in dyslexic and age-matched control children (n = 27 subjects per group; data from Experiment 1).

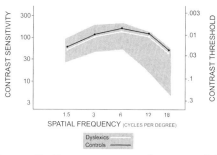

Figure 2. Contrast sensitivity functions of developmental dyslexics and age-matched control children (n = 27 subjects per group; data from Experiment 1).

et al., 2005). Written informed consent was obtained from all subjects or their parents after the procedure was fully explained. The experimental procedures were performed in accordance with the tenets of the Declaration of Helsinki.

Methods and Results

Experiment 1A: Visual Search for Orientation and Form (Complex Stimuli with Inhomogeneous Background)

The aim of the first experiment was to investigate the role of sustained attention in children with developmental dyslexia. We used highly demanding visual search tasks with com-

plex stimuli, similar to the letter material that has been shown to pose difficulties for children with developmental dyslexia. This material was used because it is known that dyslexic children typically struggle with alphanumeric material.

This experiment involved a group of 27 consecutive dyslexic and 27 control subjects, aged between 7 and 19 years. The control children were matched for age and gender to the experimental children. There were no significant differences in intelligence between the two groups. The subjects were divided into three groups by grade: grades 2–4, 5–7, and 8–13, corresponding roughly to the age ranges 8–10, 11–13, and 14–19 years.

The stimuli are shown in the insets of Figures 3–5. Stimuli were displays containing one target item (a single item differing from the distracting items by orientation, form, or form and orientation) amid an array of distracting items (total number of items on the display could be 8, 16, or 24). In half of the trials, no target was presented. In the conjunction search task, the target differed from the distractors by a combination of features (orientation and form). In both feature and conjunction tasks, the distractors could be of two types: half of them shared the shape, but were mirror images of the target; the other half shared part of the orientation of the target; we call this display "inhomogeneous" (for example, see insets in Figure 3).

The children were asked to press a predetermined computer key with the index finger of one hand for target-present trials and another key with the index finger of the other hand for target-absent trials. Half of the children used the right hand for the target-present trials, the other half for the target-absent trials. Reaction time and error rates were recorded. Feedback was given after each block of trials. All children participated in all tasks, in counterbalanced order.

As shown in Figure 3, for both target-present and target-absent trials, reaction times increased with the number of distractors,

CONJUNCTION SEARCH FOR ORIENTATION AND FORM /
INHOMOGENEOUS BACKGROUND (*n*=27/group)

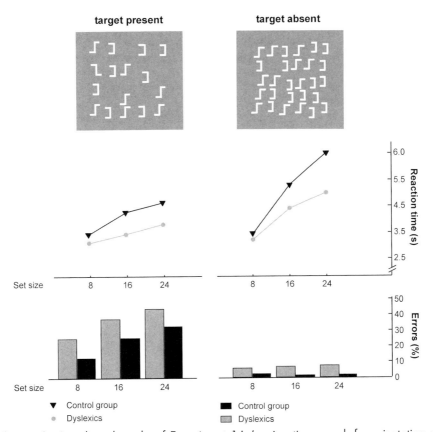

Figure 3. Stimuli and results of Experiment 1A (conjunction search for orientation and form)—effect of set size (*n* = 27 subjects/group): *upper panels:* the stimuli; *middle panels:* mean reaction times; *lower panels:* mean error rates.

indicating serial search. Reaction times for target-absent trials were much longer than those for target-present trials for both groups of subjects (see middle panels in Figure 3). Surprisingly, for both target-present and target-absent tasks, the reaction times of the dyslexic children were significantly shorter than those of the age-matched control children, indicating that the dyslexic children terminated the search prematurely. An analysis of variance (ANOVA with repeated measurements) revealed that these differences were statistically significant for both target-present ($F = 5.938$, $P = 0.018$) and target-absent trials ($F = 4.929$, $P = 0.031$).

Response latencies decreased significantly with increasing age for both groups of sub-

jects (see middle panels in Figure 4). With increasing age, the differences between the dyslexic and control children diminished significantly ($F = 6.957$, $P = 0.011$ for target-present trials and $F = 5.152$, $P = 0.028$ for target-absent trials; ANOVA with repeated measures). Dyslexic children produced significantly more errors than age-matched control subjects ($F = 11.602$, $P = 0.001$ and $F = 8.79$, $P = 0.005$, respectively). While the overall error rates diminished with age for both groups, the difference between the two groups of subjects showed a tendency to increase; this tendency did not reach statistical significance, however (see lower panels in Figure 4).

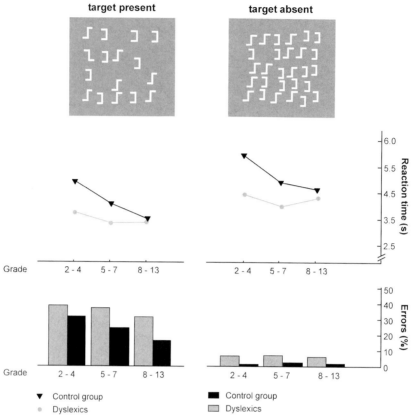

Figure 4. Stimuli and results of Experiment 1A (conjunction search for orientation and form)—effect of age (*n* = 27 subjects/group): *upper panels:* the stimuli; *middle panels:* mean reaction times; *lower panels:* mean error rates.

Experiment 1B: Feature Search for Form (Complex Stimuli with Inhomogeneous Background)

In this task, the target and distractors differed from each other in shape. The distractors were the same as in the previous experiment (inhomogeneous display; for an example, see inset in Figure 5).

In this experiment, we found that reaction times increased significantly with the number of distractors, indicating serial search ($F = 20.99$, $P < 0.0001$; middle left panel in Figure 5). However, there was no significant difference in reaction times between dyslexic and control children ($F = 0.245$, $P > 0.05$). Reaction times decreased slightly with age for both groups of

subjects; this decrease was not statistically significant (lower left panel in Figure 5). Error rates showed a tendency to be higher for the dyslexic than for the aged-matched control children (right panels in Figure 5).

Summary of Experiment 1

The results of this experiment show that children with developmental dyslexia present difficulties in complex visual search tasks involving letter-like material, but much less so if the search tasks involved single features. Still, we wondered whether the impaired performance of the dyslexics might have been due to the use of the complex, letter-like stimuli, or to

FEATURE SEARCH FOR FORM / INHOMOGENEOUS BACKGROUND (*n*=27/group)

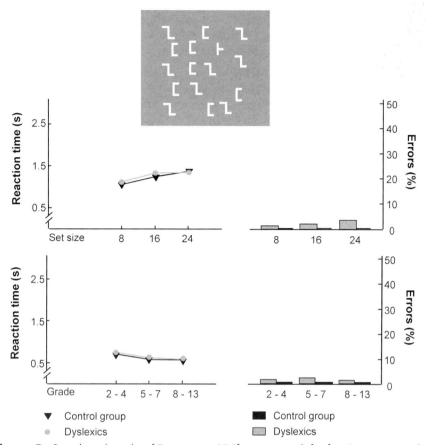

Figure 5. Stimuli and results of Experiment 1B (feature search for form): *upper panels:* the stimuli; *middle panels:* effect of set size; *lower panels:* effect of age (*n* = 27 subjects/group). *Left panels:* mean reaction times; *right panels:* mean error rates.

the combination of features. In the following experiment, we attempted to disentangle these two possibilities, by using feature and conjunction tasks with stimuli which did not resemble letter material.

Experiment 2: Feature and Conjunction Search for Color and Orientation (Homogeneous Background)

In this experiment, we tested the performance of dyslexic and control children in two feature search tasks (visual search for color or orientation) and one conjunction search task

(visual search for color and orientation). This experiment involved a group of 18 consecutive dyslexic and 18 age-matched control children (age range: 8–15 years). Selection criteria were the same as in the previous experiment. None of the children had participated in Experiment 1.

Stimuli for the three conditions were displays containing one target item (a single item differing from the distracting items by its color, by its orientation, or by its color and orientation), amid an array of distracting items (total number of items could be 1, 8, or 16). Half of the trials contained a target, in the other half, the target

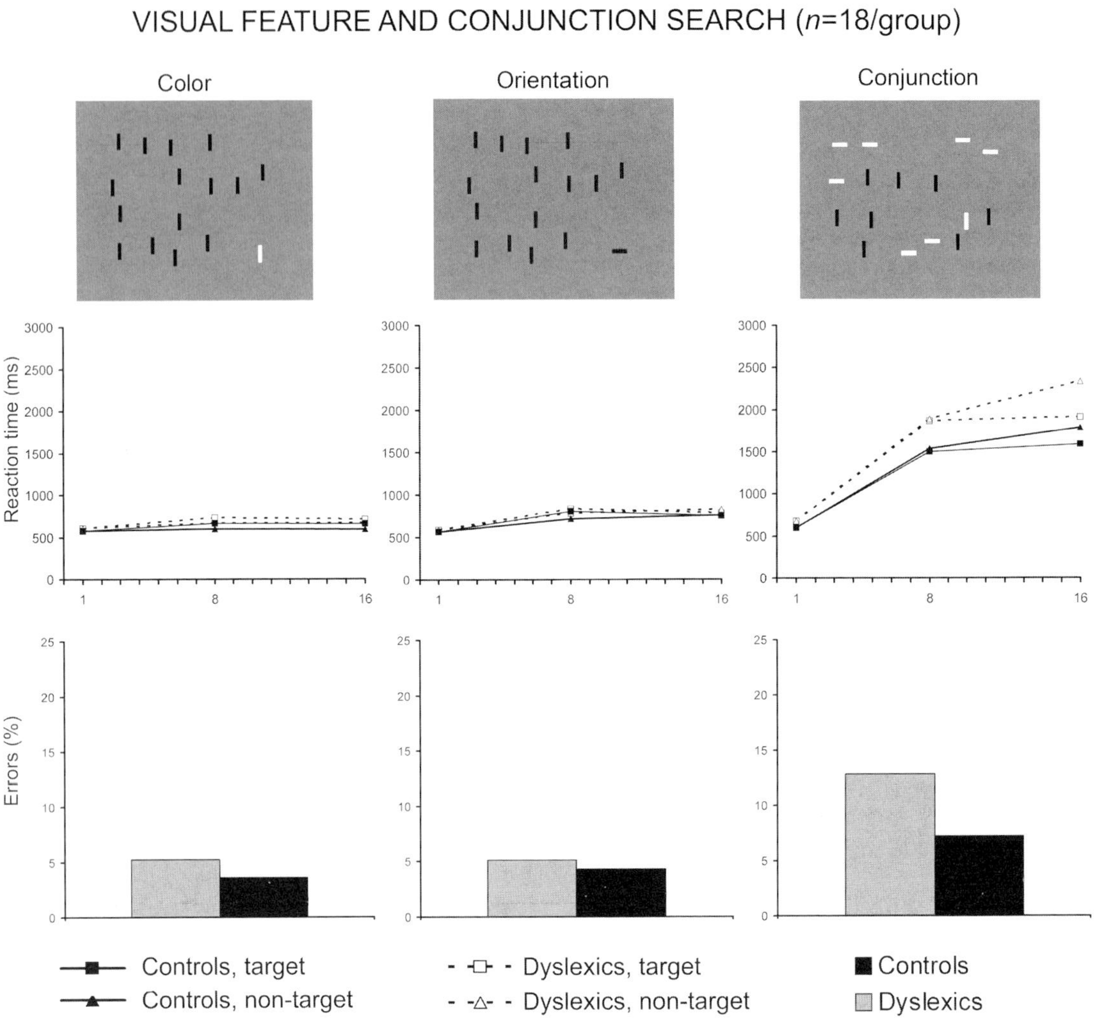

VISUAL FEATURE AND CONJUNCTION SEARCH (*n*=18/group)

Figure 6. Stimuli and results of Experiment 2 (feature and conjunction search for color and orientation) —effect of set size (*n* = 18 subjects/group): *upper panels:* the stimuli (red and green stimuli are indicated by brighter and darker shadings, respectively); *middle panels:* mean reaction times; *lower panels:* mean error rates.

was absent. The orientation of the items could be vertical or horizontal; the colors were red and green of matched luminance on a black background. In the feature tasks, the distractors were always of a single type (homogeneous background). For the conjunction task, half of the distracting items shared the color and the other half the orientation with the target item. The experimental procedure was similar to that of Experiment 1.

For both feature search tasks (color or orientation), reaction times for target-present and target-absent trials were independent of

the number of distractors, indicating parallel search. In both cases, reaction times and error rates did not differ significantly between the dyslexic children and the age-matched control children ($F = 1.445$, $P = 0.268$; $F = 0.381$, $P = 0.556$; see left and middle panels in Figure 6).

Experiment 2B: Conjunction Search for Orientation and Color

For this form of search, reaction times for both target-present and target-absent trials increased with the number of distractors, indicating serial search. Dyslexic children showed significantly ($F = 80.473$, $P < 0.000$) longer reaction times than the age-matched control children (see middle right panel in Figure 6). The error rates of the dyslexic children were significantly higher than those of the control children (12.83% versus 7.25%; $F = 6.507$, $P = 0.038$; see lower right panel in Figure 6).

Summary of Experiment 2

As in the previous experiment, dyslexic children were impaired in conjunction search, but not in the feature search tasks. Both experiments suggest that performance on feature search tasks is not impaired in dyslexic children. The accelerated response seen in the complex conjunction search in the previous experiment was not seen with the less demanding visual conjunction task of orientation and color examined here. Rather, dyslexic children showed longer reaction times than the age-matched children in the control group. As in the previous experiment, dyslexic children produced significantly more errors than the control children. These results suggest that children with developmental dyslexia show a complex pattern of deficits in tasks requiring sustained visual attention.

The question arises whether these findings might be related to the increased demand of conjunction tasks on attentional resources. To answer this question, in the next experiment, we used exclusively feature search tasks. The tasks contained both attention-dependent and attention-independent components.

Experiment 3: Pop-Out Visual Tasks

In this experiment, the subjects were tested with visual search for four basic visual search tasks ("gap," "added line," "convergence," and "tilt"). All tasks contain preattentive as well as attention-dependent components (Treisman & Gelade, 1980; Treisman & Gormican, 1988). The experiment was carried out with another

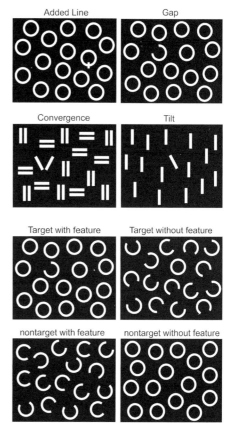

Figure 7. Stimuli of Experiment 3 (feature search for basic visual search tasks). *Upper four panels:* examples of the stimuli (target present in each case). *Lower four panels:* examples of the four possible constellations for the stimulus "gap."

group of 19 consecutive dyslexic and 19 control children matched for age and gender to the experimental children (age range: 8–15 years). Stimuli and procedures were identical to those described in Sireteanu and Rettenbach (1995, 1996, 2000) and Rettenbach, Diller, and Sireteanu (1999). In brief: the subjects were asked to locate a target item as rapidly and correctly as possible amid an array of distracting items. The distracting items were all of a single type (homogeneous display). Total number of items on the display could be 1, 4, 8, or 16. Half of the trials did not contain a target (Fig. 7).

The procedure differed from those of the previous two experiments: for target-present trials, the task of the subject was to press a button of

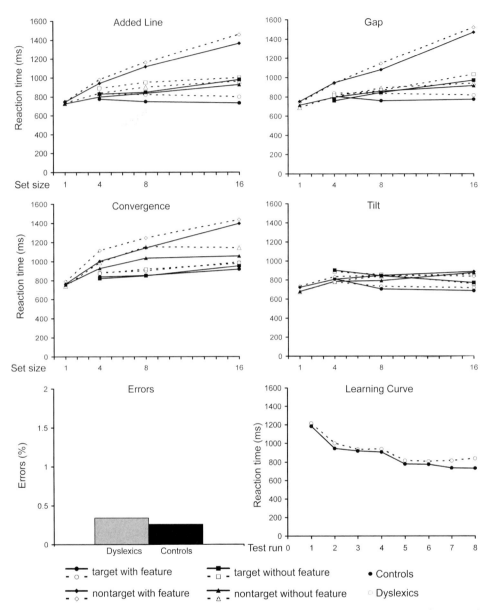

Figure 8. Results of Experiment 3 (feature search for basic visual search tasks). *Upper four panels:* effect of set size for all four search tasks (*n* = 19 subjects/group). *Lower left panel:* error rates, averaged over all tasks. *Lower right panel:* Effect of practice. Each point shows the reaction time of the group of dyslexic or control children, averaged over all tasks, for consecutive test runs.

the computer mouse and then point with the index finger of the dominant hand toward the location on the screen where the target had been presented; for target-absent trials, they were required to press the button and then raise the same hand. There was trial-by-trial feedback on the correctness of the response. Both response times and error rates were recorded. The children were tested on two consecutive days. Four test runs were included on each experimental day. In each test run, each stimulus type and each set size was presented once, in randomized order.

For all tasks, reaction times for the target-present trials were independent of the number of distractors, indicating parallel search (Fig. 8). For the tasks "gap," "added line," and "convergence," reaction times for target-absent trials increased consistently with set size, indicating serial search ($F = 84.683$; $P < 0.001$ in a 4×2 ANOVA test). For the task "tilt," reaction times did not increase with set size, thus confirming the results for the task "orientation" in Experiment 2. Dyslexic children showed longer reaction times than the control children for the serial components of the tasks; these differences approached statistical significance ($F = 0.424$, $P = 0.052$). Basic reaction times did not differ significantly between the two groups of subjects.

The error rates were much smaller than in the previous experiments (under 1% for both groups of subjects), probably because this task was much less demanding than the tasks in the previous experiments. Still, dyslexic children showed a tendency to produce more errors than the age-matched nondyslexic children; this tendency did not reach statistical significance (lower left panel in Figure 8). Both groups of children showed clear improvements with prolonged testing. Reaction times decreased continuously from one test run to the next during the two experimental days. The most dramatic improvement occurred during the first two experimental runs ($F = 63.564$, $P < 0.001$).

Summary of Experiment 3

The results of this experiment confirm that dyslexic children are similar to age-matched control children when tested with parallel visual search tasks. When tested with serial search tasks, their performance is consistently impaired.

Discussion

The purpose of this study was to investigate whether children with developmental dyslexia differ from age-matched control children in visual search tasks. The first experiment investigated the performance in highly demanding feature and conjunction tasks involving letter-like material. The second experiment used feature and conjunction tasks involving geometric items defined by orientation and color; and finally, the third experiment tested the performance for feature tasks with geometric items. All tasks contained parallel and serial components. Our hypothesis was that dyslexic children would show deficits in serial tasks involving sustained attention, but not in preattentive visual search tasks. In addition, we hypothesized that the performance of the dyslexic children would be dramatically impaired for tasks containing letter-like stimulus material.

The results of the three experiments confirmed our hypotheses. When tested with a highly demanding, serial visual search task involving letter-like material, dyslexic children respond with significantly shorter reaction times as compared to controls, but produce an exorbitant number of errors. This result suggests that the serial search tasks may have been ended prematurely, indicating a deficit in sustained visual attention. In the second experiment, the dyslexic children showed slower responses in conjunction than in feature search, together with a moderately increased number of errors. The results of the third experiment show that performance in "pop-out" tasks is only minimally impaired in dyslexic children. The dyslexic subjects tend to produce more errors, but their reaction times do not differ significantly from those of the control subjects. Both groups of subjects show clear improvements with age and practice, but dyslexic children tend to be more easily fatigued than nondyslexic children.

These findings suggest that the accelerated reaction of the dyslexic subjects in the first experiment might be specific to the very complex, letter-like stimulus material. This result might explain discrepancies between data in the literature (Casco & Prunetti, 1996; Sireteanu *et al.*, 2006; Vidyasagar & Pammer, 1999).

The absence of a statistically reliable difference in reaction times between dyslexic and typical children in visual feature search tasks might indicate that the cortical areas most likely to be responsible for solving these tasks are unlikely to be affected in developmental dyslexia. The finding of a deficit in serial search agrees with our previous finding of a left "minineglect" in dyslexia (Sireteanu *et al.*, 2005; 2006) and points toward a deficit in the right posterior parietal cortex (see also Facoetti, Lorusso, Cataneo, Galli & Molteni, 2005; Facoetti & Molteni, 2001). The deficit in sustained attention, shown by the premature termination of the highly demanding tasks in Experiment 1, suggests an additional involvement of dorsal areas in the prefrontal cortex, which are responsible for sustained attention (Courtney, Ungerleider, Keil & Haxby, 1996; Kastner & Ungerleider, 2000; Wilson, Scalaidhe, & Goldman-Rakic, 1993).

The current findings suggest that, in addition to the known deficits in the parietal and prefrontal areas on the left side of the brain, responsible for phonological and rapid auditory processing (Hansen *et al.*, 2001; Temple *et al.*, 2003), and to the deficits in the left posterior fusiform gyrus, developmental dyslexics show impairments in the network of cortical areas responsible for directing and sustaining visual attention, including areas in the right parietal and prefrontal areas. Thus, dyslexia might reflect a more generalized brain deficit, involving circuits located in the parietal and frontal areas of both sides of the brain.

Acknowledgments

Part of the experiments included in this study was supported by grants from the Deutsche Forschungsgemeinschaft (Si 344/16–1, 2). We are grateful to Wolf Singer for support, to Iris Bachert for the careful orthoptic examination of the subjects, and to our subjects for their patience. Thanks are due to Rainer Goebel and Dan H. Constantinescu for development of the software for running part of the experiments. C.G. was supported by the Evangelisches Studienwerk Villigst, eV.

Conflicts of Interest

The authors declare no conflicts of interest.

References

Ben-Yehudah, G. & M. Ahissar. 2004. Sequential spatial frequency discrimination is consistently impaired among adult dyslexics. *Vision Research* **44:** 1047–1063.

Casco, C. & E. Prunetti. 1996. Visual search of good and poor readers: effects of targets having single and combined features. *Perceptual and Motor Skills* **82**(3Pt2): 1155–1167.

Corbetta, M., G. L. Shulman, F. M. Miezin & S. E. Petersen. 1995. Superior parietal cortex activation during spatial attention shifts and visual feature conjunction. *Science* **270**(5237): 802–805.

Cornelissen, P., A. Richardson, A. Mason, S. Fowler & J. Stein. 1995. Contrast sensitivity and coherent motion detection measured at photopic luminance levels in dyslexic and controls. *Vision Research* **35**(10): 1483–1494.

Courtney, S. M., L. G. Ungerleider, K. Keil & J. V. Haxby. 1996. Object and spatial visual working memory activate separate neural systems in human cortex. *Cerebral Cortex* **6:** 39–49.

Eden, G. F., J. F. Stein & F. B. Wood. 1996. Visuospatial judgment in reading disabled and normal children. *Perceptual and Motor Skills* **82:** 155–177

Facoetti, A. & M. Molteni. 2001. The gradient of visual attention in developmental dyslexia. *Neuropsychologia* **39**(4): 352–357.

Facoetti, A., M. L. Lorusso, C. Cataneo, R. Galli & M. Molteni. 2005. Visual and auditory attentional capture are both sluggish in children with developmental dyslexia. *Acta Neurobiologiae Experimentalis (Warsaw)* **65**(1): 61–72.

Facoetti, A., P. Paganoni & M. L. Lorusso. 2000. The spatial distribution of visual attention in developmental dyslexia. *Experimental Brain Research* **132**(4): 531–538.

Facoetti, A., P. Paganoni, M. Turatto, V. Marzola & G. G. Mascetti. 2000. Visual-spatial attention in developmental dyslexia. *Cortex* **36**(1): 109–123.

Facoetti, A. & M. Turatto. 2000. Asymmetrical visual fields distribution of attention in dyslexic children: a neuropsychological study. *Neuroscience Letters* **290**(3): 216–218.

Goebel, C., D. E. Linden, R. Sireteanu, H. Lanfermann, F. E. Zanella, W. Singer, *et al.* 1997. Different attention processes in visual search tasks investigated with functional magnetic resonance imaging. *NeuroImage* **5**(4): 81.

Gross-Glenn, K., B. C. Skottun, W. Glenn, A. Kushch, R. Lingua, M. Dunbar, *et al.* 1995. Contrast sensitivity in dyslexia. *Visual Neuroscience* **12**: 153–163.

Hansen, P. C., J. F. Stein, S. R. Orde, J. L. Winter & J. B. Talcott. 2001. Are dyslexics' visual deficits limited to measures of dorsal stream function? *Neuroreport* **12**: 1527–1530.

Hari, R. & H. Renvall. 2001. Impaired processing of rapid stimulus sequences in dyslexia. *Trends in Cognitive Sciences* **5**: 525–532.

Hari, R., M. Valta & K. Uutela. 1999. Prolonged attentional dwell time in dyslexic adults. *Neuroscience Letters* **271**: 202–204.

Kastner, S. & L. G. Ungerleider. 2000. Mechanisms of visual attention in the visual cortex. *Annual Review of Neuroscience* **23**: 27–43.

Leonards, U., S. Sunaert, P. Van Hecke & G. A. Orban. 2000. Attention mechanisms in visual search: an fMRI Study. *Journal of Cognitive Neuroscience* **12**: 61–75.

Mesulam, M. M. 1999. Spatial attention and neglect: parietal, frontal and cingulate contributions to the mental representation and attentional targeting of extrapersonal events. *Philosophical Transactions of the Royal Society (London) B* **354**: 1325–1346.

Paulesu, E., J. F. Demonet, F. Fazio, E. McCrory, V. Chanoine, N. Brunswick, *et al.* 2001. Dyslexia: cultural diversity and biological unity. *Science* **291**: 2165–2167.

Rettenbach, R., G. Diller & R. Sireteanu. 1999. Do deaf people see better? Texture segmentation and visual search compensate in adult, but not in juvenile subjects. *Journal of Cognitive Neuroscience* **11**: 560–583.

Rutkowski, J. S., D. P. Crewther & S. G. Crewther. 2003. Change detection is impaired in children with dyslexia. *Journal of Vision* **3**: 95–105.

Simmers, A. J. & P. J. Bex. 2001. Deficits of visual contour integration in dyslexia. *Investigative Ophthalmology & Visual Science* **42**: 2737–2742.

Sireteanu, R., C. Goebel, R. Goertz & T. Wandert. 2006. Do children with developmental dyslexia show a selective visual attention deficit? *Strabismus* **14**(2): 85–93.

Sireteanu, R., R. Goertz, I. Bachert & T. Wandert. 2005. Children with developmental dyslexia show a left visual minineglect. *Vision Research* **45**: 25–26, 3075–3082.

Sireteanu, R. & R. Rettenbach. 1995. Perceptual learning in visual search: fast, enduring, but non-specific. *Vision Research* **35**: 2037–2043.

Sireteanu, R. & R. Rettenbach. 1996. Textursegmentierung und visuelle Suche: Entwicklung, Lernen und Plastizität. [Texture discrimination and visual search: development and plasticity.] *Klinische Monatsblätter für Augenheilkunde* **207**: 3–10.

Sireteanu, R. & R. Rettenbach. 2000. Perceptual learning in visual search generalizes over tasks, locations, and eyes. *Vision Research* **40**: 2925–2949.

Stuart, G. W., K. I. McAnally & A. Castles. 2001. Can contrast sensitivity functions in dyslexia be explained by inattention rather than a magnocellular deficit? *Vision Research* **41**: 3205–3211.

Temple, E., G. K. Deutsch, R. A. Poldrack, S. L. Miller, P. Tallal, M. M. Merzenich, *et al.* 2003. Neural deficits in children with dyslexia ameliorated by behavioural remediation: evidence from functional MRI. *Proceedings of the National Academy of Sciences USA* **100**(5): 2863–2865.

Treisman, A. & G. Gelade. 1980. A feature integration theory of visual attention. *Cognitive Psychology* **12**: 97–136.

Treisman, A. & S. Gormican. 1988. Feature analysis in early vision: evidence from search asymmetries. *Psychological Review* **95**: 15–48.

Vidyasagar, T. R. 2001. From attentional gating in macaque primary visual cortex to dyslexia in humans. *Progress in Brain Research* **134**: 297–312.

Vidyasagar, T. R. & K. Pammer. 1999. Impaired visual search in dyslexia relates to the role of the magnocellular pathway in attention. *Neuroreport* **10**(6): 1283–1287.

Williams, M. J., G. W. Stuart, A. Castles & K. I. McAnally. 2003. Contrast sensitivity in subgroups of developmental dyslexia. *Vision Research* **43**: 467–477.

Wilson, F. A., S. P. Scalaidhe & P. S. Goldman-Rakic. 1993. Dissociation of object and spatial processing domains in the primate prefrontal cortex. *Science* **260**: 1955–1958.

Structural Correlates of Implicit Learning Deficits in Subjects with Developmental Dyslexia

Deny Menghini,[a,b] Gisela E. Hagberg,[b] Laura Petrosini,[b,c] Marco Bozzali,[b] Emiliano Macaluso,[b] Carlo Caltagirone,[b,d] and Stefano Vicari[a,e]

[a] IRCCS, Children's Hospital "Bambino Gesù," Rome, Italy

[b] IRCCS, Santa Lucia Foundation, Rome, Italy

[c] Department of Psychology, University "La Sapienza," Rome, Italy

[d] University Tor Vergata, Rome, Italy

[e] University LUMSA, Rome, Italy

Several neuroimaging studies in developmental dyslexia (DD) have mainly focused on brain regions subserving phonological processes. However, additional deficits characterize subjects with DD, such as an impairment of visual and rapid stimuli processing and deficits in implicit learning (IL). Little is known about structural abnormalities in brain regions not directly related to phonology and reading processes. The aim of this study was to investigate, using voxel-based morphometry, whether subjects with DD exhibit any structural grey matter (GM) abnormalities in regions that have previously shown abnormal functional magnetic resonance imaging (fMRI) activation during an IL task. Significantly smaller GM volumes were found in the right posterior superior parietal lobule and precuneus and in the right supplementary motor area (SMA) of subjects with DD compared to controls. Moreover, a larger GM volume in parietal cortex was associated with an increase of IL effect in controls but not in subjects with DD. These structural abnormalities are consistent with functional changes and reinforce the hypothesis that an impairment of IL might play a relevant role in learning to read.

Key words: voxel based morphometry; implicit memory; developmental dyslexia; volumetric MRI; developmental disorders

Introduction

DD is defined as a specific reading disability resulting in unexpected, specific, and persistent low reading achievement despite conventional instruction, adequate intelligence, and socio-cultural opportunity (Shaywitz, 1998). From an epidemiological point of view, DD is reported as familial cases (Lyytinen *et al.*, 2004; Pennington & Gilger, 1996), and there is an in-

creasing evidence that such a disorder might be regarded as genetically determined (Fisher & DeFries, 2002). This hypothesis fits well with growing data that DD not only is associated with an isolated phonological deficit (Snowling, 2001), but also presents with additional impairments involving visual processing (Eden *et al.*, 1996, 2006) rapid processing of sensory stimuli (Tallal, Miller, & Fitch, 1993; Van Ingelghem *et al.*, 2001) and automatization skills (Nicolson & Fawcett, 1990). Recent behavioral studies suggest that a deficit of IL may also be present in subjects with DD (Vicari *et al.*, 2005; Howard, Howard, Japikse, & Eden, 2006). IL plays a central role in a number of cognitive

Address for correspondence: Deny Menghini, Ph.D., Child Neuropsychiatry Unit, Department of Neuroscience, IRCCS Children Hospital Bambino Gesù, Piazza Sant'Onofrio 4, I-00165, Roma (Italy). Voice: +39-06-68592475; menghini@opbg.net and d.menghini@hsantalucia.it

Ann. N.Y. Acad. Sci. 1145: 212–221 (2008). © 2008 New York Academy of Sciences.
doi: 10.1196/annals.1416.010

functions, such as acquisition of motor sequences, stimulus-response associations, priming effect, and classical conditioning (Clark & Squire, 1998; Chang, Dell, Bock, & Griffin, 2000; Richter *et al.*, 2004).

A complete definition of the neural network involved in IL is still a matter of investigation (Desmond & Fiez, 1998). Empirical evidence based on studies including subjects with brain damage supports the role of the basal ganglia, the cerebellum, and the frontal cortex in the implicit acquisition of motor sequences (Ferraro, Balota, & Connor, 1993; Pascual-Leone *et al.*, 1993; Jackson, Jackson, Harrison, Henderson, & Kennard, 1995; Doyon *et al.*, 1997; Knopman & Nissen, 1991). Furthermore, functional imaging studies have shown that the primary motor and supplementary motor areas are the structures most consistently activated when performing an IL task (Grafton, Hazeltine, & Ivry, 1995, 1998; Hazeltine, Grafton, & Ivry, 1997). The involvement of the premotor cortex (Jenkins, Brooks, Nixon, Frackowiak, & Passingham, 1994; Grafton *et al.*, 1995) in the IL process has also been documented and confirmed by lesion studies in nonhuman primates (Halsband & Passingham, 1985). Finally, lesion, electrophysiological, and functional neuroimaging studies produced evidence about an involvement of posterior parietal areas (Corbetta, Miezin, Shulman, & Petersen, 1993; Corbetta, 1998) and cerebellum in IL (Rauch *et al.*, 1995; Molinari *et al.*, 1997; Jueptner *et al.*, 1997; Gomez-Beldarrain, Garcia-Monco, Rubio, & Pascual-Leone, 1998; Exner, Koschack, & Irle, 2002; Torriero, Olivieri, Koch, Caltagirone, & Petrosini, 2004).

We recently studied a group of subjects with DD (DDs) and normal readers (NRs) in a paradigm of motor sequence learning using fMRI (Menghini, Hagberg, Caltagirone, Petrosini, & Vicari, 2006). A direct comparison between subjects with DD and NRs showed specific differences in activations that mainly involved the parietal cortex, SMA, and the cerebellum. This suggests a possible link between these brain structures and an IL deficit

in individuals with DD. Here we further investigated these regions using VBM to assess possible structural abnormalities underlying these physiological findings in the same population of subjects (DDs and NRs) as in the fMRI study. VBM is a spatially specific and unbiased method of analysis of MR images, reflecting the regional grey matter (GM) and white matter (WM) volume or density at a voxel scale (Ashburner & Friston, 2000). This technique has already been employed in previous studies to assess brain abnormalities in subjects with DD (Brown *et al.*, 2001; Brambati *et al.*, 2004; Silani *et al.*, 2005; Vinckenbosch, Robichon, & Eliez, 2005). These previous VBM studies have shown a prominent reduction of GM in the left parietotemporal regions of subjects with DD (Brown *et al.*, 2001; Silani *et al.*, 2005; Vinckenbosch *et al.*, 2005). Nevertheless, GM alterations have also been described outside brain regions traditionally involved in language processes, such as the superior bilateral cerebellum (Brown *et al.*, 2001) and cerebellar nuclei (Brambati *et al.*, 2004).

While some of these studies have correlated GM morphometry with behavioral measures (e.g., Silani *et al.*, 2005), none of these studies has examined morphological differences between DDs and NRs in the context of IL, a skill that is potentially impaired in DD. Specific aims of the current study were: (*a*) to investigate whether there are structural abnormalities in IL-related regions that have been shown to be functionally altered in subjects with DD; and (*b*) to evaluate possible correlations between structural MRI measures obtained from these regions and behavioral data of IL.

Methods

Study Participants

Fourteen adults with DD and 14 NRs, all right-handed, were originally recruited for the fMRI study (Menghini *et al.*, 2006). Four participants from each group were excluded

TABLE 1. Demographic Data and Reading Scores in Word and Nonword Reading Tests from "The Battery for Evaluating Dyslexia and Dysorthography"[a]

	DD ($n = 10$)	NR ($n = 10$)	$t (1, 13)$
Demographic data			
Sex (F/M)	9/1	9/1	
Mean age (SD)[range] years	40.7 (6.7) [34–51]	40.8 (7.0) [32–53]	
Median education level (range) years	17 (13–17)	17 (13–17)	
Reading score			
Speed in seconds (SD)	83.80 (13.60)	52.60 (5.13)	4.88*
No. of errors (SD)	2.10 (2.23)	0.20 (0.45)	1.85
Speed in seconds (SD)	64.20 (11.37)	33.40 (2.51)	5.88*
No. of errors (SD)	4.10 (3.70)	1.60 (0.55)	1.48

Abbreviations: DD = subjects with developmental dyslexia; NRs = normal readers; F = female; M = male; SD = standard deviation.

[a]Sartori, Job, & Tressoldi (1995).

*$P < .001$

from VBM analyses because of movement artifacts in their structural scans. All subjects with DD were recruited from the relatives of consecutive dyslexic children attending a pediatric hospital. The main demographic data for the remaining subjects (10 individuals with DD and 10 NRs) are summarized in Table 1 (column 1). All the subjects with DD met the standard *DSM IV* criteria for developmental reading disorder (American Psychiatric Association, 1994). All the NRs had no history of any reading deficits. Major systemic, psychiatric, and neurological illnesses were carefully investigated and excluded in all the studied subjects. Additionally, specific interviews were carried out to ensure that none of the recruited subjects had ever suffered from attention deficits.

Behavioral Assessments

All the studied subjects (dyslexics and controls) were assessed by a trained neuropsychologist (D.M.) before MRI acquisition. Reading abilities were evaluated using word and nonword reading from "The Battery for Evaluating Dyslexia and Dysorthography" (Sartori, Job, & Tressoldi, 1995). IL was selectively evaluated in all subjects using a classical version of the Serial Reaction Time Task

(SRTT) (Nissen & Bullemer, 1987). An extensive description of this procedure has already been reported elsewhere (Vicari *et al.*, 2005). In brief, the fMRI task consisted of a reaction-timed keypress response, which subjects were requested to perform whenever one of four visually presented empty boxes (baseline) changed its color to red (stimulus). Each box corresponded to one of four keys placed on two separate response units, one for each hand; the index and middle fingers of each hand controlled the keys. After any stimulus presentation, the response had to be as quick and accurate as possible.

The whole procedure consisted of seven blocks (total duration: 16.5 min). Two of the blocks were characterized by a pseudo-random presentation of 54 trials (blocks R1 and R2) and five of them (blocks S1-S5) by a repeated presentation of a nine-element sequence (positions: 243413231). Participants were not informed about the presence of the repeated sequence. After scanning, to exclude any potential explicit awareness effect, subjects were requested to reproduce on a keyboard any possible sequence that they believed to have detected during fMRI.

A one-way ANOVA model was employed to quantify IL in the two groups (subjects with DD and NRs) by comparing median reaction times obtained in the last two blocks of SRTT (S5-R2).

MRI Acquisition

Anatomical MRI scans were acquired at 1.5T (Siemens, Magnetom Vision, Erlangen, Germany). In a single session, a 3D T1-weighted turbo-flash magnetization-prepared rapid-acquisition gradient echo (MPRAGE) (TR/TE = 11.4/4.4 ms, TI = 300 ms, flip angle = 15°) sequence was obtained from all subjects with an isotropic 1 mm^3 voxel size.

MRI Analysis and Postprocessing

All the acquired MRI data were first assessed by visual examination to exclude from the analysis those scans that were affected by movement artifacts. The MPRAGE images were then processed using SPM 2 (Wellcome Department of Cognitive Nuerology, University College, London; http://www.fil.ion.ucl.ac.uk/spm). To optimize brain extraction and tissue segmentation, these images underwent an iterative procedure. According to the optimized VBM approach (Good *et al.*, 2001), the extracted GM in native space was normalized to the canonical GM template (using a combination of linear and nonlinear functions) included in SPM2, and the optimized transformation parameters were then applied to the original T1-volumes in native space. Finally, the normalized images were segmented again producing GM, WM, and cerebrospinal fluid (CSF) maps in normalized space. Voxel values in segmented images were multiplied by the Jacobian determinants derived from spatial normalization to provide intensity correction for induced regional volumetric changes, thus preserving within-voxel volumes that may have been altered during non-linear normalization (Ashburner & Friston, 2000). The signal intensity in every voxel of these maps represents the probability of belonging to a given class of tissue and reflects the regional volume of such a tissue. Statistical analysis of the regional GM

and WM volume was performed after smoothing the normalized and segmented images with a 12 mm^3 FWHM Gaussian kernel.

On the basis of our *a priori* anatomical hypotheses on the role for IL of supplementary and premotor cortices, parietal lobes, and cerebellum, a small volume correction procedure was employed to assign statistical threshold values, corrected for multiple comparisons (Menghini *et al.*, 2006). The volumes of interest were defined according to anatomical landmarks using an in-house-developed software (BrainShow) (Committeri *et al.*, 2004, 2007), according to landmarks defined. BrainShow uses a macroscopic anatomical parcellation of the MNI single-subject brain (Tzourio-Mazoyer *et al.*, 2002), as defined by the Brodmann map (Talairach & Tournoux, 1988) supplied with MRIcro (Rorden & Brett, 2000).

Approximately corresponding Brodmann's areas (BAs) were determined using the MRIcro software based on Talairaich and Tournoux (1988).

Statistical Analysis

An ANCOVA model was used in SPM2 to compare differences in regional GM or WM volumes between subjects with DD and NR. Global GM or WM volumes were entered as nuisance covariates to correct for potential confounds (i.e., differences in average brain volume that might account for regional differences). The 5% threshold used to assess differences between groups was corrected for multiple comparisons at the cluster level after applying a statistical threshold of $P = .005$ at the voxel level.

Furthermore, regression models considering possible links between behavioral performance in the IL task and the GM or WM volume were implemented in SPM2. These analyses correlated the regional IL effect, estimated as the difference in reaction times obtained during the last two SRTT blocks (S5-R2) with the regional GM and WM volumes. The analyses were run separately for subjects with DD and NRs, again considering supplementary and premotor cortices, parietal lobes, and cerebellum as volumes of interest.

Results

Behavioral Data

Table 1 reports the results obtained in reading tasks for subjects with DD and NRs. A statistical comparison (Student's t-test) between the two groups showed that subjects with DD were slower than NRs in both word and nonword reading tasks ($P < .001$). Consistent with our previous fMRI report, the group of 10 subjects with DD selected for the current study were impaired in IL, showing no SRTT changes between S5 and R2 (444.0 ± 73.5 and 450.0 ± 60.7 msec; one-way ANOVA: $P > .1$). In contrast, the subgroup of NRs showed an IL effect (405.2 ± 57.2 in S5 vs. 428.4 ± 52.5 msec in R2; one-way ANOVA: $P > .05$). Rauch's procedure showed an absence of declarative knowledge of the nine-element repeated sequences in any of the studied subjects ($P > .10$).

Voxel-Based Morphometry

Subjects with DD compared to NRs showed smaller GM volumes in the right posterior superior parietal lobule and precuneus (highest peak for the cluster within the Montreal Neurological Institute (MNI) coordinate system: $x = 14$; $y = -49$; $z = 63$, cluster size, voxels: 1414) and in the right SMA (highest peak for the cluster within the MNI coordinate system: $x = 8$; $y = 7$; $z = 54$, cluster size, voxels: 1540) (Fig. 1). The opposite contrast did not show any significant difference. There was no significant difference in the regional WM volume between subjects with DD and NRs.

The linear regression analysis did not yield any significant correlation between the IL effect and the regional GM or WM volumes in subjects with DD. Conversely, in the NR group the subjects with higher IL effect also showed higher GM volume in the right superior posterior parietal lobule (BA7) (Fig. 2).

Discussion

DD is generally considered as a specific learning disorder involving phonological deficits (Demonet, 2004), but deficits in other cognitive domains are increasingly reported. In the present study we investigated the morphological integrity of brain structures that have previously been associated with IL (Willingham, Salidis, & Gabrieli, 2002). We found smaller GM volumes in the right superior posterior parietal lobule, right precuneus, and right SMA in subjects with DD compared with NRs. Furthermore, we found that larger GM volume in a circumscribed region of the parietal lobule is associated with an increase in IL effect in NR. The altered brain areas in our subjects with DD play a relevant role in the IL process as supported by a number of fMRI studies (Curran, 1997; Rauch *et al.*, 1997; Grafton, Hazeltine, & Ivry, 1998).

The superior parietal lobule is a key structure in the control of visuospatial attention (Corbetta, Kincade, Ollinger, McAvoy, & Shulman, 2000; Culham & Kahnwishher, 2001). Attentional requirements are likely to be important in the early stages of implicit sequence learning, as measured with SRTT. In these early stages, attention is necessary to form the critical visuomotor association between the spatial location of visual target and the motor response (Müller, Kleinhans, Pierce, Kemmotsu, & Courchesne, 2002). Failure to establish efficient stimulus-response associations could in principle interfere with the establishment of implicit performance in these types of task. Interestingly, in the current study we found that higher GM volume of the superior parietal cortex is associated with better implicit learning performance in NR. This result reinforces the idea that the superior parietal cortex is involved in IL, and it suggests that structural abnormalities of this brain region might account, at least partially, for some behavioral manifestations of DD.

A significantly smaller GM volume was also found in the precuneus of subjects with DD.

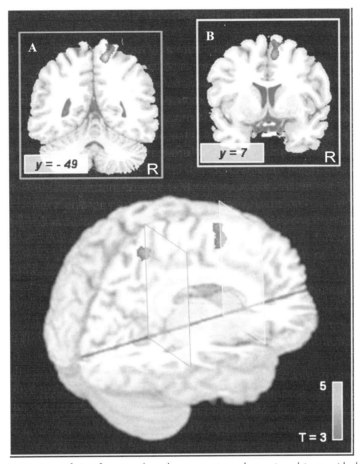

Figure 1. Regions of significant reduced grey matter volumes in subjects with developmental dyslexia compared to controls in the right posterior superior parietal lobule and precuneus (Montreal Neurological Institute coordinates: 14, −49, 63) (**A**) and in the right supplementary motor area (Montreal Neurological Institute coordinates: 8, 7, 54) (**B**).

Precuneus is believed to be specifically involved in retrieving motor sequences, especially during the intermediate stage of motor-sequences learning (Sadato, Campbell, Ibáñez, Deiber, & Hallett, 1996; Sakai *et al.*, 1998).

The abnormalities found in the SMA are consistent with the potential role of this region for the acquisition of implicit motor skills, as has been suggested by several neuroimaging studies (Grafton, Hazeltine, & Ivry, 1995). A transition from guided to generated movements should be one of the critical steps for implicit sequence learning (Hazeltine, Grafton, & Ivry, 1997). In this process, SMA would contribute specifically to representing motor sequences at an abstract level.

Although an abnormal pattern of fMRI activation was found in the cerebellum of our subjects with DD, VBM analysis did not detect any structural change at the anatomical level in these regions. This apparent inconsistency may be due to the relatively small sample size of studied subjects. Moreover, subjects with DD present with more variability in structural anatomy. It is therefore possible that some group differences remain masked as a consequence of insufficient statistical power. In any case, the dissociation of functional and structural findings in this area may be a comforting result as it suggests that functional changes did not merely arise from underlying morphometric differences.

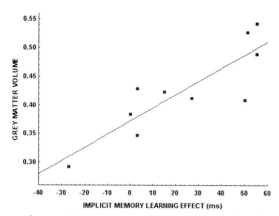

Figure 2. Correlations in normal readers between the implicit learning effect and grey matter volume in the right posterior superior parietal lobule (BA7: [Montreal Neurological Institute coordinates: 21, −67, 60]).

The present study did not find any significant increase of GM volume in subjects with DD compared to NRs. Previous neuroanatomical studies (for example, Galaburda *et al.*, 1985) investigating language areas have reported enlarged areas in the right hemisphere of DD subjects compared to controls, thus suggesting a potential compensation mechanism for reading function (Shaywitz *et al.*, 2002). In the current work we included (on the basis of fMRI data obtained with an IML paradigm) only regions that were involved in visual-motor learning abilities. The level of hemispheric lateralization for these functions is less pronounced than for language processes. Accordingly, mechanisms of interhemispheric reorganization are less likely to occur.

The pattern of IL-related structural abnormalities in DD subjects extends previous work that mainly focused on brain regions directly involved in phonological processes (Brambati *et al.*, 2004). VBM has already been used to directly investigate morphological measures targeted to brain areas with functional alterations (Silani *et al.*, 2005). In particular, altered volumes of GM and WM in brain regions involved in phonological and reading processes (such as the left middle and inferior temporal gyri and the left arcuate fasciculus) were found.

However, the interpretation of these interesting results may be hampered since the size of the selected volumes of interest, based on previous PET data (Paulesu *et al.*, 2001), was relatively small (10-mm-wide spheres), especially considering the smoothing size (10 mm) that was chosen for VBM preprocessing. A previous VBM study including the whole brain has investigated subjects with DD without any *a priori* hypothesis, albeit using poorly conservative thresholds (Brown *et al.*, 2001). The extent of GM abnormalities was widely distributed and included additional regions not strictly related to phonological deficits, suggesting a coexistence of phonological and non-phonological deficits in DD. These results support our findings of structural alterations in brain areas not strictly related to phonological processing. It may be noteworthy that the volumes of interest that we used included large portions of the brain (ranging between 34 and 60 mL), thus resulting in a reasonably conservative investigation of the underlying brain structures.

The presence of additional non-phonological deficits (Goswami, 2006) is consistent with growing evidence that DD is a genetically determined syndrome and prompts alternative theories in terms of pathophysiology. It is possible that a genetic alteration may selectively affect one or more neural networks associated with single cognitive domains. Alternatively, an involvement of neural networks of less specialized cognitive functions, underlying multiple brain modalities, might result in a wide range of more specific deficits. To support this second interpretation, several models have been proposed. For example, the double-deficit hypothesis combines the effect of two independent deficits (processing of phonemes and rapid naming of visual stimuli).

A selective deficit of IL might contribute to the understanding of several difficulties that have been reported in subjects with DD, including their characteristic disability in learning and improving reading skills. Indeed, it is reasonable to assume that IL is involved in some fundamental processes during the development of reading skills. For example an implicit knowledge of spelling conventions is likely to be already present in preschool children (Gaux & Gombert, 1999; Sperling, Lu, & Manis, 2004). When children learn to read, they undergo explicit instructions on grapheme–phoneme conversion. Afterwards, this explicit orthographic knowledge tends to progressively assume a more implicit character (Share, 1995). Consistently, there are some studies that have reported a direct correlation between IL and reading abilities (Sperling *et al.*, 2004; Howard *et al.*, 2006). IL allows motor, perceptual, and cognitive skills to be acquired and efficiently executed. Therefore, an impairment of IL may be related to visual processing inadequacy or information-processing deficits, possibly contributing also to phonological failure.

Conclusions

The present study shows smaller GM volumes in the superior posterior parietal lobule, precuneus, and SMA in subjects with DD, extending to the structural domain our previous fMRI results of impaired functioning of these regions. These structural and functional brain abnormalities support the hypothesis that a deficit in the IL process may explain some of the difficulties experienced by subjects with DD.

Acknowledgments

We thank Marta Bianciardi for help with image processing.

Conflicts of Interest

The authors declare no conflicts of interest.

References

American Psychiatric Association. 1994. *Diagnostic and statistical manual of mental disorders, 4th edition [DSM-IV]*. Washington, DC: American Psychiatric Association.

Ashburner, J., & Friston, K. J. 2000. Voxel-based morphometry: the methods. *Neuroimage*, **11:** 805–821.

Brambati, S. M., Termine, C., Ruffino, M., Danna, M., Lanzi, G., Stella, G., *et al.* 2004. Regional reductions of gray matter volume in familial dyslexia. *Neurology*, **63:** 742–745.

Brown, W. E., Eliez, S., Menon, V., Rumsey, J. M., White, C. D., & Reiss, A. L. 2001. Preliminary evidence of widespread morphological variations of the brain in dyslexia. *Neurology*, **56:** 781–783.

Chang, F., Dell, G. S., Bock, K., & Griffin, Z. M. 2000. Structural priming as implicit learning: a comparison of models of sentence production. *Journal of Psycholinguistic Research*, **29**(2): 217–229.

Clark, R. E., & Squire, L. R. 1998. Classical conditioning and brain systems: the role of awareness. *Science*, **280:** 77–81.

Committeri, G., Galati, G., Paradis, A. L., Pizzamiglio, L., Berthoz, A., & LeBihan, D. 2004. Reference frames for spatial cognition: different brain areas are involved in viewer-, object-, and landmark-centered judgments about object location. *Journal of Cognitive Neuroscience*, **16:** 1517–1535.

Committeri, G., Pitzalis, S., Galati, G., Patria, F., Pelle, G., Sabatini, U., *et al.* 2007. Neural bases of personal and extrapersonal neglect in humans. *Brain*, **130:** 431–441.

Corbetta, M. 1998. Frontoparietal cortical networks for directing attention and the eye to visual locations: identical, independent, or overlapping neural systems? *Proceedings of the National Academy of Sciences of the United States of America*, **95:** 831–838.

Corbetta, M., Kincade, J. M., Ollinger, J. M., McAvoy, M. P., & Shulman, G. L. 2000. Voluntary orienting is dissociated from target detection in human posterior parietal cortex. *Nature Neuroscience*, **3:** 292–297.

Corbetta, M., Miezin, F.M., Shulman, G.L., & Petersen, S.E. 1993. A PET study of visuospatial attention. *Journal of Neuroscience*, **13:** 1202–1226.

Culham, J. C., & Kahnwishher, N. G. 2001. Neuroimaging of cognitive functions in human parietal cortex. *Current Opinion in Neurobiology*, **11:** 157–163.

Curran, T. 1997. Implicit sequence learning from a cognitive neuroscience perspective. In M. A. Stadler & P. A. Frensch (Eds.), *Handbook of implicit learning* (pp. 365–400). Thousand Oaks, CA: Sage Publications.

Demonet, J. F. 2004. Developmental dyslexia. *Lancet*, **9419:** 1451–1460.

Desmond, J., & Fiez, J. 1998. Neuroimaging studies of the cerebellum: language, learning and memory. *Trends in Cognitive Science*, **2:** 355–362.

Doyon, J., Gaudreau, D., Laforce, R., Castonguay, M., Bédard, F., & Bouchard, J.-P. 1997. Role of the striatum, cerebellum, and frontal lobes in the learning of a visual sequence. *Brain & Cognition*, **34:** 218–245.

Eden, G. F., Howard, J. H., Jr., Howard, D. V., & Japikse, K. C. 2006. Dyslexics are impaired on implicit higher-order sequence learning, but not on implicit spatial context learning. *Neuropsychologia*, **44:** 1131–1144.

Eden, G. F., VanMeter, J. W., Rumsey, J. M., Maisog, J. M., Woods, R. P., & Zeffiro, T. A. 1996. Abnormal processing of visual motion in dyslexia revealed by functional brain imaging. *Nature*, **382:** 66–69.

Exner, C., Koschack, J., & Irle, E. 2002. The differential role of premotor frontal cortex and basal ganglia in motor sequence learning: evidence from focal basal ganglia lesions. *Learning & Memory*, **9:** 376–386.

Ferraro, F.R., Balota, D.A., & Connor, L.T. 1993. Implicit memory and the formation of new associations in nondemented Parkinson's disease individuals and individuals with senile dementia of the Alzheimer type: a serial reaction time (SRT) investigation. *Brain and Cognition*, **21:** 163–180.

Fisher, S. E., & DeFries, J. C. 2002. Developmental dyslexia: genetic dissection of a complex cognitive trait. *Nature Review of Neuroscience*, **3:** 767–780.

Galaburda, A. M., Sherman, G. F., Rosen, G. D., Aboitiz, F., & Geschwind, N. 1985. Developmental dyslexia: four consecutive patients with cortical anomalies. *Annals of Neurology*, **18:** 222–233.

Gaux, C., & Gombert, J. E. 1999. Implicit and explicit syntactic knowledge and reading in pre-adolescents. *British Journal of Developmental Psychology*, **17:** 169–188.

Gomez-Beldarrain, M., Garcia-Monco, J.C., Rubio, B., & Pascual-Leone, A. 1998. Effect of focal cerebellar lesions on procedural learning in the serial reaction time task. *Experimental Brain Research*, **120:** 25–30.

Good, C. D., Johnsrude, I. S., Ashburner, J., Henson, R. N., Friston, K. J., & Frackowiak R. S. 2001. A voxel-based morphometric study of ageing in 465 normal adult human brains. *Neuroimage*, **14:** 21–36.

Goswami, U. 2006. Sensorimotor impairments in dyslexia: getting the beat. *Developmental Science*, **9:** 257–259.

Grafton, S. T., Hazeltine, E., & Ivry, R. B. 1995. Functional mapping of sequence learning in normal humans. *Journal of Cognitive Neuroscience*, **7:** 497–510.

Grafton, S. T., Hazeltine, E., & Ivry, R. B. 1998. Abstract and effector-specific representations of motor sequences identified with PET. *Journal of Neuroscience*, **18:** 9420–9428.

Halsband, U., & Passingham, R.E. 1985. Premotor cortex and the conditions for movement in monkey (*Macaca fascicularis*). *Behavioural Brain Research*, **18:** 69–277.

Hazeltine, E., Grafton, S. T., & Ivry, R. B. 1997. Attention and stimulus characteristics determine the locus of motor-sequence encoding a PET study. *Brain*, **120:** 123–140.

Howard, J. H., Howard, D. V., Japikse, K. C., & Eden, G. F. 2006. Dyslexics are impaired on implicit higher-order sequence learning, but not on implicit spatial context learning. *Neuropsychologia*, **44:** 1131–1144.

Jackson, G.M., Jackson, S.R., Harrison, J., Henderson, L., & Kennard, C. 1995. Serial reaction time learning and Parkinson's disease: evidence for a procedural learning deficit. *Neuropsychologia*, **33:** 577–593.

Jenkins, I.H., Brooks, D.J., Nixon, P.D., Frackowiak, R.S.J., & Passingham, R.E. 1994. Motor sequence learning: a study with positron emission tomography. *Journal of Neuroscience*, **14:** 3775–3790.

Jueptner, M., Stephan, K.M., Frith, C.D., Brooks, D.J., Frackowiak, R.S.J., & Passingham, R.E. 1997. Anatomy of motor learning. II. Subcortical structures and learning by trial and error. *Journal of Neurophysiology*, **77:** 1325–1337.

Knopman, D., & Nissen, M.J. 1991. Procedural learning is impaired in Huntington's disease: evidence from the serial reaction time task. *Neuropsychologia*, **29:** 245–254.

Lyytinen, H., Aro, M., Eklund, K., Erskine, J., Guttorm, T., Laakso, M. L., *et al.* 2004. The development of children at familial risk for dyslexia: birth to early school age. *Annals of Dyslexia*, **54:** 184–220.

Menghini, D., Hagberg, G. E., Caltagirone, C., Petrosini, L., & Vicari, S. 2006. Implicit learning deficits in dyslexic adults: an fMRI study. *NeuroImage*, **33:** 1218–1226.

Molinari, M., Leggio, M.G., Solida, A., Ciorra, R., Misciagna, S., Silveri, M.C., *et al.* 1997. Cerebellum and procedural learning: evidence from focal cerebellar lesions. *Brain*, **120:** 1753–1762.

Müller, R. A., Kleinhans, N., Pierce, K., Kemmotsu, N., & Courchesne, E. 2002. Functional MRI of motor sequence acquisition: effects of learning stage and performance. *Cognitive Brain Research*, **14:** 277–293.

Nicolson, R. I., & Fawcett, A. J. 1990. Automaticity: a new framework for dyslexia research? *Cognition*, **35:** 159–182.

Nissen, M. J., & Bullemer, P. 1987. Attentional requirements of learning: evidence from performance measures. *Cognitive Psychology*, **19:** 1–32.

Pascual-Leone, A., Grafman, J., Clark, K., Steward, M., Massaquoi, S., Lou, J.-S., *et al.* 1993. Procedural learning in Parkinson's disease and cerebellar degeneration. *Annals of Neurology*, **34:** 594–602.

Paulesu, E., Démonet, J. F., Fazio, F., McCrory, E., Chanoine, V., Brunswick, N., *et al.* 2001. Dyslexia: cultural diversity and biological unity. *Science*, **291:** 2064–2065.

Pennington, B. F., & Gilger, J. W. 1996. How is dyslexia transmitted?. In C. H. Chase, G. D. Rosen, & G. F. Sherman (Eds.), *Developmental dyslexia: neural, cognitive, and genetic mechanisms* (pp. 41–61). Baltimore, MD: York Press.

Rauch, S. L. Savage, C. R., Brown, H. D., Curran, T., Alpert, N. M., Kendrick, A., *et al*. 1995. A PET investigation of implicit and explicit sequence learning. *Human Brain Mapping*, **3:** 271–286.

Rauch, S. L., Whalen, P. J., Savage, C. R., Curran, T., Kendrick, A., Brown, H. D., *et al*. 1997. Striatal recruitment during an implicit sequence learning task as measured by functional magnetic resonance imaging. *Human Brain Mapping*, **5:** 124–132.

Richter, S., Matthies, K., Ohde, T, Dimitrova, A, Gizewski, E, Beck, A., *et al*. 2004. Stimulus-response versus stimulus-stimulus-response learning in cerebellar patients. *Experimental Brain Research*, **158**(4): 438–449.

Rorden, C. & Brett, M. 2000. Stereotaxic display of brain lesions. *Behavioural Neurology*, **12:** 191–200.

Sadato, N., Campbell, G., Ibáñez, V., Deiber, M., & Hallett, M. 1996. Complexity affects regional cerebral blood flow change during sequential finger movements. *Journal of Neuroscience*, **16:** 2691–2700.

Sakai, K., Hikosaka, O., Miyachi, S., Takino, R., Sasaki, Y., & Pütz, B. 1998. Transition of brain activation from frontal to parietal areas in visuomotor sequence learning. *Journal of Neuroscience*, **18:** 1827–1840.

Sartori, G., Job, R., & Tressoldi, P. E. 1995. *Batteria per la valutazione della dislessia e della disortografia evolutiva*. Firenze: Edizioni O.S.

Share, D. L. 1995. Phonological receding and self-teaching: sine qua non of reading acquisition. *Cognition*, **55:** 151–218.

Shaywitz, B. A., Shaywitz, S. E., Pugh, K. R., Mencl, W. E., Fulbright, R. K., Skudlarski, P., *et al*. 2002. Disruption of posterior brain systems for reading in children with developmental dyslexia. *Biological Psychiatry*, **52**(2): 101–110.

Shaywitz, S. 1998. Current concepts: dyslexia. *New England Journal of Medicine*, **338:** 307–312.

Silani, G., Frith, U., Demonet, J. F., Fazio, F., Perani, D., Price, C., *et al*. 2005. Brain abnormalities underlying altered activation in dyslexia: a voxel based morphometry study. *Brain*, **23:** 1–9.

Snowling, M. J. 2001. From language to reading and dyslexia. *Dyslexia*, **7:** 37–46.

Sperling, A. J., Lu, Z. L., & Manis, F. R. 2004. Slower implicit categorical learning in adult poor readers. *Annals of Dyslexia*, **54:** 281–303.

Talairach, J., & Tournoux, P. 1988. *Co-planar stereotaxic atlas of the human brain: A 3-dimensional proportional system, an approach to cerebral imaging*. New York: Thieme.

Tallal, P., Miller, S., & Fitch, R. H. 1993. Neurobiological basis of speech: a case for the preeminence of temporal processing [review]. *Annals of the New York Academy of Sciences*, **682:** 27–47.

Torriero, S., Olivieri, M., Koch, G., Caltagirone, C., & Petrosini, L. 2004. Interference of left and right cerebellar rTMS with procedural learning. *Journal of Cognitive Neuroscience*, **16:** 1605–1611.

Tzourio-Mazoyer, N., Landeau, B., Papathanassiou, D., Crivello, F., Etard, O., Delcroix, N., *et al*. 2002. Automated anatomical labeling of activations in SPM using a macroscopic anatomical parcellation of the MNI- MRI single-subject brain. *NeuroImage*, **15:** 273–289.

Van Ingelghem, M., van Wieringen, A., Wouters, J., Vandenbussche, E., Onghena, P., & Ghesquière, P. 2001. Psychophysical evidence for a general temporal processing deficit in children with dyslexia. *Neuroreport*, **12:** 3603–3607.

Vicari, S., Finzi, A., Menghini, D., Marotta, L., Baldi, S., & Petrosini, L. 2005. Do children with developmental dyslexia have an implicit learning deficit? *Journal of Neurology, Neurosurgery, and Psychiatry*, **76:** 1392–1397.

Vinckenbosch, E., Robichon, F. & Eliez, S. 2005. Gray matter alteration in dyslexia: converging evidence from volumetric and voxel-by-voxel MRI analyses. *Neuropsychologia*, **43:** 324–331.

Willingham, D. B., Salidis, J., & Gabrieli, J. D. E. 2002. Direct comparison of neural systems mediating conscious and unconscious skill learning. *Journal of Neurophysiology*, **88:** 1451–1460.

Cerebellar Volume and Cerebellar Metabolic Characteristics in Adults with Dyslexia

Suzanna K. Laycock,[a,b] **Iain D. Wilkinson,**[b] **Lauren I. Wallis,**[b] **Gail Darwent,**[b] **Sarah H. Wonders,**[a] **Angela J. Fawcett,**[c] **Paul D. Griffiths,**[b] **and Roderick I. Nicolson**[a]

[a]*Department of Psychology, University of Sheffield, Sheffield, England, United Kingdom*

[b]*Academic Unit of Radiology, University of Sheffield, Sheffield, England, United Kingdom*

[c]*Centre for Child Research, University of Swansea, Swansea, Wales, United Kingdom*

Developmental dyslexia is associated with problems in a range of linguistic and nonlinguistic skills. Some of those problems have been attributed to dysfunction of the cerebellum and its associated neural systems. Two studies of cerebellar structure were undertaken by our group. In Study 1, white and grey matter volumes in the cerebellum were investigated in 10 dyslexic and 11 control adult male, right-handed participants using whole-brain volumetric MRI (3D-T1-weighted data sets with a spatial resolution of $0.8 \times 0.8 \times 0.8 \ mm^3$). The key finding was that the dyslexic group had a larger volume of white matter in both cerebellar hemispheres, differences that remained significant even when adjusting for total cerebellar volume. In Study 2, with the same participants, long-echo-time proton spectroscopy was used to investigate the ratios of the metabolites choline (Cho), N-acetylaspartate (NAA), and creatine (Cr) in the cerebellar hemispheres and vermis. Two significant differences were found: The dyslexic group had a lower ratio of NAA/Cho in the right cerebellar hemisphere together with a higher ratio of Cho/Cr in the left cerebellar hemisphere. Although it is difficult to interpret the volumetric and spectroscopic results unambiguously, taken together they suggest two possible interpretations: excessive connectivity or abnormal myelination.

Key words: white matter; connectivity; language; noise; spectroscopy; stereology

Introduction

Developmental dyslexia is one of the most prevalent learning disabilities in the Western world, affecting approximately 4% of children (Jorm, Share, McLean, & Matthews, 1986). Although its defining symptom is a difficulty in reading, dyslexia is a highly complex disorder with numerous cognitive and behavioral difficulties (reviewed in Demonet, Taylor, & Chaix, 2004), underpinned by altered structure in a variety of brain regions (reviewed by Eckert, 2004). There are a number of theories for the causation of dyslexia including the phonological deficit hypothesis (Snowling, 1998), which has been a long-standing theory within the field. An alternative theory suggests that an impairment in cerebellar function underlies the range of difficulties manifested (Nicolson, Fawcett, & Dean, 2001), and this has recently been broadened to include the neural systems linked to the cerebellum, which underlie procedural learning: the specific procedural learning deficit hypothesis (Nicolson & Fawcett, 2007). At a brain level, this neural systems theory involves not only specific brain regions, but also the connections between them.

Over the decades, there has been much evidence presented for abnormalities in cerebral regions. Early histological postmortem studies

Address for correspondence: Suzanna K. Laycock, Department of Psychology, University of Sheffield, Western Bank, Sheffield, S10 2TP, UK. Voice: +44-114-2226579; fax: +44-114-2766515. s.k.laycock@sheffield.ac.uk

Ann. N.Y. Acad. Sci. 1145: 222–236 (2008). © 2008 New York Academy of Sciences.
doi: 10.1196/annals.1416.002

in dyslexic adults by Galaburda and colleagues found cortical neuronal loss, myelinated scars in the cerebral cortex (Humphreys, Kaufmann, & Galaburda, 1990), polymicrogyria (Galaburda & Kemper, 1979), and ectopias (Galaburda, 1989). Evidence from a single case study suggested abnormalities in the functional cortical units, minicolumns, in Wernicke's area (Casanova, Buxhoeveden, Cohen, Switala, & Roy, 2002). More recently, neuroimaging studies have also indirectly demonstrated microscopic abnormalities; for example, voxel-based morphometry indicates increased density in the left middle temporal gyrus grey matter and decreased white matter density under Broca's area and within regions of the arcuate fasiculus (Silani *et al.*, 2005), and reduced grey matter density in the left temporal lobe and increased density in precentral gyri (Vinckenbosch, Robichon, & Eliez, 2005). Gross structural differences have shown reduced volume of the temporal (Eliez *et al.*, 2000), pars triangularis in the inferior frontal lobe (Eckert *et al.*, 2003), and the parietal lobe (Robichon, Levrier, Farnarier, & Habib, 2000). The connectivity between brain regions has also begun to be investigated through the use of an MRI technique which investigates the integrity of nerve fiber pathways—diffusion tensor imaging (DTI). DTI has shown differences in the white matter connecting into cortical language areas in the temporoparietal lobe in both adults (Klingberg *et al.*, 2000) and children (Beaulieu *et al.*, 2005; Deutsch *et al.*, 2005).

The evidence suggests that numerous cerebral regions and some pathways are abnormal in dyslexics, implying that the etiology of dyslexia cannot be ascribed to a single brain region. Indeed, it has been proposed that the abnormal brain regions correlate to parts of two reading-related neural systems (Eckert, 2004). One deals with orthography and includes the medial occipital cortex, inferior parietal cortex, fusiform gyrus, inferior frontal cortex, and superior temporal gyrus. The second neural system processes phonolog-

ical information and utilizes the auditory cortex, inferior parietal cortex, insula, and inferior frontal gyrus. Both neural systems include the cerebellum.

With regard to the cerebellum, the amount of anatomical data is not as extensive as that for the cerebrum. To the best of our knowledge, the only direct microscopic study was conducted by Finch, Nicolson, and Fawcett (2002) on the same brains studied by Galaburda and discussed above. The study demonstrated that the dyslexic cerebellums had larger Purkinje cell areas in the posterior cerebellar cortex, but no changes in cellular density. At the other end of the scale, gross differences have also been reported by a number of groups using MRI techniques; these include a smaller volume of the right anterior cerebellar lobe in both adults (Leonard *et al.*, 2001) and children (Eckert *et al.*, 2003), and less grey matter bilaterally in the semilobular lobules of the posterior lobe (Brown *et al.*, 2001). The symmetry of the cerebellar grey matter has also been reported to differ to that of controls, with dyslexics failing to show the asymmetry exhibited by control participants (Rae *et al.*, 2002). In relation to cerebellar white matter, the automated technique of voxel-based morphometry demonstrated that the right anterior cerebellar lobe had clusters of voxels with reduced volumes of white matter, in comparison to those in control participants, although this significance was lost when total white matter was controlled for (Eckert *et al.*, 2005). On the other hand, Rae and colleagues found no differences in cerebellar white matter (Rae *et al.*, 2002).

In addition to the histological and structural imaging studies, a different approach to gain information about the dyslexic brain utilizes magnetic resonance spectroscopy (MRS), which investigates metabolites in brain tissue (Talos *et al.*, 2006). In the case of proton MRS, the metabolites include N-acetylaspartate (NAA), choline (Cho), and creatine (Cr), which have different cellular localities: NAA is predominantly found in neuronal cell bodies and synapses and is considered a measure of neuronal density, Cho is a component of cell membranes, and Cr is a component of the energy cycle within mitochondria. Knowledge about metabolite variations enables inferences to be drawn about the tissue cytoarchitecture. In relation to dyslexia, the ratio of Cho/NAA was decreased in the left temporoparietal lobe, whereas the ratios of Cho/NAA and Cre/NAA were decreased in the right (Rae *et al.*, 1998). Taken together, these changes were interpreted as alterations in cell membranes and cell density. Lactate, a marker of increased glucose metabolism, was found to be higher in left cerebral anterior regions in dyslexic children during an auditory phonological task (Richards *et al.*, 2000; Richards *et al.*, 1999), suggesting the task required greater mental effort, utilizing more neuronal activity and additional glucose-driven energy.

The evidence suggests that there are a number of differences in both the cerebrum and cerebellum of the dyslexic, and it is possible that these differences relate to parts of reading-related or procedural learning–related neural systems. Because both of these neural systems involve the cerebellum, we set out to investigate its structure and metabolic characteristics in adults with dyslexia using means of high magnetic field strength. We chose to investigate the volumes of cerebellar grey and white matter separately. We attributed the information-processing capabilities of the cerebellum to the grey matter, whereas differences in the cerebellar white matter were more likely to be ascribed to its connectivity with cerebral regions and could imply abnormal neural systems utilizing the cerebellum. Based on the published literature pertaining to differences in cerebellar grey matter, a preliminary prediction would be differences in the cerebellar grey matter volume in dyslexics. Because this matter is composed predominantly of neurons, we would expect concomitant changes in the ratios of NAA/Cho and NAA/Cr to be seen spectroscopically.

Methods

Participants

Ten dyslexic and eleven control adults participated in the volumetric study. Control participants were recruited either by advertisements within the University of Sheffield or they had been part of control groups for other experiments within the Dyslexia Research Group (DRG), University of Sheffield. Dyslexic participants were either part of experimental groups for other DRG research, or had undergone a dyslexia assessment at the University of Sheffield and had stated an interest in participating in dyslexia research. Participants were sent information sheets about the study and asked to e-mail the main investigator if they wished to participate; they did not receive payment for their participation. All participants were male and right-handed. All participants, except for one dyslexic and one control, were current or former university undergraduates. Participants were required to have a full-scale IQ above 90 as measured by the WAIS-III (Wechsler, 1999) or a short form thereof. The short form included the following subtests: vocabulary, similarities, picture completion, digit span, digit-symbol coding, block design, and matrix reasoning. It was required that the control group had no known or suspected learning difficulty and did not show a dyslexic profile through the psychometric testing in this study. Members of the dyslexic group all scored an Adult Dyslexia Index (ADI) of at least 2.5 of a maximum of 4 points in their University of Sheffield dyslexia assessments (Nicolson & Fawcett, 1997). There are four aspects to the ADI score, each worth up to 1.0 point. The first aspect and 1.0 point is given if the participant had a previous (childhood/adolescent) diagnosis. The second aspect is related to spelling (Wechsler, 1993), where 1.0 point is obtained for a spelling age of 15.6 years or fewer, or 0.5 point for a score between 15.6 and 17 years. The third aspect relates

TABLE 1. Psychometric and Literacy Performance of the Two Groups

	Dyslexic ($N = 10$)	Control ($N = 11$)	Effect size	Significance (t-test)
Age (years)	21.1 ± 2.1)	22.1 (±2.8)	–	$t(19) = -1.0, P = $ ns
Full IQ[a]	126.0 (±16.1)	128 (±7.9)	–	$t(19) = -0.5, P = $ ns
Reading[b]	95.7 (±14.2)	113.0 (±5.6)[c]	−3.40	$t(13) = 2.5, P = 0.03$
Spelling[d]	93.3 (±19.9)	118.7 (±8.8)[c]	−2.89	$t(13) = 2.6, P = 0.02$
Nonsense passage reading time (sec)[e]	65.2 (±10.6)	47.4 (±9.4)[c]	1.89	$t(13) = 3.2, P = 0.007$
Nonsense passage reading time (no. of errors)[e]	9.6 (±3.3)	3.4 (±2.1)[c]	2.99	$t(13) = 3.8, P = 0.002$

Note: Expressed as mean (± standard deviation). Groups were matched for age, IQ, sex, and handedness.
[a]WAIS-III or short form thereof.
[b]One-minute reading Dyslexia Adult Screening Test (Fawcett & Nicolson, 1998).
[c]Only six of the control group underwent the tests for literacy; the remainder were recruited on the basis of reporting no problems with reading or spelling.
[d]Wechsler Objective Reading Dimension (Wechsler, 1993).
[e]Finucci Nonsense Passage (Finucci, Guthrie, Childs, Abbey, & Childs, 1976). Significance was calculated with a two-tailed independent variance t-test.

to reading of a passage of text including nonsense words (Finucci, Guthrie, Childs, Abbey, & Childs, 1976), in which 0.5 point is given for slow reading and/or 0.5 point for inaccurate reading. The fourth aspect depends on significant discrepancies (greater than 3 points) on the WAIS-III ACID subtests (Arithmetic, Digit-Symbol Coding, Information, and Digit Span) relative to the mean non-ACID performance. For one ACID subtest having a significant discrepancy, 0.5 point is given, or 1 point if more than one ACID subtest was significantly different.

A subset of the participants (six dyslexics and six controls) underwent spectroscopy. These participants formed a pilot group undergoing both spectroscopy and volumetric scans and were recruited first. The remaining participants were recruited for another imaging study but underwent the same volumetric scan as part of their array of scans.

Table 1 shows the psychometric data for the two groups. The groups were matched for sex, handedness, age, and IQ. Ethical approval was granted by the Ethics Committee of the Department of Psychology, University of Sheffield. All participants gave fully informed consent before taking part in this study.

Study 1: Volumetric MRI Measures

Image Acquisition

Anatomical MRI scans were acquired at 3T (Intera 3T, Philips Medical Systems, Holland) using a T1-weighted, 3D magnetization-prepared rapid-acquisition gradient echo (3D-MPRAGE) sequence (TR = 10.5 msec, TE = 4.8 msec, TI = 1400 msec, flip angle = 8°, NSA = 1, matrix = 256 × 256, 200 secondary phase encodes, voxel size = 0.8 × 0.8 × 0.8 mm, scan time = 11 min 47 sec). The data set was realigned to give 0.8-mm-thick coronal sections angled along the floor of the fourth ventricle (Deshmukh *et al.*, 1997).

Delineation of Region of Interest

For all of the following measures the raters were blind to the participant's group and the contrast level was set to the same value for every participant's brain scan. Unless otherwise stated, delineations were conducted on coronal oriented scans. The total intracranial volume (TICV) was defined as the volume of the cerebral hemispheres, within the dura, which was rostral to the superior colliculi of the midbrain. It included the ventricle and subdural spaces, but excluded the brain-stem caudal to the superior colliculi and excluded the cerebellum. In relation to the cerebellum, five regions of interest (ROI) were measured: the vermis, right hemisphere white and grey matter, and the left hemisphere white and grey matter. Two important delineations were required to ensure accurate cerebellar ROI volume measurements: (1) the division between the cerebellar white matter and cerebellar peduncles and (2) the division between the vermis and the lateral hemispheres. For the determination of cerebellar hemisphere white matter, the division between the deep cerebellar white matter (arbor vitae) and cerebellar peduncles was defined by the method used by Raz, Dupuis, Briggs, McGavran, and Acker (1998). Briefly stated, the division between the two regions was determined using the most anterior coronal slice containing the anterior vermis. Anterior to this slice, only the grey matter was measured, whereas posterior to this slice both the grey and white matters were measured. The vermis was the major anatomical region, which had to be delineated accurately because anything lateral to this area was considered lateral cerebellar hemisphere (Fig. 1). Because overestimation of the vermis would result in underestimation of the volume of the cerebellar hemispheres, the vermis was initially carefully delineated and traced on axial scans, where it was more visible. When the image was switched into the coronal plane, the trace lines from the original delineation appeared as "dots" (Fig. 2A), which were used as guidelines in conjunction with atlases (Duvernoy & Duvernoy, 1995; Schmahmann, 2000) to fully outline the vermis (Fig. 2B). The cerebellar hemisphere grey matter was defined as tissue lateral to the vermis.

Stereology

The volumes of the TICV, vermis, and cerebellar hemispheric grey and white matter were estimated using stereology in the coronal plane. Stereologic studies were conducted using third-party software (Analyze AVW, Mayo Foundation, Rochester, MN, USA) on a Unix workstation (Sun Ultra 30, Sun Microsystems Inc,

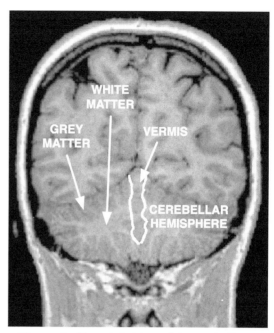

Figure 1. The subdivisions of the cerebellum into a midline vermis and two lateral cerebellar hemispheres. The latter consisted of white and grey matter.

USA). Stereology is based on the Cavalieri method (Mayhew & Olsen, 1991; Roberts, Puddephat, & McNulty, 2000). An unbiased estimate of the volume (estV) of an ROI can be determined by measuring the area (A) on a proportion (the first of every n slices) of the total number of slices. The slice increment, T, is then given by $T = n \cdot t$, where t is the thickness of any individual slice. The area may then be estimated by interpolation using the formula

$$\text{estV} = T \cdot (A_1 + A_2 + \cdots + A_m)$$

where a total of m slices have been selected. The point-counting method was used to determine the area of the ROI. In this method, a grid of crosses tessellating the region of interest is placed over the brain slice and only those crosses within the ROI are counted. Each cross corresponds to a specific area (a). The area A_i on slice i can be estimated by the formula $A_i = a \cdot P_i$ where P_i is the number of points on the ith slice. Given A_i, the estimate of the volume of the region of interest can then be calculated using the formula estV described above. Validity

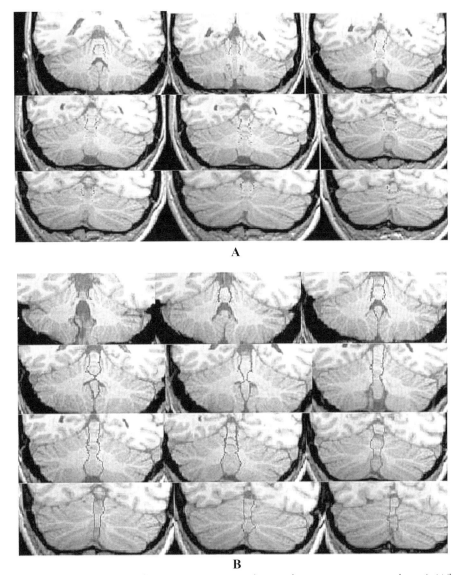

Figure 2. Delineation of the vermis (scans in the axial orientation are not shown). When images were switched into the coronal plane, they appeared as dots defining the lateral borders of the vermis (**A**). These dots were used in conjunction with atlases to outline the vermis in every coronal slice (**B**).

of the chosen parameters is ascertained using the coefficient of error, CE, which should be below 0.05 (Gundersen & Jensen, 1987)

$$CE = \sqrt{\left[(3 \sum A_i \times A_i + \sum A_i \times A_{i+2} - 4 \sum A_i \times A_{i+1}) / 12 \right] / \sum A_i}$$

The parameters for the cerebellum were a cross size of 6 × 6 voxels ($a = 23.04$ mm^2) and slice in-

crement of 2.4 mm, yielding a CE of 0.02. The cerebral volume was measured using a cross size of 25 × 25 voxels ($a = 400.00$ mm^2) and slice increment of 9.6 mm, producing a CE of 0.01. The delineation and stereology methods took approximately 3 hr per brain.

Ratings

Intra- and interobserver ratings were obtained through redelination of the cerebellar

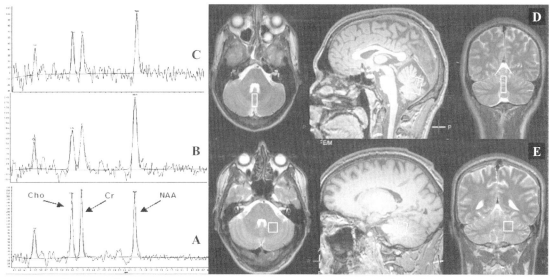

Figure 3. Long-echo-time proton MR spectroscopy. Examples of spectra from the vermis (**A**), right cerebellar hemisphere (**B**), and left cerebellar hemisphere (**C**) show the NAA, Cr, and Cho peaks at 2.0, 3.0, and 3.2 ppm, respectively. Location of the voxel in the vermis (**D**) and the left cerebellar hemisphere (**E**) are also shown. The placement in the right cerebellar hemisphere mirrors the position in the left side (not shown).

regions of interest and repeated stereological measurements on the original *n* slices. Raters were blind to the group to which the participant belonged. Intraratings were undertaken by S.K.L. and interratings by L.I.W. Interclass correlations (Shrout & Fleiss, 1979) were 0.997 and 0.948 for intra- and interratings, respectively.

Study 2: Magnetic Resonance Spectroscopy Measures

Participants

The participants were a subset of those who participated in Study 1, with six participants in each group. Mean (± SD) ages for the dyslexic and control groups were 21.2 (±0.5) years and 21.2 (±1.9) years, respectively. Mean IQ scores were 123.0 (±7.7) and 124.7 (±3.6) for the dyslexic and control groups, respectively.

Spectra Acquisition

Proton [¹H] spectroscopy was conducted on a Philips Intera 3T system (Philips Medical Systems, the Netherlands) using a point-resolved spectroscopy sequence (PRESS)

(TR = 1600 msec, TE = 144 msec, number of samples = 2048, bandwidth = 2 kHz, vermis number of signal averages [NSA] = 256, and cerebellar hemispheres NSA = 192, scan time = 7 min 20 sec [vermis] and 5 min 40 sec [per hemisphere]). After automatic first-order shimming and gradient-tuning, optimal water suppression was achieved with the addition of a chemically selective saturation (CHESS) pulse.

Spectroscopy Voxel Placement

A 1.5 × 1.5 × 1.5 cm (3.375 cm³) voxel was placed within the right and left cerebellar hemispheres and a 2 × 2 × 1 cm (4 cm³) voxel within the vermis. Voxels were placed using anatomical landmarks observed on the T1-weighted 3D-MPRAGE scan (mentioned above) and transaxial and coronal T2-weighted fast spin echo scans (TR = 4727 msec, TE = 80 msec, ETL = 21, voxel size = 0.9 × 1.0 × 4.0 mm, scan time = 1 min 6 sec). Voxels were placed by the same investigator (S.K.L.) to ensure consistency of methods between participants. The cerebellar hemisphere voxels were placed over the dentate nucleus and included both white and grey matter, and its anterior

TABLE 2. Descriptive Data for the Unadjusted Volumes

Region of interest	Dyslexic ($N = 10$)	Control ($N = 11$)	Effect size	Significance (ANOVA)
TICV	1347.07 (±69.63)	1249.05 (±126.01)	0.87	$F(1,19) = 4.72, P = 0.04$
	1297.26–1396.89	*1164.39–1333.71*		
Vermis	12.47 (±0.89)	11.53 (±1.05)	0.88	$F(1,19) = 4.83, P = 0.04$
	11.83–13.10	*10.82–12.23*		
Right hemisphere white matter	9.32 (±0.97)	7.92 (±1.06)	1.14	$F(1,19) = 9.90, P = 0.005$
	8.63–10.02	*7.21–8.63*		
Right hemisphere grey matter	54.51 (±3.42)	53.40 (±5.06)	0.26	$F(1,19) = 0.34, P = ns$
	52.06–56.96	*50.00–56.79*		
Left hemisphere white matter	9.32 (±0.96)	7.87 (±0.98)	1.21	$F(1,19) = 11.67, P = 0.003$
	8.63–10.00	*7.21–8.53*		
Left hemisphere grey matter	55.39 (±3.86)	55.36 (±4.85)	0.01	$F(1,19) = 0.00, P = ns$
	52.63–58.15	*52.10–58.62*		

Note: Expressed as mean volume (mL ± standard deviation); 95% confidence intervals are shown in *italics*. TICV = total intracranial volume. Significance was calculated with a univariate ANOVA.

border was always rostral to the anterior vermis so as not to include the cerebellar peduncle (Fig. 2E). The vermis voxel was placed towards the anterior of the vermis and did not include any of the tissue from the two lateral hemispheres (Fig. 2D). Because every participant's cerebellar shape differed, careful inspection of the voxel placements on the T1- and T2-weighted scans was conducted to ensure there was no sampling of cerebrospinal fluid, nonbrain tissue, or bone.

Spectral Analysis

Spectral analysis was performed on the MR system manufacturer's software, which automatically corrected the baseline and calculated the area under the peak at 2.0 ppm, 3.0 ppm, and 3.2 ppm, corresponding to NAA, Cr, and Cho, respectively (Fig. 2A–C). Results are presented as the three possible area ratios: NAA/Cho, NAA/Cr, and Cho/Cr.

Analyses

Statistics were calculated using SPSS version 11.0.4 (2005). For the volumetric data, a MANOVA tested the independent variable group against the dependent variables of cerebellar regions of interest. Because of the rela-

tively small group sizes, Pillai's trace has been reported. After the MANOVA, significance of individual dependent variables was tested with a univariate ANOVA. A paired-samples *t*-test compared the volumes of right-versus-left cerebellar hemisphere white matter within groups.

On account of the smaller group sizes, between-group differences in the spectroscopy data for the three ratios were assessed with Mann–Whitney *U* test. Within-group analyses in the spectroscopy data used a Wilcoxon signed-rank test.

Group effect sizes were calculated by subtracting the dyslexic sample mean from the control sample mean and dividing by the standard deviation of the combined sample (Cohen, 1988). Effect sizes may be seen as a *z*-score for the between-group differences standardized to a control mean of 0 and a standard deviation of 1.

Results

Study 1: Cerebellar MRI Volume Measures

The overall descriptive statistics are presented in Table 2. There was a significant effect of group (dyslexic vs. control) on the

TABLE 3. Descriptive Data for the Adjusted and Normalized White Matter Volumes

Region of interest	Dyslexic ($N = 10$)	Control ($N = 11$)	Effect size	Significance (ANOVA)
Adjusted cerebellar white matter (percentage of TCbV)				
Right hemisphere	6.62 (±0.75)	5.83 (±0.71)	0.98	$F(1,19) = 6.31, P = 0.004$
	6.09–7.17	*5.36–6.30*		
Left hemisphere	6.61 (±0.55)	5.79 (±0.60)	1.17	$F(1,19) = 10.50, P = 0.02$
	6.21–7.00	*5.38–6.19*		
Normalized cerebellar white matter (normalized to TICV)				
Right hemisphere	0.69 (±0.07)	0.64 (±0.08)	0.70	$F(1,19) = 2.82, P = 0.08$
	0.64–0.74	*0.58–0.69*		
Left hemisphere	0.69 (±0.07)	0.63 (±0.08)	0.76	$F(1,19) = 3.36, P = 0.11$
	0.64–0.74	*0.58–0.69*		

Note: Expressed as mean (± standard deviation); 95% confidence intervals are shown in *italics*. Adjusted volumes are divided by the total cerebellar volume (TCbV) and are expressed as a percentage. Normalized volumes are divided by the (TICV). Significance was calculated with a univariate ANOVA.

region of interest (TICV, vermis, right hemisphere grey and white matter, left hemisphere grey and white matter), $F(6,14) = 2.80$, $P = 0.05$; Pillai's trace = 0.55; partial $\eta^2 = 0.55$. Analysis of each individual dependent variable demonstrated that four variables had a significant contribution to the overall effect: vermis, $F(1,19) = 4.82$, $P < 0.05$; partial $\eta^2 = 0.20$, TICV, $F(1,19) = 4.72$, $P < 0.05$; partial $\eta^2 = 0.20$, right hemisphere white matter, $F(1,19) = 9.90$, $P = 0.005$; partial $\eta^2 = 0.34$, and left hemisphere white matter, $F(1,19) = 11.67$, $P < 0.005$; partial $\eta^2 = 0.38$. For all these variables, the dyslexic group's mean volume was larger than the control group's. Neither the right nor the left hemisphere's grey matter was significantly different between groups: right, $F(1,19) = 0.34$; $P = $ ns; partial $\eta^2 = 0.02$; left: $F(1,19) = 0.00$, $P = $ ns; partial $\eta^2 = 0.00$. When a Bonferroni adjusted alpha level of 0.008 was applied to take into account the multiple hypotheses tested, significant group differences only remained for the right and left hemisphere's white matter. In both groups, there were no between-hemisphere differences in the white matter volume, suggesting symmetrical distribution, dyslexic $t(9) = 0.1$, $P = $ ns; control $t(10) = 0.5$, $P = $ ns.

To ascertain whether the increased volume of white matter in the left and right dyslexic cerebellar hemispheres could be ascribed to an overall larger cerebellar volume, we calculated the percentage of the total cerebellar volume that the white matter constituted. The total cerebellar volume was the summation of the volumes of the vermis, right hemisphere grey and white matter, and left hemisphere grey and white matter. The descriptive statistics for these adjusted white matter volumes are presented in Table 3. There was a significant effect of group on the percentage of white matter, $F(2,18) = 5.07$, $P < 0.05$; Pillai's trace = 0.36; partial $\eta^2 = 0.36$. When a Bonferroni corrected alpha of 0.025 was applied, the dyslexic's cerebellum contained a significantly larger percentage of white matter in both hemispheres: right, $F(1,19) = 6.31$, $P < 0.025$; partial $\eta^2 = 0.25$; left: $F(1,19) = 10.50$, $P < 0.005$; partial $\eta^2 = 0.36$. The larger percentage of white matter in the dyslexic cerebellum suggests that the increased volume of white matter cannot be simply attributed to each dyslexic participant possessing a larger cerebellum.

It is standard practice with morphometric studies to normalize brain regions to the TICV in case any volume differences reflect only overall brain size (Table 3). This was achieved by dividing the unadjusted white matter volume by the TICV. The logic behind this approach is less applicable for this study of the cerebellar

TABLE 4. Spectroscopy Ratios for the Vermis and Right and Left Cerebellar Hemispheres

Cerebellar region	Ratio	Dyslexic ($N = 6$)	Control ($N = 6$)	Significance (Mann–Whitney)
Vermis	NAA/Cho	1.09 (±0.06)	1.11 (±0.09)	$U = 16.5, P =$ ns
	NAA/Cr	1.04 (±0.11)	1.05 (±0.12)	$U = 16.5, P =$ ns
	Cho/Cr	0.95 (±0.08)	0.94 (±0.09)	$U = 20.0, P =$ ns
Right hemisphere	NAA/Cho	1.78 (±0.12)	2.30 (±0.50)	$U = 3.5, P = 0.008$
	NAA/Cr	1.94 (±0.25)	2.01 (±0.33)	$U = 17.0, P =$ ns
	Cho/Cr	1.10 (±0.20)	0.90 (±0.18)	$U = 9.5, P = 0.10$
Left hemisphere	NAA/Cho	1.72 (±0.41)	1.97 (±0.37)	$U = 9.0, P =$ ns
	NAA/Cr	1.65 (±0.52)	1.61 (±0.41)	$U = 17.0, P =$ ns
	Cho/Cr	0.96 (±0.10)	0.82 (±0.12)	$U = 5.5, P = 0.05$

Note: Mean group ratios are expressed as mean (± standard deviation). Significance was calculated by the Mann–Whitney U test. NAA = N-acetylaspartate; Cho = choline; Cr = creatine.

white matter volumes, since they have already been "normalized" to the total cerebellar volume. In any case, when normalizing against TICV, the between-group differences in cerebellar white matter for the left and the right hemispheres were lost, $F(2,18) = 1.73, P =$ ns; Pillai's trace $= 0.16$; partial $\eta^2 = 0.16$.

Study 2: Cerebellar MR Spectroscopy

The ratios of NAA/Cho, NAA/Cr, and Cho/Cr were calculated separately for each individual for the vermis and the right and left cerebellar hemispheres. Group mean data are shown in Table 4. There were no significant between-group differences for the three ratios in the vermis (NAA/Cho, $U = 16.5, P =$ ns; NAA/Cr, $U = 16.5, P =$ ns; Cho/Cr, $U = 20.0, P =$ ns). However, in the right cerebellar hemisphere, the dyslexics had a significantly smaller ratio of NAA/Cho compared to the control group ($U = 3.5, P < 0.01$). There was also a possible nonsignificant trend in this hemisphere for Cho/Cr whereby the dyslexic cerebella contained a larger ratio ($U = 9.5, P = 0.10$). The ratio of NAA/Cr in the right hemisphere did not differ between groups ($U = 17.0, P =$ ns). The Cho/Cr ratio was significantly greater for the dyslexic group in the left hemisphere ($U = 5.5, P < 0.05$); however, the other two ratios did not differ significantly between groups. Neither the dyslexic nor the control groups exhibited differences in the ratios between the left and right cerebellar hemispheres (dyslexic: NAA/Cr, $z = -1.4, P =$ ns; Cho/Cr, $z = -1.8, P =$ ns; NAA/Cho, $z = -0.7, P =$ ns; control: NAA/Cr, $z = -1.9, P =$ ns; Cho/Cr, $z = -0.7, P =$ ns; NAA/Cho, $z = -1.4, P =$ ns).

Discussion

The results demonstrate certain differences between the dyslexic and nondyslexic cerebellum in adults: The dyslexics possessed a greater volume of bilateral cerebellar white matter, a smaller NAA/Cho ratio in the right cerebellar hemisphere, and a greater Cho/Cr ratio in the left cerebellar hemisphere. These novel findings contribute to the growing body of evidence demonstrating abnormalities within the cerebellum of dyslexics.

Our main finding of a greater volume of white matter, with no concomitant increase in grey matter volume in the cerebellum of the dyslexic sample, means that dyslexics possess a greater volume of white matter per unit of grey matter. This finding could not be explained simply by a larger cerebellum in the dyslexic group as the percentage of white matter remained significantly larger. These findings differ from our preliminary hypotheses, which predicted grey matter differences. Our findings are also inconsistent with previous volumetric findings in the cerebellum of adults with dyslexia that have revealed reduced volumes in the grey matter of the right cerebellar anterior lobe (Leonard *et al.*, 2001) and no changes in cerebellar white matter (Rae *et al.*, 2002). However, our data cannot be easily compared to the reported grey matter findings (Eckert *et al.*, 2003; Leonard *et al.*, 2001) as we investigated different cerebellar regions. Eckert and colleagues subdivided their cerebellum laterally into an anterior and posterior lobe, whereas we divided our cerebellum longitudinally into a midline vermis and two lateral hemispheres. The right anterior lobe would include portions of our vermis and right cerebellar hemisphere grey matter; therefore further investigation would be needed to determine whether we could replicate the data of Eckert *et al.*

With any volumetric analysis, the method used to delineate the regions of interest will have an impact on subsequent measurements. The volumes we measured for the intracranial and cerebellar regions were in line with those published by a range of groups using different MRI, delineation, and analysis methods (e.g., Brambilla *et al.*, 2001; Edwards *et al.*, 1999; Hutchinson, Lee, Gaab, & Schlaug, 2003; Luft *et al.*, 1999; Okugawa *et al.*, 2002). Of interest, our results are consistent with the finding of increased white matter volume in the cerebral cortex in other developmental disorders such as autism (Herbert *et al.*, 2004) and developmental language disorders (Herbert *et al.*, 2003). Further, in relation to dyslexia, white matter differences have been recently reported at the level of the cerebral cortex using DTI, which allows the detection of differences in the microscopic constituents of white matter. These DTI results have demonstrated that the level of fractional anisotropy (FA) differs in the left temporoparietal area of dyslexics (Beaulieu *et al.*, 2005; Deutsch *et al.*, 2005; Klingberg *et al.*, 2000). FA is thought to reflect axonal directionality and integrity (Beaulieu, 2002). A further study, investigating reading-disabled children, reported FA values in two left temporoparietal regions which correlated with word identification (Niogi & McCandliss, 2006). However, none of the forementioned experiments investigated the connectivity of the cerebellum.

While our volumetric MRI data cannot provide information about the cytoarchitectural changes that may be responsible for the increased volume of white matter, such differences are likely to be subtle (no obvious pathology or gross differences were observable in the MRI scans). Three potential causes of an increase in white matter (as discussed in Herbert *et al.*, 2004) are (1) an increased number of axons; (2) bulkier or more myelin, producing a greater ratio of myelin to axons; and (3) other factors in white matter, such as other types of glial cells. Further investigations are needed to distinguish between these possibilities. In particular, an investigation of the signal intensity of the cerebellar white matter using multiple, differently weighted MRI sequences (T1, T2, proton-density, etc.) would provide converging information about the cytoarchitecture underlying the signal intensities.

The information gained from our spectroscopy data may shed some light on the reasons for differences in the white matter volumes found between the two groups. The right cerebellar hemisphere in the dyslexic sample had a significantly smaller ratio of NAA/Cho. This could be due to a reduced level of NAA or an increased level of choline. The corresponding ratios of NAA/Cr and Cho/Cr did not differ significantly between groups, so it is difficult to state which metabolite accounts for this decreased ratio. However, given the trend in increased Cho/Cr ratio in the dyslexic group, it may be that there are higher levels of Cho in the dyslexic's right cerebellar hemisphere. On the other hand, in the left cerebellar hemisphere, the ratio of Cho/Cr was significantly larger in the dyslexics. Once again, there were no corresponding significant alterations in the NAA/Cr or NAA/Cho ratios. A small hint may lie in the fact that the mean NAA/Cho ratio was slightly smaller in the dyslexic sample. Although this observation was not statistically supported, it may again provide a clue that, just as in the right hemisphere, the dyslexic group may have increased Cho levels. This possibility will need to be investigated further using larger sample sizes as the current study may have lacked sufficient statistical power, as only six dyslexic and six control participants underwent MRS.

However, should our observation be reproducible and an increase in Cho levels prove to be the driving force behind the change in ratios, this would then be inconsistent with previous findings by Rae *et al.* (1998), who reported decreased bilateral Cho and increased NAA on the right and decreased NAA in the left cerebellum. However, it should be noted that the study by Rae and colleagues used larger spectroscopy voxels ($3 \times 3 \times 3$ cm). In comparison to the current study this is an eight times increase of the volume interrogated and is likely to have included a greater proportion of grey matter, which could explain their NAA result. While we have discussed our results in relation to increases in Cho levels, we must also acknowledge that long-echo-time spectroscopy in influenced by T2 effects. This means that the difference in the ratios between the dyslexic and control groups could reflect dissimilar chemical environments due to a difference in cytoarchitecture, rather than absolute concentration differences (Wilkinson *et al.*, 1994). Ideally, future MRS investigations of the cerebellum would include both long- and short-echo-time sequences, which would provide converging information on any underlying metabolic differences.

There are a number of alternative interpretations of our spectroscopy results, including increased membrane turnover, cellular density, and myelination (Ross & Sachdev, 2004). The spectroscopy voxel in our participants' cerebellar hemispheres included grey and white matter as well as the dentate nucleus. As Cho is a component of cell membranes, both neuronal and glial, a change in Cho may suggest a greater proportion of cell membranes in the voxels of the dyslexic cerebellar hemispheres. The increased amount of cell membrane could

be a sign of increased axon density. Alternatively, it may be related to the myelin and glial cells, such as a greater amount of myelin membrane, which would not alter the NAA levels. Finally, it may suggest increased membrane turnover with higher levels of free choline. If there are higher rates of turnover of membrane molecules, then a lack of suitable fatty acids to manufacture new lipids could produce abnormal membranes. In relation to dyslexia, deficiencies of essential fatty acids could be problematic (Cyhlarova *et al.*, 2007).

On the basis of our combined results, we propose that there are two possible interpretations: (1) excessive connectivity and (2) abnormal myelination.

Excessive connections would lead to an increased volume of white matter and an increase in Cho without altering the NAA levels. Excessive connectivity could be the result of abnormal developmental stages, specifically a lack of synaptic or axon pruning (Low & Cheng, 2006), perhaps implying delayed development. One of the final stages in the development of the cerebellum is the refinement of course connectivity maps through pruning (Sotelo, 2004) to produce the shortest and most efficient communication route between cortico-cerebellar regions. A larger communication route, due to excessive connections, would lead to increased information transmission time, which could generate physiological "noise" and a reduced signal-to-noise ratio (Buzsái, 2006). This could generate difficulties integrating information from numerous brain regions.

However, the increased numbers of axons would have to originate from the mossy and climbing fiber inputs and deep cerebellar nuclei outputs, as opposed to an increased number of Purkinje cell axons from the cerebellar cortex. The latter would require more neurons in the cerebellar cortex, leading to a larger volume of grey matter and an increase in NAA. The increased volume of white matter lost significance when normalized to the dyslexic TICV (which tended to be larger in the dyslexic group).

This suggests that the larger cerebrum may be generating more input fibers to cerebellum via the pontine nuclei. As the pontine nuclei relay inputs from the cerebrum to the cerebellar cortex, it would be interesting to investigate this structure in dyslexics. At this stage we cannot rule out disordered cerebellar connections, but the disorderliness would need to increase volumes and Cho ratios. Examination of cerebellar white matter with DTI would shed further light into the microscopic changes underlying the white matter differences. If the white matter results relate to excessive or disordered inputs, it implies that the neural systems involving this structure are different in dyslexics. Turning to the second possible interpretation of our results, we need to consider the glial component of white matter. The cerebellum is one of the last structures to fully develop and be myelinated, with this process continuing in the lateral cerebellar hemispheres and inputs from the pontine nuclei until at least four months after birth (Triulzi, Parazzini, & Righini, 2005). An increase in the ratio of myelin to axons or the number of oligodendrocytes would increase the volume of white matter, and once again this would increase the overall amount of cell membrane relative to the number of neurons (the NAA/Cho ratio). As myelin increases the conduction speed of action potentials, the concept of more myelin being problematic, rather than beneficial, seems counterintuitive. However, a possible explanation could relate to abnormal compaction during the final stages of myelin formation, which would produce mature myelin that does not act as a neuronal insulator as efficiently as normal myelin (Boison & Stoffel, 1994). Herbert and colleagues found increased white matter in autistic children and children with developmental language disorders, and they suggest that because oligodendrocytes are responsive to neuronal activity, myelin increase could be a secondary consequence of increased physiological "noise"—in other words, in an attempt to overcome excessive noise during axonal transmission, the myelin has thickened.

Taken together, these two explanations are not mutually exclusive, but both require further study. Whatever the etiology of the increase in white matter (as well as the changes that account for the altered chemical ratios), in the light of either of the above discussed interpretations, there is the potential for generating physiological noise. This would in turn engender difficulties with neural timing, information processing, and integration of information—neuronal processes essential for accurate skill acquisition.

Acknowledgments

We wish to thank David Capener, radiographer, for his suggestions for improving the MRI sequences, and assistance with the MRI scanning and Dr. Jacqui Graham for her advice on the stereology method.

Conflict of Interest

The authors declare the following potential conflicts of interest:

Suzanna K. Laycock receives half of her Ph.D. maintenance grant from the Dore Foundation, a charity associated with Dore Achievement Centres. The Dore Foundation and Dore Achievement Centres have had no input into the goal of the study, the methodology, the analysis of the results, or the interpretation of the data.

References

Beaulieu, C. 2002. The basis of anisotropic water diffusion in the nervous system: a technical review. *NMR Biomedicine*, **15**(7–8): 435–455.

Beaulieu, C., Plewes, C., Paulson, L. A., Roy, D., Snook, L., Concha, L., *et al*. 2005. Imaging brain connectivity in children with diverse reading ability. *NeuroImage*, **25**(4): 1266–1271.

Boison, D., & Stoffel, W. 1994. Disruption of the compacted myelin sheath of axons of the central nervous system in proteolipid protein-deficient mice. *Proceedings of the National Academy of Sciences of the United States of America*, **91**(24): 11709–11713.

Brambilla, P., Harenski, K., Nicoletti, M., Mallinger, A. G., Frank, E., Kupfer, D. J., *et al*. 2001. MRI study of posterior fossa structures and brain ventricles in bipolar patients. *Journal of Psychiatric Research*, **35**(6): 313–322.

Brown, W. E., Eliez, S., Menon, V., Rumsey, J. M., White, C. D., & Reiss, A. L. 2001. Preliminary evidence of widespread morphological variations of the brain in dyslexia. *Neurology*, **56**(6): 781–783.

Buzsái, G. 2006. Structure defines function. In *Rhythms of the brain* (pp. xiv). New York: Oxford University Press.

Casanova, M. F., Buxhoeveden, D. P., Cohen, M., Switala, A. E., & Roy, E. L. 2002. Minicolumnar pathology in dyslexia. *Annals of Neurology*, **52**(1): 108–110.

Cohen, J. 1988. *Statistical power analysis for the behavioral sciences* (2nd ed.). New York: Academic Press.

Cyhlarova, E., Bell, J. G., Dick, J. R., Mackinlay, E. E., Stein, J. F., & Richardson, A. J. 2007. Membrane fatty acids, reading and spelling in dyslexic and non-dyslexic adults. *European Neuropsychopharmacology*, **17**(2): 116–121.

Demonet, J. F., Taylor, M. J., & Chaix, Y. 2004. Developmental dyslexia. *Lancet*, **363**(9419): 1451–1460.

Deshmukh, A. R., Desmond, J. E., Sullivan, E. V., Lane, B. F., Lane, B., Matsumoto, B., *et al*. 1997. Quantification of cerebellar structures with MRI. *Psychiatry Research*, **75**(3): 159–171.

Deutsch, G. K., Dougherty, R. F., Bammer, R., Siok, W. T., Gabrieli, J. D. E., & Wandell, B. 2005. Children's reading performance is correlated with white matter structure measured by diffusion tensor imaging. *Cortex*, **41**(3): 354–363.

Duvernoy, H. M., & Duvernoy, H. M. 1995. *The human brain stem and cerebellum: surface, structure, vascularization, and three-dimensional sectional anatomy with MRI*. Vienna and New York: Springer-Verlag.

Eckert, M. A. 2004. Neuroanatomical markers for dyslexia: a review of dyslexia structural imaging studies. *Neuroscientist*, **10**(4): 362–371.

Eckert, M. A., Leonard, C. M., Richards, T. L., Aylward, E. H., Thomson, J., & Berninger, V. W. 2003. Anatomical correlates of dyslexia: frontal and cerebellar findings. *Brain*, **126**: 482–494.

Eckert, M. A., Leonard, C. M., Wilke, M., Eckert, M., Richards, T., Richards, A., *et al*. 2005. Anatomical signatures of dyslexia in children: Unique information from manual and voxel based morphometry brain measures. *Cortex*, **41**(3): 304–315.

Edwards, S. G., Gong, Q. Y., Liu, C., Zvartau, M. E., Jaspan, T., Roberts, N., *et al*. 1999. Infratentorial atrophy on magnetic resonance imaging and disability in multiple sclerosis. *Brain*, **122**(Pt 2): 291–301.

Eliez, S., Rumsey, J. M., Giedd, J. N., Schmitt, J. E., Patwardhan, A. J., & Reiss, A. L. 2000. Morphological alteration of temporal lobe gray matter in dyslexia: An MRI study. *Journal of Child Psychology and Psychiatry and Allied Disciplines*, **41**(5): 637–644.

Fawcett, A. J., & Nicolson, R. I. 1998. *The dyslexia adult screening test*. London: The Psychological Corporation.

Finch, A. J., Nicolson, R. I., & Fawcett, A. J. 2002. Evidence for a neuroanatomical difference within the olivo-cerebellar pathway of adults with dyslexia. *Cortex*, **38**(4): 529–539.

Finucci, J. M., Guthrie, J. T., Childs, A. L., Abbey, H., & Childs, B. 1976. Genetics of specific reading-disability. *Annals of Human Genetics*, **40**(Jul): 1–23.

Galaburda, A. M. 1989. Ordinary and extraordinary brain development: anatomical variation in developmental dyslexia. *Annals of Dyslexia*, **39**.

Galaburda, A. M., & Kemper, T. L. 1979. Cytoarchitectonic abnormalities in developmental dyslexia: a case study. *Annals of Neurology*, **6:** 94–100.

Gundersen, H. J., & Jensen, E. B. 1987. The efficiency of systematic sampling in stereology and its prediction. *Journal of Microscopy*, **147**(Pt 3): 229–263.

Herbert, M. R., Ziegler, D. A., Makris, N., Bakardjiev, A., Hodgson, J., Adrien, K. T., *et al*. 2003. Larger brain and white matter volumes in children with developmental language disorder. *Developmental Science*, **6**(4): F11-F22.

Herbert, M. R., Ziegler, D. A., Makris, N., Filipek, P. A., Kemper, T. L., Normandin, J. J., *et al*. 2004. Localization of white matter volume increase in autism and developmental language disorder. *Annals of Neurology*, **55**(4): 530–540.

Humphreys, P., Kaufmann, W. E., & Galaburda, A. M. 1990. Developmental dyslexia in women: neuropathological findings in three patients. *Annals of Neurology*, **28**(6): 727–738.

Hutchinson, S., Lee, L. H., Gaab, N., & Schlaug, G. 2003. Cerebellar volume of musicians. *Cerebral Cortex*, **13**(9): 943–949.

Jorm, A. F., Share, D. L., McLean, R., & Matthews, D. 1986. Cognitive factors at school entry predictive of specific reading retardation and general reading backwardness: a research note. *Journal of Child Psychology and Psychiatry and Allied Disciplines*, **27:** 45–54.

Klingberg, T., Hedehus, M., Temple, E., Salz, T., Gabrieli, J. D. E., Moseley, M. E., *et al*. 2000. Microstructure of temporo-parietal white matter as a basis for reading ability: evidence from diffusion tensor magnetic resonance imaging. *Neuron*, **25**(2): 493–500.

Leonard, C. M., Eckert, M. A., Lombardino, L. J., Oakland, T., Kranzler, J., Mohr, C. M., *et al*. 2001. Anatomical risk factors for phonological dyslexia. *Cerebral Cortex*, **11**(2): 148–157.

Low, L. K., & Cheng, H. J. 2006. Axon pruning: an essential step underlying the developmental plasticity of neuronal connections. *Philosophical Transactions of the Royal Society of London, Series B: Biological Sciences,* **361**(1473): 1531–1544.

Luft, A. R., Skalej, M., Schulz, J. B., Welte, D., Kolb, R., Burk, K., *et al.* 1999. Patterns of age-related shrinkage in cerebellum and brainstem observed in vivo using three-dimensional MRI volumetry. *Cerebral Cortex,* **9**(7): 712–721.

Mayhew, T. M., & Olsen, D. R. 1991. Magnetic resonance imaging (MRI) and model-free estimates of brain volume determined using the Cavalieri principle. *Journal of Anatomy,* **178:** 133–144.

Nicolson, R. I., & Fawcett, A. 1997. Development of objective procedures for screening and assessment of dyslexic students in higher education. *Journal of Research in Reading,* **20**(1): 77–83.

Nicolson, R. I., & Fawcett, A. J. 2007. Procedural learning difficulties: re-uniting the developmental disorders? *Trends in Neurosciences,* **30**(4): 135–141.

Nicolson, R. I., Fawcett, A. J., & Dean, P. 2001. Developmental dyslexia: the cerebellar deficit hypothesis. *Trends in Neurosciences,* **24**(9): 508–511.

Niogi, S. N., & McCandliss, B. D. 2006. Left lateralized white matter microstructure accounts for individual differences in reading ability and disability. *Neuropsychologia,* **44**(11): 2178–2188.

Okugawa, G., Sedvall, G., Nordstrom, M., Andreasen, N., Pierson, R., Magnotta, V., *et al.* 2002. Selective reduction of the posterior superior vermis in men with chronic schizophrenia. *Schizophrenia Research,* **55**(1–2): 61–67.

Rae, C., Harasty, J. A., Dzendrowskyj, T. E., Talcott, J. B., Simpson, J. M., Blamire, A. M., *et al.* 2002. Cerebellar morphology in developmental dyslexia. *Neuropsychologia,* **40**(8): 1285–1292.

Rae, C., Lee, M. A., Dixon, R. M., Blamire, A. M., Thompson, C. H., Styles, P., *et al.* 1998. Metabolic abnormalities in developmental dyslexia detected by H-1 magnetic resonance spectroscopy. *Lancet,* **351:** 1849–1852.

Raz, N., Dupuis, J. H., Briggs, S. D., McGavran, C., & Acker, J. D. 1998. Differential effects of age and sex on the cerebellar hemispheres and the vermis: a prospective MR study. *AJNR. American Journal of Neuroradiology,* **19**(1): 65–71.

Richards, T. L., Corina, D., Serafini, S., Steury, K., Echelard, D. R., Dager, S. R., *et al.* 2000. Effects of a phonologically driven treatment for dyslexia on lactate levels measured by proton MR spectroscopic imaging. *AJNR. American Journal of Neuroradiology,* **21**(5): 916–922.

Richards, T. L., Dager, S. R., Corina, D., Serafini, S., Heide, A. C., Steury, K., *et al.* 1999. Dyslexic children have abnormal brain lactate response to reading-related language tasks. *AJNR. American Journal of Neuroradiology,* **20**(8): 1393–1398.

Roberts, N., Puddephat, M. J., & McNulty, V. 2000. The benefit of stereology for quantitative radiology. *British Journal of Radiology,* **73**(871): 679–697.

Robichon, F., Levrier, O., Farnarier, P., & Habib, M. 2000. Developmental dyslexia: atypical cortical asymmetries and functional significance. *European Journal of Neurology,* **7**(1): 35–46.

Ross, A. J., & Sachdev, P. S. 2004. Magnetic resonance spectroscopy in cognitive research. *Brain Research. Brain Research Review,* **44**(2–3): 83–102.

Schmahmann, J. D. 2000. *MRI atlas of the human cerebellum.* San Diego, CA: Academic Press.

Shrout, P. E., & Fleiss, J. L. 1979. Intraclass correlations: uses in assessing rater reliability. *Psychological Bulletin,* **86**(2): 420–428.

Silani, G., Frith, U., Demonet, J. F., Fazio, F., Perani, D., Price, C., *et al.* 2005. Brain abnormalities underlying altered activation in dyslexia: a voxel based morphometry study. *Brain,* **128**(Pt 10): 2453–2461.

Snowling, M. 1998. Dyslexia as a phonological deficit: evidence and implications. *Child and Adolescent Mental Health,* **3**(1): 4–11.

Sotelo, C. 2004. Cellular and genetic regulation of the development of the cerebellar system. *Progress in Neurobiology,* **72**(5): 295–339.

SPSS. 2005. *SPSS for Mac OS X, version 11.0.4.* Chicago, IL: SPSS Inc.

Talos, I. F., Mian, A. Z., Zou, K. H., Hsu, L., Goldberg-Zimring, D., Haker, S., *et al.* 2006. Magnetic resonance and the human brain: anatomy, function and metabolism. *Cellular and Molecular Life Sciences,* **63**(10): 1106–1124.

Triulzi, F., Parazzini, C., & Righini, A. 2005. MRI of fetal and neonatal cerebellar development. *Seminars in Fetal & Neonatal Medicine,* **10**(5): 411–420.

Vinckenbosch, E., Robichon, F., & Eliez, S. 2005. Gray matter alteration in dyslexia: converging evidence from volumetric and voxel-by-voxel MRI analyses. *Neuropsychologia,* **43**(3): 324–331.

Wechsler, D. 1993. *Wechsler Objective Reading Dimension (WORD).* London: The Psychological Corporation.

Wechsler, D. 1999. *Wechsler Adult Intelligence Scale* (3rd UK edition). Oxford, UK: Harcourt Assessment.

Wilkinson, I. D., Paley, M., Chong, W. K., Sweeney, B. J., Shepherd, J. K., Kendall, B. E., *et al.* 1994. Proton spectroscopy in HIV infection: relaxation times of cerebral metabolites. *Magnetic Resonance Imaging,* **12**(6): 951–957.

A Meta-analysis of Functional Neuroimaging Studies of Dyslexia

José M. Maisog,[a] Erin R. Einbinder,[a] D. Lynn Flowers,[a,b] Peter E. Turkeltaub,[c] and Guinevere F. Eden[a]

[a]*Center for the Study of Learning, Georgetown University Medical Center, Washington, DC, USA*

[b]*Wake Forest University School of Medicine, Winston-Salem, North Carolina, USA*

[c]*Department of Neurology, University of Pennsylvania Health System, Philadelphia, PA, USA*

Reading and phonological processing deficits have been the primary focus of neuroimaging studies addressing the neurologic basis of developmental dyslexia, but to date there has been no objective assessment of the consistency of these findings. To address this issue, spatial coordinates reported in the literature were submitted to two parallel activation likelihood estimate (ALE) meta-analyses. First, a meta-analysis including 96 foci from nine publications identified regions where typical readers are likely to show greater activation than dyslexics: two left extrastriate areas within BA 37, precuneus, inferior parietal cortex, superior temporal gyrus, thalamus, and left inferior frontal gyrus. Right hemisphere ALE foci representing hypoactivity in dyslexia were found in the fusiform, postcentral, and superior temporal gyri. To identify regions in which dyslexic subjects reliably show greater activation than controls, 75 foci from six papers were entered into a second meta-analysis. Here ALE results revealed hyperactivity associated with dyslexia in right thalamus and anterior insula. These findings suggest that during the performance of a variety of reading tasks, normal readers activate left-sided brain areas more than dyslexic readers do, whereas dyslexia is associated with greater right-sided brain activity. The most robust result was in left extrastriate cortex, where hypoactivity associated with dyslexia was found. However, the ALE maps provided no support for cerebellar dysfunction, nor for hyperactivity in left frontal cortex in dyslexia, suggesting that these findings, unlike those described above, are likely to be more varied in terms of their reproducibility or spatial location.

Key words: meta-analysis; dyslexia; functional imaging

Introduction

Developmental dyslexia is a common reading disorder which accounts for 80% of all learning disabilities in the United States (Lerner, 1989; Lyon, 1995a). The cognitive deficits associated with developmental dyslexia have been intensely studied over the last 40 years (for review see Vellutino, Fletcher, Snowling, & Scanlon, 2004). Behavioral studies of dyslexia suggest that a core deficit in phonological processing, specifically phonemic awareness, underlies problems in the decoding of text (Bruck, 1992; Fletcher *et al.*, 1994; Flowers, 1995; Liberman & Shankweiler, 1991; Morris *et al.*, 1998; Ramus, 2003; Shankweiler, Liberman, Mark, Fowler, & Fischer, 1979; Shaywitz *et al.*, 1999; Shaywitz *et al.*, 2003; Stanovich & Siegel, 1994; Torgesen, 1995; Wagner & Torgesen, 1987). In addition to language, several other domains, such as the visual, auditory, and motor systems, are affected (Eden *et al.*, 1996; Fawcett & Nicolson, 1992; Lovegrove, Heddle, & Slaghuis, 1980; Tallal, 1980).

Address for correspondence: José M. Maisog, M.D., Center for the Study of Learning, Department of Pediatrics, Georgetown University Medical Center, Box 571406, Suite 150, Building D, 4000 Reservoir Road, NW, Washington, DC 20057, USA. jmm97@georgetown.edu

Although the criteria that define dyslexia have been refined over time and are now well established (Lyon, 1995b; Lyon, Shaywitz, & Shaywitz, 2003; Shaywitz, Fletcher, & Shaywitz, 1995), the underlying pathology of dyslexia remains uncertain. Neuroimaging technologies provide one approach to determine the neural basis of dyslexia; following the lines of behavioral studies in dyslexia, research using these newer modalities have focused primarily on the study of reading and phonological processing. Neuroimaging methods such as functional magnetic resonance imaging (fMRI), positron emission tomography (PET), event-related potentials (ERP), and magnetoencephalography (MEG) have been used in different countries to provide evidence of hypoactivation of the left posterior language system in dyslexia, across different languages (Brunswick, McCrory, Price, Frith, & Frith, 1999; Helenius, Tarkiainen, Cornelissen, Hansen, & Salmelin, 1999; Horwitz, Rumsey, & Donohue, 1998; Ingvar *et al.*, 2002; Paulesu *et al.*, 2001; Rumsey *et al.*, 1992; Rumsey *et al.*, 1997b; Salmelin, 1996; Shaywitz *et al.*, 2002; Temple *et al.*, 2000). This hypoactivity has been localized to left posterior parietal cortex (Brunswick *et al.*, 1999; Eden *et al.*, 2004; Flowers *et al.*, under review; Pugh *et al.*, 2000; Rumsey *et al.*, 1997b; Shaywitz *et al.*, 2002; Simos *et al.*, 2000a; Simos *et al.*, 2000b; Temple *et al.*, 2001), inferior occipitotemporal cortex (Brunswick *et al.*, 1999; McCrory, Mechelli, Frith, & Price, 2005; Paulesu *et al.*, 2001; Shaywitz *et al.*, 2002), and superior temporal gyrus (Flowers *et al.*, under review; Paulesu *et al.*, 2001; Paulesu *et al.*, 1996; Rumsey *et al.*, 1997b).

On the other hand, there is some disagreement in the literature regarding certain brain regions. For example, left inferior frontal cortex has been reported by some investigators to be more active in dyslexics (Brunswick *et al.*, 1999; Grünling *et al.*, 2004; Shaywitz *et al.*, 1998), and compensatory mechanisms have been suggested to account for this observation (Shaywitz & Shaywitz, 2005). However, other studies have not found this hyperactivation in

dyslexia (Eden *et al.*, 2004; Rumsey *et al.*, 1994), and there are even reports of hypoactivity in left inferior frontal regions, relative to controls (Flowers *et al.*, under review; Georgiewa *et al.*, 1999; Paulesu *et al.*, 1996; Rumsey *et al.*, 1997b; Shaywitz *et al.*, 2002). Some of the studies showing an absence of frontal hyperactivation in dyslexia were conducted in children and could suggest that dyslexia leads to compensatory mechanisms once adulthood is reached (Shaywitz *et al.*, 2002). However, this age-specific theory does not account for the left inferior frontal gyrus hypoactivity reported for adults in other studies (Flowers *et al.*, under review; Georgiewa *et al.*, 1999; Paulesu *et al.*, 1996; Rumsey *et al.*, 1997b; Shaywitz *et al.*, 2002).

Another area of intense investigation in reading and dyslexia involves the role of the cerebellum. Although traditionally not considered a participant in language, more recent evidence suggests that the cerebellum might play a significant role in reading (Fiez & Petersen, 1998), and that its activity may differ during reading and word repetition tasks in individuals with dyslexia (Brunswick *et al.*, 1999; McCrory, Frith, Brunswick, & Price, 2000). Combined with evidence of cerebellar dysfunction from the behavioral (Nicolson, Fawcett, & Dean, 2001), metabolic (Rae *et al.*, 1998), anatomical (Rae *et al.*, 2002) and functional literature (Nicolson *et al.*, 1999), the cerebellum is considered to play a potential role in reading disability (Ramus, 2003).

In general, discrepancies in the published literature are most likely explained by subtle differences in task paradigms. The neural basis of reading is known to be influenced by task parameters such as duration and frequency of the word presentation (Price, Moore, & Frackowiak, 1996). Subject selection (severity of dyslexia, bilingualism in the subjects, etc.) and proficiency of task performance are also believed to play a role. There have been some investigations into the role of a language's orthography, particularly the consistency by which mapping of sound to print occurs. Notably, Paulesu *et al.* showed that aberrant activity in left inferior posterior temporal regions was common to French, Italian, and English dyslexics, suggesting that the orthography of the language cannot account for differences in neural activity during reading, at least in alphabetic languages (Paulesu *et al.*, 2001). However, the functional anatomy of dyslexia has proven to be somewhat different in some studies of Asian languages. Siok and colleagues in China found that dyslexia in nonalphabetic languages may have a neural signature distinct from dyslexia in alphabetic languages (Siok, Perfetti, Jin, & Tan, 2004). In sum, the particular population studied, the cognitive tasks employed, and differences in methodology influence functional neuroimaging results. These study-specific factors lead to variable results. Despite this variability, a solid understanding of the neurologic basis of dyslexia can be obtained if an objective approach is employed, which identifies the most robust and consistent functional differences.

Using the terminology of Koretz (2002), a "narrative review" of the literature has thus far been the only method by which the findings from neuroimaging studies of dyslexia have been summarized. Such reviews are based on findings that are most dependable across multiple studies (Eden & Zeffiro, 1998; McCrory, 2004; Shaywitz & Shaywitz, 2005; Temple, 2002). However, narrative reviews are susceptible to biases (Koretz, 2002). This problem is compounded by the fact that the choice of anatomic labels applied in studies of brain imaging is somewhat subjective. To address this issue, meta-analytic approaches have recently been applied to published brain imaging findings (Chein, Fissell, Jacobs, & Fiez, 2002; Turkeltaub, Eden, Jones, & Zeffiro, 2002). As in other fields, meta-analyses are a post-hoc combination of results from independent studies, allowing for a better estimation of parameters of interest. To this end, statistically significant effects from different studies are pooled to estimate the spatial location of activation likelihood for specific cognitive functions. For example, Turkeltaub *et al.* developed an objective, quantitative meta-analytic method to determine consistency across neuroimaging studies, and employed it to identify regions commonly seen during reading in adults (Turkeltaub *et al.*, 2002). This method generates an activation likelihood estimate (ALE) at each voxel. There are numerous advantages to such "systematic reviews" (Koretz, 2002), which have been described in detail by Fox and colleagues (Fox, Laird, & Lancaster, 2005b; Laird *et al.*, 2005b).

Of importance, meta-analytic approaches aid the estimation of concordance across multiple published brain imaging findings and present a principled way of assessing spatial reproducibility. The ALE method and similar methods (Chein *et al.*, 2002) have been used to identify common cortical networks for a range of cognitive functions (Bolger, Perfetti, & Schneider, 2005; Buchsbaum, Greer, Chang, & Berman, 2005; Derrfuss, Brass, Neumann, & von Cramon, 2005; Farrell, Laird, & Egan, 2005; Fox *et al.*, 2005a; Grosbras, Laird, & Paus, 2005; Laird *et al.*, 2005b; Neumann, Lohmann, Derrfuss, & von Cramon, 2005; Owen, McMillan, Laird, & Bullmore, 2005; Petacchi, Laird, Fox, & Bower, 2005; Price, Devlin, Moore, Morton, & Laird, 2005; Tan, Laird, Li, & Fox, 2005). In addition to conducting meta-analysis in alphabetic writing systems (Turkeltaub *et al.*, 2002), the ALE approach has also been used to determine regions of the brain that are universally engaged in readers of English, Chinese and Japanese (Bolger *et al.*, 2005). However, the ALE approach has only recently been implemented to examine and compare findings across the published literature in clinical populations, namely those with stuttering and schizophrenia (Brown, Ingham, Ingham, Laird, & Fox, 2005; Glahn *et al.*, 2005).

The present ALE meta-analysis aims to derive an objective conclusion about the most commonly reported differences in the dyslexic population during tasks involving reading of alphabetic languages. The method employed here includes all coordinates from an eligible experimental contrast, not just regions of particular interest based on trends in the literature. The studies chosen employ PET or fMRI, and compare dyslexics and typical readers engaged in linguistic tasks that involve the visual presentation of words or letters. This provides a good degree of task consistency across studies, suitable for the meta-analytical approach.

The primary objective of the meta-analysis is to identify the most robust regions of hypo- and hyperactivation in dyslexia. The inclusion of studies that reported on hyper- and hypoactivity in dyslexia using the same paradigms made this possible. We expected to find cross-study agreement for hypoactivity in dyslexia in areas of left posterior brain regions, including parietal cortex, inferior occipitotemporal, and superior temporal gyri. Areas revealed by this meta-analysis can serve the purpose of determining acquisition and analysis strategies in future studies. For example, the location of these areas might be used to conduct region-of-interest analyses, aid in selecting voxels that serve as a "seed" for whole-brain correlations, and help to model the neural correlates predicted for mechanisms of compensation.

Methods

Criteria for Papers Included in the Meta-analysis

We performed a MEDLINE search to identify published fMRI or PET studies comparing dyslexics and normal readers. We limited studies to those using tasks involving reading of alphabetic languages, with visually presented words, pseudowords, or letters in the subjects' native language. Only studies involving healthy postpubertal dyslexic or nondyslexic teens and adults, with no history of neurologic or psychiatric disorders, matched for age and handedness, were allowed into the analysis. The following studies were excluded: those which did not present stereotactic Talairach (Talairach & Tournoux, 1988) or Montreal Neurological Institute (MNI) coordinates of local maxima (x, y, z) for a direct comparison between normal readers and dyslexics, those that used a region-of-interest rather than voxel-wise analysis, and

those studies whose subjects were prepubertal age.

Nine papers (Brunswick *et al.*, 1999; Flowers *et al.*, under review; Georgiewa *et al.*, 1999; Grünling *et al.*, 2004; Ingvar *et al.*, 2002; McCrory *et al.*, 2005; Paulesu *et al.*, 2001; Paulesu *et al.*, 1996; Rumsey *et al.*, 1997b) met the selection criteria and provided 96 activation foci from a combined total of 171 subjects, in which controls exhibited greater activity than dyslexics. Six of the nine papers reported 75 foci from 159 subjects in which dyslexics showed greater activity than controls.

Summaries of Papers Included in the Meta-analysis

The paradigms employed in the studies included here were generally of two types: either those requiring decisions about visually presented letters, words, and pseudowords; or those requiring explicit reading of visually presented words and pseudowords. Some papers report using both approaches. One meta-analysis included two reports that employed a decision-making task only (Studies 1 and 2 described below), three reports that utilized both a decision-making task and an explicit reading task (Studies 3 to 5), and four reports (Studies 6 to 9) that relied only on paradigms involving explicit reading. Within each meta-analysis the tasks and contrasts between the dyslexic and nondyslexic groups were identical, allowing for easy comparison and clear interpretation of the resultant ALE maps. Each report is described in more detail next.

(1) A study by Paulesu *et al.* represents the earliest neuroimaging work included in this meta-analysis on the neural basis of dyslexia (Paulesu *et al.*, 1996). PET was used to measure regional cerebral blood flow (rCBF) in five partially compensated adult dyslexics with residual phonological deficits and five control subjects. Subjects made a manual response to specifically defined target stimuli. In the rhyming

paradigm included in this meta-analysis, subjects directed a joystick to indicate when visually presented letters rhymed with "B." In a short-term memory task employed in the same study, but not included in our meta-analysis, subjects were instructed to indicate whether a probe consonant was present in a preceding group of six consonants. The dyslexics showed reduced activation in Broca's area (left inferior frontal, BA 6/44) and Wernicke's area (left superior temporal gyrus, BA 21/22) during the short-term memory task and the rhyming task, respectively. During both tasks, dyslexics showed less activity in the left insula compared to the control group, who activated all three areas during both tasks. Paulesu *et al.* proposed a "disconnection" deficit model for dyslexia in which the insula is critical to integrate anterior and posterior systems for the processing of linguistic stimuli.

(2) Grünling *et al.* combined data from fMRI and EEG to assess differences between dyslexics and controls (Grünling *et al.*, 2004). Seventeen dyslexics and 21 controls performed a variety of matching tasks, involving letter strings, high frequency words, and pseudowords, similar to the paradigms previously used by Shaywitz and colleagues (Shaywitz *et al.*, 1998). fMRI data gathered when subjects had to decide whether two visually presented pseudowords rhymed (contrasted to letter-string matching) were submitted to the meta-analysis. Grünling and colleagues reported this contrast to reveal hyperactivity in the dyslexics in left and right frontal areas, and hypoactivity in left middle temporal gyrus (BA 21), right superior frontal gyrus (BA 10), and left cuneus (BA 18) compared with controls. The investigators also reported differences in timing of neuronal processing (EEG) between dyslexics and controls.

(3) In a study using PET-rCBF measurements, Rumsey *et al.* (1997b) examined

17 adult male dyslexics with persistent reading deficits and 14 matched controls during performance of two explicit reading tasks, one phonological (reading aloud of pseudowords such as "chirl"), and the other orthographic (reading aloud of real "exception" words such as "choir"), as well as two decision-making tasks, again one phonological (given two pseudowords such as "bape" and "baik," which would sound like a read word when spoken) and the other orthographic (given a word and its pseudohomophone such as "hoal" and "hole," which is a real word) (Rumsey *et al.*, 1997b). The task paradigm was designed to place varying demands on the main deficit thought to account for impaired word recognition in dyslexics, that is, phonological processing. Regions in which dyslexics showed reduced blood flow relative to controls for either the phonological explicit reading or phonological decision-making tasks included bilateral parietal areas (BA 40) and temporal regions (including BA 37, 39, 20, 21, 22, and 42), right pre/postcentral gyrus, and bilateral precuneus. Areas of hyperactivation in the dyslexic group during either the phonological explicit reading or phonological decision-making tasks were found in left inferior occipital gyrus (BA 18), left medial temporal cortex, right insula, left pre/postcentral gyrus, right frontal (BA 10/46), and several subcortical and cerebellar regions. Dyslexics had relative deactivations compared to controls in left inferior frontal cortex (BA 44/45 and 47) for both orthographic tasks. In contrast to the findings from Paulesu *et al.* (1996), Rumsey *et al.* (1997b) found hyperactivation of the left insula in the dyslexic group during real and pseudoword reading. On the basis of the dyslexics' poor performance during reading, Rumsey *et al.* proposed a compensation hypothesis for the increased activity seen in the left insula in dyslexics as compared to controls.

(4) In an attempt to address methodological concerns regarding potential performance confounds in earlier studies comparing dyslexics and typical readers, Brunswick *et al.* (1999) designed two reading experiments. Their first experiment, an explicit reading task in which subjects read real or pseudowords aloud was administered. In their second experiment a decision-making "implicit reading" task was used, in which subjects indicated by button press whether or not a real or pseudoword contained an "ascender" letter (for example, l, f, d, or t); a false font condition was used as an active baseline. By including both explicit and implicit reading paradigms, the researchers hoped to differentiate between compensatory activity during explicit reading of words or pseudowords and abnormal activations during implicit processing of these words, respectively. PET was used to measure rCBF in 12 compensated dyslexics with persistent reading deficits and 12 controls (12 in each experiment). During both studies, subjects were exposed to the same number of phonologically simple stimuli designed to minimize performance differences between the two groups. During explicit reading (regardless of word type), several areas showed reduced activation in dyslexics compared to controls, including posterior regions such as left posterior inferior temporal cortex/fusiform gyrus (in and around BA 37) and bilateral medial extrastriate cortex, left subcortical regions, and cerebellum. Left premotor cortex (BA 6/44, Broca's area), was more active in the dyslexic group relative to controls. Given these findings, Brunswick *et al.* hypothesized that dyslexics may compensate for underactivation of medial extrastriate cortex, a region that may be important for whole-word processing, with increased sublexical articulation mediated by the premotor cortex. Since the second experiment did not require vocalization, the investigators did not predict a similar effect in premotor cortex for implicit reading. Consistent with that hypothesis, the results of the second experiment (based on the decision-making task) were notable for an absence of frontal hyperactivity in dyslexics. Reduced activation was seen only in posterior areas, such as posterior inferior and middle temporal cortex (BA 37/20/21), as well as inferior parietal cortex (BA 40/7).

(5) In a later paper, Paulesu *et al.* (2001) used PET-rCBF measurements to compare dyslexics and controls during the same explicit and implicit reading paradigm employed by Brunswick and colleagues in order to elucidate specific neurobiological deficits that are consistent across languages with varying orthographic depth (English and French have a deep orthography as the mapping is not as direct as for Italian, which has a shallow orthography). The investigators scanned a group of 12 dyslexics and 12 well-matched controls from three countries: Italy, France, and the UK. Half of the subjects from each country performed the explicit reading task (reading words and pseudowords aloud) and the other half performed an implicit reading task that involved decision-making regarding the presence or absence of an ascender. Although Italian dyslexics performed better than English and French dyslexics on reading measures, dyslexics from each country were equally impaired relative to their respective control groups. Combining the data from the explicit reading study and the decision-making study, four left hemisphere areas proved to be more active in controls compared to dyslexics regardless of word type, task, or language: superior temporal gyrus (BA 22), middle temporal gyrus (BA 21), inferior temporal gyrus (BA 37), and middle occipital gyrus (BA 37). Paulesu *et al.* concluded that dyslexia has a universal

neurobiological basis across alphabet-based languages, but that the behavioral manifestations depend on orthographic depth.

(6) Georgiewa *et al.* used fMRI to examine brain activity in dyslexics and controls during several tasks designed to place varying demands on phonological skills (Georgiewa *et al.*, 1999). Seventeen adolescent dyslexics and seventeen matched controls performed three silent reading tasks during scanning: letter strings, pseudowords, real words, and a phonological transformation task (similar to pig Latin). Scans from these three conditions were contrasted with passively viewing letter strings. During the tasks which placed the heaviest demands on phonological processing (pseudoword reading and phonological transformation, included in our meta-analysis), reduced activation was seen in left inferior frontal gyrus (BA 44) and thalamus in dyslexics compared with controls. Dyslexics activated the lingual gyrus (BA 18) during real-word reading and superior temporal gyrus (BA 22) during both real- and pseudoword reading to a greater extent than controls. It should be noted that the brain was scanned only within a limited region along the vertical axis (Talairach Z level restricted to the range −15 mm to +15 mm), introducing a regional bias to this study. However, the nature of the meta-analytic technique does not preclude the usefulness or validity of the between-group differences reported here, and so available data meeting the inclusion criteria were included.

(7) To examine differences between dyslexics and controls during language processing, Ingvar *et al.* (200) measured rCBF using PET in 9 adult Swedish-speaking male dyslexics and 9 matched controls. Swedish has a shallower orthography than English. Aloud and silent reading tasks of real words and pseudowords were compared with a resting baseline. During silent real-word reading versus fixation, dyslexics showed more activity than controls in right occipitotemporal cortex (BA 37), whereas controls showed more activity than dyslexics in right dorsolateral prefrontal cortex (BA 10) and right angular gyrus (BA 39). Ingvar suggested that these results support a separate functional compensational processing pathway in dyslexia.

(8) McCrory *et al.* (2005) sought to identify an abnormal pattern of neural activation in dyslexics common to both reading and naming. During PET scanning, 8 adult dyslexics and 10 controls performed a real-word reading- and picture-naming task (the latter task was not included in the present meta-analysis). Results revealed less activity in left occipitotemporal cortex (BA 37) in dyslexics compared to controls during both tasks, suggesting that reading disability in dyslexia may be related to an underlying deficit in the assignment of phonology to any visual stimuli, and thus may not be specific to words.

(9) In a recent study, Flowers *et al.* (under review) used fMRI to examine decoding ability in 12 adult dyslexics and 14 matched controls during aloud pseudoword and real-word reading. A direct contrast of the two activation conditions revealed that both dyslexics and controls increase activity in left parietal and bilateral inferior frontal cortex during the more phonologically demanding task, pseudoword reading, whereas left inferior temporal cortex was more active during real-word reading. Regardless of word type (real or pseudowords), compared to controls, dyslexics underactivated bilateral inferior frontal gyri (BA 47), left parietal cortices (BA 40/2), and left inferior temporal cortex (BA 37/20), as well as several right hemisphere regions, including superior temporal gyrus (BA 22), post central gyrus (BA 40/2), and

cerebellum. Orbitofrontal gyrus (47/11), anterior temporal pole (BA 38), right inferior frontal gyrus (BA 44/45), and bilateral thalamus were found to be more active in dyslexics. The results from this main effects analysis were submitted to the meta-analysis. The group-by-task interaction (which was not included in the present meta-analysis) revealed that bilateral parietal and premotor regions as well as left inferior, middle, and superior frontal cortices were more active in controls during pseudoword reading compared with those of dyslexics.

Activation Likelihood Estimate Method

We used the activation likelihood estimate (ALE) method to perform the meta-analyses (Turkeltaub *et al.*, 2002). To ensure that all input coordinates were in the same standard anatomical space, we avoided mixing Talairach coordinates with MNI coordinates (Brett, Christoff, Cusack, & Lancaster, 2001; Brett, Johnsrude, & Owen, 2002). We treated the foci of activity as coordinates of MNI space if a study (1) used a version of SPM (Wellcome Department of Cognitive Neurology, London, UK) that officially employs the MNI templates (SPM96 or later) and did not apply a conversion to Talairach space, or (2) used some other template-based software with an MNI template to perform spatial normalization (e.g., Automated Image Registration [AIR] of Woods, Grafton, Watson, Sicotte, & Mazziotta, 1998). All coordinates thought to be reported using the Talairach coordinates were converted to MNI space (Brett, 1999), thereby bringing all studies into a common coordinate system.

With all foci in MNI space, we submitted the coordinates to two separate ALE meta-analyses: one to identify locations in the brain where control groups showed greater task-related activity than the dyslexic groups (Controls > Dyslexics: 96 foci from 9 papers,

14 contrasts; Table 1), and a second analysis to reveal the reverse, that is, where dyslexics demonstrated more activity than controls (Dyslexics > Controls: 75 foci from 6 papers, 10 contrasts; Table 2). For each of these two meta-analyses, a spatial smoothing factor of 14.1 mm FWHM was used. Ten thousand (10,000) randomizations were performed to estimate the null ALE distribution (Turkeltaub *et al.*, 2002). To account for multiple comparisons, an ALE threshold was selected by controlling the false discovery rate at a level of 0.0001 (Genovese, Lazar, & Nichols, 2002; Laird *et al.*, 2005a).

After thresholding each ALE map, local maxima were identified, their MNI coordinates converted to Talairach coordinates (Brett, 1999), and their anatomical labels were assigned using the atlas of Talairach and Tournoux (Talairach & Tournoux, 1988). The relative contribution of each study to each ALE local maximum was calculated (Tables 3 and 4). For visualization purposes, the thresholded ALE maps were overlaid on a structural MRI scan in MNI space and displayed in 2D (axial slices captured in MEDx) as well as 3D volume renderings (VolView, Kitware, Clifton Park, NY, USA).

Results

Controls > Dyslexics

The meta-analysis for Controls > Dyslexics revealed nine distinct clusters of suprathreshold voxels in the ALE map, the largest of which had two local maxima (Table 5). The local maxima in the left hemisphere were located in precuneus (BA 31), middle occipital gyrus (BA 37), fusiform gyrus (BA 37), inferior parietal lobule (BA 40), superior temporal gyrus (BA 22), thalamus (pulvinar), and inferior frontal gyrus (BA 47/11). In the right hemisphere, the ALE analysis identified foci in fusiform gyrus (BA 20), postcentral gyrus (BA 2), and superior temporal gyrus (BA 21). 2D slices at the level of the

TABLE 1. Characteristics of the Nine Papers Included in the Meta-analysis for Controls > Dyslexics

	Study	Year	Imaging	Task type	Response modality	Word type	Baseline	# of foci	Uncorrected threshold	Dyslexics (N)				Controls (N)				Native language
										Total	Male	RH	Mean age	Total	Male	RH	Mean Age	
1	Paulesu	1996	PET	Decision (rhyme)	Button press	Single letters	Korean shape decision	6	$P < .05$	5	5	5	25.2	5	5	5	27.2	English
2	Grünling	2004	fMRI	Decision (rhyme)	Button press	Pseudo	Letter-string matching	3	$P < .01$	17	NA	17	14	21	NA	21	13	German
3a	Rumsey	1997	PET	Decision (phonological)	Button press	2 pseudo	Fixation	12	$P < .01$	17	17	17	27	14	14	14	25	English
				Decision (orthographic)	Button press	1 real 1 pseudo	Fixation	11	$P < .01$	17	17	17	27	14	14	14	25	English
4a	Brunswick	1999	PET	Decision (ascender)	Button press	Real + pseudo	False font	6	$P < .001$	6	6	6	24.5	6	6	6	24.5	English
5	Paulesu	2001	PET	Explicit + decision	Both	Real + pseudo	Rest + false font	4	$P < .001$	12 / 12 / 12	12 / 12 / 12	12 / 12 / 12	~24	12 / 12 / 12	12 / 12 / 12	12 / 12 / 12	~24	English / French / Italian
3b	Rumsey	1997	PET	Explicit phonological	Aloud	Pseudo	Fixation	14	$P < .01$	17	17	17	27	14	14	14	25	English
				Explicit orthographic	Aloud	Exception real	Fixation	11	$P < .01$	17	17	17	27	14	14	14	25	English
4b	Brunswick	1999	PET	Explicit reading	Aloud	Real + pseudo	Rest (eyes closed)	14	$P < .01$	6	6	6	23	6	6	6	23.2	English
6	Georgiewa	1999	fMRI	Explicit reading	Silent	Pseudo	Letter-string reading	2	$p < .001$	17	8	17	13.6	17	8	17	14.4	German
				Transformation	Silent	Real	Letter-string reading	2	$P < .001$	17	8	17	13.6	17	8	17	14.4	German
7	Ingvar	2002	PET	Explicit reading	Silent	Teal	Rest (eyes open)	3	$P < .001$	9	9	9	20-26	9	9	9	20-28	Swedish
8	McCrory	2005	PET	Explicit reading	Aloud	Real	False font (saying "yes")	1	$P < .001$	8	8	8	20	10	10	10	20	English
9	Flowers	Under review	fMRI	Explicit reading	Aloud	Real + pseudo	Fixation	18	$P < .001$	12	9	10	43.7	14	10	13	40.7	English

TABLE 2. Characteristics of the Six Papers Included in the Meta-analysis for Dyslexics > Controls

	Study	Year	Imaging	Task type	Response modality	Word type	Baseline	# of foci	Uncorrected threshold	Dyslexics (N)				Controls (N)				Native language
										Total	Male	RH	Mean age	Total	Male	RH	Mean Age	
1	Grünling	2004	fMRI	Decision (rhyme)	Button press	Pseudo	Letter-string matching	31	$P < .01$	17	?	17	14	21	?	21	13	German
2a	Rumsey	1997	PET	Decision phonological	Button press	2 pseudo	Fixation matching	10	$P < .01$	17	17	17	27	14	14	14	25	English
				Decision orthographic	Button press	1 real; 1 pseudo	Fixation	6	$P < .01$	17	17	17	27	14	14	14	25	English
2b	Rumsey	1997	PET	Explicit phonological	Aloud	Pseudo	Fixation	7	$P < .01$	17	17	17	27	14	14	14	25	English
				Explicit orthographic	Aloud	Exception real	Fixation	8	$P < .01$	17	17	17	27	14	14	14	25	English
3	Brunswick	1999	PET	Explicit reading	Aloud	Real + pseudo	Rest (eyes closed)	1	$P < .001$	6	6	6	23	6	6	6	23.2	English
4	Georgiewa	1999	fMRI	Explicit reading	Silent	Pseudo	Letter-string reading	1	$P < .01$	17	8	17	13.6	17	8	17	14.4	German
				Transformation	Silent	Real	Letter-string reading	2	$P < .01$	17	8	17	13.6	17	8	17	14.4	German
5	Ingvar	2002	PET	Explicit reading	Silent	Real	Rest (eyes open)	3	$P < .001$	9	9	9	20–26	9	9	9	20–28	Swedish
6	Flowers	Under review	fMRI	Explicit reading	Aloud	Real + pseudo	Fixation	18	$P < .001$	12	9	10	43.7	14	10	13	40.7	English

TABLE 3. Relative Contributions of Each Contrast to Each ALE Local Maximum for Controls > Dyslexics

	Precuneus (BA 31)	Left inferior temporal gyrus (BA 37)	Left fusiform gyrus (BA 37)	Left inferior parietal lobule (BA 40)	Left superior temporal gyrus (BA 22)	Left thalamus	Left inferior frontal gyrus (BA 47/11)	Right fusiform gyrus (BA 20)	Right postcentral gyrus (BA 2)	Right superior temporal gyrus (BA 21)
1 Paulesu, 1996					(1%)					
2 Grünling, 2004					9%					26%
3a Rumsey, 1997	34%	(1%)	32%	36%	33%		32%	33%		25%
4a Brunswick, 1999		18%	36%	36%	(2%)		41%			
5 Paulesu, 2001		32%	19%	(1%)	(1%)					
3b Rumsey, 1997	47%	(4%)	(1%)		24%		27%	36%	60%	27%
4b Brunswick, 1999	19%	34%	(5%)	26%	29%	46%		31%	39%	22%
6 Georgiewa, 1999						27%				
7 Ingvar, 2002						27%				
8 McCrory, 2005		11%	(5%)						(1%)	
9 Flowers			(1%)							
Experiments	3	4	3	3	4	3	3	3	2	4

Note: Values in parentheses are below the cutoff of 7%.

TABLE 4. Relative Contributions of Each Contrast to Each ALE Local Maximum for Dyslexics > Controls

		Right thalamus	Right insula (BA 13)
1	Grünling, 2004		14%
2a	Rumsey, 1997	(8%) 20%	33 %
2b	Rumsey, 1997	35%	20% 33%
3	Brunswick, 1999		
4	Georgiewa, 1999		
5	Ingvar, 2002		
6	Flowers	38%	
	Experiments	3	4

Note: Values in parentheses are below the cutoff of 10%.

maxima are shown in Figure 1, and 3D volume renderings are shown in Figure 2. The relative contributions of the fourteen contrasts to each of these local maxima are shown in Table 3. Ideally, each local maximum would have been derived from equal contributions from all contrasts (Turkeltaub *et al.*, 2002), each providing 1/14th of the total probability at the local maximum; therefore, values less than 7% are shown in parentheses in Table 3.

Dyslexics > Controls

The meta-analysis results for Dyslexics > Controls showed only two distinct clusters of suprathreshold voxels in the ALE map, one in the right insula (BA 13) and the other in the right thalamus. The estimated locations for the local maxima are shown in Table 6. 2D slices at the level of the two local maxima are shown in Figure 3, and a 3D volume rendering of the right hemisphere is shown in Figure 4. The relative contributions of the ten contrasts are shown in Table 4; values less than 1/10 are shown in parentheses.

Discussion

Altogether, the two meta-analyses examining differences in brain activity during reading

TABLE 5. The Ten Local Maxima Found after Thresholding the ALE Map for Controls > Dyslexics

Estimated localization of local maximum	MNI coordinates of local maximum			ALE local maximum within cluster (10^{-3})	Cluster size (voxels)
	X	Y	Z		
Left precuneus (BA 31)	−4	−76	28	5.55	32
Left inferior temporal gyrus (BA 37)	−48	−58	−10	7.52	843
Left fusiform gyrus (BA 37)	−48	−42	−22	7.01	
Left inferior parietal lobule (BA 40)	−46	−44	26	5.82	42
Left superior temporal gyrus (BA 22)	−52	−36	8	7.29	155
Left thalamus	−18	−24	10	7.09	133
Left inferior frontal gyrus (BA 47/11)	−22	32	−4	5.68	30
Right fusiform gyrus (BA 20)	48	−34	−26	6.28	51
Right postcentral gyrus (BA 2)	50	−26	32	5.76	30
Right superior temporal gyrus (BA 21)	44	−22	−4	8.49	190

Note: The two local maxima in left inferior temporal gyrus and left fusiform gyrus were both located in the largest cluster of contiguous suprathreshold voxels, which contained 843 voxels.

between dyslexics and controls, revealed twelve foci that distinguished these two diagnostic groups. The Controls > Dyslexics meta-analysis confirmed that dyslexic readers tend to underactivate numerous regions in left hemisphere posterior cortex as well as three regions in the right hemisphere. Specifically, in the left hemisphere, ALE maps suggest that dyslexic readers showed hypoactivity in portions of the extrastriate (BA 37 and 31), inferior parietal (BA 40) and inferior frontal (BA 47/11) cortices, as well as the pulvinar of the thalamus. Dyslexic readers also underactivated bilateral superior temporal cortex (BA 21 and 22) as well as right hemisphere post central gyrus (BA 2), and right fusiform gyrus (BA20). In the second meta-analysis, examining Dyslexics > Controls, ALE maps revealed a high likelihood of overactivation in two right hemisphere regions in the dyslexics: anterior insula (BA 13) and lateral posterior thalamus.

In addition to the location of these foci, the ALE analysis also provides information on the statistical significance of the ALE value, its spatial extent and the number of studies that contributed to the focus. These will be taken into consideration next, as our findings are discussed in the context of the functional anatomy of reading.

Posterior Ventral Regions Postulated to Mediate Addressed Phonology

Many studies have suggested that portions of the left ventral visual processing stream, including the inferior temporal and lingual/fusiform gyri, have a role in the direct mapping of orthographic information to the corresponding phonological representation (Binder *et al.*, 2003; Brunswick *et al.*, 1999; Fiebach, Friederici, Muller, & von Cramon, 2002; Hagoort *et al.*, 1999; Herbster, Mintun, Nebes, & Becker, 1997; Rumsey *et al.*, 1997b). Indeed, some call a large area of the extrastriate region the "visual word form area" (Cohen *et al.*, 2000; McCandliss *et al.*, 2003). However, it is debatable whether the function of this region is confined to the processing of words and word-like stimuli, and there is recent evidence that its overall function is phonological retrieval, whether of language-related or object stimuli (McCrory *et al.*, 2005; Price & Devlin, 2003). Nevertheless, a frequent finding has been of relatively less activity (including deactivation relative to a contrast condition) among dyslexics as compared to controls in the left ventral extrastriate region (Brunswick *et al.*, 1999; Flowers *et al.*, under review; Georgiewa *et al.*, 1999; Paulesu *et al.*, 2001; Rumsey *et al.*, 1997b).

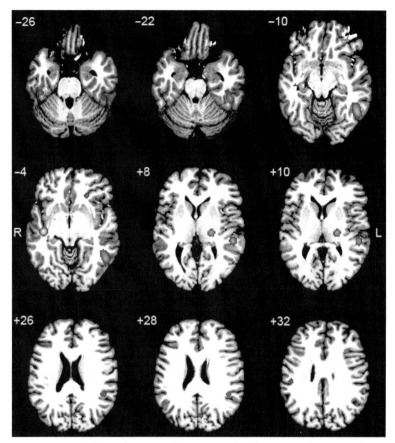

Figure 1. 2D axial slices depicting the ten ALE local maxima for Controls > Dyslexics (Table 5). All images are presented in radiologic convention (subject left = image right) and MNI coordinates in the inferior-superior (Z) plane are provided in the upper left corners of each image. The ALE maps reveal differences in left hemisphere precuneus (BA 31), middle occipital gyrus (BA 37), fusiform gyrus (BA 37), inferior parietal lobule (BA 40), superior temporal gyrus (BA 22), thalamus (pulvinar), and inferior frontal gyrus (BA 47/11). In the right hemisphere, the ALE analysis identified foci in fusiform gyrus (BA 20), postcentral gyrus (BA 2), and superior temporal gyrus (BA 21).

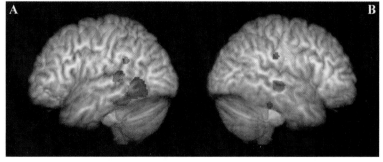

Figure 2. 3D volume rendering of the thresholded ALE map for Controls > Dyslexics, seen from the left (**A**) and right (**B**) sides. ALE values located closer to the surface (which are more lateral) appear as a more solid red, whereas those further away (more medial) appear as a lighter red.

TABLE 6. The Two Local Maxima Found after Thresholding the ALE Map for Controls > Dyslexics

Estimated localization of local maximum	MNI coordinates of local maximum			ALE local maximum within cluster ($\times 10^{-3}$)	Cluster size (voxels)
	X	Y	Z		
Right thalamus	14	−20	12	6.09	66
Right insula (BA 13)	34	18	2	7.10	113

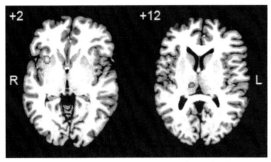

Figure 3. 2D axial slices revealing the location of the two local maxima for the Dyslexics > Controls meta-analysis: right insula (BA 13) and right thalamus (for corresponding coordinates see Table 6; subject left = image right).

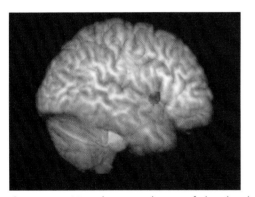

Figure 4. 3D volume rendering of the thresholded ALE map for Dyslexics > Controls, seen from the right side.

In the Control > Dyslexic meta-analysis, seven experiments were identified where dyslexics underactivated the left ventral extrastriate cortex (BA 37). Three of these contrasts contributed to the left fusiform gyrus finding, and four to the left inferior temporal gyrus finding, making this the most robust outcome of the analysis. The contrasts that elicited these findings were varied, and included implicit and explicit reading of words and pseudowords as well as orthographic and phonologic decisions. This task-invariant hypoactivity has also been linked to a robust difference in brain structure within this region in individuals with dyslexia drawn from a variety of different countries (Silani *et al.*, 2005). A significant ALE value in the left precuneus (BA31/23) suggests that hypoactivity in dyslexia during reading in some instances extends to the medial aspect of the left posterior cortex.

Underactivation by dyslexics in a more anterior portion of the fusiform region (BA 20) was also found, but this time in the right hemisphere (contributed by three experiments), suggesting the presence of right as well as left ventral extrastriate deficiency associated with dyslexia. This result is consistent with a finding of right BA 20 hypoactivity in dyslexia during an auditory sound manipulation task (Eden *et al.*, 2004). It is possible that the ventral streams of both hemispheres are compromised in dyslexia, with a behavioral deficit attributed to the right hemisphere (e.g. face processing, which is more subtle than that observed for word processing) (Tarkiainen, Helenius, & Salmelin, 2003).

Posterior Dorsal Regions Postulated to Mediate Assembled Phonology

Grapheme–phoneme correspondence, the mapping of the written representations of words onto their associated sounds ("assembled phonology"), is the principal defining characteristic of dyslexia and found to be impaired throughout the lifespan (Bruck, 1992; Fletcher *et al.*, 1994; Flowers, 1995; Liberman & Shankweiler, 1991; Lyon, 1995b; Lyon *et al.*,

2003; Morris *et al.*, 1998; Ramus, 2003; Shankweiler *et al.*, 1979; Shaywitz *et al.*, 1995; Shaywitz *et al.*, 1999; Shaywitz *et al.*, 2003; Stanovich & Siegel, 1994; Torgesen, 1995; Wagner & Torgesen, 1987). Several functional imaging studies of dyslexia entered into the meta-analysis have independently reported underactivation in superior/middle temporal and inferior parietal regions believed to mediate assembled phonology. For example, dyslexics were found to have reduced activation in the left superior temporal gyrus/inferior parietal lobule (usually incorporating the supramarginal gyrus, BA 40) during implicit reading of either real words or pseudowords relative to false font strings or during overt word reading relative to visual fixation (Brunswick *et al.*, 1999). The same observation has also been made during overt pseudoword reading, relative to real-word reading (Flowers *et al.*, under review), and during phonological and orthographic overt reading as well as during silent decision making (relative to visual fixation) (Rumsey *et al.*, 1997b).

Our meta-analytic results are consistent with the converging findings of the literature. In an early rCBF study, the posterior superior temporal cortex was reported to be underactivated in dyslexics who carried out an orthographic task (Flowers, Wood, & Naylor, 1991). Subsequently, others have reported similar findings in superior and middle temporal gyri (BAs 21, 22, 42). For example, underactivation by dyslexics has been found during either a rhyming task relative to a shape-similarity task or during word reading relative to baseline (Paulesu *et al.*, 1996), when contrasting rhyming pseudowords with letter strings (Grünling *et al.*, 2004), and during phonological or orthographic reading or decision-making tasks compared to a visual fixation baseline (Rumsey *et al.*, 1997b). However, the meta-analytic results are incongruent with reports of greater activation in the superior and middle temporal gyri in dyslexics (Georgiewa *et al.*, 1999), suggesting that there may be variability in this region as a function of task demands or language of the participants.

In the meta-analysis, three contrasts from one paper (Rumsey *et al.*, 1997b) accounted for the majority of the contribution to the meta-analytic finding in the left inferior parietal lobe, and therefore this cannot be considered a consistent finding across the nine papers. Also, as Rumsey *et al.* pointed out, the dyslexic participants in their study exhibited markedly impaired behavioral performance, leading to a much more widespread pattern of activation and deactivation. Thus, contrast maps between their dyslexic and nondyslexic groups must be interpreted with caution. As has been discussed extensively by McCrory and others (e.g., 2004), it is unclear how impaired behavioral performance and variable performance as a consequence of self-paced tasks affects the activation results. If control subjects were to perform the same tasks at a lower level of accuracy and with slower reaction times, the task-related activity is likely to be somewhat different. This has been demonstrated in studies where inter-stimulus intervals were parametrically modulated (Price *et al.*, 1996).

It is noteworthy that in the study by Rumsey and colleagues, two of the tasks employed were orthographic in nature, suggesting that the inferior parietal region is involved in both phonological and orthographic processes. As pointed out by Rumsey and colleagues in a study of typical readers (Rumsey *et al.*, 1997a), the attempts to distinguish separate pathways that subserve the "direct" orthographic route versus the "indirect" phonological route have not been as successful as might be predicted by theoretical models of reading (Coltheart, Curtis, Atkins, & Haller, 1993). Nevertheless, these results suggest that during reading, dyslexic readers are deficient in recruiting essential left hemisphere language-related regions around the temporoparietal junction.

Turning to the opposite hemisphere, while some studies have previously shown right inferior parietal (BA 40) (Rumsey *et al.*, 1997b), angular gyrus (BA 39), or superior parietal region (BA 7) (Grünling *et al.*, 2004) to be underactivated by dyslexics, our meta-analysis found no robust concordance in this region. Instead, we found a high likelihood for hypoactivity in dyslexics in the right superior temporal gyrus (BA 21). This result is consistent with those observed in studies of dyslexia that involve reading of printed words (Flowers *et al.*, under review) and repetition of spoken words (McCrory *et al.*, 2000).

Neither ALE analysis revealed differences in the cerebellum, suggesting that even if the cerebellum is involved in linguistic tasks (Fiez & Petersen, 1998), there is no robust evidence of a cerebellar deficit in dyslexia during reading as has been found for motor learning (Nicolson *et al.*, 1999).

Anterior Regions Postulated to Mediate Word Production and Semantic Processing

The left inferior frontal gyrus has been proposed to mediate articulatory recoding of phonological information, and activation of this area during a variety of reading and phonological processing tasks has been widely reported. Dorsal and ventral subdivisions are implicated for phonological processes and semantic processes, respectively (Brunswick *et al.*, 1999; Fiez, Balota, Raichle, & Petersen, 1999; Hagoort *et al.*, 1999; Herbster *et al.*, 1997; Poldrack *et al.*, 1999; Pugh *et al.*, 1996; Rumsey *et al.*, 1997b; Zurowski *et al.*, 2002). The inferior frontal region, and specifically Broca's area (BA 44/45/46), is more commonly related to prevocalization programs for word production (Brunswick *et al.*, 1999; Dietz, Jones, Gareau, Zeffiro, & Eden, 2005; Hagoort *et al.*, 1999; Xu *et al.*, 2001). The left ventral inferior frontal gyrus (BA 47) is believed to be involved in the retrieval and maintenance of semantic representations, making semantic decisions, and holding semantic material in working memory (Brunswick *et al.*, 1999; Rumsey *et al.*, 1997b; Shaywitz *et al.*, 1998).

Both under- and overactivation of the left inferior frontal cortex have been reported in dyslexia. Overactivation in BA 44/45 and BA 44/6 (premotor cortex) in dyslexics compared to controls during phonological decision-making tasks has been proposed to represent compensation to counteract deficits in phonological processing normally mediated by posterior cortical regions (Brunswick *et al.*, 1999; Grünling *et al.*, 2004; Shaywitz *et al.*, 1998). However, reading aloud has been associated with under activation in the left and simultaneous overactivation in the right frontal cortex by dyslexics (Flowers *et al.*, under review; Georgiewa *et al.*, 1999). Still other studies have found no differences in activation between dyslexics and controls in the inferior frontal gyrus during rhyming (Paulesu *et al.*, 1996), reading aloud of words and pseudowords (Brunswick *et al.*, 1999), and phonological and orthographic tasks (Rumsey *et al.*, 1997b). In our meta-analysis of Controls > Dyslexics, three of the four contrasts from a single paper (Rumsey *et al.*, 1997b) made the majority contribution to underactivation in the left inferior frontal gyrus associated with dyslexia (see Table 3). It is noteworthy that the original study reported several regions within the left frontal cortex that demonstrated relative "deactivations" in the dyslexic group when contrasting the orthographic tasks with the resting baseline (Rumsey *et al.*, 1997b). Since this region is located in the ventral subdivision associated with semantic processes (BA 47/11), the result of the meta-analysis suggests that dyslexics underutilize semantic processes when reading, perhaps because of a lifelong history of insufficient reading experience. There was no evidence of over-activation in the left inferior frontal gyrus, a finding that in previous reports has been suggested to be "compensatory" (Shaywitz *et al.*, 1998). Nor did the ALE maps suggest any areas of relatively enhanced activity located in regions homotopic to those left hemispheric areas that demonstrated hypoactivity in the dyslexics.

The meta-analyses revealed overactivation by dyslexics in the right insula; four contrasts from two papers (Rumsey *et al.*, 1997b; Grünling *et al.*, 2004) contributed to this finding

(Table 4). One interpretation for an increased likelihood for dyslexics to engage the anterior insula is the aversive nature of reading for individuals who have continuously suffered reading failure. The anterior insula, which receives input from the autonomic nervous system, has been shown to increase activity in response to aversive visual stimuli (Kosslyn *et al.*, 1996). This theory could be tested directly by examining task-related activity in dyslexics during the processing of words and adverse stimuli. Neither of the two meta-analyses revealed differences in the left insular area. Previous reports in this region have been mixed, with Paulesu and colleagues (1996) reporting left insular underactivation thought to represent an anterior-posterior connectivity failure, whereas Rumsey *et al.* (1997b) proposed that the overactivation observed in the left anterior insula by dyslexics during overt reading represented compensation.

Although the meta-analytic findings in the left inferior frontal gyrus (Table 3) may be consistent with the literature, this focus was derived mostly from a single paper (Rumsey *et al.*, 1997b). Further, the dyslexic participants in this study did not perform the task to the same level of proficiency as the nondyslexics, again leading to the same problems of data interpretation as discussed above for the left inferior parietal cortex. Task performance was not considered as a criterion for inclusion during the selection process for the meta-analysis, but it is known to play a potential role in modulating brain activity, especially in studies of clinical populations (Price & Friston, 1999).

Subcortical Grey Matter

Both over- and underactivation in the thalamus has been reported during reading and phonological tasks. Brunswick *et al.* (1999) found that dyslexics had reduced activation relative to control subjects in the left thalamus during implicit reading, regardless of word type (real words or pseudowords). For both phonological processing (nonwords versus letter strings) as well as phonological awareness (phonological transformation versus letter strings), Georgiewa *et al.* reported left thalamic signal decreases in dyslexics compared to controls (Georgiewa *et al.*, 1999). Conversely, several studies have reported greater activation in the left thalamus in dyslexics when reading either real words or pseudowords (Flowers *et al.*, under review), when reading real words silently (Ingvar *et al.*, 2002), or during phonological pronunciation (Rumsey *et al.*, 1997b).

The Controls > Dyslexics meta-analysis identified the pulvinar region of the left thalamus as an area underactivated by dyslexics, as a result of two contributing papers (Table 3). The pulvinar of the thalamus is connected to striate and extrastriate cortex (Bender, 1981) and the superior temporal cortex (Galaburda & Eidelberg, 1982), consistent with underactivation in those regions. The second meta-analysis examining Dyslexics > Controls identified the lateral posterior region of the thalamus in the opposite (right) hemisphere to be relatively more active in dyslexics. This is a region that is connected to medial parietal cortex, but its role in dyslexia is harder to explain. Further, the ALE meta-analytic method together with the spatial smoothing applied in the original analyses do not result in resolution sufficient to justify a strong neuroanatomical interpretation of a small structure such as the thalamus. Rumsey and colleagues' (1997b) orthographic decision-making result contributed 20% to the meta-analytic finding in right thalamus. Two tasks from the same paper resulted in activations near the right caudate, which also contributed to the meta-analytic finding in right thalamus: 8% from the phonological decision-making task and 35% from the orthographic pronunciation task. The remainder (38%) was contributed by a right thalamic finding from a study in our group (Flowers *et al.*, under review). Although the opposite polarity of the ALE values for the left and right thalami are intriguing, the interpretation of these findings, based on the size of the thalamus, altogether require some caution.

Studies Not Included in the Meta-analysis

As described in the Methods section, there were several PET or fMRI studies of dyslexic and typical readers engaged in reading tasks that did not meet the criteria for inclusion in this meta-analysis. Although the exclusions were largely made on the basis of age (postpubertal, for the purpose of increasing the homogeneity among the studies) and on technical constraints (published spatial coordinates were necessary to enter the data in the meta-analysis), it is worth considering whether the ALE maps reported here reflect the findings from those studies that were not included. Only two studies using visual word presentation in adults were excluded (Gross-Glenn *et al.*, 1991; Shaywitz *et al.*, 1998). These generally demonstrated underactivity in dyslexics in the left occipital regions (including lingual and fusiform gyri) and the angular gyrus, and overactivity of the right parietal and inferior occipital temporal cortex. These findings are consistent with the generally held view of left hemisphere deficits of assembled and addressed phonology and right hemisphere compensation in dyslexia (Pugh *et al.*, 2000).

The studies described so far have focused on reading, and they therefore employed visually presented words. Since dyslexics have difficulties in isolating and manipulating the constituent sounds of spoken language, several investigations have used auditory stimuli. These studies, five conducted in adults (Eden *et al.*, 2004; Flowers *et al.*, 1991; Ruff, Marie, Celsis, Cardebat, & Demonet, 2003; Rumsey *et al.*, 1992; Temple *et al.*, 2000) and one in children (Corina, San Jose-Robertson, Guillemin, High, & Braun, 2003), largely employed rhyming paradigms. Two of these reported underactivation in dyslexia in right inferior frontal regions (Ruff *et al.*, 2003; Rumsey *et al.*, 1992), but they differed in their findings in the right extrastriate cortex: one study demonstrated overactivity (Rumsey *et al.*, 1992) and another underactivity in dyslexics (Eden *et al.*, 2004). Of importance,

none of the adult studies using auditory stimuli demonstrated differences between dyslexics and controls in the left extrastriate region, even though this brain region is the site of greatest difference in dyslexia when visually presented paradigms are used. The only pediatric study of dyslexia using an auditory tasks found left extrastriate overactivation in dyslexics during a phonological judgment task (Corina *et al.*, 2001).

While our ALE results are based on adult subjects and cannot be generalized to pediatric populations, we can informally examine the concordance with the published literature of children with dyslexia. Five studies in which children performed reading or phonological (largely rhyming) tasks in response to visually presented stimuli yielded widespread activation differences (Aylward *et al.*, 2003; Backes *et al.*, 2002; Georgiewa *et al.*, 2002; Shaywitz *et al.*, 2002; Temple *et al.*, 2001): dyslexics underactivated multiple left frontal, temporal, and parietal regions *as well as* their right hemisphere homologues. This symmetry differs from the largely left-lateralized findings of the adult meta-analysis. In addition, one study reported left posterior occipital hypoactivity in dyslexia (Shaywitz *et al.*, 2002). A finding consistent with our meta-analysis in adults was a finding of greater activation in the left thalamus in non-impaired children (Temple *et al.*, 2001). Finally, numerous regions were found to be overly active in dyslexics compared to controls, especially in the left inferior frontal/anterior insular/anterior superior temporal regions, and in the right inferior posterior regions (Aylward *et al.*, 2003; Georgiewa *et al.*, 2002; Temple *et al.*, 2001).

Together, the studies not included in the meta-analysis are consistent with the more focused findings generated by meta-analyses. The most salient difference is that studies of children report more widespread differences in activation, including the right hemisphere. This might be predicted from developmental studies of reading (Turkeltaub, Gareau, Flowers, Zeffiro, & Eden, 2003) and could be investigated in future meta-analyses once sufficient numbers of pediatric studies are available.

Conclusions

The ALE method, a coordinate-based, voxel-wise meta-analytic method, has been used widely to identify the most robust findings regarding the primary neuroanatomical substrates for a variety of cognitive tasks. Here we used the ALE approach to examine published studies of adults with dyslexia. The likelihood for controls to show more task-related activity compared to dyslexics was greatest in left hemisphere posterior ventral, inferior parietal/temporal, and inferior frontal cortices, as well as the right fusiform, postcentral, and superior temporal gyri. The highest ALE values and greatest convergence among studies for this comparison was found in left extrastriate cortex (inferior temporal gyrus) in BA 37. The Dyslexics > Controls meta-analysis revealed a right hemisphere overactivation by dyslexics in the right thalamus, and a less robust finding in the anterior aspect of the right insula. We found no evidence for hyperactivation in left frontal cortex in adult dyslexia, nor for cerebellar differences. Future meta-analyses in studies involving children will help elucidate age-specific effects that distinguish dyslexic and nondyslexic readers.

Acknowledgments

This work was supported by the National Institute of Child Health and Human Development (Grants HD36461 and HD40095) and by the National Institute of Mental Health (Grant MH6500), National Institutes of Health, as well as by the Latham Trust. The results of this meta-analysis were presented at the Annual Conference of the Society for Neuroscience, 2005.

Conflicts of Interest

The authors declare no conflicts of interest.

References

Aylward, E. H., Richards, T. L., Berninger, V. W., Nagy, W. E., Field, K. M., Grimme, A. C., *et al.* 2003. Instructional treatment associated with changes in brain activation in children with dyslexia. *Neurology* **61**(2): 212–219.

Backes, W., Vuurman, E., Wennekes, R., Spronk, P., Wuisman, M., van Engelshoven, J., *et al.* 2002. Atypical brain activation of reading processes in children with developmental dyslexia. *Journal of Child Neurology* **17**(12): 867–871.

Bender, D. B. 1981. Retinotopic organization of macaque pulvinar. *Journal of Neurophysiology* **46**(3): 672–693.

Binder, J. R., McKiernan, K. A., Parsons, M. E., Westbury, C. F., Possing, E. T., Kaufman, J. N., *et al.* 2003. Neural correlates of lexical access during visual word recognition. *Journal of Cognitive Neuroscience* **15**(3): 372–393.

Bolger, D. J., Perfetti, C. A., & Schneider, W. 2005. Cross-cultural effect on the brain revisited: universal structures plus writing system variation. *Human Brain Mapping* **25**(1): 92–104.

Brett, M. 1999. *The MNI brain and the Talairach atlas.* Cambridge Imagers. Retrieved October 16, 2008, from http://imaging.mrc-cbu.cam.ac.uk/;imaging/MniTalairach.

Brett, M., Christoff, K., Cusack, R., & Lancaster, J. 2001. Using the Talairach atlas with the MNI template. *NeuroImage* **13**(6): S85.

Brett, M., Johnsrude, I. S., & Owen, A. M. 2002. The problem of functional localization in the human brain. *Nature Reviews Neuroscience* **3**(3): 243–249.

Brown, S., Ingham, R. J., Ingham, J. C., Laird, A. R., & Fox, P. T. 2005. Stuttered and fluent speech production: an ALE meta-analysis of functional neuroimaging studies. *Human Brain Mapping* **25**(1): 105–117.

Bruck, M. 1992. Persistence of dyslexics' phonological awareness deficits. *Developmental Psychology* **28**(5): 874–886.

Brunswick, N., McCrory, E., Price, C. J., Frith, C. D., & Frith, U. 1999. Explicit and implicit processing of words and pseudowords by adult developmental dyslexics: a search for Wernicke's Wortschatz? *Brain* **122**(10): 1901–1917.

Buchsbaum, B. R., Greer, S., Chang, W. L., & Berman, K. F. 2005. Meta-analysis of neuroimaging studies of the Wisconsin card-sorting task and component processes. *Human Brain Mapping* **25**(1): 35–45.

Chein, J. M., Fissell, K., Jacobs, S., & Fiez, J. A. 2002. Functional heterogeneity within Broca's area during verbal working memory. *Psychology and Behavior* **77**: 636–639.

Cohen *et al.* 2000. The visual word form area: spatial and temporal characterization of an initial stage of reading in normal subjects and posterior split-brain patients. *Brain* **123**(pt 2): 291–307.

Coltheart, M., Curtis, B., Atkins, P., & Haller, M. 1993. Models of reading aloud: dual-route and parallel-distributed-processing approaches. *Psychological Review* **100**(4): 589–608.

Corina, D. P., Richards, T. L., Serafini, S., Richards, A. L., Steury, K., Abbott, R. D., *et al*. 2001. fMRI auditory language differences between dyslexic and able reading children. *Neuroreport* **12**(6): 1195–1201.

Corina, D. P., San Jose-Robertson, L., Guillemin, A., High, J., & Braun, A. R. 2003. Language lateralization in a bimanual language. *Journal of Cognitive Neuroscience* **15**(5): 718–730.

Derrfuss, J., Brass, M., Neumann, J., & von Cramon, D. Y. 2005. Involvement of the inferior frontal junction in cognitive control: meta-analyses of switching and Stroop studies. *Human Brain Mapping* **25**(1): 22–34.

Dietz, N. A., Jones, K. M., Gareau, L., Zeffiro, T. A., & Eden, G. F. 2005. Phonological decoding involves left posterior fusiform gyrus. *Human Brain Mapping* **26**(2): 81–93.

Eden, G. F., Jones, K. M., Cappell, K., Gareau, L., Wood, F. B., Zeffiro, T. A., *et al*. 2004. Neural changes following remediation in adult developmental dyslexia. *Neuron* **44**(3): 411–422.

Eden, G. F., VanMeter, J. W., Rumsey, J. M., Maisog, J. M., Woods, R. P., & Zeffiro, T. A. 1996. Abnormal processing of visual motion in dyslexia revealed by functional brain imaging. *Nature* **382**(6586): 66–69.

Eden, G. F., & Zeffiro, T. A. 1998. Neural systems affected in developmental dyslexia revealed by functional neuroimaging. *Neuron* **21**(2): 279–282.

Farrell, M. J., Laird, A. R., & Egan, G. F. 2005. Brain activity associated with painfully hot stimuli applied to the upper limb: a meta-analysis. *Human Brain Mapping* **25**(1): 129–139.

Fawcett, A. J., & Nicolson, R. I. 1992. Automatisation deficits in balance for dyslexic children. *Perceptual and Motor Skills* **75**(2): 507–529.

Fiebach, C. J., Friederici, A. D., Muller, K., & von Cramon, D. Y. 2002. fMRI evidence for dual routes to the mental lexicon in visual word recognition. *Journal of Cognitive Neuroscience* **14**(1): 11–23.

Fiez, J. A., Balota, D. A., Raichle, M. E., & Petersen, S. E. 1999. Effects of lexicality, frequency, and spelling-to-sound consistency on the functional anatomy of reading. *Neuron* **24**: 205–218.

Fiez, J. A., & Petersen, S. E. 1998. Neuroimaging studies of word reading. *Proceedings of the National Academy of Sciences of the United States of America* **95**(3): 914–921.

Fletcher, J. M., Shaywitz, S. E., Shankweiler, D. P., Katz, L., Liberman, I. Y., Stuebing, K. K., *et al*. 1994. Cognitive profiles of reading disability: Comparisons of discrepancy and low achievement definitions. *Journal of Educational Psychology* **86**(1): 6–23.

Flowers, D. L. 1995. Neuropsychological profiles of persistent reading disability and reading improvement. In C. K. J. Leong, R.M. (Eds.), *Developmental and acquired dyslexia* (pp. 61–77). Dordrecht, Netherlands: Kluwer Academic Publishers.

Flowers, D. L., Maisog, J. M., Einbinder, E., Curran, E., Jones, K., Cappell, K., *et al*. (under review). Pseudoword reading in adult developmental dyslexia. *Annals of Neurology*.

Flowers, D. L., Wood, F. B., & Naylor, C. E. 1991. Regional cerebral blood flow correlates of language processes in reading disability. *Archives of Neurology* **48**(6): 637–643.

Fox, P. T., Laird, A. R., Fox, S. P., Fox, P. M., Uecker, A. M., Crank, M., *et al*. 2005a. BrainMap taxonomy of experimental design: description and evaluation. *Human Brain Mapping* **25**(1): 185–198.

Fox, P. T., Laird, A. R., & Lancaster, J. L. 2005b. Coordinate-based voxel-wise meta-analysis: dividends of spatial normalization: report of a virtual workshop. *Human Brain Mapping* **25**(1): 1–5.

Galaburda, A. M., & Eidelberg, D. 1982. Symmetry and asymmetry in the human posterior thalamus. II. Thalamic lesions in a case of developmental dyslexia. *Archives of Neurology* **39**(6): 333–336.

Genovese, C. R., Lazar, N. A., & Nichols, T. 2002. Thresholding of statistical maps in functional neuroimaging using the false discovery rate. *NeuroImage* **15**(4): 870–878.

Georgiewa, P., Rzanny, R., Gaser, C., Gerhard, U. J., Vieweg, U., Freesmeyer, D., *et al*. 2002. Phonological processing in dyslexic children: a study combining functional imaging and event related potentials. *Neuroscience Letters* **318**(1): 5–8.

Georgiewa, P., Rzanny, R., Hopf, J. M., Knab, R., Glauche, V., Kaiser, W. A., *et al*. 1999. fMRI during word processing in dyslexic and normal reading children. *Neuroreport* **10**(16): 3459–3465.

Glahn, D. C., Ragland, J. D., Abramoff, A., Barrett, J., Laird, A. R., Bearden, C. E., *et al*. 2005. Beyond hypofrontality: a quantitative meta-analysis of functional neuroimaging studies of working memory in schizophrenia. *Human Brain Mapping* **25**(1): 60–69.

Grosbras, M. H., Laird, A. R., & Paus, T. 2005. Cortical regions involved in eye movements, shifts of attention, and gaze perception. *Human Brain Mapping* **25**(1): 140–154.

Gross-Glenn, K., Duara, R., Barker, W. W., Loewenstein, D., Chang, J. Y., Yoshii, F., *et al*. 1991. Positron emission tomographic studies during serial word-reading by normal and dyslexic adults. *Journal of Clinical and Experimental Neuropsychology* **13**(4): 531–544.

Grünling, C., Ligges, M., Huonker, R., Klingert, M., Mentzel, H. J., Rzanny, R., *et al.* 2004. Dyslexia: the possible benefit of multimodal integration of fMRI- and EEG-data. *Journal of Neural Transmission* **111**(7): 951–969.

Hagoort, P., Indefrey, P., Brown, C., Herzog, H., Steinmetz, H., & Seitz, R. J. 1999. The neural circuitry involved in the reading of German words and pseudowords: a PET study. *Journal of Cognitive Neuroscience* **11**: 383–398.

Helenius, P., Tarkiainen, A., Cornelissen, P., Hansen, P. C., & Salmelin, R. 1999. Dissociation of normal feature analysis and deficient processing of letter-strings in dyslexic adults. *Cerebral Cortex* **9**(5): 476–483.

Herbster, A. N., Mintun, M. A., Nebes, R. D., & Becker, J. T. 1997. Regional cerebral blood flow during word and nonword reading. *Human Brain Mapping* **5:** 84–92.

Horwitz, B., Rumsey, J. M., & Donohue, B. C. 1998. Functional connectivity of the angular gyrus in normal reading and dyslexia. *Proceedings of the National Academy of Sciences of the United States of America* **95**(15): 8939–8944.

Ingvar, M., af Trampe, P., Greitz, T., Eriksson, L., Stone-Elander, S., & von Euler, C. 2002. Residual differences in language processing in compensated dyslexics revealed in simple word reading tasks. *Brain and Language* **83**(2): 249–267.

Koretz, R. L. 2002. Methods of meta-analysis: an analysis. *Current Opinion in Clinical Nutrition and Metabolic Care* **5**(5): 467–474.

Kosslyn, S. M., Shin, L. M., Thompson, W. L., McNally, R. J., Rauch, S. L., Pitman, R. K., *et al.* 1996. Neural effects of visualizing and perceiving aversive stimuli: a PET investigation. *Neuroreport* **7**(10): 1569–1576.

Laird, A. R., Fox, P. M., Price, C. J., Glahn, D. C., Uecker, A. M., Lancaster, J. L., *et al.* 2005a. ALE meta-analysis: controlling the false discovery rate and performing statistical contrasts. *Human Brain Mapping* **25**(1): 155–164.

Laird, A. R., McMillan, K. M., Lancaster, J. L., Kochunov, P., Turkeltaub, P. E., Pardo, J. V., *et al.* 2005b. A comparison of label-based review and ALE meta-analysis in the Stroop task. *Human Brain Mapping* **25**(1): 6–21.

Lerner, J. W. 1989. Educational interventions in learning disabilities. *Journal of the American Academy of Child and Adolescent Psychiatry* **28**(3): 326–331.

Liberman, I. Y., & Shankweiler, D. 1991. Phonology and beginning to read: a tutorial. In L. Rieben, & C. A. Perfetti (Eds.), *Learning to read: Basic research and its implications* (pp. 3–18). Hillsdale, NJ: Lawrence, Erlbaum.

Lovegrove, W. J., Heddle, M., & Slaghuis, W. 1980. Reading disability: spatial frequency specific deficits in visual information store. *Neuropsychologia* **18**(1): 111–115.

Lyon, G. R. 1995a. Research initiatives in learning disabilities: contributions from scientists supported by the National Institute of Child Health and Human Development. *Journal of Child Neurology* **10**(Suppl 1): S120–S126.

Lyon, G. R. 1995b. Toward a definition of dyslexia. *Annals of Dyslexia* **45**(1): 3–27.

Lyon, G. R., Shaywitz, S. E., & Shaywitz, B. A. 2003. A definition of dyslexia. *Annals of Dyslexia* **53**(1): 1–14.

MsCindliss *et al.* 2003. The visual word form area: expertise for reading in the fusiform gyrus. *Trends in Cognitive Sciences* **7**(7): 293–299.

McCrory, E., Frith, U., Brunswick, N., & Price, C. 2000. Abnormal functional activation during a simple word repetition task: A PET study of adult dyslexics. *Journal of Cognitive Neuroscience* **12**(5): 753–762.

McCrory, E. J. 2004. The neurocognitive basis of developmental dyslexia. In R. S. J. Frackowiack, K. J. Friston, C. D. Frith, R. J. Dolan, C. J. Price, S. Zeki, *et al.* (Eds.), *Human brain function* (2nd ed., pp. 563–582). San Diego, CA: Academic Press.

McCrory, E. J., Mechelli, A., Frith, U., & Price, C. J. 2005. More than words: a common neural basis for reading and naming deficits in developmental dyslexia? *Brain* **128**(Pt 2): 261–267.

Morris, R. D., Stuebing, K. S., Fletcher, J. M., Shaywitz, S. E., Lyon, G. R., Shankweiler, D. P., *et al.* 1998. Subtypes of reading disability: variability around a phonological core. *Journal of Educational Psychology* **90**(3): 347–373.

Neumann, J., Lohmann, G., Derrfuss, J., & von Cramon, D. Y. 2005. Meta-analysis of functional imaging data using replicator dynamics. *Human Brain Mapping* **25**(1): 165–173.

Nicolson, R. I., Fawcett, A. J., Berry, E. L., Jenkins, I. H., Dean, P., & Brooks, D. J. 1999. Association of abnormal cerebellar activation with motor learning difficulties in dyslexic adults. *Lancet* **353**(9165): 1662–1667.

Nicolson, R. I., Fawcett, A. J., & Dean, P. 2001. Developmental dyslexia: the cerebellar deficit hypothesis. *Trends in Neuroscience* **24**(9): 508–511.

Owen, A. M., McMillan, K. M., Laird, A. R., & Bullmore, E. 2005. N-back working memory paradigm: a meta-analysis of normative functional neuroimaging studies. *Human Brain Mapping* **25**(1): 46–59.

Paulesu, E., Demonet, J.-F., Fazio, F., McCrory, E., Chanoine, V., Brunswick, N., *et al.* 2001. Dyslexia: cultural diversity and biological unity. *Science* **291**(5511): 2165.

Paulesu, E., Frith, C., Snowling, M., Gallagher, A., Morton, J., Frackowiak, R. S. J., *et al.* 1996. Is developmental dyslexia a disconnection syndrome?

Evidence from PET scanning. *Brain* **119**(Pt 1): 143–157.

Petacchi, A., Laird, A. R., Fox, P. T., & Bower, J. M. 2005. Cerebellum and auditory function: an ALE meta-analysis of functional neuroimaging studies. *Human Brain Mapping* **25**(1): 118–128.

Poldrack, R. A., Wagner, A. D., Prull, M. W., Desmond, J. E., Glover, G. H., & Gabrieli, J. D. 1999. Functional specialization for semantic and phonological processing in the left inferior prefrontal cortex. *NeuroImage* **10**(1): 15–35.

Price, C. J., & Devlin, J. T. 2003. The myth of the visual word form area. *NeuroImage* **19**(3): 473–481.

Price, C. J., Devlin, J. T., Moore, C. J., Morton, C., & Laird, A. R. 2005. Meta-analyses of object naming: effect of baseline. *Human Brain Mapping* **25**(1): 70–82.

Price, C. J., & Friston, K. J. 1999. Scanning patients with tasks they can perform. *Human Brain Mapping* **8**(2–3): 102–108.

Price, C. J., Moore, C. J., & Frackowiak, R. S. 1996. The effect of varying stimulus rate and duration on brain activity during reading. *NeuroImage* **3**(1): 40–52.

Pugh, K. R., Mencl, W. E., Shaywitz, B. A., Shaywitz, S. E., Fulbright, R. K., Constable, R. T., *et al*. 2000. The angular gyrus in developmental dyslexia: task-specific differences in functional connectivity within posterior cortex. *Psychological Science* **11**(1): 51–56.

Pugh, K. R., Shaywitz, B. A., Shaywitz, S. E., Constable, R. T., Skudlarski, P., Fulbright, R. K., *et al*. 1996. Cerebral organization of component processes in reading. *Brain* **119**(Pt 4): 1221–1238.

Rae, C., Harasty, J. A., Dzendrowskyj, T. E., Talcott, J. B., Simpson, J. M., Blamire, A. M., *et al*. 2002. Cerebellar morphology in developmental dyslexia. *Neuropsychologia* **40**(8): 1285–1292.

Rae, C., Lee, M. A., Dixon, R. M., Blamire, A. M., Thompson, C. H., Styles, P., *et al*. 1998. Metabolic abnormalities in developmental dyslexia detected by 1H magnetic resonance spectroscopy. *Lancet* **351**(9119): 1849–1852.

Ramus, F. 2003. Developmental dyslexia: specific phonological deficit or general sensorimotor dysfunction? *Current Opinions in Neurobiology* **13**(2): 212–218.

Ruff, S., Marie, N., Celsis, P., Cardebat, D., & Demonet, J. F. 2003. Neural substrates of impaired categorical perception of phonemes in adult dyslexics: an fMRI study. *Brain and Cognition* **53**(2): 331–334.

Rumsey, J. M., Andreason, P., Zametkin, A. J., Aquino, T., King, A. C., Hamburger, S. D., *et al*. 1992. Failure to activate the left temporopareital cortex in dyslexia. *Archives of Neurology* **49**(5): 527–534.

Rumsey, J. M., Horwitz, B., Donohue, B. C., Nace, K., Maisog, J. M., & Andreason, P. 1997a. Phonological and orthographic components of word recognition: a PET-rCBF study. *Brain* **120**(Pt 5): 739–759.

Rumsey, J. M., Nace, K., Donohue, B., Wise, D., Maisog, J. M., & Andreason, P. 1997b. A positron emission tomographic study of impaired word recognition and phonological processing in dyslexic men. *Archives of Neurology* **54**(5): 562–573.

Rumsey, J. M., Zametkin, A. J., Andreason, P., Hanahan, A. P., Hamburger, S. D., Aquino, T., *et al*. 1994. Normal activation of frontotemporal language cortex in dyslexia, as measured with oxygen 15 positron emission tomography. *Archives of Neurology* **51**(1): 27–38.

Salmelin, R. 1996. Impaired visual word processing in dyslexia revealed with magnetoencephalography. *Annals of Neurology* **40**(2): 157–162.

Shankweiler, D., Liberman, I. Y., Mark, L. S., Fowler, C. A., & Fischer, F. W. 1979. The speech code and learning to read. *Journal of Experimental Psychology. Human Learning and Memory* **5**(6): 531–545.

Shaywitz, B. A., Fletcher, J. M., & Shaywitz, S. E. 1995. Defining and classifying learning disabilities and attention-deficit/hyperactivity disorder. *Journal of Child Neurology* **10**(Suppl 1): S50–S57.

Shaywitz, B. A., Shaywitz, S. E., Pugh, K. R., Mencl, W. E., Fulbright, R. K., Skudlarski, P., *et al*. 2002. Disruption of posterior brain systems for reading in children with developmental dyslexia. *Biological Psychiatry* **52**(2): 101–110.

Shaywitz, S. E., Fletcher, J. M., Holahan, J. M., Shneider, A. E., Marchione, K. E., Stuebing, K. K., *et al*. 1999. Persistence of dyslexia: the Connecticut Longitudinal Study at adolescence. *Pediatrics* **104**(6): 1351–1359.

Shaywitz, S. E., & Shaywitz, B. A. 2005. Dyslexia (specific reading disability). *Biological Psychiatry* **57**(11): 1301–1309.

Shaywitz, S. E., Shaywitz, B. A., Fulbright, R. K., Skudlarski, P., Mencl, W. E., Constable, R. T., *et al*. 2003. Neural systems for compensation and persistence: young adult outcome of childhood reading disability. *Biological Psychiatry* **54**(1): 25–33.

Shaywitz, S. E., Shaywitz, B. A., Pugh, K. R., Fulbright, R. K., Constable, R. T., Mencl, W. E., *et al*. 1998. Functional disruption in the organization of the brain for reading in dyslexia. *Proceedings of the National Academy of Sciences of the United States of America* **95**(5): 2636–2641.

Silani, G., Frith, U., Demonet, J. F., Fazio, F., Perani, D., Price, C., *et al*. 2005. Brain abnormalities underlying altered activation in dyslexia: a voxel based morphometry study. *Brain* **128**(Pt 10): 2453–2461.

Simos, P. G., Breier, J. I., Fletcher, J. M., Foorman, B. R., Bergman, E., Fishbeck, K., *et al*. 2000a. Brain activation profiles in dyslexic children during nonword reading: a magnetic source imaging study. *Neuroscience Letters* **290**(1): 61–65.

Simos, P. G., Breier, J. I., Wheless, J. W., Maggio, W. W., Fletcher, J. M., Castillo, E. M., *et al.* 2000b. Brain mechanisms for reading: the role of the superior temporal gyrus in word and pseudoword naming. *Neuroreport* **11**(11): 2443–2447.

Siok, W. T., Perfetti, C. A., Jin, Z., & Tan, L. H. 2004. Biological abnormality of impaired reading is constrained by culture. *Nature* **431**(7004): 71–76.

Stanovich, K. E., & Siegel, L. S. 1994. Phenotypic performance profile of children with reading disabilities: a regression-based test of the phonological-core variable-difference model. *Journal of Educational Psychology* **86**(1): 24–53.

Talairach, J., & Tournoux, P. 1988. *Co-planar stereotaxic atlas of the human brain: an approach to medical cerebral imaging.* Stuttgart and New York: Thieme Medical Publishers.

Tallal, P. 1980. Auditory temporal perception, phonics, and reading disabilities in children. *Brain and Language* **9**: 182–198.

Tan, L. H., Laird, A. R., Li, K., & Fox, P. T. 2005. Neuroanatomical correlates of phonological processing of Chinese characters and alphabetic words: a meta-analysis. *Human Brain Mapping* **25**(1): 83–91.

Tarkiainen, A., Helenius, P., & Salmelin, R. 2003. Category-specific occipitotemporal activation during face perception in dyslexic individuals: an MEG study. *NeuroImage* **19**(3): 1194–1204.

Temple, E. 2002. Brain mechanisms in normal and dyslexic readers. *Current Opinions in Neurobiology* **12**(2): 178–183.

Temple, E., Poldrack, R. A., Protopapas, A., Nagarajan, S., Salz, T., Tallal, P., *et al.* 2000. Disruption of the neural response to rapid acoustic stimuli in dyslexia: evidence from functional MRI. *Proceedings of the National Academy of Sciences of the United States of America* **97**(25): 13907–13912.

Temple, E., Poldrack, R. A., Salidis, J., Deutsch, G. K., Tallal, P., Merzenich, M. M., *et al.* 2001. Disrupted

neural responses to phonological and orthographic processing in dyslexic children: an fMRI study. *Neuroreport* **12**(2): 299–307.

Torgesen, J. K. 1995. *Phonological awareness: A critical factor in dyslexia.* Baltimore: International Dyslexia Association.

Turkeltaub, P. E., Eden, G. F., Jones, K. M., & Zeffiro, T. A. 2002. Meta-analysis of the functional neuroanatomy of single-word reading: method and validation. *NeuroImage* **16**(3 Pt 1): 765–780.

Turkeltaub, P. E., Gareau, L., Flowers, D. L., Zeffiro, T. A., & Eden, G. F. 2003. Development of neural mechanisms for reading. *Nature Neuroscience* **6**(7): 767–773.

Vellutino, F. R., Fletcher, J. M., Snowling, M. J., & Scanlon, D. M. 2004. Specific reading disability (dyslexia): what have we learned in the past four decades? *Journal of Child Psychology and Psychiatry* **45**(1): 2–40.

Wagner, R. K., & Torgesen, J. K. 1987. The nature of phonological processing and its causal role in the acquisition of reading skills. *Psychological Bulletin* **101**(2): 192–212.

Woods, R. P., Grafton, S. T., Watson, J. D., Sicotte, N. L., & Mazziotta, J. C. 1998. Automated image registration: II. Intersubject validation of linear and nonlinear models. *Journal of Computer Assisted Tomography* **22**(1): 153–165.

Xu, B., Grafman, J., Gaillard, W. D., Ishii, K., Vega-Bermudez, F., Pietrini, P., *et al.* 2001. Conjoint and extended neural networks for the computation of speech codes: the neural basis of selective impairment in reading words and pseudowords. *Cerebral Cortex* **11**(3): 267–277.

Zurowski, B., Gostomzyk, J., Gron, G., Weller, R., Schirrmeister, H., Neumeier, B., *et al.* 2002. Dissociating a common working memory network from different neural substrates of phonological and spatial stimulus processing. *NeuroImage* **15**: 45–57.

Impact of Cerebellar Lesions on Reading and Phonological Processing

Gal Ben-Yehudah[a,c,d] and Julie A. Fiez[a,b,c,d]

[a]*Department of Psychology,* [b]*The Center for Neuroscience,* [c]*The Center for the Neural Basis of Cognition, and the* [d]*Learning Research and Development Center, University of Pittsburgh, Pittsburgh, Pennsylvania, USA*

The relationship between cerebellar function and reading abilities is unclear. One theory of developmental dyslexia implicates the cerebellum in this reading disorder. Neuroimaging studies in normal readers consistently show cerebellar activation in tasks that involve reading. However, neuropsychological evidence for a relationship between cerebellar function and skilled reading is sparse. To further examine the role of the cerebellum in reading, we assessed reading skills and phonological processing in a group of patients with focal damage to the cerebellum. The patients' accuracy in naming single words and nonwords and their reading fluency and comprehension did not differ from that of age- and education-matched healthy controls. The patients' performance on phonological awareness and phonological memory tasks was also within the range of the control group, although their performance was highly variable. In contrast, cerebellar damage did significantly compromise performance in two other tasks associated with phonological processing. In a visual rhyme judgment task, a subset of the patient group was impaired on items with a mismatch between orthographic and phonological information. On a verbal working memory task, the cerebellar compared to the control group recalled fewer items from a list of nonwords, but not from lists of familiar items. On the basis of the patients' pattern of behavioral impairments, we propose that cerebellar damage affects an articulatory monitoring process. Our findings indicate that intact cerebellar function is not necessary for skilled reading; however, we cannot exclude the potential contribution of the cerebellum to reading acquisition.

Key words: rhyme judgment; working memory; monitoring

Introduction

Reading is a cognitive skill that involves segmentation, association, and integration of information both within and between different levels of representation (visual, phonological, semantic, and linguistic). Despite the highly complex nature of these skills, children typically learn to read within a year of explicit instruction (Seymour, Aro, & Erskine, 2003), and for many adults reading is an effortless task. This is not the case for the 5–10% of the population who suffer from a specific reading disorder (Shaywitz, 1998). First documented more than 100 years ago, developmental dyslexia is characterized by slow and erroneous reading, spelling mistakes, and phonological impairments, some of which persist into adulthood (Pennington, Van Orden, Smith, Green, & Haith, 1990; Wilson & Lesaux, 2001).

Although the predominant explanation for developmental dyslexia is a deficit in phonological processes (Ramus, 2003; Snowling, 2000), some research has suggested that broader perceptual or motor deficits may be at the core of this reading disorder (Nicolson & Fawcett, 1990; Stein & Walsh, 1997; Tallal, 1980). One theory of developmental dyslexia proposed that abnormal processing in the cerebellum could cause reading difficulties as well as a range of

Address for correspondence: Gal Ben-Yehudah, Ph.D., 640 Learning Research and Development Center, 3939 O'Hara St., Pittsburgh, PA 15260. Voice: +412-624-4920; fax: +412-624-9149. galb@pitt.edu

Ann. N.Y. Acad. Sci. 1145: 260–274 (2008). © 2008 New York Academy of Sciences.
doi: 10.1196/annals.1416.015

mild perceptual and motor impairments associated with dyslexia (Nicolson & Fawcett, 1990). An updated account of this "cerebellar deficit hypothesis" (Nicolson, Fawcett, & Dean, 2001) claimed that 80% of dyslexic children had motor and nonmotor impairments similar to those of patients with cerebellar damage. For instance, the dyslexic children had poor balance and muscle tone (Fawcett & Nicolson, 1999), as well as a difficulty estimating differences in the duration of consecutive tones (Nicolson, Fawcett, & Dean, 1995).

The cerebellar deficit hypothesis explains the causal relationship between cerebellar function and reading abilities by considering two motor functions to which the cerebellum is thought to contribute: the automation of skills and the production of inner speech. The former function relates to the long-standing theory that the cerebellum associates, through trial and error, a sequence of movements with a specific behavioral context; thus, over time motor execution of learned actions becomes rapid and automatic (also see Laycock *et al.*, this volume) (Albus, 1971; Marr, 1969). The latter function relates to a recent idea that the cerebellum may contribute to cognitive processes that rely on internal speech (Ackermann, Mathiak, & Ivry, 2004). For instance, verbal working memory is a cognitive process that relies on an articulatory rehearsal mechanism to maintain verbal items in a memory buffer (Baddeley, 2003). Poor verbal working memory is a well-known characteristic of developmental dyslexia (Pennington *et al.*, 1990; Wilson & Lesaux, 2001). The cerebellar deficit hypothesis suggests that impairments in these functions may lead to difficulties automating word recognition processes and to impoverished phonological representations.

While the cerebellar deficit account of dyslexia provides a logical framework for the involvement of the cerebellum in reading, support for this hypothesis has been mixed. Some researchers have argued against the cerebellar deficit hypothesis of dyslexia, proposing that the cerebellum receives input from and projects to perisylvian cortical regions that show anatomic abnormalities; thus, deficient cerebellar function may just as well reflect disordered processing in the cortex (Zeffiro & Eden, 2001). Others have suggested that abnormal development of the cerebellum is common to several neurodevelopmental disorders and therefore may be a correlate and not a cause of specific reading disorders (Ivry & Justus, 2001). Moreover, only a subset of the findings reported by Nicolson and colleagues (Nicolson *et al.*, 2001) have been observed by other research groups that examined motor and perceptual deficits in dyslexic individuals (Ramus, Pidgeon, & Frith, 2003).

If the cerebellum contributes to reading, then it should be possible to find evidence in support of the cerebellar deficit account by turning to studies of normal readers and the impact of acquired cerebellar damage on reading abilities. Initially, functional imaging studies of normal readers and neuropsychological studies focused on cerebellar involvement in cognitive functions such as language and memory (Desmond & Fiez, 1998; Ivry & Fiez, 2000). However, these studies also incidentally examined the role of the cerebellum in reading because they used written words as stimuli. One of the first studies to report cerebellar activity during higher-level language processing found increased blood flow to the right lateral cerebellum that was specific to the generation of verbs for presented nouns (Petersen, Fox, Posner, Mintun, & Raichle, 1989). More medial and bilateral cerebellar regions, on the other hand, were active during a range of tasks that involved reading. These findings were consistent with a neuropsychological report of a patient with right cerebellar damage who was impaired on a similar verb generation task, but did not experience difficulties in reading (Fiez, Petersen, Cheney, & Raichle, 1992). Although this case study suggested that the cerebellum was not involved in skilled reading, later neuroimaging studies consistently observed bilateral and paravermal cerebellar activity in adults during tasks that involved reading (Mechelli,

Gorno-Tempini, & Price, 2003; Turkeltaub, Eden, Jones, & Zeffiro, 2002).

One way to reconcile these seemingly contradictory findings of cerebellar involvement in reading is to acknowledge that the cerebellum is a large brain structure that contains about half of the number of neurons in the brain (Zagon, McLaughlin, & Smith, 1977). Therefore some cerebellar regions may be involved in reading, whereas others are not. Moreover, different lobules of the cerebellum may contribute to different aspects of reading, as suggested by findings that reading aloud engages different cerebellar regions depending on the characteristics of the stimuli (Fiez, Balota, Raichle, & Petersen, 1999). Specifically, bilateral medial and paramedial cerebellar regions were similarly active for reading both words (varying with frequency and consistency) and nonwords, whereas the right lateral cerebellum was active more for nonwords than words.

Neuropsychological studies provide another method to examine the relationship between cerebellar function and reading skills. To our knowledge, only one study has been designed to directly test this relationship, and it was conducted with a group of 10 Italian patients with lesions to the vermis and the paravermis regions (Moretti, Bava, Torre, Antonello, & Cazzato, 2002). This study found a significant increase in the number of errors that patients made when reading words, nonwords, sentences, and a passage relative to the errors made by the control group. The patients' elevated number of errors was most pronounced in the sentence and passage-reading conditions. Across all of the reading conditions, the most frequent types of errors in the patient group were anticipations (e.g., "tortrino" for "tortino") and regularizations (e.g., "catrame" for "catrumo"). These acquired reading errors are different from those typically described in the developmental dyslexia literature, in which reading words in context improves accuracy, and regularization errors are less prevalent (Ellis, McDougall, & Monk, 1996; Nation & Snowling, 1998).

In summary, one theory of developmental dyslexia implicates the cerebellum in this reading disorder despite mixed findings in the literature (Nicolson *et al.*, 2001). To date, only one neuropsychological study has investigated the relationship between cerebellar damage and reading abilities (Moretti *et al.*, 2002). One limitation of that study was that the patients' lesions were confined to vermial/paravermial regions. Functional imaging studies of reading typically observe activation in several cerebellar lobules. Therefore, to fully understand the relationship between cerebellar function and reading, it is important to examine reading skills in patients with damage to cerebellar regions other than the vermis. In the present study we assessed a range of reading skills in patients with lesions to the lateral cerebellar hemispheres relative to an age- and education-matched healthy control group. We also evaluated phonological abilities known to be impaired in developmental dyslexia, such as phonological awareness and verbal working memory. A finding that damage to the cerebellum in adults without a history of reading disorders results in impaired reading (particularly of unfamiliar words) and poor phonological abilities would provide strong support for the cerebellar deficit hypothesis of dyslexia. Null findings, on the other hand, would suggest that skilled reading does not depend on the cerebellum, although its involvement in the acquisition of reading skill could not be excluded.

Methods

Participants

Six patients with focal damage to the cerebellum, and six healthy controls participated in this study. The patient and the control groups were carefully matched on age (respectively, 63.5 and 59.7 years; $t[10] = -0.5, P > 0.5$) and education (respectively, 12.2 and 12.5 years, $t[10] = 0.6, P > 0.5$). All of the participants scored in the normal range (>23 points) on the Mini-Mental State Exam (Folstein, Folstein, &

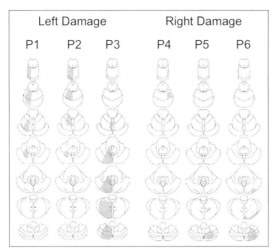

Figure 1. Location of focal unilateral damage to the cerebellum (denoted by the grey regions) shown on a cerebellar template in the six patients studied. Patients are grouped by hemispheric lateralization of their lesion (P1–P3 left cerebellar lesions; P4–P6 right cerebellar lesions). (From Ravizza *et al.*, 2006. Modified by permission.)

McHugh, 1975), which assesses general cognitive competence (patients' average score 27.6 and range 26–30; controls' average score 29.2 and range 26–30). A speech pathologist present at the time of testing indicated that the patients did not suffer from speech deficits, as assessed by the Frenchay Dysarthria Battery (Enderby, 1983). The control participants did not report any history of neurologic abnormalities or current cognitive difficulties. The patients did not report any reading difficulties prior to the cerebellar damage. The neurologic damage resulted from an ischemic event to the left ($n = 3$) or right ($n = 3$) cerebellar hemisphere that occurred at least 3 years before this study. Laterality of the cerebellar damage as well as the lobular localization and extent of this damage was determined from the medical magnetic resonance imaging (MRI) or computed tomography (CT) scans of each patient (Fig. 1; Table 1). The patients described in this study are a subset of the patients who participated in a previous study, and therefore additional details on the lesion analysis method are described in Ravizza *et al.* (2006). All of

the participants gave their informed consent to participate in this study and were compensated for their time.

Reading, Phonology, and Working Memory Tests

We administered a large battery of standardized and custom-made tests to assess reading skills, phonological processing, and working memory abilities in all of the participants. Reading skills were assessed with the standardized Woodcock Reading Mastery Tests–Revised (WRMT-R, form H; Woodcock, 1998), which provides a comprehensive assessment of single word and nonword reading (word identification and word attack subtests, respectively) and comprehension of words (i.e., generation of synonyms, antonyms, and analogies) and passages. Reading fluency was measured using a college-level passage from the Nelson–Denny Comprehension Test (form E, passage five; Brown, Bennett, & Hanna, 1981). Participants were asked to accurately read the passage aloud at their normal reading pace. Once they finished reading, the passage was removed and the participants had to answer a simple comprehension question from memory. Fluency was defined as the reading rate in words per minute, irrespective of the number of reading errors, but contingent upon a correct response to the comprehension question. All of the participants answered the comprehension question correctly and the groups did not differ in their reading accuracy (data not shown).

Phonological processing was assessed with two tests of phonological awareness and a standardized test of phonological memory. One measure of phonological awareness was rhyme judgment. In this custom-made test, 24 pairs of words were presented in upper case, each pair on a separate note card. The word pairs varied in their orthographic and phonological similarity, which resulted in four categories of stimuli: orthographic and phonologically similar (SAIL-PAIL, 9 pairs), orthographic

TABLE 1. Characteristics of the Cerebellar Damage of Each Patient

Patient	Laterality	% Lesion (total)	% Lesion (lobules I–V)	% Lesion (lobules VI–VII)	% Lesion lobules (VIII–X)
P1	Left	25.54	70.05	21.63	0.0
P2	Left	24.43	64.46	32.30	0.0
P3	Left	18.90	0.0	6.08	60.61
P4	Right	7.15	7.98	6.69	0.0
P5	Right	13.69	0.0	0.0	28.27
P6[a]	Right	—	—	—	43.14

[a]Only partial image available for analysis.

and phonologically dissimilar (RUN-FIND, 6 pairs), orthographically dissimilar but phonologically similar (THIGH-FLY, 4 pairs), and orthographically similar but phonologically dissimilar (FEAR-BEAR, 5 pairs). Participants were asked to say "yes" if the words rhymed and "no" if the words did not rhyme. Ample time was given to respond. The second measure of phonological awareness was a spoonerism test, adapted from Brunswick, McCrory, Price, Frith, and Frith (1999). In this test, participants listened to 12 pairs of unrelated words (e.g., basket-lemon). After hearing each pair, they were asked to swap the initial sounds in each word and say aloud the resulting nonword (e.g., lasket-bemon). Details on the stimuli and the administration procedure are described in Brunswick *et al.* (1999). The spoonerism test requires manipulation at the phonemic level, as well as maintenance of items in working memory. Therefore, this test is considered a more difficult task than rhyme judgment and a better measure of phonological awareness in adults (Walton & Brooks, 1995). Finally, phonological memory was assessed with the nonword repetition subtest from the standardized Comprehensive Test of Phonological Processing (CTOPP; Wagner, Torgesen, & Rashotte, 1999). In this test, participants listened to one nonword at a time and then repeated it aloud. The test items gradually increased in length from one to seven syllables. Prior to the commencement of each phonological processing test, detailed instructions and a number of practice items

were given. All of the participants understood the instructions and were able to complete the practice items, except for two patients and one control subject who could not do the practice items for the spoonersim test. Their data on this test are not included in the group averages reported in the Results section.

Working memory span was measured for both verbal and visuospatial items using, respectively, the digit span and the visual memory span subtests from the standardized Wechsler Memory Scale–Revised test battery (WMS-R, Wechsler, 1987). Administration followed standard testing procedures, in which a list of digits were spoken or a series of blocks were tapped in a spatial pattern at a rate of one per second. Participants were then required to immediately recall the digits (or tap the blocks) in forward or backward (reverse) order. We further assessed verbal working memory with two custom-made tests whose stimuli were either an open set of one-syllable words (word span) or pronounceable nonwords (nonword span). The word stimuli were not related semantically, and each item began with a different phoneme to avoid phonological confusions. The nonwords were generated from the items used in the word span test by switching initial consonants (or consonant clusters) between items. The administration procedure of the custom-made span tests followed the forward recall protocol of the standardized digit span subtest. Each set size had two trials, beginning with a set size of two items and gradually increasing in length

TABLE 2. Cerebellar Patients' and Control Group's Mean Scores (and Standard Deviation) on the Reading and Phonological Processing Tests

	Control	Patient	*P*-value
1. Basic reading skills[a]			
Word identification	106.0 (12.9)	98.2 (10.8)	n.s.
Word attack	110.7 (13.0)	99.0 (10.1)	n.s.
2. Comprehension[a]			
Words	105.8 (12.1)	98.0 (14.0)	n.s.
Passage	102.5 (7.5)	98.8 (20.3)	n.s.
3. Reading fluency[b]	109.9 (29.5)	113.3 (29.5)	n.s.
4. Phonological processing[c]			
Rhyme judgment	96.7 (4.7)	84.9 (10.2)	.037
Spoonerism	75.0 (21.2)	56.3 (41.6)	n.s.
Nonword repetition	62.0 (7.4)	54.6 (18.1)	n.s.

P-values for significant group differences are noted for a two-tailed *t*-test between independent samples.
[a]Standard scores on WRMT-R subtests (population mean = 100, SD = 15).
[b]Reading rate in words per minute.
[c]Accuracy on phonological processing tests in percent correct.

until the participant failed on both trials of a set size.

To determine significant differences in performance between the cerebellar patient group and the control group, we applied a set of *t*-tests between independent samples. Since we had no *a priori* hypothesis about group differences on reading measures, we used two-tailed *t*-tests to determine the significance of group effects. On the basis of previous findings, we hypothesized that cerebellar patients would have lower verbal working memory spans; however we choose a conservative approach and examined group differences in verbal working memory using two-tailed *t*-tests between independent samples. We had several measures of verbal working memory, in which we manipulated the type of stimuli (digits, words, nonwords) and recall paradigm (forward versus backward). To assess the effect of these variables on verbal working memory performance, we conducted a series of repeated-measures analyses of variance.

Results

Table 2 summarizes the performance of the cerebellar patient group and the control group on the reading and the phonological processing tests. The patients' basic reading skills and reading comprehension abilities did not differ from those of the control group. On the various subtests, the mean WRMT-R standard score in both groups was less than 1 standard deviation from the mean of the general population (mean = 100, SD = 15). These mean scores are expected from the groups' self-reports of a high-school education. Cerebellar damage can cause dysfluent speech (Duffy, 1995) and thus have an impact on reading fluency. To assess fluency, participants read aloud a college-level passage for comprehension. The mean reading rate of the cerebellar patient group did not differ from that of the control group. Furthermore, the two groups did not differ in their reading accuracy or basic comprehension of the passage, thus indicating that there was no speed–accuracy tradeoff.

Cerebellar damage had a differential influence on performance in the phonological processing tasks (Table 2). Accuracy on the rhyme judgment task was significantly worse in the patient group relative to the control group ($t[7.01] = 2.6$, $P < 0.05$). An error analysis showed that mistakes in both groups were limited to the word pairs that contained a

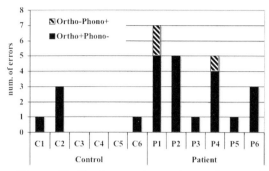

Figure 2. The type and prevalence of errors in the rhyme judgment task are shown for each participant in the patient and the control groups. *Solid bars* indicate errors on items that shared orthography, but not phonology (e.g., FEAR-BEAR, Ortho+Phono−). *Hatched bars* indicate errors on items that did not share orthography, but did rhyme (e.g., THIGH-FLY, Ortho-Phono+).

mismatch between orthography and phonology (i.e., FEAR-BEAR and THIGH-FLY). Half of the patients made an erroneous response to almost all of the stimuli (mean of 4.6 items out of five) that were orthographically similar, but did not rhyme (ortho+phono−, Fig. 2). Only one control subject (C2) judged incorrectly three of the five items in this category. Of interest, the patients (P1, P2, P4) with severe difficulties on the rhyme judgment task had cerebellar lesions that were located in the anterior and superior lobules (including medial damage), whereas patients with performance in the normal range had damage that was limited to the inferior cerebellar lobules. There was no evidence that hemispheric lateralization of the lesions was related to the patients' performance on the rhyme judgment task.

In contrast to the significant group difference found on the rhyme judgment task, the patient and control groups did not differ in their performance on the spoonerism task. This finding is surprising because a spoonerism is considered to be a more sensitive measure of phonological awareness in this age group (Walton & Brooks, 1995). In both groups, there was a large variance in the accuracy scores (patient accuracy range: 0–100% correct; control accuracy range: 0–92% correct), although it

was larger in the patient group. Unfortunately, the high degree of variability makes it difficult to determine the effect of cerebellar damage on performance in this task.

Phonological memory, as measured by the CTOPP nonword repetition subtest, did not differ between the patient and control groups. On average, participants in both groups could accurately repeat nonwords that were four syllables long, but could not repeat longer nonwords. The patients' variance on this task, however, was more than twice that of the control group (patient SD 18.1, control SD 7.4). In general, the patients showed a tendency toward larger variability in their performance on the spoonerism and nonword repetition tasks. This variability may reflect the presence of different subtypes of patients in the group we assessed, although we did not find a clear association between performance on these tasks and the anatomic location of the cerebellar lesions.

Table 3 summarizes the performance of the cerebellar patient group and the control group on the verbal and spatial working memory tests. The dependent measure on these tests is working memory span, which is the largest number of items that can be immediately recalled in the order of presentation (forward) or in the reverse order of presentation (backward). Memory span for verbal items showed the characteristic pattern of significantly larger spans for familiar verbal items relative to unfamiliar items (digits > words > nonwords; $F[2,20] = 62.2$, $P < 0.001$). This pattern was similar across both groups, although there was a trend for a group difference ($F[1,10] = 3.8$, $P = 0.08$) that resulted from the patients' significantly smaller spans for unfamiliar verbal items compared to the control group (nonword-forward, $t[10] = 2.24$, $P < 0.05$). Digit span in both groups, as assessed by the WMS-R subtest, also showed the typical pattern of significantly larger spans for the forward condition compared to the backward condition ($F[1,10] = 72.0$, $P < 0.001$). Although there was no significant group difference, there was a trend toward a smaller mean span in the patient

TABLE 3. Cerebellar Patients' and Control Group's Mean Span (and Standard Deviation) on the Working Memory Tests

	Control	Patient	P-value
1. Verbal span[a]			
Digit – forward	6.7 (0.8)	6.2 (1.0)	n.s.
Digit – backward	5.0 (1.3)	3.8 (0.8)	0.081
Word – forward	4.5 (0.8)	4.2 (0.4)	n.s.
Nonword – forward	3.8 (1.0)	2.7 (0.8)	0.049
2. Spatial span[b]			
Spatial – forward	6.0 (1.3)	5.2 (0.8)	n.s.
Spatial – backward	4.8 (0.8)	4.3 (0.8)	n.s.

P-values for significant group differences are noted for a two-tailed t-test between independent samples.
[a]Maximum number of verbal items accurately recalled in the correct order.
[b]Maximum number of blocks tapped in the correct order.

group for the more difficult digit-backward condition ($t[10] = 1.94$, $P = 0.08$). Memory span for the spatial order of nonverbal items, on the other hand, did not differ between the two groups for either the forward or backward recall conditions. To summarize, patients did not differ from controls in their ability to recall familiar verbal items (digits and words) in order of presentation, but their performance deteriorated when the verbal items were unfamiliar (nonwords) or the order of recall was reversed. In contrast to the patients' mild verbal working memory deficit, spatial working memory was not affected by overall cerebellar damage or hemispheric lateralization of the lesion.

Discussion

Neuroimaging studies typically observe cerebellar activation during tasks that require reading (Mechelli *et al.*, 2003; Turkeltaub *et al.*, 2002). Motor and nonmotor symptoms associated with cerebellar damage have been observed in children with developmental reading disorders (Nicolson *et al.*, 2001). These disparate findings suggest that the cerebellum may be involved in some aspects of reading. Indeed, patients with cerebellar damage to vermial/paravermial regions have reading impairments (Moretti *et al.*, 2002), but the spectrum of these impairments is not similar to that seen in developmental dyslexia. To further investigate cerebellar contributions to reading, we examined the performance of patients with lateral cerebellar lesions relative to age- and education-matched healthy controls on a range of reading and phonological tasks. We found that in adults who reported normal reading abilities prior to an ischemic event, cerebellar damage did not affect reading abilities such as naming familiar and unfamiliar words, reading fluency, and comprehension at both the word and the passage level. Phonological awareness, as assessed by a spoonerism task, and phonological memory (i.e., nonword repetition) were also intact in the cerebellar patient group although the high degree of variability observed in both the patient and control groups complicates the interpretation of these null effects. Performance on a rhyme judgment task was compromised, particularly for patients with anterior/superior cerebellar lesions, and most noticeably for items in which there was a mismatch between orthographic and phonological information.

Rhyme judgment and spoonerism tasks are commonly used to assess phonological awareness in different age groups (Treiman & Zukowski, 1991). The rhyme judgment task is typically used to assess young children's awareness of onset-rime structure of words (e.g. N-AP vs. CL-AP) (Lenel & Cantor, 1981). The ability to identify phonological similarity at the level of the rime unit is one factor that predicts the development of reading abilities in children (Bradley & Bryant, 1983; Bryant, MacLean, Bradley, & Crossland, 1990; Gathercole, Willis, & Baddeley, 1991). Spoonerism, on the other hand, requires both segmentation and manipulation at the phonemic level. This is a sensitive measure of phonological awareness in adults, particularly those with a history of reading disorders (Brunswick *et al.*, 1999). It is therefore surprising that the cerebellar patients were impaired on the easier rhyme judgment but not on the more challenging spoonerism task, though their highly variable performance on the latter task permits only limited speculation regarding performance differences.

For preschool children, the rhyme judgment task is administered using an auditory presentation of word pairs. In our study, the word pairs were written (visual) and presented as a pair until the subject made a judgment. In contrast, the word pairs in the spoonerism task were spoken (auditory) sequentially and then subjects produced a response without a time limit. It is possible that presentation modality is an important fact in the performance of a rhyme judgment. Rhyme judgment becomes difficult when a word's spelling induces conflict between regular and exceptional pronunciations of a rime unit (e.g., /int/ as in MINT versus PINT) (Johnston & McDermott, 1986). The ability to resolve this conflict may invoke an articulatory process supported by the cerebellum, which we speculate upon in the following sections.

Further support for the view that rhyme judgment, possibly more so with visual presentation, can require an additional process to resolve conflict between orthographic and phonological information comes from findings in both normal and impaired readers. In normal readers, visual rhyme judgment is slower and more error prone than auditory rhyme judgment for items with a mismatch between orthographic and phonological infor-

mation (McPherson, Ackerman, & Dykman, 1997). Dyslexic adolescents are extremely impaired on a visual relative to an auditory rhyme judgment, particularly for items that share orthography but not phonology (McPherson *et al.*, 1997). The similarity between dyslexics' and cerebellar patients' item-specific impairments on visual rhyme judgment supports the involvement of the cerebellum in an aspect of phonological processing. However, a comparison across these populations is limited because our study did not assess rhyme judgment with an auditory presentation.

Another main finding of our study was the patients' specific difficulty in recalling a list of nonwords relative to their intact recall of familiar items (i.e., digits and words). Although previous case studies investigating the impact of cerebellar lesions on verbal working memory have reported mixed findings (Fiez *et al.*, 1992; Silveri, Di Betta, Filippini, Leggio, & Molinari, 1998), a recent study with a large sample of cerebellar patients found mild but significant impairments on standard digit span tasks and a significant group effect for the written recall of visually presented lists of words and nonwords (Ravizza *et al.*, 2006). According to a predominant theory of verbal working memory, this cognitive construct has two components: (1) a temporary buffer that stores verbal information in a phonological code and (2) a maintenance mechanism that relies on subvocal rehearsal to refresh a decaying memory trace (Baddeley, 1986). Subvocal rehearsal is thought to involve prefrontal cortical regions that support articulatory planning (e.g., inferior frontal and premotor cortex) and subcortical regions such as the cerebellum (Baddeley, 2003). Although the role of the cerebellum in verbal working memory remains unclear, we proposed that existing neuroimaging and neuropsychological findings support an articulatory monitoring function of the cerebellum (Ben-Yehudah, Guediche, & Fiez, 2007), which we discuss in more detail in the following sections. Thus, our finding that recall of nonwords, but not digits or real words, was significantly worse in the patient compared to the control group suggests that unfamiliar items may benefit more than familiar items from such an articulatory monitoring process. Consistent with this idea are neuroimaging findings of increased prefrontal and cerebellar activation for nonwords relative to words during verbal working memory tasks (Fiez *et al.*, 1996; see Chein & Fiez, 2001, however) and rhyme judgments (Burton, LoCasto, Krebs-Noble, & Gullapalli, 2005; Xu *et al.*, 2001). Future studies are needed to determine whether tasks that use nonwords as stimuli are more sensitive to the cognitive consequences of cerebellar damage.

To summarize, cerebellar damage in adults did not affect reading skills, but it did impair visual rhyme judgment and immediate recall of nonwords. These neuropsychological findings suggest that rhyme judgment and verbal working memory may share a common process that is supported by the cerebellum. In the following sections we present evidence for a common articulatory process and speculate about its role in the acquisition of skilled reading.

A Common Articulatory Process?

In considering the potential for a common process that underlies the patients' impaired performance on rhyme judgment and some verbal working memory tasks, we were struck by the similarity between concurrent articulation effects on these tasks and that of cerebellar damage. In a concurrent articulation paradigm, the participant continuously speaks irrelevant information (e.g. "the, the, the . . .") while performing a primary task, such as deciding whether two words rhyme or remembering a list of items. When performance on a primary task has been disrupted by concurrent articulation, this disruption is attributed to the engagement of the articulatory system by both the primary and secondary tasks. To explore the hypothesis that damage to the cerebellum could result in the concurrent articulation effect—and therefore disruption of the articulatory process—we first turn to the rich literature

on concurrent articulation and its influence on rhyme judgment and verbal working memory.

A large number of behavioral studies have established that concurrent articulation interferes with rhyme judgments on visually presented pairs of words or nonwords (Barron & Baron, 1977; Besner, Davies, & Daniels, 1981; Johnston & McDermott, 1986; Kleiman, 1975; Wilding & White, 1985). Since rhyme judgment requires a comparison of phonological representations, early studies suggested that concurrent articulation interferes with the generation (or retrieval) of phonology for a given visual form (Barron & Baron, 1977; Kleiman, 1975). However, later studies showed that concurrent articulation does not disrupt tasks that explicitly require the generation of phonology, such as homophony judgment (e.g., do AIL-ALE have the same sound?) or phonological lexical decision (e.g., does FORREN sound like a real word?) (Baddeley, Eldridge, & Lewis, 1981; Besner *et al.*, 1981). On the basis of these findings, Besner and colleagues (1981) proposed that concurrent articulation impairs a phonological segmentation process that occurs after the retrieval of whole-word phonology. This hypothesis accounts for the cerebellar patients' normal reading abilities because reading requires generation of phonology and not a postlexical segmentation process. However, this hypothesis does not explain the patients' item-specific impairments on the rhyme judgment task.

Verbal working memory studies attribute the detrimental effect of concurrent articulation on recall to the limited resources of the articulatory system (Baddeley, Lewis, & Vallar, 1984; Baddeley, Thomson, & Buchanan, 1975). Specifically, Baddeley (1986) proposed that concurrent articulation interferes with verbal working memory because it engages articulatory mechanisms that also support subvocal rehearsal, an inner speech process that maintains verbal items in a short-term store. This hypothesis attributes the cerebellar patients' mild verbal working memory deficits to impaired subvocal rehearsal. Recent findings that patients with cerebellar damage continue to use rehearsal to maintain items in working memory challenge this hypothesis (Ravizza *et al.*, 2006). Furthermore, this hypothesis fails to easily account for our finding that the patients' recall of unfamiliar items was disproportionately impaired relative to their ability to recall familiar items; however, it is possible that access to long-term lexical representations reduces the burden on subvocal rehearsal for familiar items as compared to nonwords (Gathercole, Pickering, Hall, & Peaker, 2001).

In summary, the effect of concurrent articulation on rhyme judgment and verbal working memory has been ascribed to different sources of interference. Rhyme judgment studies suggest that concurrent articulation disrupts a postlexical segmentation process, whereas verbal working memory studies attribute this interference to joint reliance on articulatory mechanisms. In our study, the patients' item-specific impairments on these tasks pose a problem for both hypotheses. Although we agree with the view that concurrent articulation interferes with an articulatory process, we believe that it is possible to refine this general hypothesis by examining the role of the cerebellum in monitoring errors in motor and nonmotor tasks.

Articulatory Monitoring

We propose that verbal working memory and rhyme judgment are both impaired in our patient group because these tasks rely on a common articulatory process supported by the cerebellum. To account for the patients' poor performance on specific items, we now turn to a motor theory of cerebellar function that has evolved into the idea that the cerebellum monitors errors in performance. One predominant theory of the cerebellum is that it is involved in motor learning through a trial-and-error process that detects and corrects errors in motor commands (Ramnani, 2006). Motor learning theories in the early 1970s attributed the automatic execution of an ac-

tion to experience-dependent learning in cerebellar circuits (Albus, 1971; Marr, 1969). In essence, a sequence of movements becomes associated over time with a specific behavioral context. Experience-dependent learning occurs by modifying the synaptic strength between Purkinje and granule cells in the cerebellum. These synaptic changes are guided by error signals that are conveyed by climbing fibers from the inferior olive (De Zeeuw & Yeo, 2005; Ito, 1993). A recent computational implementation of experience-dependent learning is based on the idea that the cerebellum consists of "internal models" that simulate motor commands and their predicted sensory consequences (e.g., visual, tactile) (Wolpert, Miall, & Kawato, 1998). In this model, an error signal results from a mismatch between the predicted and the actual sensory consequence of an action. These error signals continuously refine the internal model and can potentially inform the motor system about an execution error before it occurs.

Monitoring is essential to a wide range of motor tasks, including speech production (Guenther, 2006). Recently, the cerebellum has been implicated in cognitive functions that rely on inner speech (Ackermann *et al.*, 2004), possibly because of its role in monitoring articulatory plans for errors (Ben-Yehudah *et al.*, 2007). Rhyme judgment and verbal working memory may both rely on inner speech. Subvocal rehearsal used to maintain items in verbal working memory is akin to an inner speech process (Baddeley, 2003). Rhyme judgment may also engage an inner speech process to silently reiterate word pairs. During inner speech, the cerebellum may simulate the sensory consequences of this subvocal articulation and compare these consequences to input from phonological representations (Desmond, Gabrieli, Wagner, Ginier, & Glover, 1997). Cerebellar damage that prevents this simulation interferes with articulatory monitoring. Verbal items susceptible to pronunciation errors will be affected more by impaired articulatory monitoring. Indeed, the patients' errors in rhyme judgment and serial recall were limited to items that had either inconsistent or unfamiliar pronunciations.

Specifically, the patients' ability to judge whether two words rhymed was impaired on items that had a mismatch between orthography and phonology. Rhyme judgment was particularly difficult on items in which one word had a consistent spelling–sound correspondence (e.g., FEAR) and the other word had an inconsistent correspondence (e.g., BEAR). Findings from word identification studies suggest that once a word is encountered, activation spreads to orthographic neighbors that share the rime unit but not necessarily the pronunciation (e.g., HEAR) (Grainger, Muneaux, Farioli, & Ziegler, 2005). Activation of several phonological forms for the same rime unit results in conflict, which impairs speed and accuracy of judgments (Johnston & McDermott, 1986). Behavioral and computational findings suggest that the amount of conflict is a function of both the number and the frequency of a word's orthographic neighbors (Jared, 2002). One way to reduce conflict during rhyme judgments of this type is to articulate the word pair several times. This articulation (overt or covert) may provide input to a monitoring mechanism that detects errors in pronunciation, thus amplifying the correct (or suppressing the incorrect) pronunciation. In the case of cerebellar damage, we propose that articulatory monitoring is impaired and the consistent pronunciation overrides the inconsistent one resulting in a mistaken judgment. Our study shows that damage to the anterior/superior cerebellar lobules has a detrimental effect on rhyme judgments of items with orthographic–phonological mismatches, suggesting that this cerebellar region is involved in articulatory monitoring.

We found that verbal working memory for familiar items (e.g., words and digits) was not impaired in our cerebellar patient group (though see Ravizza *et al.*, 2006). However, the patients' memory span for nonwords was significantly reduced compared to the control group. Nonwords are more prone to articula-

tion errors because they do not have preexisting lexical knowledge to support their decaying memory trace and consequently their accurate recall (Gathercole, Frankish, Pickering, & Peaker, 1999; Gathercole et al., 2001). Serial recall of nonwords, therefore, would benefit more from articulatory monitoring. Evidence supporting this claim comes from a study by Besner and Davelaar (1983), in which serial recall of pseudohomophones (e.g., PHOOD) was less impaired by concurrent articulation compared to serial recall of nonwords (e.g., BEUED).

Taken together, an articulatory monitoring hypothesis can account for the patients' item-specific deficits in the visual rhyme judgment and serial recall tasks. Furthermore, this hypothesis predicts that skilled readers would not rely on articulatory monitoring as much as beginning readers because they make few pronunciation errors. Our finding that skilled readers who suffered from cerebellar damage did not show reading impairments is consistent with this prediction. Although an intact cerebellum may not be necessary to maintain an adequate level of skilled reading in adults, we cannot exclude the possibility that the cerebellum may contribute to the acquisition of reading.

One model of speech production proposes that the cerebellum functions as a feedforward control system that monitors errors in articulatory plans by receiving input from inferior frontal representations of speech sounds and then projecting back to the motor cortex (Guenther, 2006). Drawing from this model to reading, we speculate that such a feedforward control system may bootstrap reading in its early stages. For instance, a beginning reader has to associate arbitrary symbols with sounds and then blend these sounds into a meaningful phonological unit. Blending errors result in inaccurate articulatory plans that could benefit from adjustments by a monitoring process. Indeed, a comparison of two teaching strategies in preschool children suggests that a focus on blending by not pausing between successive sounds improves word identification more than an emphasis on phonetic segmentation by inducing artificial pauses between sounds (Weisberg & Savard, 1993). An articulatory monitoring process may require a certain degree of blending before it can boost reading; therefore, this process could apply to the former, but not the latter teaching strategy. As readers become more proficient at blending speech sounds and directly mapping visual forms to their corresponding phonological representation, the role of articulatory monitoring may diminish so that skilled reading is unaffected by cerebellar damage. Future studies that examine reading acquisition in children with acquired cerebellar damage may help to refine this hypothesis and inform our understanding of the cerebellum's role in reading.

Acknowledgments

This research was funded by Grant RO1MH59256 from the National Institute of Mental Health to J.A.F. and by Grant F32HD051390 from the National Institute of Child Health and Human Development to G.B. We wish to thank Cristin McCormick for her invaluable assistance in assessing the patient's speech production and in data collection.

Conflicts of Interest

The authors declare no conflicts of interest.

References

Ackermann, H., K. Mathiak & R. B. Ivry. 2004. Temporal organization of "internal speech" as a basis for cerebellar modulation of cognitive functions. *Behavioral and Cognitive Neuroscience Reviews* **3**(1): 14–22.

Albus, J. S. 1971. A theory of cerebellar function. *Mathematical Biosciences* **10**: 25–61.

Baddeley, A. 2003. Working memory: looking back and looking forward. *Nature Reviews Neuroscience* **4**(10): 829–839.

Baddeley, A., M. Eldridge & V. Lewis. 1981. The role of subvocalization in reading. *Quarterly Journal of Experimental Psychology* **33A**: 439–454.

Baddeley, A. D. 1986. *Working memory*. New York: Oxford University Press.

Baddeley, A. D., V. Lewis & G. Vallar. 1984. Exploring the articulatory loop. *Quarterly Journal of Experimental Psychology: Human Experimental Psychology* **36A**(2): 233–252.

Baddeley, A. D., N. Thomson & M. Buchanan. 1975. Word length and the structure of short-term memory. *Journal of Verbal Learning and Verbal Behavior* **14**(6): 575–589.

Barron, R. W. & J. Baron. 1977. How children get meaning from printed words. *Child Development* **48**: 587–594.

Ben-Yehudah, G., S. Guediche & J. A. Fiez. 2007. Cerebellar contributions to verbal working memory: beyond cognitive theory. *The Cerebellum* **6**(3): 193–201.

Besner, D. & E. Davelaar. 1983. Seudohomofoan effects in visual word recognition: evidence for phonological processing. *Canadian Journal of Psychology* **37**: 300–305.

Besner, D., J. Davies & S. Daniels. 1981. Reading for meaning: the effects of concurrent articulation. *Quarterly Journal of Experimental Psychology: Human Experimental Psychology* **33A**(4): 415–437.

Bradley, L. & P. E. Bryant. 1983. Categorising sounds and learning to read: a causal connection. *Nature* **310**: 419–421.

Brown, J. I., J. M. Bennett & G. Hanna. 1981. *The Nelson-Denny reading test*. Chicago: Riverside Publishing Company.

Brunswick, N., E. McCrory, C. J. Price, C. D. Frith & U. Frith. 1999. Explicit and implicit processing of words and pseudowords by adult developmental dyslexics: a search for Wernicke's wortschatz? *Brain* **122**(Pt 10): 1901–1917.

Bryant, P. E., M. MacLean, L. Bradley & J. Crossland. 1990. Rhyme and alliteration, phoneme detection and learning to read. *Developmental Psychology* **26**: 429–438.

Burton, M. W., P. C. LoCasto, D. Krebs-Noble & R. P. Gullapalli. 2005. A systematic investigation of the functional neuroanatomy of auditory and visual phonological processing. *NeuroImage* **26**: 647–661.

Chein, J. M. & J. A. Fiez. 2001. Dissociation of verbal working memory system components using a delayed serial recall task. *Cerebral Cortex* **11**(11): 1003–1014.

De Zeeuw, C. I. & C. H. Yeo. 2005. Time and tide in cerebellar memory formation. *Current Opinion in Neurobiology* **15**: 667–674.

Desmond, J. E. & J. A. Fiez. 1998. Neuroimaging studies of the cerebellum: language, learning and memory. *Trends in Cognitive Sciences* **2**(9): 355–358.

Desmond, J. E., J. D. Gabrieli, A. D. Wagner, B. L. Ginier & G. H. Glover. 1997. Lobular patterns of cerebellar activation in verbal working-memory and finger-tapping tasks as revealed by functional MRI. *Journal of Neuroscience* **17**(24): 9675–9685.

Duffy, J. R. 1995. *Motor speech disorders*. St. Louis, MO: Mosby.

Ellis, A. W., S. McDougall & A. F. Monk. 1996. Are dyslexics different? I. A comparison between dyslexics, reading age controls, poor readers and precocious readers. *Dyslexia* **2**: 31–58.

Enderby, P. M. 1983. *Frenchay dysarthria assessment*. San Diego: College Hill Press.

Fawcett, A. J. & R. I. Nicolson. 1999. Performance of dyslexic children on cerebellar and cognitive tests. *Journal of Motor Behavior* **31**(1): 68–78.

Fiez, J., D. A. Balota, M. Raichle & S. Petersen. 1999. Effects of lexicality, frequency, and spelling-to-sound consistency on the functional anatomy of reading. *Neuron* **24**(1): 205–218.

Fiez, J., E. Raife, D. Balota, J. Schwarz, M. Raichle & S. Petersen. 1996. A positron emission tomography study of the short-term maintenance of verbal information. *Journal of Neuroscience* **16**: 808–822.

Fiez, J. A., S. E. Petersen, M. K. Cheney & M. E. Raichle. 1992. Impaired non-motor learning and error detection associated with cerebellar damage: a single case study. *Brain* **115**(Pt 1): 155–178.

Folstein, M. F., S. E. Folstein & P. R. McHugh. 1975. Mini-mental state: A practical method for grading the cognitive state of patients for the clinician. *Journal of Psychiatric Research* **12**: 189–198.

Gathercole, S. E., C. R. Frankish, S. J. Pickering & S. Peaker. 1999. Phonotactic influences on short-term memory. *Journal of Experimental Psychology: Learning, Memory, and Cognition* **25**(1): 84–95.

Gathercole, S. E., S. J. Pickering, M. Hall & S. M. Peaker. 2001. Dissociable lexical and phonological influences on serial recognition and serial recall. *Quarterly Journal of Experimental Psychology: Human Experimental Psychology* **54**(1): 1–30.

Gathercole, S. E., C. R. Willis & A. D. Baddeley. 1991. Differentiating phonological memory and awareness of rhyme: reading and vocabulary development in children. *British Journal of Psychology* **82**: 387–406.

Grainger, J., M. Muneaux, F. Farioli & J. C. Ziegler. 2005. Effects of phonological and orthographic neighbourhood density interact in viusal word recognition. *Quarterly Journal of Experimental Psychology: Human Experimental Psychology* **58**(6): 981–998.

Guenther, F. H. 2006. Cortical interactions underlying the production of speech sounds. *Journal of Communication Disorders* **39**: 350–365.

Ito, M. 1993. Synaptic plasticity in the cerebellar cortex and its role in motor learning. *Canadian Journal of Neurological Science* **20**: S70–S74.

Ivry, R. B. & J. A. Fiez. 2000. Cerebellar contributions to cognition and imagery. In M. S. Gazzaniga (Ed.), *The new cognitive neurosciences* (pp. 999–1011). Cambridge, MA: MIT Press.

Ivry, R. B. & T. C. Justus. 2001. A neuronal instantiation of the motor theory of speech. *Trends in Neurosciences* **24**(9): 513–515.

Jared, D. 2002. Spelling-sound consistency and regularity effects in word naming. *Journal of Memory and Language* **46**(4): 723–750.

Johnston, R. S. & E. A. McDermott. 1986. Suppression effects in rhyme judgement tasks. *Quarterly Journal of Experimental Psychology: Human Experimental Psychology* **38**(1-A): 111–124.

Kleiman, G. M. 1975. Speech recoding in reading. *Journal of Verbal Learning and Verbal Behavior* **24**: 323–339.

Lenel, J. C. & J. H. Cantor. 1981. Rhyme recognition and phonemic perception in young children. *Journal of Psycholinguistic Research* **10**: 57–68.

Marr, D. 1969. A theory of cerebellar cortex. *Journal of Physiology* **202**: 437–470.

McPherson, W. B., P. T. Ackerman & R. A. Dykman. 1997. Auditory and visual rhyme judgements reveal differences and similarities between normal and disabled adolescent readers. *Dyslexia* **3**: 63–77.

Mechelli, A., M. L. Gorno-Tempini & C. J. Price. 2003. Neuroimaging studies of word and pseudoword reading: consistencies, inconsistencies, and limitations. *Journal of Cognitive Neuroscience* **15**: 260–271.

Moretti, R., A. Bava, P. Torre, R. M. Antonello & G. Cazzato. 2002. Reading errors in patients with cerebellar vermis lesions. *Journal of Neurology* **49**: 461–468.

Nation, K. & M. J. Snowling. 1998. Individual differences in contextual facilitation: evidence from dyslexia and poor reading comprehension. *Child Development* **69**(4): 996–1011.

Nicolson, R. I. & A. J. Fawcett. 1990. Automaticity: a new framework for dyslexia research? *Cognition* **35**(2): 159–182.

Nicolson, R. I., A. J. Fawcett & P. Dean. 1995. Time-estimation deficits in developmental dyslexia – evidence for cerebellar involvement. *Proceedings of the Royal Society: Biological Science* **259**: 43–47.

Nicolson, R. I., A. J. Fawcett & P. Dean. 2001. Developmental dyslexia: the cerebellar deficit hypothesis. *Trends in Neurosciences* **24**(9): 508–511.

Pennington, B. F., G. C. Van Orden, D. S. Smith, P. A. Green & M. M. Haith. 1990. Phonological processing skills and deficits in adult dyslexics. *Child Development* **61**: 1753–1778.

Petersen, S. E., P. T. Fox, M. I. Posner, M. Mintun & M. E. Raichle. 1989. Positron emission tomographic studies of the processing of single words. *Journal of Cognitive Neuroscience* **1**(2): 153–170.

Ramnani, N. 2006. The primate cortico-cerebellar system: anatomy and function. *Nature Reviews* **7**: 511–522.

Ramus, F. 2003. Developmental dyslexia: specific phonological deficit or general sensorimotor dysfunction? *Current Opinion in Neurobiology* **13**(2): 212–218.

Ramus, F., E. Pidgeon & U. Frith. 2003. The relationship between motor control and phonology in dyslexic children. *J Child Psychol Psychiatry* **44**(5): 712–722.

Ravizza, S. M., C. A. McCormick, J. Schlerf, T. Justus, R. B. Ivry & J. A. Fiez. 2006. Cerebellar damage produces selective deficits in verbal working memory. *Brain* **129**: 306–320.

Seymour, P. H., M. Aro & J. M. Erskine. 2003. Foundation literacy acquisition in european orthographies. *British Journal of Psychology* **94**: 143–174.

Shaywitz, S. E. 1998. Dyslexia. *New England Journal of Medicine* **338**: 307–312.

Silveri, M., A. Di Betta, V. Filippini, M. Leggio & M. Molinari. 1998. Verbal short-term store-rehearsal system and the cerebellum: evidence from a patient with a right cerebellar lesion. *Brain* **121**: 2175–2187.

Snowling, M. J. 2000. *Dyslexia* (2nd ed.). Oxford, UK: Blackwell.

Stein, J. & V. Walsh. 1997. To see but not to read; the magnocellular theory of dyslexia. *Trends in Neurosciences* **20**(4): 147–152.

Tallal, P. 1980. Auditory temporal perception, phonics, and reading disabilities in children. *Brain and Language* **9**: 182–198.

Treiman, R. & A. Zukowski. 1991. *Levels of phonological awareness*. Hillsdale, NJ: Erlbaum.

Turkeltaub, P. E., G. F. Eden, K. M. Jones & T. A. Zeffiro. 2002. Meta-analysis of the functional neuroanatomy of single-word reading: method and validation. *NeuroImage* **16**(3 Pt 1): 765–780.

Wagner, R. K., J. K. Torgesen & C. A. Rashotte. 1999. *Comprehensive test of phonological processing*. Manual. Austin, TX: Pro-Ed, Inc.

Walton, D. & P. Brooks. 1995. The spoonerism test. *Educational and Child Psychology* **12**(1): 50–52.

Wechsler, D. 1987. *Wechsler memory scale–revised*. Manual. New York: Psychological Corporation.

Weisberg, P. & C. F. Savard. 1993. Teaching preschoolers to read: don't stop between the sounds when segmenting words. *Education and Treatment of Children* **16**(1): 1–18.

Wilding, J. M. & W. White. 1985. Impairment of rhyme judgments by silent and overt articulatory suppression. *Quarterly Journal of Experimental Psychology: Human Experimental Psychology* **37**(1-A): 95–107.

Wilson, A. M. & N. K. Lesaux. 2001. Persistence of phonological processing deficits in college students with dyslexia who have age-appropriate reading skills. *Journal of Learning Disabilities* **34**(5): 394–400.

Wolpert, D. M., R. C. Miall & M. Kawato. 1998. Internal models in the cerebellum. *Trends in Cognitive Sciences* **2**(9): 338–346.

Woodcock, R. 1998. *Woodcock reading mastery tests–revised/normative update*. Circle Pines, MN: American Guidance Service.

Xu, B., J. Grafman, W. D. Gaillard, K. Ishii, F. Vega-Bermudez, P. Pietrini, *et al.* 2001. Conjoint and extended neural networks for the computation of speech codes: the neural basis of selective impairment in reading words and pseudowords. *Cerebral Cortex* **11**(3): 267–277.

Zagon, I. S., P. J. McLaughlin & S. Smith. 1977. Neural populations in the human cerebellum: estimations from isolated cell nuclei. *Brain Research* **127**: 279–282.

Zeffiro, T. & G. F. Eden. 2001. The cerebellum and dyslexia: perpetrator or innocent bystander? *Trends in Neurosciences* **24**(9): 512–513.

Morphosyntax and Phonological Awareness in Children with Speech Sound Disorders

Jennifer Mortimer and Susan Rvachew

School of Communication Sciences and Disorders, McGill University, Montreal, Quebec, Canada, H3G 1A8

The goals of the current study were to examine concurrent and longitudinal relationships of expressive morphosyntax and phonological awareness in a group of children with speech sound disorders. Tests of phonological awareness were administered to 38 children at the end of their prekindergarten and kindergarten years. Speech samples were elicited and analyzed to obtain a set of expressive morphosyntax variables. Finite verb morphology and inflectional suffix use by prekindergarten children were found to predict significant unique variance in change in phonological awareness a year later. These results are consistent with previous research showing finite verb morphology to be a sensitive indicator of language impairment in English.

Key words: speech sound disorders; language impairment; morphosyntax; phonological awareness; phonological disorder; phonological processing

Introduction

Morphosyntax and Phonological Awareness in Children with Speech Sound Disorders

Children with speech sound disorders (SSDs) (also referred to as phonological disorders) produce speech that is characterized by a greater number of misarticulations and lower intelligibility than is expected for their age. Recent research suggests that there is etiological and symptomatic overlap between dyslexia and SSDs. Specifically, these groups share a common "core deficit" in the area of phonological processing, as indicated by numerous investigations of the phonological processing skills of children with speech sound disorders (Bird, Bishop, & Freeman, 1995; Grawburg, 2004; Larrivee & Catts, 1999; Leitao & Fletcher, 2004; Leitao, Hogben, & Fletcher, 1997; Nathan, Stackhouse, Goulandris, & Snowling, 2004; Raitano, Pennington, Tunick, Boada, &

Shriberg, 2004; Rvachew, Ohberg, Grawburg, & Heyding, 2003). Furthermore, it has been shown that these phonological awareness difficulties are associated with poorly encoded phonological representations for spoken speech input, as indexed by performance on nonword repetition and speech perception tasks (Larrivee & Catts, 1999; Rvachew & Grawburg, 2006).

While it is evident that children with SSDs have difficulties with phonological processing as a group, it is also clear that not all children with SSDs are equally at risk. For example, Rvachew and Grawburg (2006) found that only 50% of a sample of 95 children with SSDs performed below normal limits on a test of implicit phonological awareness skills. Subsequently, it was found that those children with concomitant difficulties in the areas of speech perception, phonological awareness, and speech production accuracy at age 4 years showed poorer nonword reading skills relative to control group children when reassessed at age 7 years. Many studies have attempted to identify additional risk factors that will serve to predict which children with SSDs are most likely to demonstrate difficulties with phonological processing and thus be at risk for

Address for correspondence: Jennifer Mortimer, Beatty Hall, 1266 Pine Avenue West, Montreal, Quebec, Canada, H3G 1A8. Voice: 514-398-4137; fax.: 514-398-8123. jennifer.mortimer@mail.mcgill.ca

Ann. N.Y. Acad. Sci. 1145: 275–282 (2008). © 2008 New York Academy of Sciences.
doi: 10.1196/annals.1416.011

reading disability. Two possible factors have been suggested in particular: severity of the speech impairment and the co-occurrence of language disability (Justice, Invernizzi, & Meier, 2002).

Severity of the SSD (when indexed by the number of speech errors produced) does appear to be correlated with phonological awareness and reading difficulties in this population. For example, Bird *et al.* (1995) followed children who had SSDs at school entry until second grade. Compared with good readers, children who had poor reading abilities in the second grade had produced significantly more consonant errors in their speech 2 years earlier. However, subsequent investigations indicated that this correlation was spurious, with the relationship being mediated by phonological processing skills (Larrivee & Catts, 1999; Rvachew, 2006; Rvachew & Grawburg, 2006). Some researchers have suggested that the types of errors that the children produce may be a better indicator of which children are likely to have phonological awareness difficulties (Broomfield & Dodd, 2004; Leitao & Fletcher, 2004; Rvachew, Chiang, & Evans, 2007). More precisely, within the SSD population, children with delayed phonological awareness skills tend to produce more atypical error patterns than do children with good phonological awareness skills. However, all of these studies demonstrate that patterns of speech error are not a reliable predictor of phonological awareness difficulties. In summary, it is now evident that phonological awareness difficulties can be observed in children with SSDs regardless of the severity of their speech delay whether measured by the number or type of speech errors produced.

The findings related to concomitant language impairment are not as clear. Bird *et al.* (1995) found that phonological awareness skills were equally impaired for children with SSDs with or without concomitant language delay relative to typically developing controls. Major and Bernhardt (1998) also found that language skills did not explain variation in phonological

awareness skills among children with SSDs. On the other hand, Nathan *et al.* (2004) and Raitano *et al.* (2004) reported that children with concomitant SSDs and language impairment achieved poorer phonological awareness performance than did children with SSDs alone. These studies used different global measures of language ability. The relationship between language and phonological awareness in children with SSDs may become clearer if more specific aspects of language performance are examined.

The current study focuses on the role of morphosyntactic skills because impaired morphosyntax is a recognized marker for specific language impairment, another communication disorder that is associated with heightened risk for reading disability (Bishop & Adams, 1990). Proposed explanations as to why specific aspects of morphosyntax appear to be particularly susceptible to disturbance among English-speaking children with specific language impairment (SLI) are numerous and fiercely contested, and cannot be discussed in any depth within the limited scope of this paper (Leonard, 1998, provides a detailed review of the major hypotheses). Epidemiological data from general population samples suggest that the proportion of English-speaking children with speech delay who also have SLI is rather low—approximately 11 to 15% (Shriberg, Tomblin, & McSweeney, 1999).

Given that there is some question as to whether the presence of language impairment increases the likelihood of poor phonological awareness skills in children with SSDs, the goals of the current study were to examine concurrent and longitudinal relationships of expressive morphosyntax and phonological awareness in this population. Children with SSDs were first assessed during the year prior to kindergarten entry. Speech samples were recorded and a variety of morphology and syntactic variables associated with language impairment were analyzed. The relationship between these variables and growth in phonological awareness skills during the kindergarten year was examined.

TABLE 1. Descriptive Statistics by Assessment Time

	Age (months)	GFTA-2 (percentile)	PPVT-III (ss)	No. of utterances per language sample
Prekindergarten				
Mean	57.21	9.66	108.42	67.00
SD	3.18	10.99	12.16	18.97
Range	53.00–66.00	1.00–59.00	85.00–138.00	36.00–116.00
Kindergarten				
Mean	69.18	18.89	111.05	
SD	3.50	17.16	10.95	
Range	63.00–78.00	1.00–65.00	84.00–132.00	

Abbreviations: GFTA-2 = Goldman-Fristoe Test of Articulation, 2nd ed. (Goldman & Fristoe, 2000); PPVT-III (ss) = Peabody Picture Vocabulary Test–III standard scores (Dunn & Dunn, 1997).

Methods

Participants

Results for the 38 children in this study were obtained from a project on the longitudinal development of speech, language, and reading skills in children with SSDs.[a]

Children were 4- and 5-year-olds with a primary diagnosis of speech delay of unknown origin who were referred to the project by speech language pathologists. All children performed below the 16th percentile on a standardized measure of articulation skills. Oral-motor function and hearing, as assessed by the child's clinician prior to referral, were within normal range. Children with sensory-neural hearing loss, Down syndrome, cerebral palsy, or cleft palate were not considered for the study, although children were not excluded on the basis of concomitant language impairment or suspected dyspraxia of speech. All participants spoke English as a primary language. A Blishen score (Blishen, Carroll, & Moore, 1987) for each child, based on parental occupation and level of education, showed middle class socioeconomic status for all children. There were 14 female and 24 male children.

Procedures

Participants were tested on a set of speech and language measures at prekindergarten age and again a year later at kindergarten age. At each testing time, measures were administered in one session of approximately 75 minutes or two sessions of approximately 45 minutes. Examiners were speech-language pathologists or graduate students in speech-language pathology under the supervision of a certified speech-language pathologist. Participants' ages at pre-kindergarten and kindergarten are presented in Table 1, as are articulation scores (Goldman-Fristoe Test of Articulation, 2nd ed.; Goldman & Fristoe, 2000) and receptive vocabulary scores (Peabody Picture Vocabulary Test – III; Dunn & Dunn, 1997).

Phonological Awareness

The phonological awareness test that was developed by Bird *et al.* (1995) was administered to all participants. This test consisted of three subtests: rime matching, onset matching, and onset segmentation and matching. The first subtest administered to each child was rime matching. The child listened to the name of a puppet and then selected from an array of four pictures the one whose name rhymed with the name of the puppet. For example, the child was shown a puppet named "Dan." They were then told, "Dan likes things that sound like his

---

[a]Children were selected on the basis of a complete set of transcribed language results at the time of the 25th Rodin Remediation Academy Conference.

name" and asked which Dan would like from "house," "boat," "car," and "van." The pictures were named for the child, and the child was required to point to the picture of the word that matched the rime of the puppet's name. For the onset matching subtest, the child was shown a puppet and told that everything it owned began with the same sound. The relevant sound was produced in isolation by the examiner and then the child was asked to select the picture whose name began with that sound. Finally, for onset segmentation and matching, the child was again told the puppet's name and then asked to point to the picture whose name "began with the same sound as the puppet's name." In this case, the child was given the puppet's name but was not told the specific target sound. Before each of the three sections, the children were given five practice questions with feedback. The instructions were repeated and the response alternatives named for every item on the test. There were 34 test items in total across the three subtests (14 rime awareness, 10 onset awareness, 10 onset segmentation), involving the target rimes /æn, ʌg, æt, æp/ and target onsets /p, tʃ, m, t, s/. The test items and administration procedures and instructions were exactly as described in Bird *et al.* (1995) except that we replaced the item *settee* with *soap*. Split-half reliability for total test score for 87 randomly selected samples was .98.

Language Samples

A picture book description task was used to elicit language samples from each child. Children were shown a copy of *Carl Goes Shopping* (Day, 1989) and requested to "talk about the pictures." Broad questions such as "What is happening here?" and "What do you think is going to happen next?" were used to encourage quiet children. Samples were recorded in stereo on a Sony MiniDisc using a Portable MiniDisc recorder MZ-B3 and transcribed according to the Systematic Analysis of Language Transcripts protocol (SALT; Miller &

Chapman, 1996). SALT was used to calculate the mean length of utterance in morphemes (MLUm) and in words (MLUw) for each sample. The language samples were further analyzed to obtain indices of morphological and syntactic development.

Finite Verb Morphology Composite

This composite is the percent correct production of copula and auxiliary "be," present third person singular "-s," and past tense "-ed" in obligatory contexts (Goffman & Leonard, 2000; Leonard, Miller, & Gerber, 1999). Difficulty with finite verb morphology is considered by many to be a clinical marker of specific language impairment in English (Rice & Wexler, 1996).

Inflectional Suffix Ratio

The inflectional suffix ratio score centers on the use of the following grammatical morphemes: plural "-s," possessive "-'s," present tense third person singular "-s," and past tense "-ed." These morphophonemes are described by Paul and Shriberg (1982) as being phonetically complex in that appending these affixes to a verb or noun stem may create consonant clusters (e.g., "walked"). Additionally, they may trigger voicing assimilation processes (e.g. /kæts/ versus /dɔgz/).

The percentage of complex inflectional suffixes used in obligatory contexts was calculated. Since some of the children showed evidence of eliminating word-final consonants as a result of their speech difficulties, the percentage of word-final consonants correctly used in noninflected words was also calculated. The percentage of inflectional suffixes correct was then divided by the percentage of word-final consonants correct, forming a ratio. If a child experienced difficulties with inflectional suffix production over and above a tendency to drop word-final consonants, the value of the ratio approached zero. If the production of inflectional affixes was commensurate with the production of word-final consonants, the value of the ratio approached one.

Subject Pronoun Composite

Children with specific language impairment (SLI) are more likely to omit subject case markings on pronouns than are their typically developing language-matched peers, producing utterances such as "him go" (Loeb & Leonard, 1991). The percentage of third person singular pronouns "he" and "she" and third person plural pronoun "they" accurately marked for case was determined for each speech sample. Subject pronoun case-marking errors are comparatively easy to identify in the speech of children with SSD and are not explicable in terms of an articulation deficit.

Developmental Sentence Score

Developmental Sentence Scores (DSS; Lee, 1974) for the five most complex sentences in each language sample were averaged. The DSS analyzes speech samples in terms of eight different linguistic constructs (negatives, conjunctions, wh-questions, interrogative reversals, indefinite pronouns or noun modifiers, personal pronouns, main verbs, and secondary verbs). Each construct is subcategorized into multiple stages across longitudinal language development. A weighted score is assigned to a child's utterance if it shows an appropriate example of a linguistic construct at a particular developmental stage. The DSS correlates well with other measures of productive syntax (Rice, Redmond, & Hoffman, 2006).

Results

Table 2 presents the correlations among the phonological awareness, morphology, and syntax scores at prekindergarten, and the phonological awareness scores at kindergarten. Nonparametric analyses indicated that suffix ratio at prekindergarten was weakly but significantly correlated with phonological aware-

TABLE 2. Correlations among Phonological Awareness and Morphosyntax Variables

	PA—p kindergarten	PA— kindergarten
MLUm pre-k	.375*	.184
MLUw pre-k	.381*	.178
FVM pre-k	.241	.387*
Suffix R pre-k	.328*	.432**
Pronoun pre-k	.002	.036
DSS pre-k	.063	.235

Abbreviations: PA = phonological awareness; MLUm = mean length of utterance in morphemes; MLUw = mean length of utterance in words; FVM = finite verb morphology composite; Suffix R = inflectional suffix ratio; pre-k = prekindergarten; Pronoun = pronoun composite; DSS = developmental sentence score.

*Correlation is significant at the 0.05 level (two-tailed).
**Correlation is significant at the 0.01 level (two-tailed).

ness at the same age; likewise there was a significant relationship between prekindergarten mean length of utterance (in morphemes and in words) and contemporaneous phonological awareness. The prekindergarten suffix ratio was also correlated with phonological awareness a year later. In addition, prekindergarten finite verb morphology and kindergarten phonological awareness were significantly correlated.

Multiple hierarchical regression analyses with kindergarten phonological awareness as the dependent variable indicated that the suffix ratio predicted unique variance after prekindergarten phonological awareness and receptive vocabulary scores were accounted for. (Size of vocabulary store has been linked to degree of sophistication of phonological representations; Metsala & Walley, 1998; Rvachew & Grawburg, 2006.) Similar findings were obtained for finite verb morphology and the developmental sentence score when these were again entered into the model last. Neither MLU (in words or morphemes) nor pronoun use predicted significant unique variance in kindergarten phonological awareness scores. Results are listed in Table 3.

TABLE 3. Relationships between Prekindergarten Morphosyntax and Kindergarten Phonological Awareness Skills Assessed by Hierarchical Multiple Regression Analyses

Step	Variable	R^2 change	F change	P
1	PA pre-k	.236	11.109	.002**
2	Receptive Vocabulary pre-k	.099	5.182	.029*
3	MLUm pre-k	.014	.746	.394
3	MLUw pre-k	.010	.511	.479
3	DSS pre-k	.073	4.219	.048*
3	Pronoun pre-k	.008	.425	.519
3	Suffix R pre-k	.094	5.404	.026*
3	FVM pre-k	.077	4.472	.042*

Abbreviations: PA = phonological awareness; MLUm = mean length of utterance in morphemes; MLUw = mean length of utterance in words; DSS = developmental sentence score; pre-k = prekindergarten; Pronoun = pronoun composite; Suffix R = inflectional suffix ratio; FVM = finite verb morphology composite.

*$P < .05$.

**$P < .01$.

Discussion

Of the six morphosyntactic variables investigated, the finite verb morphology composite and the suffix ratio score were the most reliably associated with kindergarten phonological awareness outcomes. Concurrent correlations among prekindergarten phonological awareness, mean length of utterance, and suffix ratio were more modest. In particular, scores on the inflectional suffix ratio in prekindergarten predicted advances in phonological awareness development over the next year, with lesser amounts of variance predicted by the finite verb morphology composite and the developmental sentence score, respectively.

Finite verb morphology is considered to be a particularly sensitive measure of language impairment in English. Use of these morphemes has been found to discriminate well between children with specific language impairment and children with typical development (Bedore & Leonard, 1998). Two of the four inflectional affixes included in the suffix ratio were finite verb inflections, and the finite verb morphology composite was the best predictor of development in phonological awareness after the suffix ratio. It is possible that children with weaker language skills, as indexed by their performance on finite verb morphology, may be expected to have more difficulty with phonological awareness.

A second consideration is the degree to which the inflectional affixes examined in this study and finite verb morphology draw on phonological processes (such as voicing assimilation and the creation of consonant clusters). Several hypotheses have been proposed to explain difficulties in finite verb morphology among individuals with language impairment, and it would be premature to categorically link problems with verb morphology in this population to a phonological processing deficit (however, for a discussion of this issue, see Joanisse & Seidenberg, 1998). Nevertheless, with regard to individuals with SSDs, for whom atypical phonological processing is widely recognized, performance on finite verb morphology and inflectional suffixes may reflect in part the degree of development of the child's phonological system, particularly for cases in which expressive morphosyntax is linked to phonological awareness. However, it might be said that any theory which attempts to pinpoint a single underlying cause for the association between morphosyntax and phonological awareness in this population will be confounded by evidence that not all children with SSDs acquire poor phonological awareness skills, and comparatively few children with SSDs demonstrate concomitant SLI (Shriberg *et al.*, 1999). The data may perhaps be better understood as illustrating how a confluence of risk factors might lead to increased susceptibility of weakness in phonological awareness in some children (see Raitano *et al.*, 2004). The current results indicate that preschool-aged children with SSDs and poor morphosyntax demonstrated slower growth in PA skills during the kindergarten year than their peers with SSDs but relatively good morphosyntactic abilities.

Conclusions

Results in the present study were consistent with findings by Nathan *et al.* (2004) and Raitano *et al.* (2004) indicating a link between language difficulties and phonological awareness in individuals with SSDs. However, the link found in this study may be specific to a particular aspect of expressive morphosyntax. This study supports previous research on the usefulness of the finite verb morphology composite as a clinical tool. It extends the application of this composite from the domain of language acquisition to literacy development. Further research to broaden current understanding of the expressive language processes contributing to phonological awareness should benefit literacy acquisition research.

Acknowledgments

This research was supported by funding from the Canadian Language and Literacy Research Network, the Alberta Children's Hospital Foundation, the Fonds de la Recherche en Santé du Québec, and the Centre for Research on Language, Mind and Brain. We would like to thank the children who participated in this study, and their families. We are grateful to the students and assistants who were involved in the data collection and processing, including Geneviève Cloutier, Myra Cox, Marie Desmarteau, Meghann Grawburg, Natalia Evans, Joan Heyding, Debbie Hughes, Catherine Norsworthy, Alyssa Ohberg, Alysha Serviss, and Rishanthi Sivakumaran. We also thank the speech-language pathologists at the Alberta Children's Hospital and the Children's Hospital of Eastern Ontario for their assistance with recruitment of children.

Conflicts of Interest

The authors declare no conflicts of interest.

References

Bedore, L. M., & Leonard, L. 1998. Specific language impairment and grammatical morphology: a discriminant function analysis. *Journal of Speech, Language and Hearing Research*, **41**: 1185–1192.

Bird, J., Bishop, D. V. M., & Freeman, N. H. 1995. Phonological awareness and literacy development in children with expressive phonological impairments. *Journal of Speech and Hearing Research*, **38**: 446–462.

Bishop, D. V. M., & Adams, C. 1990. A prospective study of the relationship between specific language impairment, phonological disorders, and reading retardation. *Journal of Child Psychology and Psychiatry*, **31**: 1027–1050.

Blishen, B. R., Carroll, W. K., & Moore, C. 1987. The 1981 Socioeconomic Index for Occupations in Canada. *Canadian Review of Sociology and Anthropology*, **24**: 465–487.

Broomfield, J., & Dodd, B. 2004. Children with speech and language disability: caseload characteristics. *International Journal of Language and Communication Disorders*, **39**(3): 303–324.

Day, A. 1989. *Carl goes shopping*. New York: Farrar Straus Giroux.

Dunn, L. M., & Dunn, L. M. 1997. *Peabody Picture Vocabulary Test* (3rd ed.). Circle Pines, MN: American Guidance Service.

Goffman, L., & Leonard, J. 2000. Growth of language skills in children with specific language impairment: implications for assessment and intervention. *American Journal of Speech-Language Pathology*, **9**: 151–161.

Goldman, R., & Fristoe, M. 2000. *Goldman-Fristoe Test of Articulation* (2nd ed.). Circle Pines, MN: American Guidance Service.

Grawburg, M. 2004. *The role of implicit phonemic perception skills in the acquisition of explicit phonological awareness skills*. Montreal, Quebec, Canada: McGill University.

Joanisse, M. F., & Seidenberg, M. S. 1998. Specific language impairment: a deficit in grammar or processing? *Trends in Cognitive Sciences*, **2**: 240–247.

Justice, L. M., Invernizzi, M. A., & Meier, J. D. 2002. Designing and implementing an early literacy screening protocol: suggestions for the speech-language pathologist. *Language, Speech, and Hearing Services in Schools*, **33**: 84–101.

Larrivee, L. S., & Catts, H. W. 1999. Early reading achievement in children with expressive phonological disorders. *American Journal of Speech-Language Pathology*, **8**: 118–128.

Lee, L. 1974. *Developmental sentence analysis*. Evanston, IL: Northwestern University Press.

Leitao, S., & Fletcher, J. 2004. Literacy outcomes for students with speech-language impairment: long-term follow-up. *International Journal of Language and Communication Disorders*, **29**(2): 245–256.

Leitao, S., Hogben, J. H., & Fletcher, J. 1997. Phonological processing skills in speech and language impaired children. *European Journal of Disorders of Communication*, **32**: 73–93.

Leonard, L. 1998. *Children with specific language impairment*. Cambridge, MA: MIT Press.

Leonard, L. B., Miller, C., & Gerber, E. 1999. Grammatical morphology and the lexicon in children with specific language impairment. *Journal of Speech, Language, and Hearing Research*, **42**: 678–689.

Loeb, D. F., & Leonard, L. B. 1991. Subject case marking and verb morphology in normally developing and specifically language-impaired children. *Journal of Speech and Hearing Research*, **34**: 340–346.

Major, E. M., & Bernhardt, B. H. 1998. Metaphonological skills of children with phonological disorders before and after phonological and metaphonological intervention. *International Journal of Language and Communication Disorders*, **33**: 413–444.

Metsala, J. L., & Walley, A. C. 1998. Spoken vocabulary growth and the segmental restructuring of lexical representations: Precursors to phonemic awareness and early reading ability. In J. L. Metsala & L. C. Ehri (Eds.), *Word recognition in beginning literacy* (pp. 89–120). Mahwah, NJ: Erlbaum.

Miller, J. F., & Chapman, R. S. 1996. Systematic Analysis of Language Transcripts [computer software]. Madison: Language Analysis Laboratory, University of Wisconsin.

Nathan, L., Stackhouse, J., Goulandris, N., & Snowling, M. J. 2004. The development of early literacy skills among children with speech difficulties: a test of the "critical age hypothesis." *Journal of Speech, Language, and Hearing Research*, **47**: 377–391.

Paul, R., & Shriberg, L. D. 1982. Associations between phonology and syntax in speech-delayed children. *Journal of Speech and Hearing Research*, **25**: 536–547.

Raitano, N. A., Pennington, B. F., Tunick, B. F., Boada, R., & Shriberg, L. D. 2004. Pre-literacy skills of subgroups of children with speech sound disorders. *Journal of Child Psychology and Psychiatry*, **45**(4): 821–835.

Rice, M. L., Redmond, S. M., & Hoffman, L. 2006. Mean length of utterance in children with specific language impairment and in younger control children shows concurrent validity and stable and parallel growth trajectories. *Journal of Speech, Language, and Hearing Research*, **49**: 793–808.

Rice, M. L., & Wexler, K. 1996. Toward tense as a clinical marker of specific language impairment in English-speaking children. *Journal of Speech and Hearing Research*, **39**: 678–689.

Rvachew, S. 2006. Longitudinal prediction of implicit phonological awareness skills. *American Journal of Speech-Language Pathology*, **15**: 165–176.

Rvachew, S., Chiang, P., & Evans, N. 2007. Characteristics of speech errors produced by children with and without delayed phonological awareness skills. *Language, Speech, and Hearing Services in Schools*, **38**: 60–71.

Rvachew, S., & Grawburg, M. 2006. Correlates of phonological awareness in preschoolers with speech sound disorders. *Journal of Speech, Language, and Hearing Research*, **49**: 74–87.

Rvachew, S., Ohberg, A., Grawburg, M., & Heyding, J. 2003. Phonological awareness and phonemic perception in 4-year-old children with delayed expressive phonology skills. *American Journal of Speech-Language Pathology*, **12**: 463–471.

Shriberg, L. D., Tomblin, J. B., & McSweeney, J. L. 1999. Prevalence of speech delay in 6-year-old children and comorbidity with language impairment. *Journal of Speech, Language, and Hearing Research*, **42**: 1461–1481.

Brain Mechanisms for Social Perception

Lessons from Autism and Typical Development

Kevin A. Pelphrey[a] and Elizabeth J. Carter[b]

[a]*Yale Child Study Center, Yale University, New Haven, Connecticut, USA*

[b]*Department of Psychology, Carnegie Mellon University, Pittsburgh, Pennsylvania, USA*

In this review, we summarize our research program, which has as its goal charting the typical and atypical development of the social brain in children, adolescents, and adults with and without autism. We highlight recent work using virtual reality stimuli, eye tracking, and functional magnetic resonance imaging that has implicated the superior temporal sulcus (STS) region as an important component of the network of brain regions that support various aspects of social cognition and social perception. Our work in typically developing adults has led to the conclusion that the STS region is involved in social perception via its role in the visual analysis of others' actions and intentions from biological-motion cues. Our work in high-functioning adolescents and adults with autism has implicated the STS region as a mechanism underlying social perception dysfunction in this neurodevelopmental disorder. We also report novel findings from a study of biological-motion perception in young children with and without autism.

Key words: autism; fMRI; superior temporal sulcus

Introduction

Humans are deeply social creatures. They have existed for millennia in highly collective environments in which each person is dependent upon other individuals, including larger families and societal entities. *Social cognition*, broadly construed, is the term we use to refer to the fundamental abilities to perceive, categorize, remember, analyze, reason with, and behave toward other conspecifics. The extent to which such processes work successfully helps determine the fate of individual humans. A potential path to examine the neural basis of social cognition is to understand what separates those individuals who "do" social cognition effectively from those who do not. Our research program adopts this approach in two ways. We

first study typically developing children, adolescents, and adults at different points along the developmental pathway toward mature social cognition abilities. Just as biology is gaining immeasurably from examinations of organisms in development, so it is with mental phenomena. In order to understand the neural basis of typical and atypical social cognition, it is important to understand the normative development of social cognition in children, because such a focus can provide the crucially needed early view of intricate mental processes during their formation. Advances in techniques for imaging the developing brain have provided exciting opportunities for studying the mechanisms involved in the development of social cognition abilities. We also compare brain function and brain development in individuals with and without autism, a disorder that limits social cognition. The use of functional neuroimaging to study abnormal brain function provides an approach in which brain differences can inform us about disease processes and also help us

Address for correspondence: Kevin A. Pelphrey, Ph.D., Yale Child Study Center, 203 South Frontage Road, Yale University, New Haven, CT 06520. Voice: +203-785-3486. kevin.pelphrey@yale.edu

Ann. N.Y. Acad. Sci. 1145: 283–299 (2008). © 2008 New York Academy of Sciences.
doi: 10.1196/annals.1416.007

to better understand normal brain functioning and development.

For much of the twentieth century, psychologists produced theories and a wealth of empirical evidence concerning the basic building blocks of social cognition. This understanding is beginning to benefit from the use of noninvasive brain imaging techniques, including functional magnetic resonance imaging (fMRI), to identify a network of brain regions that support various facets of social cognition in humans. In the past decade, studies of how we think about ourselves and other minds, how we mimic and change, and how we regulate our emotions and perceive emotions in other people have allowed us to learn about the various components of social cognition. However, this work has focused on the mature minds of adult humans almost exclusively. Little work has been conducted to explore patterns of brain development as they relate to the emergence and refinement of social cognition abilities, leaving this area wide open for investigation.

Through the lens of recent social neuroscience research, it is increasingly clear that social cognition abilities depend upon specialized brain systems for processes which include rapidly recognizing the faces of others, interpreting the actions of others through an analysis of biological-motion cues, and determining others' emotional states via inspection of facial expression. Various proposals have been put forth describing the brain regions involved in social cognition. One early and influential model was outlined by Brothers (1990), who conceived of social cognition as the processing of information that culminates in the accurate analysis of the dispositions and intentions of other individuals and proposed the involvement of the amygdala, orbitofrontal cortex (OFC), and superior temporal sulcus (STS) region as key nodes of the primate "social brain." In this and other models of the social brain, components of the neural circuitry supporting social cognition consist of mechanisms that are relatively old in evolutionary terms. The social world in which the human brain carries out its functions, however, has changed dramatically over a relatively short period. For example, a child born 50,000 years ago would have had similar mental powers as a child today, but a decidedly different set of demands, aspirations, and opportunities, not to mention rights, responsibilities, chances of survival, and definitions of success.

Work in our laboratory has focused on identifying and characterizing the development of psychological and brain mechanisms supporting a relatively simple aspect of social cognition, social perception, which refers to the initial stages of evaluating the emotions, actions, and intentions of others using their gaze direction, body movements, hand gestures, facial expressions, and other biological-motion cues (Allison, Puce, & McCarthy, 2000). We have employed virtual-reality character animation, behavioral, eye-tracking, and fMRI techniques to explore normal and abnormal development of brain mechanisms for social perception. In particular, we have focused on the use of biological-motion cues to interpret others' actions. We will describe some of the key recent findings from this research program regarding the role of the STS region in neurologically normal adults and in typically developing children. Then, we will consider how these advances have informed, and have been informed by, our understanding of the brain mechanisms underlying social-perception dysfunction in autism.

Defining the Social Brain

As illustrated in Figure 1, neuroscientists have described several brain regions that comprise the neural circuitry supporting various aspects of social cognition and social perception. These include:

(*1*) The lateral fusiform gyrus or "fusiform face area," which is important for structural encoding of faces in the environment and for rapid face recognition (Kanwisher, McDermott, & Chun, 1997; Puce, Allison, Asgari, Gore, & McCarthy, 1996).

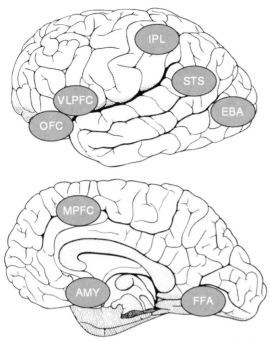

Figure 1. Some of the brain regions involved in various aspects of social cognition and social perception. VLPFC = ventral lateral prefrontal cortex; IPL = inferior parietal lobule; STS = superior temporal sulcus; OFC = orbital frontal cortex; MPFC = medial prefrontal cortex; EBA = extrastriate body area; AMY = amygdale; FFA = fusiform face area.

(2) The posterior STS region, which has been implicated in processing dynamic expressions of emotion and in the interpretation of the actions and intentions of others through visual analysis of biological-motion cues (Bonda, Petrides, Ostry, & Evans, 1996; LaBar, Crupain, Voyvodic, & McCarthy, 2003; Pelphrey *et al.*, 2003a; Pelphrey, Morris, & McCarthy, 2004a; Pelphrey, Singerman, Allison, & McCarthy, 2003b; Pelphrey, Viola, & McCarthy, 2004b). In humans, the *STS region* is a term used to describe the STS proper, portions of the superior and middle temporal gyri, and areas of the angular gyrus near the ascending limb of the STS (Allison *et al.*, 2000).

(3) The amygdala and interconnected frontal-limbic regions. These regions have been implicated in determining the emotional states of others through analysis of facial expressions (Adolphs, Tranel, Damasio, & Damasio, 1995;

Morris *et al.*, 1996) and play a central and complex role in multiple aspects of emotion (Davis & Whalen, 2001; Kluver & Bucy, 1997; LeDoux, 1992).

(4) The extrastriate body area (EBA), which has been implicated in the visual perception of human bodies (Downing, Jiang, Shuman, & Kanwisher, 2001).

(5) A set of regions involving portions of the parietal cortex, including the inferior and superior parietal lobules, the anterior intraparietal sulcus, and frontal cortical regions, including the inferior frontal gyrus (IFG). This set of regions has been dubbed the "mirror system" in humans because the regions activate equally to the execution of a motor action and the observation of a motor action by another person (Buccino *et al.*, 2001; Iacoboni *et al.*, 2001; Iacoboni *et al.*, 1999; Rizzolatti, Fadiga, Gallese, & Fogassi, 1996).

(6) The orbitofrontal cortex (OFC), which has been implicated in the processing of reward and social reinforcement (Bechara, Damasio, Damasio, & Anderson, 1994; Rolls, 2000). While the OFC has been most commonly implicated in "low-level" representation of reward or punishment values (O'Doherty, Kringelbach, Rolls, Hornak, & Andrews, 2001), the more lateral (i.e., ventral and dorsal) prefrontal cortices (VLPFCs) have been implicated in facilitating relatively more complex adaptive behavioral responses to changes in reward or punishment values (Cools, Clark, Owen, & Robbins, 2002).

(7) The medial prefrontal cortex (MPFC), which has been implicated in the making of inferences about other people's intentions and mental states (Castelli, Frith, Happe, & Frith, 2002; Frith & Frith, 1999; Gregory *et al.*, 2002) as well as the attribution of emotion to self and others (Ochsner *et al.*, 2004).

To date, cognitive neuroscientists have emphasized the identification of the unique contribution of each region to social cognition and social perception. This analytic perspective has helped provide a framework for organizing our emerging understanding of the social brain, but this approach does not fully reflect the complexity of interactions among these neuroanatomical structures. It is likely that, as our field evolves, these structures will be better understood as components in a network of regions subserving social cognition and social perception.

Brain Studies of Social Perception in Adults

We have established a program of research that has as its major goal the identification and definition of the neural systems involved in social perception and the study of those systems in typically and atypically developing children, adolescents, and adults. We began our research on the neurobiology of social perception in humans with the intention of further specifying the role of the STS region. This work was initiated to test the hypothesis that the STS region plays an important role in social perception via its involvement in interpreting the actions and social intentions of other people from an analysis of biological-motion cues (Allison *et al.*, 2000). This proposition was based on the available human neuroimaging evidence as well as elegant work in nonhuman primates demonstrating the sensitivity of neurons in the STS to various socially relevant cues, including head and gaze direction (Perrett *et al.*, 1985). Here, we describe selected experiments that addressed this question using fMRI and virtual-reality techniques with typically developing, adult participants.

Are There Specialized Brain Regions for the Perception of Biological Motion?

The STS region was identified early on as playing a role in biological motion perception (for a review, see Allison *et al.*, 2000). We define *biological motion* as the visual perception of a living being performing a recognizable action or movement such as dancing, waving, and talking. Our visual system can identify oth-

ers engaging in such activities even in the absence of visual form detail. For example, many researchers have created stimuli by affixing a number of small lights to the joints of actors and filming these individuals while they perform various movements. Experimental participants viewing these stimuli are able to describe correctly the actors, their emotions, and their activities (Johannson, 1973). Most of these prior studies used point-light displays as stimuli. For instance, Bonda and colleagues (1996) demonstrated that the perception of point-light displays conveying recognizable hand movements activated the STS region more than did random motion of lights. This left open the possibility that the response from the STS region was being driven by the fact that biological motion was more familiar, recognizable, and nameable than random motion. It is possible that coordinated and meaningful nonbiological motion might also activate the STS region, and this called into question the specificity of this region for processing biological motion.

To address this issue, we conducted an event-related fMRI study to compare the responses from the STS region to four different types of motion conveyed via animated virtual-reality characters. As illustrated in the top panel of Figure 2, participants viewed walking, a biological motion conveyed by a robot (Robot) or a human (Human). They also viewed a nonmeaningful but complex nonbiological motion in the form of a disjointed mechanical figure (Mechanical) and a complex, meaningful, and nameable, nonbiological motion involving the movements of a grandfather clock (Clock) (Pelphrey *et al.*, 2003a). Our design addressed the critical question of whether the STS region is specialized for the perception of biological motion. As shown in the bottom panel of Figure 2, we observed strong and equivalent activity in the right hemisphere STS region to the Human and Robot conditions. This result ruled out the possibility that the STS region was merely responding to the presence of a human form. Overall, the response to biological

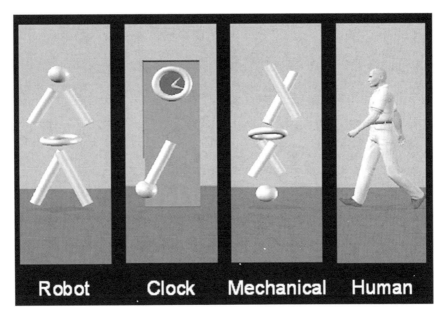

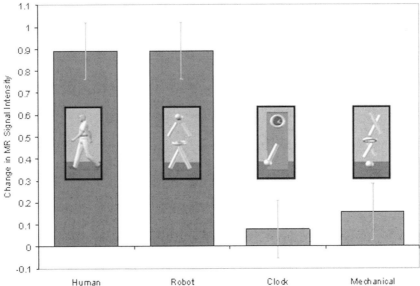

Figure 2. Stimuli (*top*) and results (*bottom*) from a study of biological-motion perception in typically developing adults. The STS region responded more strongly to the biological than to nonbiological motion (*bottom*).

motion was far greater than that to the moving clock and the mechanical figure. Critically, not every brain region showed this pattern of effects. For instance, MT or V5 (MT/V5), which is known to respond to various kinds of motion (Puce *et al.*, 1995; Watson *et al.*, 1993; Zeki *et al.*, 1991), responded strongly to all four types of motion. From these results, we concluded that biological motion selectively activates the STS region. Thus, we began to view the STS region as a node of the neural system supporting social perception via its role in the detection and perception of human actions.

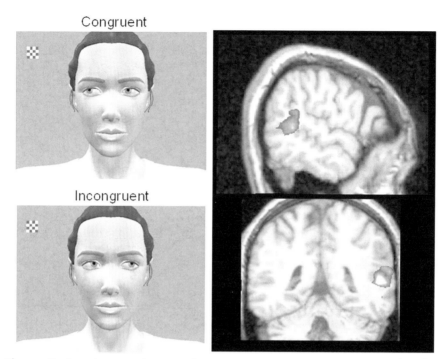

Figure 3. Experiment to determine brain activation in response to expected and unexpected gaze shifts on the part of another person (*left*) and corresponding brain activation to biological motion (observed human movements; *right*). Incongruent trials evoked greater right hemisphere STS activity than did congruent trials, demonstrating the sensitivity of the STS region to the intentions conveyed by eye-gaze shifts. (From Pelphrey and Morris, 2006, reprinted with permission.)

Is the STS Region Involved in Representing the Intentions of Other People?

Our prior study demonstrated that the STS region is involved selectively in the perception of biological motion. Given this finding, we next sought to determine whether the STS region represents the intentions of other people. That is, we evaluated whether the STS region is sensitive to the goals and intentions of observed actions—in this case, the movement of a character's eyes to be consistent or inconsistent with a subject's expectation about what the virtual character "ought" to do in a particular context.

Inside the MRI scanner, our subjects watched an animated character as a small checkerboard appeared and flickered in her visual field (Fig. 3, left). On congruent trials, the character looked toward the checkerboard

(Fig. 3, top left), acting in accordance with the subject's presumed expectation. On incongruent trials, the character looked away from the checkerboard at a different part of her visual field (Fig. 3, bottom left), thereby violating expectations. We had suspected that the STS region would be sensitive to these differences in intentionality and that this region would therefore differentiate between the congruent and incongruent conditions. This would suggest that this area is involved in monitoring expectations about the goals of others. Activity in the STS region was greater for incongruent than for congruent gaze shifts, demonstrating a need for different levels of processing for observed goal-directed and non-goal-directed observed actions.

This study advanced our understanding of the social brain by demonstrating that the activity in the STS region is modulated by the perceived intentions of actions. Thus, we concluded that the STS region participates in social perception beyond its role in the perception of biological motion: it is also involved in the visual analysis of other people's actions and intentions. We note that the pattern of effects (incongruent > congruent) is not specific to eye movements, because it is also observed when subjects view congruent and incongruent reaching-to-grasp movements of the hand and arm (Pelphrey *et al*., 2004a).

Does the STS Region Serve as a Mechanism for the Detection of Socially Relevant Gaze Shifts?

Our prior fMRI study of gaze processing established that the STS region is sensitive to at least one aspect of the context within which an action is observed (i.e., goal-directedness vs. non-goal-directedness). Here, we conducted an fMRI study to evaluate whether the STS region is also sensitive to overtly social messages regarding approach and avoidance conveyed via mutual and averted gaze. Gaze direction can serve as a powerful social cue, with mutual gaze often signaling threat or approach and averted gaze conveying submission or avoidance (Argyle & Cook, 1976). Of all the primate species, humans have the most prominent eyes (largest and brightest sclera), which facilitates the determination of gaze direction (Kobayashi & Kohshima, 1997). This and other findings support the "cooperative eye" hypothesis put forward by Tomasello and colleagues (Tomasello, Hare, Lehmann, & Call, 2007). They suggest that particularly visible eyes have made it increasingly easy throughout evolution to coordinate close-range collaborative activities, promoting the understanding the attentional focus and plans of others. One prediction of this hypothesis is that the primate social brain should include mechanisms for the detection of socially relevant gaze shifts.

In order to further examine the roles played by gaze in social interactions, we created a virtual-reality scenario wherein characters would approach the participant and either meet or avoid his or her eyes (Fig. 4, top). Participants viewed these stimuli through virtual-reality goggles in an MRI scanner. We predicted greater activity for mutual compared to averted gaze, reflecting the demand for greater social processing in the case of mutual gaze. As illustrated in the bottom panel of Figure 4, we saw this pattern of response for the approach and associated gaze shift in the STS region. However, there was a functional dissociation between the STS and the right fusiform gyrus wherein the fusiform gyrus did not differentiate between mutual and averted gaze. This suggests a more straightforward role of the right fusiform gyrus in face detection, but a more specific function for the STS region in gaze comprehension.

These two studies of eye-gaze perception illustrate a role for the STS region in the detection and processing of eye movements in order to interpret the attentional foci and goals of others during social interactions. They also support the hypothesis that a social brain component can be influenced by the context of an action, even during passive observation of others. Also, this research suggests that such processing occurs prior to such higher-level executive functions as decision making, response selection, and the perception of novelty, which largely take place in prefrontal regions. More broadly, our findings regarding contextual influences on brain activity fit well within social psychology findings regarding the behavioral effects that result from situational and contextual factors. Thus, the principles of situational and contextual influence operate at multiple levels of the organism, including the individual's behavior in social situations and localized brain activity.

Summary of the Characteristics of the STS Region

In summary, the studies reviewed above, together with others not discussed here, have allowed us to characterize the STS region as a

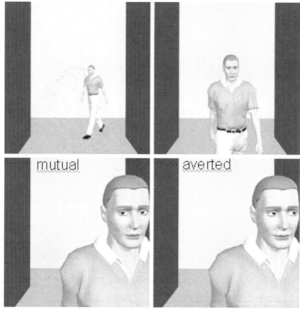

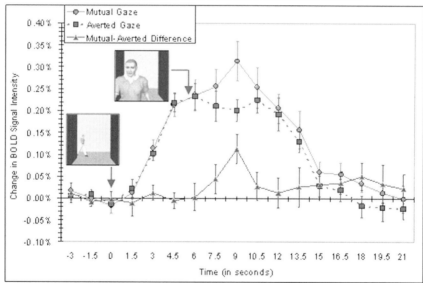

Figure 4. Stimuli (*top*) and findings (*bottom*) from an experiment measuring brain activation in response to a stranger initiating or avoiding social interaction. Participants viewed an animated character approaching down a virtual hallway, who shifted his gaze either toward or away from the subject. In both situations, the animated sequence evoked activation in the right STS region. The graph at *bottom* shows the time courses of activation (indicated as average blood oxygenation level–dependent contrast, or BOLD, signal changes) from the right STS region in response to the passerby's gaze movements. The mutual and averted gaze conditions are plotted along with a plot of their difference (mutual minus averted gaze). Note that the change in activity begins with the appearance of the character in the hallway and increases again at the moment the gaze shift occurs. (From Pelphrey and Morris, 2006, reprinted with permission.)

node in the social brain. To date, we know that: (*a*) The STS region demonstrates a preferential response to biological motion relative to non-biological motion (Pelphrey *et al.*, 2003a). (*b*)The STS region is multimodal, responding to auditory and visual stimuli and exhibiting polysensory interactions (Wright, Pelphrey, Allison, McKeown, & McCarthy, 2003). Also, this region is sensitive to the goals or intentions (social and nonsocial) conveyed by biological-motion cues (Mosconi, Mack, McCarthy, & Pelphrey, 2005; Pelphrey *et al.*, 2004a; Pelphrey, Morris, Michelich, Allison, & McCarthy, 2005b; Pelphrey *et al.*, 2003b; Pelphrey *et al.*, 2004b). (*c*) The STS region exhibits a roughly somatotopic organization (Pelphrey *et al.*, 2005b).

Given the emerging portrait of the role of the STS region in social perception, it is not surprising that this neuroanatomical structure has become a focus of research for several groups seeking to understand brain mechanisms in autism, a disorder that features profound deficits in several aspects of social perception and social cognition. We now turn to a discussion of our laboratory's work in this area.

Neural Basis of Social Perception Dysfunction in Autism

Defining the Phenotype: Social Perception Dysfunction in Autism

Autism is a complex, behaviorally defined, neurodevelopmental disorder characterized by severe and pervasive deficits in social functioning and communication as well as restricted, repetitive behaviors and a distinctive developmental course (American Psychiatric Association, 2000). Affected individuals differ in the extent to which they demonstrate each of these impairments, but the core disability appears to revolve around social functioning (Kanner, 1943; Waterhouse *et al.*, 1996). As highlighted by Kanner (1943), the "inability to interact in the ordinary way" is a cardinal feature of autism and is pathognomonic of this neurodevelop-

mental disorder. In Kanner's (1943) first description of 11 children with "infantile autism," he described the children as lacking the necessary skills for normal social functioning, with a particular impairment in social interactions. To wit, "We must, then, assume that these children have come into the world with innate inability to form the usual, biologically provided affective contact with other people, just as other children come into the world with innate physical or intellectual handicaps." (p. 250). In his view, the most notable social difficulties were a lack of variation in emotional expression, withdrawn interest in other people, detachment, and inaccessibility in social interactions, and the preference for objects over people. Although each individual varied along a spectrum, they all shared an inherent lack of understanding of social situations and an inability to offer an emotional connection when interacting with others. The uniqueness of social behavior in autism led Kanner (1943) to characterize this disorder as a "disturbance of affective contact." In a 30-year follow-up of these same children, Kanner (1973) found little improvement in affective contact with people, and he concluded that they lacked the appropriate biological mechanisms for such contact. These brief highlights from Kanner's original observations of autism confirm the same spectrum of autism observed today and the multiple facets of social dysfunction in autism.

Viewing the World through the Eyes of Autism

Our laboratory's first foray into the study of autism provided a striking illustration of the social perception deficits that characterize this neurodevelopmental disorder. As displayed in Figure 5, we used eye tracking to evaluate the visual scanpaths of high-functioning adults with autism while they viewed faces displaying various expressions of emotion. Neurologically normal adults (Fig. 5, right) spent most of their time viewing the core, socially informative features of the faces (i.e., the eyes, nose, and mouth). In

Autism

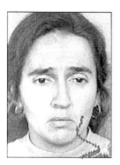

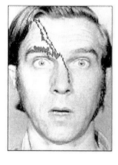

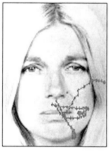

Typical

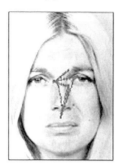

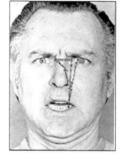

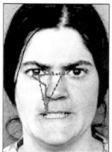

Figure 5. Sample scanpaths from an eye-tracking study of high-functioning adults with autism (*left column*) and IQ, gender, and age-matched, typically developing comparison subjects (*right column*). (From Pelphrey *et al.*, 2002, reprinted with permission.)

stark contrast, individuals with autism (Fig. 5, left) did not look at the eyes or the other core features of the faces. Instead, they scanned the faces in a seemingly random fashion, suggesting a failure to understand the significance of the features for social understanding.

The STS Region and Social Dysfunction in Autism

Along with the scanpath differences we reported, individuals with autism have been char-

acterized as possessing deficits in using gaze information to understand the intentions and mental states of others as well as to coordinate joint attention (Baron-Cohen, 1995; Baron-Cohen *et al.*, 1999; Dawson, Meltzoff, Osterling, Rinaldi, & Brown, 1998; Frith & Frith, 1999; Leekam, Hunnisett, & Moore, 1998; Leekam, Lopez, & Moore, 2000; Loveland & Landry, 1986; Mundy, Sigman, Ungerer, & Sherman, 1986). Such deficits are seen very early in development. Joint attention can be learned in some cases, using gaze information to infer mental states and intentions, and is consistently impaired even in high-functioning adults with autism (Baron-Cohen, Wheelwright, Hill, Raste, & Plumb, 2001). Note that it is not that these individuals cannot detect gaze direction, but rather that they cannot use such information to infer others' mental states and behaviors. On the basis of our prior findings and knowledge of these deficits, we decided to explore the role of the STS in gaze processing dysfunction in autism. To do so, we utilized our checkerboard paradigm. We knew that typically developing individuals should show an increased response for incongruent versus congruent gaze shifts in the STS and other social brain regions, showing expectations of intentionality. However, although we found activity in the same brain regions in individuals with autism, we saw no such differentiation in brain activity based on condition. This suggests an absence of contextual influence on the STS region, which is a possible mechanism underlying the gaze-processing deficits reported behaviorally in autism. Hypoactivation of the STS and reduced functional connectivity between the STS and portions of the inferior occipital gyrus (visual area V3) have also been reported in individuals with autism during tasks involving attribution of intentions to moving geometric figures (Castelli, Frith, Happe, & Frith, 2002).

One of the most interesting aspects of our findings was the observation that dysfunction in the STS region was strongly and specifically correlated with the level of social impairment exhibited by individual subjects. Recall that as a group, activity in the STS region in the subjects with autism did not differ significantly for incongruent and congruent gaze shifts. However, just as autism is heterogeneous in severity, there were clear individual differences in the degree of STS dysfunction. To explore whether these individual differences were related to the severity of autism, we computed correlations between the scores on several algorithmic domains of the Autism Diagnostic Interview–Revised (ADI-R; Lord, Rutter, & Le Couteur, 1994), which is used to support the diagnosis of autism, and the magnitude of the incongruent versus congruent differentiation in the right STS region. We assumed that lower levels of incongruent versus congruent differentiation (i.e., incongruent minus congruent difference scores) in the STS region would indicate greater cortical dysfunction. Higher scores on aspects of the ADI-R can indicate greater severity of autism. Strikingly, the magnitude of the incongruent versus congruent difference score was strongly, negatively correlated with scores in the Reciprocal Social Interaction Domain ($r = -0.78$, $P = 0.004$). However, it was not significantly correlated with impairments in the Communication Domain or the Restricted, Repetitive and Stereotyped Patterns of Behavior Domain. These findings suggest that the degree of neurofunctional impairment in the right STS region is related to the severity of specific core features of the autism phenotype.

Another deficit reported in the behaviors of individuals with autism is that of speech- and language-processing difficulties, including speech perception. The STS has also been shown to play a role in these processes. Reports from neuroimaging studies have suggested abnormal laterality during speech perception (Boddaert *et al.*, 2002) as well as abnormal responses in the STS region to human voices (Gervais *et al.*, 2004) and a lack of response to vocal sounds (Belin, Zatorre, Lafaille, Ahad, & Pike, 2000) in individuals with autism. Note, however, that these individuals showed typical auditory cortex responses to nonvocal sounds. We decided to further explore speech perception deficits by using audiovisual speech displays in individuals with autism and neurologically normal controls (Collins & Pelphrey, unpublished thesis data). When perceiving the simultaneous auditory and visual speech displays, the STS region showed bilateral activation. In typically developing individuals, there was a greater level of activity in this region when the auditory and visual displays matched than when they did not match or when auditory or visual information was presented in isolation. However, the individuals with autism exhibited hypoactivation in the STS region for all conditions and no differentiation between matching and mismatching speech presentations. These results suggest failed integration of auditory and visual speech.

Neurobiology of Social Perception Development in Children with and without Autism

While cognitive neuroscientists have generated a wealth of information regarding the brain regions involved in social perception and social cognition, very little work has been conducted to evaluate the development of the social brain in typically or atypically developing children. Several early studies focused on the amygdala and its response to fearful faces. First, Baird and colleagues (1999) demonstrated amygdala activation to fearful faces in children ages 12 to 17 years. Thomas and colleagues (2001) reported that adults demonstrated greater amygdala activation to fearful facial expressions, whereas 11-year-old children showed greater amygdala activation to neutral faces. It may be that the neutral faces were seen as more ambiguous than fearful facial expressions, with resulting increases in amygdala activation. Sex differences in amygdala development have been reported in children and adolescents (Killgore, Oki, & Yurgelun-Todd, 2001). Whereas the left amygdala responded to fearful facial expressions in all children, its activity decreased over the adolescent period in females but not in males. In a follow-up study, Killgore and Yurgelun-Todd (2004) compared children, adolescents, and adults during the perception of fearful faces. They reported that males and females differed in the asymmetry of activation of the amygdala and prefrontal cortex (PFC) across the three age groups. For males, activation within the dorsolateral PFC was bilateral in childhood, right lateralized in adolescence, and bilateral in adulthood, whereas females showed a monotonic relationship with age, with older females showing more bilateral activation than younger ones. In contrast, amygdala activation was similar for both sexes, with bilateral activation in childhood, right-lateralized activation in adolescence, and bilateral activation in adulthood. Finally, Lobaugh, Gibson, and Taylor (2006) reported that fear, disgust, and sadness recruit distinct neural systems in 10-year-old children similarly to adults (Phan, Wager, Taylor, & Liberzon, 2002). Other studies have examined the role of the lateral fusiform gyrus (FFG) in face processing in children, with studies using fMRI and ERPs beginning to provide important information. Thus far, it is known that some degree of FFG specialization for faces is apparent early in development (e.g., Tzourio-Mazoyer et al., 2002), and this specialization continues to develop throughout infancy and into late childhood and adolescence (Aylward *et al.*, 2005; Mosconi *et al.*, 2005; Taylor, Edmonds, McCarthy, & Allison, 2001). Studies have found similar mirror neuron activity in children between 10 and 12 years of age, as had been identified previously in adults, but patterns of activity in these areas have not yet been explored in younger children (Dapretto *et al.*, 2006; Ohnishi et al., 2004).

Acquisition of neuroimaging data from children involves a number of methodological challenges. Perhaps the most noteworthy of these is the child's compliance with the requirement to remain motionless during the scanning session. A key methodological advance in our laboratory's efforts to establish a program of child functional neuroimaging research was been to develop "mock scanning" facilities. We completed construction of an MRI simulator for use in acclimating children to the scanner environment and for training these subjects to minimize head motion. Specifically, children are trained using operant conditioning procedures implemented with custom-written software that receives input from a head-motion sensor and uses this input to direct the operation of a video player. The child watches a movie, and the movie is halted whenever the child exhibits head motion above a progressively stricter threshold. We have successfully used this system to prepare children ages 4 to 12 years for fMRI sessions (Cantlon, Brannon, Carter, & Pelphrey, 2006; Carter & Pelphrey, 2006; Mosconi *et al.*, 2005).

The Neural Basis of Gaze Perception in Typically Developing Children

Building upon our work on the role of the STS region in adults with and without autism, we have initiated a series of studies to examine the neurofunctional development of this region in children with and without autism. We first examined the neural circuitry involved in school-aged children (Mosconi *et al.*, 2005). Using our incongruent versus congruent gaze paradigm (Fig. 2, left), we investigated the sensitivity of brain regions involved in processing gaze and the intentions conveyed by shifts in eye gaze in typically developing children between 7 and 10 years old. On the basis of our prior findings using this and similar fMRI paradigms in adults (Pelphrey *et al.*, 2003b, 2004b, 2005), we hypothesized that STS activity would differentiate congruent and incongruent trials, reflecting the ability of typically developing 7-year-old children to link the perception of the gaze shift with its mentalistic significance. Our results confirmed our prediction and indicated that the STS region was sensitive to the intentions underlying the stimulus character's eye movements. These findings suggest that the neural circuitry underlying the processing of eye gaze and the detection of intentions from gaze in children in this age range is very similar to that of adults.

Functional Neuroimaging of Biological Motion Perception in Children with and without Autism

More recently, we examined the degree to which the STS region is selective for biological as compared to nonbiological motion in 6- to 10-year-old children with and without autism. In an elegant behavioral study, Blake, Turner, Smoski, Pozdol, and Stone (2003) demonstrated that children (ages 8–10 years) with autism are significantly impaired at recognizing biological motion from point-light displays relative to IQ-matched neurologically normal children. We sought to identify the brain correlates of these biological-motion perception deficits in children with autism. We employed our prior design with four different motion conditions: a walking man, a walking robot, a disjointed mechanical figure with the same components as the robot, and a grandfather clock (Pelphrey *et al.*, 2003a). In this way, we were able to control for whether the figure was biological, whether the motion was biological, and whether the motion was organized. As reviewed above, we had previously shown that the STS region in neurologically normal adults was activated more by the biological-motion conditions (human and robot) than by the nonbiological motion conditions (clock and mechanical figure). As illustrated in the left panel of Figure 6, we identified a network of brain regions in our sample of 7- to 10-year-old typically developing children that had greater responses evoked by biological than by nonbiological motion, including the STS region and portions of the purported human mirror neuron system, including the inferior frontal gyri, the precentral gyri, and middle and superior frontal gyri (Carter & Pelphrey, 2006). Additionally, we found a developmental change that suggested increasing specificity

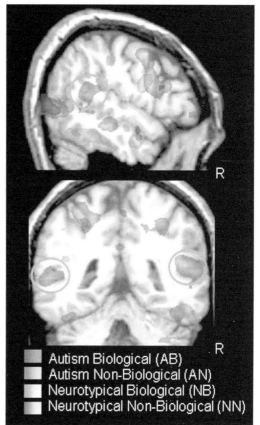

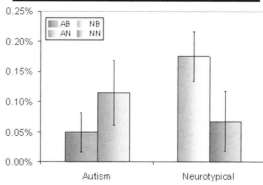

Figure 6. Summary activations from participants with and without autism viewing biological and non-biological motion (*top*). The graph at the *bottom* shows the response from the STS region as a function of condition and participant group.

for biological motion with age in the STS region. Specifically, the magnitude of the biological greater than non-biological difference score was positively correlated with age in the right STS region ($r = .64$, $P < .03$, two-tailed), with age accounting for approximately 41% of the variance in the biological greater than non-biological difference scores.

As shown in the right panel of Figure 6, when we used this same paradigm with 7- to 10-year-old high-functioning children with autism ($N = 5$), we found that they did not have different STS activity for biological and non-biological motion. Critically, not every brain region showed these patterns of effects: the motion-sensitive visual area MT/V5 was equally activated by both motion types in children with and without autism. This functional dissociation suggests that the STS and other social brain regions are specific for biological motion in typically developing children, but not in children with autism. We did not observe reduced activity in all brain areas investigated, indicating that the effect we observed was not being driven by a general reduction in the fMRI signal.

These findings are particularly interesting in light of theoretical perspectives that emphasize the importance of biological motion in the development of theory-of-mind abilities. For example, Frith and Frith (1999) suggested that the ability to distinguish between biological and nonbiological figures and their actions is one of the likely evolutionary and developmental precursors to theory of mind. Thus, early biological-motion detection abilities could allow children to develop the ability to use knowledge about the actions and intentions of others to infer mental states and thus to develop full-fledged theory-of-mind abilities. The findings from our fMRI study of biological-motion perception in children with and without autism suggest that children with autism do not possess one of the basic building blocks believed to underlie theory of mind. It is noteworthy that these individuals also show pronounced deficits on theory-of-mind tasks (Baron-Cohen, Leslie, & Frith, 1985; Perner, Frith, Leslie, & Leekam, 1989).

Conclusion

Prior functional neuroimaging studies of autism have focused on the adolescent and adult age ranges, with the average age of samples in fMRI studies of adults with autism at 21 years and the youngest age group at 12 years. There are several reasons why it is critical to adopt a developmental perspective for studies of the brain mechanisms underlying emotion-processing deficits in autism. First, many of the neuroimaging findings from adults with autism could represent either actual causes of autism and/or compensatory changes in the brains of people with autism. Group differences in imaging data from adults might represent a causal factor or an effect on the brain of having autism. Recognizing the manifestations of compensatory effects in people with autism will be critical to understanding neuroimaging findings and may lead to novel treatments. Second, autism has its onset in the earliest years of childhood and its symptoms change over ontogeny. Neuroimaging studies of autism that take into account these psychological and behavioral continuities and discontinuities will better inform us of the neurobiological mechanisms in autism than studies that provide only a static picture in adults. Third, functional brain correlates of autism in children may prove useful in early diagnosis, and the elucidation of developmental trajectories of the neural circuitry supporting emotion processing might inform the design of more effective treatments. Fourth, a developmental perspective can be a useful tool for unraveling the interaction between seemingly disparate levels of organization, such as those among the molecular biology of gene expression, the structure and function of the brain, and the development of cognitive abilities. Ultimately, only prospective, longitudinal studies of children at risk for developing autism will be able to clarify the relationship between brain abnormalities and the course of the disorder.

Acknowledgments

The studies reviewed herein were supported in part by grants from the National Institute of Mental Health, the John Merck Scholars

Fund, the National Institute of Child Health and Human Development, the Veterans Affairs Administration, the National Alliance for Autism Research/Autism Speaks, and the National Institute for Neurological Disorders and Stroke. Kevin Pelphrey is supported by a Career Development Award from the National Institutes of Health, NIMH Grant MH071284. Elizabeth Carter is supported by a predoctoral fellowship from the National Alliance for Autism Research/Autism Speaks. We gratefully acknowledge our collaborators, especially Gregory McCarthy, James Morris, and Truett Allison. We are grateful to Jaime Doyle for assistance with manuscript preparation.

Conflicts of Interest

The authors declare no conflicts of interest.

References

Adolphs, R., Tranel, D., Damasio, H., & Damasio, A. R. 1995. Fear and the human amygdala. *Journal of Neuroscience*, **15**(9): 5879–5891.

Allison, T., Puce, A., & McCarthy, G. 2000. Social perception from visual cues: role of the STS region. *Trends in Cognitive Science*, **4**(7): 267–278.

American Psychiatric Association. 2000. *Diagnostic and statistical manual of mental disorders (text rev.)*. Washington, DC: Author.

Argyle, M., & Cook, M. 1976. *Gaze and mutual gaze*. Cambridge: Cambridge University Press.

Aylward, E. H., Park, J. E., Field, K. M., Parsons, A. C., Richards, T. L., Cramer, S. C., *et al.* 2005. Brain activation during face perception: evidence of a developmental change. *Journal of Cognitive Neuroscience*, **17**(2): 308–319.

Baird, A. A., Gruber, S. A., Fein, D. A., Maas, L. C., Steingard, R. J., Renshaw, P. F., *et al.* 1999. Functional magnetic resonance imaging of facial affect recognition in children and adolescents. *Journal of the American Academy of Child and Adolescent Psychiatry*, **38**(2): 195–199.

Baron-Cohen, S. 1995. *Mindblindness: an essay on autism and "theory of mind."* Cambridge, MA: MIT Press.

Baron-Cohen, S., Leslie, A. M., & Frith, U. 1985. Does the autistic child have a "theory of mind"? *Cognition*, **231:** 37–46.

Baron-Cohen, S., Ring, H. A., Wheelwright, S., Bullmore, E. T., Brammer, M. J., Simmons, A., *et al*. 1999. Social intelligence in the normal and autistic brain: an fMRI study. *European Journal of Neuroscience*, **11**(6): 1891–1898.

Baron-Cohen, S., Wheelwright, S., Hill, J., Raste, Y., & Plumb, I. 2001. The "Reading the Mind in the Eyes" Test revised version: a study with normal adults, and adults with Asperger syndrome or high-functioning autism. *Journal of Child Psychology and Psychiatry*, **42**(2): 241–251.

Bechara, A., Damasio, A. R., Damasio, H., & Anderson, S. W. 1994. Insensitivity to future consequences following damage to human prefrontal cortex. *Cognition*, **50**(1–3): 7–15.

Belin, P., Zatorre, R. J., Lafaille, P., Ahad, P., & Pike, B. 2000. Voice-selective areas in human auditory cortex. *Nature*, **403**(6767): 309–312.

Blake, R., Turner, L. M., Smoski, M. J., Pozdol, S. S., & Stone, W. L. 2003. Visual recognition of biological motion is impaired in children with autism. *Psychological Science*, **14:** 151–157.

Boddaert, N., Chabane, N., Barthelemy, C., Bourgeois, M., Poline, J. B., Brunelle, F., *et al*. 2002. [Bitemporal lobe dysfunction in infantile autism: positron emission tomography study]. *Journal de Radiologie*, **83**(12 Pt 1): 1829–1833.

Bonda, E., Petrides, M., Ostry, D., & Evans, A. 1996. Specific involvement of human parietal systems and the amygdala in the perception of biological motion. *Journal of Neuroscience*, **16**(11): 3737–3744.

Brothers, L. 1990. The social brain: a project for integrating primate behavior and neurophysiology in a new domain. *Concepts in Neuroscience*, **1**: 27–51.

Buccino, G., Binkofski, F., Fink, G. R., Fadiga, L., Fogassi, L., Gallese, V., *et al*. 2001. Action observation activates premotor and parietal areas in a somatotopic manner: an fMRI study. *European Journal of Neuroscience*, **13**(2): 400–404.

Cantlon, J. F., Brannon, E. M., Carter, E. J., & Pelphrey, K. A. 2006. Functional imaging of numerical processing in adults and 4-y-old children. *PLoS Biol*, **4**(5): e125.

Carter, E. J., & Pelphrey, K. A. 2006. School-aged children exhibit domain-specific responses to biological motion. *Social Neuroscience*, **1**(3–4): 396–411.

Castelli, F., Frith, C., Happe, F., & Frith, U. 2002. Autism, Asperger syndrome and brain mechanisms for the attribution of mental states to animated shapes. *Brain*, **125**(Pt 8): 1839–1849.

Cools, R., Clark, L., Owen, A. M., & Robbins, T. W. 2002. Defining the neural mechanisms of probabilistic reversal learning using event-related functional magnetic resonance imaging. *Journal of Neuroscience*, **22**(11): 4563–4567.

Dapretto, M., Davies, M. S., Pfeifer, J. H., Scott, A., Sigman, M., Bookheimer, S. Y., *et al.* 2006. Understanding emotions in others: mirror neuron dysfunction in children with autism spectrum disorders. *Nature Neuroscience*, **9**: 28–30.

Davis, M., & Whalen, P. J. 2001. The amygdala: vigilance and emotion. *Molecular Psychiatry*, **6**(1): 13–34.

Dawson, G., Meltzoff, A. N., Osterling, J., Rinaldi, J., & Brown, E. 1998. Children with autism fail to orient to naturally occurring social stimuli. *Journal of Autism and Developmental Disorders*, **28**(6): 479–485.

Downing, P. E., Jiang, Y., Shuman, M., & Kanwisher, N. 2001. A cortical area selective for visual processing of the human body. *Science*, **293**(5539): 2470–2473.

Frith, C. D., & Frith, U. 1999. Interacting minds: a biological basis. *Science*, **286**(5445): 1692–1695.

Gervais, H., Belin, P., Boddaert, N., Leboyer, M., Coez, A., Sfaello, I., *et al.* 2004. Abnormal cortical voice processing in autism. *Nature Neuroscience*, **7**(8): 801–802.

Gregory, C., Lough, S., Stone, V., Erzinclioglu, S., Martin, L., Baron-Cohen, S., *et al.* 2002. Theory of mind in patients with frontal variant frontotemporal dementia and Alzheimer's disease: theoretical and practical implications. *Brain*, **125**(Pt 4): 752–764.

Iacoboni, M., Koski, L. M., Brass, M., Bekkering, H., Woods, R. P., Dubeau, M. C., *et al.* 2001. Reafferent copies of imitated actions in the right superior temporal cortex. *Proceedings of the National Academy of Sciences of the Unites States of America*, **98**(24): 13995–13999.

Iacoboni, M., Woods, R. P., Brass, M., Bekkering, H., Mazziotta, J. C., & Rizzolatti, G. 1999. Cortical mechanisms of human imitation. *Science*, **286**(5449): 2526–2528.

Johannson, G. 1973. *Visual perception of biological motion and a model for its analysis.* (Vol. 14).

Kanner, L. 1943. Autistic disturbances of affective contact. *Nervous Child*, **2**(2): 217–230.

Kanner, L. 1973. Historical perspective on developmental deviations. *Journal of Autism and Childhood Schizophrenia*, **3**(3): 187–198.

Kanwisher, N., McDermott, J., & Chun, M. M. 1997. The fusiform face area: a module in human extrastriate cortex specialized for face perception. *Journal of Neuroscience*, **17**(11): 4302–4311.

Killgore, W. D., Oki, M., & Yurgelun-Todd, D. A. 2001. Sex differences in amygdala activation during the perception of facial affect. *Neuroreport*, **12**(11): 2543–2547.

Killgore, W. D., & Yurgelun-Todd, D. A. 2004. Sex-related developmental differences in the lateralized activation of the prefrontal cortex and amygdala during perception of facial affect. *Perception and Motor Skills*, **99**(2): 371–391.

Kluver, H., & Bucy, P. C. 1997. Preliminary analysis of functions of the temporal lobes in monkeys. 1939. *Jouranl of Neuropsychiatry and Clinical Neuroscience*, **9**(4): 606–620.

Kobayashi, H., & Kohshima, S. 1997. Unique morphology of the human eye. *Nature*, **387**(6635): 767–768.

LaBar, K. S., Crupain, M. J., Voyvodic, J. T., & McCarthy, G. 2003. Dynamic perception of facial affect and identity in the human brain. *Cerebral Cortex*, **13**(10): 1023–1033.

LeDoux, J. E. 1992. Brain mechanisms of emotion and emotional learning. *Current Opinion in Neurobiology*, **2**(2): 191–197.

Leekam, S. R., Hunnisett, E., & Moore, C. 1998. Targets and cues: gaze-following in children with autism. *Journal of Child Psychology and Psychiatry*, **39**(7): 951–962.

Leekam, S. R., Lopez, B., & Moore, C. 2000. Attention and joint attention in preschool children with autism. *Developmental Psychology*, **36**(2): 261–273.

Lobaugh, N. J., Gibson, E., & Taylor, M. J. 2006. Children recruit distinct neural systems for implicit emotional face processing. *Neuroreport*, **17:** 215–219.

Lord, C., Rutter, M., & Le Couteur, A. 1994. Autism Diagnostic Interview-Revised: a revised version of a diagnostic interview for caregivers of individuals with possible pervasive developmental disorders. *Journal of Autism and Developmental Disorders*, **24**(5): 659–685.

Loveland, K. A., & Landry, S. H. 1986. Joint attention and language in autism and developmental language delay. *Journal of Autism and Developmental Disorders*, **16**(3): 335–349.

Morris, J. S., Frith, C. D., Perrett, D. I., Rowland, D., Young, A. W., Calder, A. J., *et al.* 1996. A differential neural response in the human amygdala to fearful and happy facial expressions. *Nature*, **383**(6603): 812–815.

Mosconi, M. W., Mack, P. B., McCarthy, G., & Pelphrey, K. A. 2005. Taking an "intentional stance" on eye-gaze shifts: a functional neuroimaging study of social perception in children. *Neuroimage*, **27**(1): 247–252.

Mundy, P., Sigman, M., Ungerer, J., & Sherman, T. 1986. Defining the social deficits of autism: the contribution of non-verbal communication measures. *Journal of Child Psychology and Psychiatry*, **27**(5): 657–669.

O'Doherty, J., Kringelbach, M. L., Rolls, E. T., Hornak, J., & Andrews, C. 2001. Abstract reward and punishment representations in the human orbitofrontal cortex. *Nature Neuroscience*, **4**(1): 95–102.

Ochsner, K. N., Knierim, K., Ludlow, D. H., Hanelin, J., Ramachandran, T., Glover, G., *et al.* 2004. Reflecting upon feelings: an fMRI study of neural systems supporting the attribution of emotion to self and other. *Journal of Cognitive Neuroscience*, **16**(10): 1746–1772.

Ohnishi, T., Moriguchi, Y., Matsuda, H., Mori, T., & Makiko, K. 2004. The neural network for the mirror system and mentalizing in normally developed children: an fMRI study. *Neuroreport*, **15**(9): 1483–1487.

Pelphrey, K. A., Mitchell, T. V., McKeown, M. J., Goldstein, J., Allison, T., & McCarthy, G. 2003a. Brain activity evoked by the perception of human walking: controlling for meaningful coherent motion. *Journal of Neuroscience*, **23**(17): 6819–6825.

Pelphrey, K. A., & Morris, J. P. 2006. Brain mechanisms for interpreting the actions of others from biological-motion cues. *Current Directions in Psychological Science*, **15**: 136–140.

Pelphrey, K. A., Morris, J. P., & McCarthy, G. 2004a. Grasping the intentions of others: the perceived intentionality of an action influences activity in the superior temporal sulcus during social perception. *Journal of Cognitive Neuroscience*, **16**(10): 1706–1716.

Pelphrey, K. A., Morris, J. P., Michelich, C. R., Allison, T., & McCarthy, G. 2005. Functional anatomy of biological motion perception in posterior temporal cortex: an FMRI study of eye, mouth and hand movements. *Cerebral Cortex*, **15**(12): 1866–1876.

Pelphrey, K. A., Singerman, J. D., Allison, T., & McCarthy, G. 2003b. Brain activation evoked by perception of gaze shifts: the influence of context. *Neuropsychologia*, **41**(2): 156–170.

Pelphrey, K. A., Sasson, N. J., Reznick, J. S., Paul, G., Goldman, B., & Piven, J. 2002. Visual scanning of faces in autism. *Journal of Autism and Developmental Disorders*, **32**(4): 249–261.

Pelphrey, K. A., Viola, R. J., & McCarthy, G. 2004b. When strangers pass: processing of mutual and averted social gaze in the superior temporal sulcus. *Psychological Science*, **15**(9): 598–603.

Perner, J., Frith, U., Leslie, A. M., & Leedham, S. 1989. Exploration of the autistic child's theory of mind: knowledge, belief, and communication. *Child Development*, **60**(33): 689–700.

Perrett, D. I., Smith, P. A., Potter, D. D., Mistlin, A. J., Head, A. S., Milner, A. D., *et al*. 1985. Visual cells in the temporal cortex sensitive to face view and gaze direction. *Proceedings of the Royal Society of London. Series B, Containing papers of a Biological character. Royal Society (Great Britian)*, **223**(1232): 293–317.

Phan, K. L., Wager, T., & Taylor, S. F. 2002. Functional neuroanatomy of emotion: a meta-analysis of emotion activation studies in PET and fMRI. *NeuroImage*, **16**(2): 331–348.

Puce, A., Allison, T., Asgari, M., Gore, J. C., & McCarthy, G. 1996. Differential sensitivity of human visual cortex to faces, letterstrings, and textures: a functional magnetic resonance imaging study. *Journal of Neuroscience*, **16**(16): 5205–5215.

Puce, A., Constable, R. T., Luby, M. L., McCarthy, G., Nobre, A. C., Spencer, D. D., *et al*. 1995. Functional magnetic resonance imaging of sensory and motor cortex: comparison with electrophysiological localization. *Journal of Neurosurgery*, **83**(2): 262–270.

Rizzolatti, G., Fadiga, L., Gallese, V., & Fogassi, L. 1996. Premotor cortex and the recognition of motor actions. *Brain Research. Cognitive Brain Research*, **3**(2): 131–141.

Rolls, E. T. 2000. The orbitofrontal cortex and reward. *Cerebral Cortex*, **10**(3): 284–294.

Taylor, Edmonds, McCarthy, & Allison 2001.

Thomas, K. M., Drevets, W. C., Whalen, P. J., Eccard, C. H., Dahl, R. E. Ryan, N. D., *et al*. 2001. Amygdala response to facial expressions in children and adults. *Biological Psychiatry*, **49**(4): 309–316.

Tomasello, M., Hare, B., Lehmann, H., & Call, J. 2007. Reliance on head versus eyes in the gaze following of great apes and human infants: the cooperative eye hypothesis. *Journal of Human Evolution*, **52**(3): 314–320.

Tzourio-Mazoyer, N., De Schonen, S., Crivello, F., Reutter, B., Aujard, Y., & Mazoyer, B. 2002. Neural correlates of woman face processing by 2-monthy-old infants. *NeuroImage*, **15**(2): 454–461.

Waterhouse, L., Morris, R., Allen, D., Dunn, M., Fein, D., Feinstein, C., *et al*. 1996. Diagnosis and classification in autism. *Journal of Autism and Developmental Disorders*, **26**(1): 59–86.

Watson, J. D., Myers, R., Frackowiak, R. S., Hajnal, J. V., Woods, R. P., Mazziotta, J. C., *et al*. 1993. Area V5 of the human brain: evidence from a combined study using positron emission tomography and magnetic resonance imaging. *Cerebral Cortex*, **3**(2): 79–94.

Wright, T. M., Pelphrey, K. A., Allison, T., McKeown, M. J., & McCarthy, G. 2003. Polysensory interactions along lateral temporal regions evoked by audiovisual speech. *Cerebral Cortex*, **13**(10): 1034–1043.

Zeki, S., Watson, J. D., Lueck, C. J., Friston, K. J., Kennard, C., & Frackowiak, R. S. 1991. A direct demonstration of functional specialization in human visual cortex. *Journal of Neuroscience*, **11**(3): 641–649.

From Loci to Networks and Back Again

Anomalies in the Study of Autism

Ralph-Axel Müller

Brain Development Imaging Laboratory, Department of Psychology, San Diego State University, San Diego, California, USA
Department of Cognitive Science, University of California, San Diego, California USA

Recent developments in functional imaging as well as the emergence of new anatomical imaging techniques suited for the study of white matter have shifted investigational paradigms from a localized to a more holistic network approach. Aside from detecting local activity, functional MRI can be applied to the study of connectivity. However, the concept of "functional connectivity" remains broad, and specific designs and analyses may affect the results. In addition, connectivity cannot be viewed in isolation. Rather, from a developmental perspective, connectivity and local cortical architecture are intimately related. Therefore, combined approaches examining local organization and connectivity are the most promising avenues for elucidating disturbances of neurofunctional organization in developmental disorders. Here this approach is illustrated via data obtained from autism research that suggest impaired local cortical architecture and reduced long-range connectivity between cerebral regions.

Key words: localization, functional connectivity, developmental disorders, autism

Introduction

From Loci to Networks

In his *Structure of Scientific Revolutions*, Thomas Kuhn (1962) describes how the progress of a science may be characterized by "paradigm shifts." In his view, a field of research would be dominated by a fixed set of assumptions about an object of study or a set of questions for potentially long periods of time until "anomalies," that is, findings that cannot be reconciled with these assumptions, reach a critical threshold. At this point, the field may undergo a sudden "revolution" or "paradigm shift," resulting in a completely new approach with a new set of fixed assumptions.

In the history of neuropsychology, events have not been as dramatic. One could indeed make the point that the conflict between localizing and holistic approaches to the study of brain function has had a long history through the centuries (Clarke & Dewhurst, 1972). Nonetheless, localizing approaches have been overall dominant, at least since the times of Paul Broca. The reasons are largely methodological. The dominant and most productive techniques of neuropsychology have been ones that naturally lent themselves to conclusions about localized function. Thus Broca's description (Broca, 1861) of expressive speech loss in patient Leborgne found to be associated with what was then considered as a localized lesion in left inferior frontal cortex was among the first of thousands of cases in which presumably localized lesions in a patient or a group of patients was related to a circumscribed pattern of cognitive or behavioral deficit (see Shallice, 1988, for a methodological review). It is of note that a later reexamination of Leborgne's brain by

Address for correspondence: Ralph-Axel Müller, Ph.D., Department of Psychology, San Diego State University, 6363 Alvarado Ct., #225 E, San Diego, CA 92120-1863. Voice: +619-594-5276; fax: +619-594-8707. amueller@sciences.sdsu.edu, http://www.sci.sdsu.edu/~amueller/index.html

Signoret *et al.* (1984) showed much more extensive damage.

In the history of neuropsychology, voices of caution—from Hughlings-Jackson (1878) to Henry Head (1926) or Jason Brown (1988)—have been mostly met with puzzled respect. Certainly, anyone with a basic knowledge of the brain could tell just by appreciating the vast volumes of connecting white matter that the cooperation of regions in large networks was highly likely. However, incorporating lesion data into holistic or distributed models was less than straightforward, whereas localizing models could generate clear and falsifiable hypotheses, often considered the hallmark of true science (Popper, 1965).

The more recent history of functional neuroimaging has been characterized by a similar methodological bias. The two most important techniques for activation mapping, [^{15}O]-water positron emission tomography (PET) and functional magnetic resonance imaging (fMRI) detect signals based on increased blood flow and blood oxygenation in regions of enhanced synaptic transmission. The signal arises almost exclusively from gray matter. Indeed, effects in white matter are often discarded as artifactual by definition. Although these techniques have almost unlimited ability to detect multiple concurrent activation sites, the function of white matter remains literally in the dark. Not surprisingly, the localizationist program, though much more refined than in the times of the phrenologists (Gall & Spurzheim, 1810) or classical localizationists (Lichtheim, 1885; Wernicke, 1874), has progressed greatly since the emergence of functional neuroimaging. An impressive example is the review by Cabeza and Nyberg (2000) of 275 PET and fMRI studies in which they identify loci of activation sorted by Brodmann areas for a large number of cognitive domains and types of tasks. At the end of this tour de force, Cabeza and Nyberg emphasize that network approaches, although not included in the review, are supported by the finding that any type of task performance appears to rely on multiple brain regions.

This insight may imply that the massive attempt at localizing components of cognitive and sensorimotor function in many thousands of current functional imaging studies of the healthy adult brain has been leading to its own demise, reminiscent of what Kuhn described as a paradigm shift. The added driving forces in this process are the methodological advances in neuroimaging technology. Among these are noninvasive methods of studying white matter integrity (in MR spectroscopy [MRS] and diffusion tensor imaging [DTI]) and fiber tracts (in DTI tractography) on the anatomical side and functional connectivity MRI (fcMRI) on the functional side.

In this review, I will examine how the change in perspective described above—from local specialization to distributed network organization—affects the study of developmental disorders. The exemplary disorder to be discussed will be autism, but many of the issues raised will likely apply to other disorders, such as developmental dyslexia.

"Functional Connectivity"

One of the pioneers of the study of functional connectivity in developmental disorders, Barry Horwitz, who in the late 1980s was the first to study regional cross-correlations of PET data of glucose metabolism in autism (Horwitz *et al.*, 1988), titled a recent review (Horwitz, 2003) "The elusive concept of brain connectivity." While our concept of anatomical connectivity may be straightforward, relating to axons and the tissue compartments containing them (white matter), the definition of *functional connectivity* is much less clear. In electrophysiological studies, phase coherence has been applied as a measure of functional connectivity and its changes in childhood have been described (Thatcher *et al.*, 1987). Animal studies, in which electrical currents were recorded directly from cortex, suggest that phase-locked synchronization of spiking in distal neurons may reflect perceptual binding (Nase *et al.*, 2003). Temporal coherence is found in high-frequency domains, in particular in the beta (15–30 Hz) and gamma bands (30–80 Hz, Uhlhaas & Singer, 2006). Electrophysiological approaches to functional connectivity have been applied to autism in only a few studies. Grice and colleagues (2001) reported reduced modulation of gamma band activity associated with face orientation (upright and inverted) in autistic adults. One additional study by Brown and colleagues (2005) found atypical gamma peaks in autistic adolescents during viewing of illusory shapes, which the authors interpreted as reduced signal-to-noise ratio due to impaired inhibition. Wilson *et al.* (2007) recently reported reduced gamma band power of magnetoencephalographic responses to acoustic stimuli in the left hemisphere of 10 children with autism, whereas gamma power in the right hemisphere was close to normal.

While EEG coherence studies of functional connectivity in autism are still very scarce, some recent studies have applied functional connectivity MRI (fcMRI), which is characterized by lower temporal but higher spatial resolution. Analogous to conventional activation fMRI, fcMRI relies on the blood oxygenation level–dependent (BOLD) signal, which indirectly reflects complex physiological changes associated with local neuronal activity (Ances *et al.*, 2008). Instead of modeling the variance of BOLD time series in terms of task on–off blocks or trial sequences as in conventional fMRI activation analysis, fcMRI measures interregional cross-correlations of the BOLD signal. Yet, as pointed out in the review by Horwitz (2003), there is no general consensus on what *functional connectivity* exactly means. The term has been defined by Friston *et al.* (1993) as "observed temporal correlations between spatially remote neurophysiological events"—in contrast with *effective connectivity*, defined as "the influence one neural system exerts over another." However, this dichotomy is clearer conceptually than it may be in actual research applications. Of course, there is a difference between studies exploring time-series correlations without making assumptions about underlying anatomical connectivity and those that model correlations only between selected regions assumed to affect each other through anatomical connectivity as known from animal studies. The distinction is not unlike the two different approaches in statistical activation analyses of fMRI or [^{15}O]-water PET data, which can be tested either on a voxel-wise basis throughout the brain or with regard to predetermined regions of interest (ROIs, each containing many voxels). However, no one would assume that functional connectivity, as originally defined by Friston or more recently by Rippon and colleagues (2007) as a "temporal relationship between two or more neuronal assemblies acting synchronously, measured by cross-correlating time series," could exist in the absence of effective connectivity and anatomical connections.

In actual research practice, the lines between functional and effective connectivity are therefore often not as distinct. For example, Castelli and colleagues (2002) reported reduced activation associated with a "theory of mind" condition (observing triangles that appeared to interact like human beings) in superior temporal sulcus (STS), basal temporal cortex (close to the amygdala), and medial prefrontal cortex of the right hemisphere in adults with autism spectrum disorders (ASDs). Their connectivity analysis focused on these regions, which were activated in the control group, and extrastriate cortex, which was activated in both groups. They found that connectivity between extrastriate cortex and STS was reduced in the autism group. Since connectivity analyses were limited to ROIs, they may be considered as related to effective connectivity. Although the authors did not explicitly establish the existence of anatomical connectivity between the ROIs, the assumption is almost trivial in view of the density and abundance of anatomical connectivity in the brain (Schmahmann & Pandya, 2006). This is particularly so, because the low temporal resolution of PET and fcMRI does not warrant any assumption about observed connectivity being monosynaptic. The ease with which anatomical connections, through which brain regions may affect each other functionally, can be established for just about any interregional functional signal correlation thus softens the dichotomy between functional and effective connectivity. The dichotomy appears to be more related to the investigator's approach than to an actual biological distinction.

There is an important additional issue already alluded to in the previous example, in which ROIs were selected on the basis of activation findings. Many variants of connectivity studies consider functional or effective connectivity a derivation of task-driven activation effects. For example, dynamic causal modeling includes effects of experimental conditions on connectivity (Lee *et al.*, 2006). This stands in contrast to the evidence that first jumpstarted fcMRI. Biswal and colleagues (1995) identified primary motor cortex using a simple finger movement paradigm. Using the observed activation cluster in left motor cortex as a seed volume, they demonstrated BOLD time-series cross-correlations specifically in other brain regions considered part of a motor network (e.g., homotopic contralateral primary motor cortex and supplementary motor areas). Remarkably, these correlations were seen during rest, that is, in the absence of any task or stimulation. Furthermore, such correlations have been predominantly observed at very low frequencies below 0.1 Hz (Cordes *et al.*, 2001). This suggests that there are components in BOLD time series that reflect neural network organization and that are not driven by stimulation or cognitive challenge. There are two implications, one promising, the other problematic. First, low-frequency BOLD correlations promise to open a window onto functional brain organization that may be orthogonal to conventional activation imaging, providing an entirely independent set of useful evidence. Second, however, since these low-frequency correlations cannot be explained by hemodynamic responses to task challenge, it is not clear what their functional and neurophysiological basis is. There is some evidence suggesting that these fcMRI effects

may reflect low-frequency fluctuations in local field potentials, possibly driven by thalamocortical afferents (Leopold *et al.*, 2003).

Despite the lack of a comprehensive physiological model, there are growing numbers of studies supporting the validity of low-frequency BOLD correlations for mapping out functionally specialized networks. These include, for example, studies mapping out complex distributed functional networks, such as the motor network (Xiong *et al.*, 1999), perisylvian language areas (Hampson *et al.*, 2002), or regions cooperating on a spatial working memory task (Lowe *et al.*, 2000) as well as some intriguing clinical studies. One study in patients with callosal agenesis showed disrupted interhemispheric BOLD correlations between homotopic regions, such as left and right superior temporal cortex, which are robustly correlated in healthy controls (Quigley *et al.*, 2003). Another study reported that a promotor polymorphism of the serotonin transporter gene implicated in anxiety disorders and depression was associated with changes in BOLD signal correlation between amygdala and perigenual anterior cingulate cortex (Pezawas *et al.*, 2005). Functional connectivity between these two regions was also a much stronger predictor of harm avoidance scores than BOLD activation or gray matter volume in either of the two regions.

Anatomical Evidence on Connectivity in Autism

Before turning to applications of functional connectivity in a developmental disorder such as autism, the question arises why such an endeavor would be reasonable. The very general considerations about a "paradigm change" in cognitive neuroscience towards network models alone would be a rather slim rationale for investing in such studies of a developmental disorder. However, there are several lines of independent evidence suggesting that connectivity approaches will indeed be useful in autism research. The first relates to neuroanatomical studies.

Although some reports may have suggested specific and potentially localizing impairments in brain regions such as the posterior cerebellar vermis (Courchesne *et al.*, 1988) or the amygdala (Baron-Cohen *et al.*, 2000), the structural MRI and postmortem literature on autism, not unlike that of developmental dyslexia, is extremely diverse, with findings in many regions, such as frontal (Herbert *et al.*, 2004), temporal (Kwon *et al.*, 2004; Rojas *et al.*, 2005), and parietal lobes (Courchesne *et al.*, 1993), cingulate gyrus (Haznedar *et al.*, 1997; Thakkar *et al.*, 2008), corpus callosum (Vidal *et al.*, 2006), hippocampus and amygdala (Otsuka *et al.*, 1999), thalamus (Tsatsanis *et al.*, 2003), basal ganglia (Hollander *et al.*, 2005), and brainstem (Rodier, 2002). This diversity of findings may be partly attributed to heterogeneity within the population that meets diagnostic criteria and the existence of multiple etiological pathways linking genetic and epigenetic risk with phenotypic impairment (Folstein & Rosen-Sheidley, 2001; Herbert *et al.*, 2006). In addition, however, it likely reflects the truly distributed nature of brain involvement in autism (see Müller, 2007a, for review). Support for this distributed view of anatomical impairment comes from studies showing abnormal growth patterns in autism with early postnatal overgrowth followed by reduced growth (Courchesne *et al.*, 2001; Hazlett *et al.*, 2005; Sparks *et al.*, 2002). These growth defects affect both gray and white matter throughout the brain (with the possible exception of the occipital lobe, Carper *et al.*, 2002). Such widely distributed brain growth abnormalities could relate to atypical profiles of brain growth factors that were observed in neonates later diagnosed with autism (Nelson *et al.*, 2006).

It should be noted that some MR volumetric and voxel-based morphometry studies have not yielded significant findings of white matter abnormalities (Hazlett *et al.*, 2005; McAlonan *et al.*, 2005). However, the profile of early overgrowth and subsequently reduced growth, as mentioned above and reviewed in Redcay and Courchesne (2005), may explain such null findings in older autistic children and adults. From this perspective, apparently normal brain volume may not necessarily reflect normally developed and organized fiber tracts, but may be the outcome of a sequence of disturbances with inverse polarity. In addition, some studies examining more specific aspects of white matter have identified abnormalities. One highly replicated finding of reduced white matter volume in autism concerns the corpus callosum (Alexander *et al.*, 2007; Chung *et al.*, 2004; Egaas *et al.*, 1995; Piven *et al.*, 1997; Vidal *et al.*, 2006; Waiter *et al.*, 2005).

Volumetric MRI studies examine white matter solely with regard to size. As mentioned, normal size can conceal qualitative white matter compromise affecting interregional cooperation. A study by Hendry and colleagues (2006) observed increased transverse (T2) relaxation times in frontal, parietal, and occipital white matter, which may indicate atypically increased tissue water content. While most MR spectroscopy (MRS) studies have measured large voxels with partial volume effects (including both gray and white matter), Friedman and coworkers (2006) found that in young children with autism *N*-acetylaspartate (NAA) and *Myo*-inositol, respectively considered to be markers of neuronal and membrane integrity, were reduced in the white matter. However, a similar reduction was also seen in nonautistic children with developmental delays, suggesting that this finding was not specific to autism. A further MRS study of white matter in older autistic children failed to replicate atypically reduced NAA (Fayed & Modrego, 2005).

MRS, however, can detect only a limited set of metabolites. Null findings therefore do not confirm white matter integrity. An alternative approach to the study of white matter is provided by diffusion-tensor imaging (DTI), which measures the effects of the movement of water molecules on magnetic resonance. In white matter, axonal membranes and myelin sheaths prevent water molecules from diffusing freely in all directions (isotropically). Fractional anisotropy, which can be detected by DTI, is therefore considered a measure of white matter integrity (Le Bihan, 2003). A DTI study in male autistic adolescents by Barnea-Goraly *et al*. (2004) found atypically reduced fractional anisotropy (FA) in all four forebrain lobes and in the corpus callosum. Some of the DTI findings were consistent with previous evidence implicating anterior portions of the corpus callosum and ventromedial prefrontal cortex. Other sites of reduced FA in occipital and pericentral regions were less expected. In a more recent DTI study, Alexander and colleagues (2007) reported reduced volume and fractional anisotropy accompanied by increased diffusivity in the corpus callosum, suggesting white matter compromise affecting interhemispheric connections in children and adults with autism. Keller and colleagues (2007) found several small foci of significantly reduced FA in or close to the callosum and in the corona radiata in children and adults with autism. In most of these sites, reductions in FA were age-independent and persisted into midadulthood.

The findings reviewed above indicate that although white matter volume may be in the normal range in many individuals with autism (with the possible exception of children under the age of 5 years), several MR modalities that examine organization and integrity, rather than volume alone, point at significant compromise. It is therefore reasonable to expect functional reflections of compromised anatomical connectivity in autism. I will now turn to studies examining functional connectivity in autism more directly.

Functional Connectivity in Autism

The field of fcMRI research on developmental disorders remains quite limited. Concluding from fcMRI findings in a study on sentence comprehension in high-functioning autistic adults, Just and colleagues (2004) formulated an "underconnectivity theory" of autism. They observed that in autistic participants BOLD signal cross-correlations associated with task performance (determining the agent or recipient in a sentence) was slightly reduced between a large number of paired (mostly cortical) regions of interest. Consistent findings have been reported by the same group of investigators in studies on verbal working memory (Koshino *et al*., 2005), response inhibition (Kana, Keller, Minshew, & Just, 2007), comprehension of narratives requiring theory of mind (Mason, Williams, Kana, Minshew, & Just, 2008), and executive processing on the Tower of London task (Just *et al*., 2007). In some of these studies, interesting correlations between reduced functional connectivity and other measures were found. For example, Just and colleagues (2007) found that functional connectivity associated with their executive task was not only reduced overall in their autism group, but also positively correlated with the size of the callosal genu area and negatively correlated with the total score on the Autism Diagnostic Observation Schedule (ADOS; Lord *et al*., 2001).

In view of this series of studies, it would be tempting to conclude that the autistic brain is characterized by generalized underconnectivity affecting long-range fibers. However, this conclusion is less obvious when considering the autism literature on functional connectivity in its entirety (see also Murias, Webb, Greenson, & Dawson, 2007, for relevant electroencephalographic data). In one study, which included 13 adult autism spectrum disorder (ASD) participants, Welchew and colleagues (2005) analyzed Pearson correlation matrices for 90 cortical and subcortical ROIs. While they observed reduced connectivity for the amygdala and parahippocampal gyrus (in their comparison with matched control participants), generalized underconnectivity was not seen. In fact, many ROI pairings showed greater functional connectivity in their autism sample compared to the control group. Furthermore, since participants were scanned while viewing faces with fearful expressions, findings in the medial temporal lobe may have been driven by group differences in activation effects rather than by functional connectivity effects in the strict sense (as discussed previously).

fcMRI results from our own group have also not been consistent with a generalized underconnectivity hypothesis. In one study (Villalobos *et al.*, 2005), functional connectivity of primary visual cortex was examined. Data were acquired during simple conditions of visuomotor coordination, but task effects were minimized through orthogonal regressors (smoothed task-control boxcars). The context of this study was the hypothesis of defects in the mirror neuron system (associated with impaired imitation and action understanding) in autism (Williams *et al.*, 2001). The main focus was therefore on functional connectivity with inferior frontal cortex (one of the presumed sites of mirror neurons (Rizzolatti & Craighero, 2004), which was indeed significantly reduced bilaterally. However, functional connectivity between V1 and temporal and parietal lobes was not found to be significantly reduced.

Two other fcMRI studies of autism recently examined connectivity between subcortex and cerebral cortex. In the first one (Mizuno *et al.*, 2006), seed volumes were placed in the thalamus because thalamic abnormalities in autism have been observed in a number of studies. These include an early PET study showing reduced correlation of glucose metabolic rates between thalamus and fronto-parietal cortex (Horwitz *et al.*, 1988) and more recent studies demonstrating reduced neuronal integrity in the autistic thalamus (Friedman *et al.*, 2003), reduced thalamic perfusion (Ryu *et al.*, 1999; Starkstein *et al.*, 2000), and reduced thalamic volume (Tsatsanis *et al.*, 2003). Contrary to expectations, however, the fcMRI study by Mizuno *et al.* (2006) showed partially greater than normal functional connectivity between thalami and cortex, particularly in bilateral pericentral as well as inferior frontal and insular regions. In a second study, Turner and colleagues (2006) examined connectivity between caudate nuclei and cerebral cortex in autism. This study was motivated by structural

and metabolic findings indicating abnormalities in the caudate nuclei in autism (Levitt *et al.*, 2003; Sears *et al.*, 1999). Similar to the study on thalamocortical connectivity, we found partial overconnectivity between caudate nuclei and cerebral cortex in autism, again primarily in or close to perirolandic sensorimotor regions.

In summary, while many studies of anatomical and functional connectivity are consistent with a hypothesis of underconnectivity in autism proposed by Just and colleagues (2004), nonreplications in several studies are puzzling. One potential explanation relates to the question of activation effects in fcMRI analyses, as discussed earlier. It is possible that interregional correlations found to be reduced in ASD in the studies by Just and colleagues were partly driven by activational effects, whereas in the studies showing partially increased functional connectivity, activation effects were minimized by orthogonal task regressors and low-pass temporal filtering. As discussed above, functional connectivity effects were originally detected in the absence of a task and in frequencies below 0.1 Hz (Biswal *et al.*, 1995). An alternative—less technical and more biological—interpretation of the current findings might suggest predominant cortico-cortical underconnectivity and predominant subcortico-cortical overconnectivity. Fiber tract anomalies reflected in fcMRI results may relate to recent findings of early developmental abnormalities in white matter growth (Carper *et al.*, 2002).

The findings of atypically increased subcortico-cortical fcMRI effects in the studies by Mizuno and colleagues (2006) and by Turner *et al.* (2006) should, however, not be considered evidence for "overconnectivity" in any functionally beneficial way. Instead, it is conceivable that these effects reflect atypically diffuse connectivity. Thalamocortical connectivity, for example, is highly organized and functionally segregated in the typical brain, with most thalamic nuclei connecting to specific cortical regions (Sherman & Guillery, 2001). Although the study by Mizuno *et al.* (2006) did not have sufficient spatial resolution to identify functional connectivity for individual thalamic nuclei, the results may suggest atypically undifferentiated connectivity between thalamus and cerebral cortex in autism. In the final section, I will therefore turn to the developmental roots of potential connectivity defects.

Developmental Links between Connectivity and Local Architecture

Early in this review, I referred to "anomalies" in localizing approaches to the neurofunctional organization of the adult brain. Such anomalies are even more prevalent in localizing models of developmental disorders (Thomas & Karmiloff-Smith, 2002). In development, the relevance of connectivity goes beyond the cooperation of brain regions. Connections are established and retracted in response to activity (Kandel *et al.*, 2000). Regions in distal parts of the brain may affect each other's functional and structural organization through connectivity, for example, through transfer of activity, as seen in developing thalamocortical connectivity (O'Leary & Nakagawa, 2002; Sur *et al.*, 2002). Connectivity therefore plays a larger role than just allowing a collection of mature and specialized regions to "talk" to each other. Staying with the metaphor, developing connectivity may help each region to learn how to "talk intelligibly."

From a microscopic and cellular point of view, this outcome is completely expected. Connections are established by axons and their synaptic terminals, that is, by processes of neurons whose somata and dendrites populate gray matter. The common procedure of tissue segmentation in neuroimaging, separating white matter from gray matter "compartments," is a useful (though misleading) artifact of technical limitations that prevents us from examining individual cells in the human brain *in vivo*. In reality, white matter is largely constituted by the processes of nerve cell bodies in gray matter. White matter and the connectivity it affords

are thus correlates of the architecture of gray matter rather than a distinct or "segmentable" tissue compartment. Therefore, any change of perspective in the study of developmental disorders from local specialization to network organization cannot imply that local architecture is irrelevant. It would be foolish to conclude that the search for functional specializations in cytoarchitectonic regions initiated by Korbinian Brodmann at the turn of the 20th century was fruitless and is now to be succeeded by the exclusive study of connectivity.

Developmentally speaking, connectivity and local architecture are outcomes of neuronal migration and differentiation, that is, two aspects of the same set of events. It is known from animal studies that afferent input can have dramatic effects on the functional differentiation of cortex. For example, Sur and colleagues (1990) "rewired" retinal afferents in newborn ferrets to the medial geniculate nucleus of the thalamus, which in turn connects to primary auditory cortex in the superior temporal lobe. They could show that because of modified thalamic afferent input, "auditory" cortex responded to visual stimuli and indeed became functionally involved in behavioral responses to visual stimuli (von Melchner *et al.*, 2000). While these results—or findings by Schlaggar and O'Leary (1991) suggesting similar changes due to thalamocortical afferents in transplanted occipital cortex—are usually considered evidence of developmental cross-modal plasticity, they highlight the intimate links between connectivity and the differentiation of local functional architecture in cortex. Such principles are harder to demonstrate in the living human brain although studies of cross-modal plasticity in early deaf and early blind people are entirely consistent (Amedi *et al.*, 2004; Finney *et al.*, 2001; Sadato *et al.*, 2002).

What are the implications for the study of developmental disorders such as autism? In the previous section, I laid out some of the evidence of defects in connectivity in ASDs. However, these intriguing and important findings should not suggest that we turn away from the study of local architecture and local functional differentiation because the true causes for cognitive impairments in ASDs lie solely in connectivity. The evidence from developmental neuroscience referred to above underscores that local specificity and connectivity are really only two aspects of the same set of developmental processes. Activation mapping by means of PET and fMRI has indeed revealed a large number of brain regions with suspected local abnormality, such as the fusiform gyrus (Pierce & Courchesne, 2001; Schultz *et al.*, 2000) or the medial prefrontal cortex (Castelli *et al.*, 2002; Happé *et al.*, 1996). Aside from some nonreplications (Hadjikhani *et al.*, 2004; Pierce *et al.*, 2004), such findings do not necessarily indicate locally compromised cortical function, but they may be indicative of experiential effects (as discussed in detail in Müller, 2007a, 2007b). Absence of significant activation effects in a group analysis may also reflect greater variability of activation sites in individuals of a group (e.g., Pierce *et al.*, 2001). Very few autism fMRI studies have presented findings on a single-subject level. In one study, we (Müller *et al.*, 2001) found that what appeared to be reduced motor-related activity in a group analysis of an autism sample was in fact explained by atypical scatter of activation effects in several individuals with autism, which contrasted with consistent, rather focal activity in primary motor cortex seen in matched control individuals. However, given the low contrast-to-noise ratio of single-subject analyses, it remains hard to determine whether these results truly indicate an interesting aspect of compromised cortical architecture, such as "hierarchical crowding." The term *hierarchical crowding* is adapted from the concept of crowding (cf. Lidzba *et al.*, 2006), according to which reorganization of language into the right hemisphere in children with early left hemisphere damage results secondarily in lowered visuospatial function because these typical right hemisphere functions are "crowded out" of right hemisphere regions typically crucial for visuospatial cognition. Hierarchical crowding in autism refers to the hypothesis that be-

cause of early compromise of cortical architecture and reduced processing efficiency, early developing relatively simple sensorimotor functions occupy atypically large cortical territories at the expense of later developing polymodal and executive functions (Müller *et al.*, 2003). In general, the spatial resolution of PET and of common fMRI protocols is too low to identify more microscopic abnormalities of cortical architecture. In the remainder of this section, I will therefore examine techniques more appropriate for the study of local architecture in autism.

In one *in vivo* study, Hardan and colleagues (2004) used structural MRI data to calculate a gyrification index for the frontal lobes, reflecting cortical folding. The index was significantly increased for the left frontal lobe in children (but not adults) with ASDs, which may be consistent with abnormal growth profiles discussed earlier. The results may be developmentally relevant because cortical folding may be considered a result of neuronal migration. Migrational disturbances possibly reflected in increased cortical folding would probably affect the layered architecture of emerging neocortex in the fetal brain.

While such conclusions from *in vivo* findings remain speculative, postmortem studies permit a more direct examination of local cytoarchitecture. However, just as in studies of dyslexia, postmortem studies in autism are limited by small sample sizes, large demographic and clinical variability of deceased subjects, and often by availability of only small parts of the brain to a given group of researchers. Nonetheless, it is clear that abnormalities in cellular organization are quite common in autism, although findings may vary individually (see reviews in Bauman & Kemper, 2005; Palmen *et al.*, 2004; Pickett & London, 2005). Among the more consistent findings have been cellular abnormalities in the limbic system, such as reduced neuronal size and increased cell packing density (Bauman & Kemper, 1994; Raymond *et al.*, 1996) or reduced numbers of neurons (Schumann & Amaral, 2006) in the medial temporal lobe (amygdala, hippocampus, etc.) and possibly in the anterior cingulate gyrus (Bauman & Kemper, 2005). Relatively consistent has also been the finding of decreased numbers (Bailey *et al.*, 1998; Ritvo *et al.*, 1986) or size (Fatemi *et al.*, 2002; Fehlow *et al.*, 1993) of cerebellar Purkinje cells.

Other cytoarchitectonic findings have been less widely replicated. Brain-stem abnormalities affecting superior (Rodier *et al.*, 1996) and inferior (Bailey *et al.*, 1998) olives have been noted in a few cases. Bailey and colleagues (1998) also reported various patterns of cortical dysgenesis or neuronal ectopias in six cases, mostly in the frontal lobe. A recent study of cortical layering in autism (Hutsler *et al.*, 2007) also found more frequent cases of supernumerary neurons in layer I (which usually contains no nerve cell bodies in the mature brain) and in the subplate (below layer VI). However, these findings were qualitative, whereas no statistically significant differences in cortical thickness and layering were observed between eight autism and eight control brains (in subjects aged 14–45 years).

Casanova and colleagues (2002b) reported that cortical minicolumns were smaller, more numerous, and more dispersed in fronto-temporal areas (9, 21, 22) of nine autistic brains (in subjects aged 5–28 years). Analogous findings in two patients with Asperger's disorder (aged 22 and 79 years) were also reported (Casanova *et al.*, 2002a). This pattern of minicolumnar abnormalities has been seen in one additional case, in a 3-year-old child with autism, throughout the frontal cortex and accompanied by laminar disorganization (cf. Courchesne & Pierce, 2005). It has been argued that minicolumnar abnormalities may be one of the correlates of atypical developmental trajectories of serotonin synthesis (Chandana *et al.*, 2005).

Minicolumns are considered to derive from ontogenetic columns (Buxhoeveden & Casanova, 2002), which in turn reflect the vertical migration of neurons from the ventricular zone into the cortical plate along radial glial cells (Rakic *et al.*, 2004). This would suggest that neuronal migration in the second gestational trimester may be affected in autism. Suspected minicolumnar abnormalities also tie in with another line of evidence implicating thalamocortical connections. As discussed above, there is some evidence for abnormal thalamocortical connectivity in ASDs. Additional indirect evidence consistent with thalamocortical compromise in autism includes findings of reduced serotonin synthesis capacity in thalamus and middle frontal gyrus (Chugani *et al.*, 1997) and reduced beta spectral amplitude during REM sleep, considered to reflect atypical thalamocortical connectivity (Daoust *et al.*, 2004).

Potential compromise of thalamocortical connections in autism is relevant because these connections play an important role in regional functional differentiation of developing neocortex. According to Rakic's widely accepted radial unit and protomap hypotheses (Rakic, 1988; Rakic *et al.*, 2004), cortical columns derive from neuronal clones migrating vertically along radial glial cells. Guidance molecules for thalamocortical afferents are expressed by neurons in the subplate according to their progenitors' spatial position in the ventricular zone or "protomap" (O'Leary & Borngasser, 2006). Thalamocortical connections are thus intimately and interactively tied to neocortical functional differentiation. Besides being guided by chemical information in the subplate of developing cortex, it was already discussed above that thalamocortical afferents in turn have substantial impact on the emerging functional specificity of initially pluripotential cortex (O'Leary & Nakagawa, 2002; Schlaggar & O'Leary, 1991; Sur *et al.*, 2002).

Fundamental disturbances of cortical circuitry in autism probably go beyond minicolumnar anomalies described above. For example, Rubenstein and Merzenich (2003) proposed a model of generally increased excitation/inhibition ratio in the autistic brain. Support comes from cognitive findings of autistic impairments that may reflect "noisy processing," clinical evidence of increased prevalence

of epileptiform EEG, as well as genetic and
molecular evidence implicating excitatory (glu-
tamatergic) and inhibitory (GABAergic) systems (as reviewed in Rubenstein & Merzenich,
2003). GABAergic disturbances may in turn be
related to serotonergic anomalies that are well
documented in autism (Betancur *et al.*, 2002;
Chugani, 2004).

Conclusions

Although findings of compromised local architecture and of abnormal connectivity in the
autism literature are largely derived from separate lines of research using different methodological approaches, they are likely to reflect
two aspects of overlapping sets of developmental disturbances. In other developmental disorders, such as dyslexia, the nature and timing
of developmental disturbances will differ and
so will the patterns of compromise in local architecture and connectivity. However, considerations regarding autism reviewed here will
likely apply in similar ways because they are
based on general principles of developmental
neuroscience, through which locally differentiated architecture and functional specialization
are intimately tied to the connectivity and the
transfer of activity in emerging networks.

Acknowledgments

Preparation of this review was supported by
the National Institutes of Health Grants R01-
NS43999 and R01-DC006155.

Conflicts of Interest

The authors declare no conflicts of interest.

References

Alexander, A. L., Lee, J. E., Lazar, M., Boudos, R.,
Dubray, M. B., Oakes, T. R., *et al.* 2007. Diffusion
tensor imaging of the corpus callosum in autism.
NeuroImage, **34**(1): 61–73.

Amedi, A., Floel, A., Knecht, S., Zohary, E., & Cohen,
L. G. 2004. Transcranial magnetic stimulation of
the occipital pole interferes with verbal processing in
blind subjects. *Nature Neuroscience*, **7**(11): 1266–1270.

Ances, B. M., Leontiv, O., Perthen, J. E., Liang, C.,
Lansing, A. E., & Buxton, R. B. 2008. Regional
differences in the coupling of cerebral blood flow
and oxygen metabolism changes in response to activation: implications for BOLD-fMRI. *NeuroImage*,
39(4): 1510–1521.

Bailey, A., Luthert, P., Dean, A., Harding, B., Janota, I.,
Montgomery, M., *et al.* 1998. A clinicopathological
study of autism. *Brain*, **121**: 889–905.

Barnea-Goraly, N., Kwon, H., Menon, V., Eliez, S., Lotspeich, L., & Reiss, A. L. 2004. White matter structure in autism: preliminary evidence from diffusion
tensor imaging. *Biological Psychiatry*, **55**(3): 323–326.

Baron-Cohen, S., Ring, H. A., Bullmore, E. T., Wheelwright, S., Ashwin, C., & Williams, S. C. 2000. The
amygdala theory of autism. *Neuroscience and Biobehavioral Reviews*, **24**(3): 355–364.

Bauman, M. L., & Kemper, T. L. 1994. Neuroanatomic
observations of the brain in autism. In M. L. Bauman & T. L. Kemper (Eds.), *The neurobiology of autism*
(pp. 119–145). Baltimore: Johns Hopkins University
Press.

Bauman, M. L., & Kemper, T. L. 2005. Neuroanatomic
observations of the brain in autism: a review and
future directions. *International Journal of Developmental
Neuroscience*, **23**(2–3): 183–187.

Betancur, C., Corbex, M., Spielewoy, C., Philippe, A.,
Laplanche, J. L., Launay, J. M., *et al.* 2002. Serotonin transporter gene polymorphisms and hyper-
serotonemia in autistic disorder. *Molecular Psychiatry*,
7(1): 67–71.

Biswal, B., Yetkin, F. Z., Haughton, V. M., & Hyde, J.
S. 1995. Functional connectivity in the motor cor-
tex of resting human brain using echo-planar MRI.
Magnetic Resonance in Medicine, **34**(4): 537–541.

Broca, P. 1861. Remarques sur le siège de la faculté du lan-
gage articulé, suivies d'une observation d'aphémie
(perte de la parole). *Bulletins et Mémoires de la Société
Anatomique de Paris*, **36**: 330–357.

Brown, C., Gruber, T., Boucher, J., Rippon, G., & Brock,
J. 2005. Gamma abnormalities during perception of
illusory figures in autism. *Cortex*, **41**(3): 364–376.

Brown, J. W. 1988. Introduction: microgenetic theory.
In J. W. Brown (Ed.), *The life of the mind* (pp. 1–26).
Hillsdale, NJ: Lawrence Erlbaum.

Buxhoeveden, D. P., & Casanova, M. F. 2002. The mini-
column hypothesis in neuroscience. *Brain*, **125**(Pt 5):
935–951.

Cabeza, R., & Nyberg, L. 2000. Imaging cognition II:
an empirical review of 275 PET and fMRI studies.
Journal of Cognitive Neuroscience, **12**: 1–47.

Carper, R. A., Moses, P., Tigue, Z. D., & Courchesne, E. 2002. Cerebral lobes in autism: early hyperplasia and abnormal age effects. *NeuroImage*, **16**(4): 1038–1051.

Casanova, M. F., Buxhoeveden, D. P., Switala, A. E., & Roy, E. 2002a. Asperger's syndrome and cortical neuropathology. *Journal of Child Neurology*, **17**(2): 142–145.

Casanova, M. F., Buxhoeveden, D. P., Switala, A. E., & Roy, E. 2002b. Minicolumnar pathology in autism. *Neurology*, **58**(3): 428–432.

Castelli, F., Frith, C., Happe, F., & Frith, U. 2002. Autism, Asperger syndrome and brain mechanisms for the attribution of mental states to animated shapes. *Brain*, **125**(Pt 8): 1839–1849.

Chandana, S. R., Behen, M. E., Juhasz, C., Muzik, O., Rothermel, R. D., Mangner, T. J., *et al*. 2005. Significance of abnormalities in developmental trajectory and asymmetry of cortical serotonin synthesis in autism. *International Journal of Developmental Neuroscience*, **23**(2–3): 171–182.

Chugani, D. C. 2004. Serotonin in autism and pediatric epilepsies. *Mental Retardation and Developmental Disabilities Research Review*, **10**(2): 112–116.

Chugani, D. C., Muzik, O., Rothermel, R. D., Behen, M. E., Chakraborty, P. K., Mangner, T. J., *et al*. 1997. Altered serotonin synthesis in the dentato-thalamo-cortical pathway in autistic boys. *Annals of Neurology*, **14**: 666–669.

Chung, M. K., Dalton, K. M., Alexander, A. L., & Davidson, R. J. 2004. Less white matter concentration in autism: 2D voxel-based morphometry. *NeuroImage*, **23**(1): 242–251.

Clarke, E., & Dewhurst, K. 1972. *An illustrated history of brain function*. Oxford: Sanford.

Cordes, D., Haughton, V. M., Arfanakis, K., Carew, J. D., Turski, P. A., Moritz, C. H., *et al*. 2001. Frequencies contributing to functional connectivity in the cerebral cortex in "resting-state" data. *AJNR. American Journal of Neuroradiology*, **22**(7): 1326–1333.

Courchesne, E., Karns, C. M., Davis, H. R., Ziccardi, R., Carper, R. A., Tigue, Z. D., *et al*. 2001. Unusual brain growth patterns in early life in patients with autistic disorder: an MRI study. *Neurology*, **57**(2): 245–254.

Courchesne, E., & Pierce, K. 2005. Why the frontal cortex in autism might be talking only to itself: local over-connectivity but long-distance disconnection. *Current Opinion in Neurobiology*, **15**(2): 225–230.

Courchesne, E., Press, G. A., & Yeung-Courchesne, R. 1993. Parietal lobe abnormalities detected with MR in patients with infantile autism. *American Journal of Roentgenology*, **160**(2): 387–393.

Courchesne, E., Yeung-Courchesne, R., Press, G. A., Hesselink, J. R., & Jernigan, T. L. 1988. Hypoplasia of cerebellar vermal lobules VI and VII in autism. *New England Journal of Medicine*, **318**(21): 1349–1354.

Daoust, A. M., Limoges, E., Bolduc, C., Mottron, L., & Godbout, R. 2004. EEG spectral analysis of wakefulness and REM sleep in high functioning autistic spectrum disorders. *Clinical Neurophysiology*, **115**(6): 1368–1373.

Egaas, B., Courchesne, E., & Saitoh, O. 1995. Reduced size of corpus callosum in autism. *Archives of Neurology*, **52**(8): 794–801.

Fatemi, S. H., Halt, A. R., Realmuto, G., Earle, J., Kist, D. A., Thuras, P., *et al*. 2002. Purkinje cell size is reduced in cerebellum of patients with autism. *Cellular and Molecular Neurobiology*, **22**(2): 171–175.

Fayed, N., & Modrego, P. J. 2005. Comparative study of cerebral white matter in autism and attention-deficit/hyperactivity disorder by means of magnetic resonance spectroscopy. *Academic Radiology*, **12**(5): 566–569.

Fehlow, P., Bernstein, K., Tennstedt, A., & Walther, F. 1993. Autismus infantum und exzessive Aerophagie mit symptomatischem Magakolon und Ileus bei einem Fall von Ehlers-Danlos-Syndrom [Infantile autism and excessive aerophagy with symptomatic megacolon and ileus in a case of Ehlers-Danlos syndrome]. *Pädiatrie und Grenzgebiete*, **31**(4): 259–267.

Finney, E. M., Fine, I., & Dobkins, K. R. 2001. Visual stimuli activate auditory cortex in the deaf. *Nature Neuroscience*, **4**(12): 1171–1173.

Folstein, S. E., & Rosen-Sheidley, B. 2001. Genetics of autism: complex aetiology for a heterogeneous disorder. *Nature Review Genetics*, **2**(12): 943–955.

Friedman, S. D., Shaw, D. W., Artru, A. A., Dawson, G., Petropoulos, H., & Dager, S. R. 2006. Gray and white matter brain chemistry in young children with autism. *Archives of General Psychiatry*, **63**(7): 786–794.

Friedman, S. D., Shaw, D. W., Artru, A. A., Richards, T. L., Gardner, J., Dawson, G., *et al*. 2003. Regional brain chemical alterations in young children with autism spectrum disorder. *Neurology*, **60**(1): 100–107.

Friston, K. J., Frith, C. D., & Frackowiak, R. S. J. 1993. Time-dependent changes in effective connectivity measured with PET. *Human Brain Mapping*, **1**: 69–79.

Gall, F. J., & Spurzheim, K. 1810. *Anatomie und Physiologie des Nervensystems im allgemeinen, und des Gehirnes insbesondere*. Paris: Schoell.

Grice, S. J., Spratling, M. W., Karmiloff-Smith, A., Halit, H., Csibra, G., de Haan, M., *et al*. 2001. Disordered visual processing and oscillatory brain activity in autism and Williams syndrome. *Neuroreport*, **12**(12): 2697–2700.

Hadjikhani, N., Joseph, R. M., Snyder, J., Chabris, C. F., Clark, J., Steele, S., *et al*. 2004. Activation of the fusiform gyrus when individuals with autism spectrum disorder view faces. *NeuroImage*, **22**(3): 1141–1150.

Hampson, M., Peterson, B. S., Skudlarski, P., Gatenby, J. C., & Gore, J. C. 2002. Detection of functional connectivity using temporal correlations in MR images. *Human Brain Mapping*, **15**(4): 247–262.

Happé, F., Ehlers, S., Fletcher, P. C., Frith, U., Johansson, M., Gillberg, C., *et al.* 1996. "Theory of mind" in the brain: evidence from a PET scan study of Asperger syndrome. *Neuroreport*, **8**: 197–201.

Hardan, A. Y., Jou, R. J., Keshavan, M. S., Varma, R., & Minshew, N. J. 2004. Increased frontal cortical folding in autism: a preliminary MRI study. *Psychiatry Research*, **131**(3): 263–268.

Hazlett, H. C., Poe, M., Gerig, G., Smith, R. G., Provenzale, J., Ross, A., *et al.* 2005. Magnetic resonance imaging and head circumference study of brain size in autism: birth through age 2 years. *Archives of General Psychiatry*, **62**(12): 1366–1376.

Haznedar, M. M., Buchsbaum, M. S., Metzger, M., Solimando, A., Spiegel-Cohen, J., & Hollander, E. 1997. Anterior cingulate gyrus volume and glucose metabolism in autistic disorder. *American Journal of Psychiatry*, **154**: 1047–1050.

Head, H. 1926. *Aphasia and kindred disorders of speech*. Cambridge: Cambridge University Press.

Hendry, J., DeVito, T., Gelman, N., Densmore, M., Rajakumar, N., Pavlosky, W., *et al.* 2006. White matter abnormalities in autism detected through transverse relaxation time imaging. *NeuroImage*, **29**(4): 1049–1057.

Herbert, M. R., Russo, J. P., Yang, S., Roohi, J., Blaxill, M., Kahler, S. G., *et al.* 2006. Autism and environmental genomics. *Neurotoxicology*, **27**(5): 671–684.

Herbert, M. R., Ziegler, D. A., Makris, N., Filipek, P. A., Kemper, T. L., Normandin, J. J., *et al.* 2004. Localization of white matter volume increase in autism and developmental language disorder. *Annals of Neurology*, **55**(4): 530–540.

Hollander, E., Anagnostou, E., Chaplin, W., Esposito, K., Haznedar, M. M., Licalzi, E., *et al.* 2005. Striatal volume on magnetic resonance imaging and repetitive behaviors in autism. *Biological Psychiatry*, **58**(3): 226–232.

Horwitz, B. 2003. The elusive concept of brain connectivity. *NeuroImage*, **19**(2 Pt 1): 466–470.

Horwitz, B., Rumsey, J. M., Grady, C. L., & Rapoport, S. I. 1988. The cerebral metabolic landscape in autism: intercorrelations of regional glucose utilization. *Archives of Neurology*, **45**: 749–755.

Hughlings-Jackson, J. 1878. On affections of speech from disease of the brain. *Brain*, **1**: 304–330.

Hutsler, J. J., Love, T., & Zhang, H. 2007. Histological and magnetic resonance imaging assessment of cortical layering and thickness in autism spectrum disorders. *Biological Psychiatry*, **61**(4): 449–457.

Hyde, J. S., & Biswal, B. B. 1999. Functionally related correlation in the noise. In C. T. W. Moonen & P. A. Bandettini (Eds.), *Functional MRI* (pp. 263–275). New York: Springer.

Just, M. A., Cherkassky, V. L., Keller, T. A., Kana, R. K., & Minshew, N. J. 2007. Functional and anatomical cortical underconnectivity in autism: evidence from an fMRI study of an executive function task and corpus callosum morphometry. *Cerebral Cortex*, **17**(4): 951–961.

Just, M. A., Cherkassky, V. L., Keller, T. A., & Minshew, N. J. 2004. Cortical activation and synchronization during sentence comprehension in high-functioning autism: evidence of underconnectivity. *Brain*, **127**(Pt 8): 1811–1821.

Kana, R. K., Keller, T. A., Cherkassky, V. L., Minshew, N. J., & Just, M. A. 2006. Inhibitory control in high-functioning autism: decreased activation and underconnectivity in inhibition networks. *Biological Psychiatry*, **62**(3): 198–206.

Kandel, E. R., Jessell, T. M., & Sanes, J. R. 2000. Sensory experience and the fine tuning of synaptic connections. In E. R. Kandel, J. H. Schwartz & T. M. Jessell (Eds.), *Principles of neural science* (4th ed., pp. 1115–1130). New York: Elsevier.

Keller, T. A., Kana, R. K., & Just, M. A. 2007. A developmental study of the structural integrity of white matter in autism. *Neuroreport*, **18**(1): 23–27.

Koshino, H., Carpenter, P. A., Minshew, N. J., Cherkassky, V. L., Keller, T. A., & Just, M. A. 2005. Functional connectivity in an fMRI working memory task in high-functioning autism. *NeuroImage*, **24**(3): 810–821.

Kuhn, T. 1962. *The structure of scientific revolutions*. Chicago: University of Chicago Press.

Kwon, H., Ow, A. W., Pedatella, K. E., Lotspeich, L. J., & Reiss, A. L. 2004. Voxel-based morphometry elucidates structural neuroanatomy of high-functioning autism and Asperger syndrome. *Developmental Medicine and Child Neurology*, **46**(11): 760–764.

Le Bihan, D. 2003. Looking into the functional architecture of the brain with diffusion MRI. *Nature Reviews. Neuroscience*, **4**(6): 469–480.

Lee, L., Friston, K., & Horwitz, B. 2006. Large-scale neural models and dynamic causal modelling. *NeuroImage*, **30**(4): 1243–1254.

Leopold, D. A., Murayama, Y., & Logothetis, N. K. 2003. Very slow activity fluctuations in monkey visual cortex: implications for functional brain imaging. *Cerebral Cortex*, **13**(4): 422–433.

Levitt, J. G., O'Neill, J., Blanton, R. E., Smalley, S., Fadale, D., McCracken, J. T., *et al.* 2003. Proton magnetic resonance spectroscopic imaging of the brain in childhood autism. *Biological Psychiatry*, **54**(12): 1355–1366.

Lichtheim, L. 1885. On aphasia. *Brain*, **7:** 433–484.

Lidzba, K., Staudt, M., Wilke, M., & Krageloh-Mann, I. 2006. Visuospatial deficits in patients with early left-hemispheric lesions and functional reorganization of language: Consequence of lesion or reorganization? *Neuropsychologia*, **44**(7): 1088–1094.

Lord, C., Rutter, M., DiLavore, P., & Risi, S. 2001. *Autism diagnostic observation schedule*. Los Angeles: Western Psychological Services.

Lowe, M. J., Dzemidzic, M., Lurito, J. T., Mathews, V. P., & Phillips, M. D. 2000. Correlations in low-frequency BOLD fluctuations reflect cortico-cortical connections. *NeuroImage*, **12**(5): 582–587.

Mason, R. A., Williams, D. L., Kana, R. K., Minshew, N., & Just, M. A. 2008. Theory of mind disruption and recruitment of the right hemisphere during narrative comprehension in autism. *Neuropsychologia*, **46**(1): 269–280.

McAlonan, G. M., Cheung, V., Cheung, C., Suckling, J., Lam, G. Y., Tai, K. S., *et al.* 2005. Mapping the brain in autism: a voxel-based MRI study of volumetric differences and intercorrelations in autism. *Brain*, **128**(Pt 2): 268–276.

Mizuno, A., Villalobos, M. E., Davies, M. M., Dahl, B. C., & Müller, R.-A. 2006. Partially enhanced thalamocortical functional connectivity in autism. *Brain Research*, **1104**(1): 160–174.

Müller, R.-A. (2007a). Functional neuroimaging of developmental disorders: lessons from autism research. In F. D. Hillary & J. DeLuca (Eds.), *Functional neuroimaging in clinical populations* (pp. 145–184). New York: Guilford Press. Guilford.

Müller, R.-A. 2007b. The study of autism as a distributed disorder. *Mental Retardation and Developmental Disabilities Research Review*, **13**: 85–95.

Müller, R.-A., Kleinhans, N., Kemmotsu, N., Pierce, K., & Courchesne, E. 2003. Abnormal variability and distribution of functional maps in autism: an fMRI study of visuomotor learning. *American Journal of Psychiatry*, **160**: 1847–1862.

Müller, R.-A., Pierce, K., Ambrose, J. B., Allen, G., & Courchesne, E. 2001. Atypical patterns of cerebral motor activation in autism: a functional magnetic resonance study. *Biological Psychiatry*, **49**: 665–676.

Murias, M., Webb, S. J., Grenson, J., & Dawson, G. 2007. Resting state cortical connectivity reflected in EEG coherence in individuals with autism. *Biological Psychiatry*, **62**(3): 270–273.

Nase, G., Singer, W., Monyer, H., & Engel, A. K. 2003. Features of neuronal synchrony in mouse visual cortex. *Journal of Neurophysiology*, **90**(2): 1115–1123.

Nelson, P. G., Kuddo, T., Song, E. Y., Dambrosia, J. M., Kohler, S., Satyanarayana, G., *et al.* 2006. Selected neurotrophins, neuropeptides, and cytokines: developmental trajectory and concentrations in neonatal blood of children with autism or Down syndrome. *International Journal of Developmental Neuroscience*, **24**(1): 73–80.

O'Leary, D. D., & Borngasser, D. 2006. Cortical ventricular zone progenitors and their progeny maintain spatial relationships and radial patterning during preplate development indicating an early protomap. *Cerebral Cortex*, **16**(Suppl 1): i46–i56.

O'Leary, D. D., & Nakagawa, Y. 2002. Patterning centers, regulatory genes and extrinsic mechanisms controlling arealization of the neocortex. *Current Opinions in Neurobiology*, **12**(1): 14–25.

Otsuka, H., Harada, M., Mori, K., Hisaoka, S., & Nishitani, H. 1999. Brain metabolites in the hippocampus-amygdala region and cerebellum in autism: an ^{1}H-MR spectroscopy study. *Neuroradiology*, **41**(7): 517–519.

Palmen, S. J., van Engeland, H., Hof, P. R., & Schmitz, C. 2004. Neuropathological findings in autism. *Brain*, **127**(Pt 12): 2572–2583.

Pezawas, L., Meyer-Lindenberg, A., Drabant, E. M., Verchinski, B. A., Munoz, K. E., Kolachana, B. S., *et al.* 2005. 5-HTTLPR polymorphism impacts human cingulate-amygdala interactions: a genetic susceptibility mechanism for depression. *Nature Neuroscience*, **8**(6): 828–834.

Pickett, J., & London, E. 2005. The neuropathology of autism: a review. *Journal of Neuropathology and Experimental Neurology*, **64**(11): 925–935.

Pierce, K., & Courchesne, E. 2001. Evidence for a cerebellar role in reduced exploration and stereotyped behavior in autism. *Biological Psychiatry*, **49:** 655–664.

Pierce, K., Haist, F., Sedaghat, F., & Courchesne, E. 2004. The brain response to personally familiar faces in autism: findings of fusiform activity and beyond. *Brain*, **127**(Pt 12): 2703–2716.

Pierce, K., Müller, R.-A., Ambrose, J. B., Allen, G., & Courchesne, E. 2001. Face processing occurs outside the "fusiform face area" in autism: evidence from functional MRI. *Brain*, **124:** 2059–2073.

Piven, J., Bailey, J., Ranson, B. J., & Arndt, S. 1997. An MRI study of the corpus callosum in autism. *American Journal of Psychiatry*, **154**(8): 1051–1055.

Popper, K. R. 1965. *Conjectures and refutations: The growth of scientific knowledge*. New York: Routledge & Kegan Paul.

Quigley, M., Cordes, D., Turski, P., Moritz, C., Haughton, V., Seth, R., *et al.* 2003. Role of the corpus callosum in functional connectivity. *AJNR. American Journal of Neuroradiology*, **24**(2): 208–212.

Rakic, P. 1988. Specification of cerebral cortical areas. *Science*, **241**(4862): 170–176.

Rakic, P., Ang, E. S. B. C., & Breunig, J. 2004. Setting the stage for cognition: genesis of the primate cerebral cortex. In M. S. Gazzaniga (Ed.), *The cognitive neurosciences* (3rd ed.; pp. 33–49). Cambridge, MA: MIT Press.

Raymond, G. V., Bauman, M. L., & Kemper, T. L. 1996. Hippocampus in autism: a Golgi analysis. *Acta Neuropathologica*, **91**(1): 117–119.

Redcay, E., & Courchesne, E. 2005. When is the brain enlarged in autism? A meta-analysis of all brain size reports. *Biological Psychiatry*, **58**(1): 1–9.

Rippon, G., Brock, J., Brown, C., & Boucher, J. 2007. Disordered connectivity in the autistic brain: Challenges for the "new psychophysiology." *International Journal of Psychophysiology*, **63**(2): 164–172.

Ritvo, E. R., Freeman, B. J., Scheibel, A. B., Duong, T., Robinson, H., Guthrie, D., *et al*. 1986. Lower Purkinje cell counts in the cerebella of four autistic subjects: initial findings of the UCLA-NSAC autopsy research report. *American Journal of Psychiatry*, **143:** 862–866.

Rizzolatti, G., & Craighero, L. 2004. The mirror-neuron system. *Annual Review of Neuroscience*, **27:** 169–192.

Rodier, P. M. 2002. Converging evidence for brain stem injury in autism. *Development and Psychopathology*, **14**(3): 537–557.

Rodier, P. M., Ingram, J. L., Tisdale, B., Nelson, S., & Romano, J. 1996. Embryological origin for autism: developmental anomalies of the cranial nerve motor nuclei. *Journal of Comparative Neurology*, **370:** 247–261.

Rojas, D. C., Camou, S. L., Reite, M. L., & Rogers, S. J. 2005. Planum temporale volume in children and adolescents with autism. *Journal of Autism and Developmental Disorders*, **35**(4): 479–486.

Rubenstein, J. L., & Merzenich, M. M. 2003. Model of autism: increased ratio of excitation/inhibition in key neural systems. *Genes, Brain, and Behavior*, **2**(5): 255–267.

Ryu, Y. H., Lee, J. D., Yoon, P. H., Kim, D. I., Lee, H. B., & Shin, Y. J. 1999. Perfusion impairments in infantile autism on technetium-99m ethyl cysteinate dimer brain single-photon emission tomography: comparison with findings on magnetic resonance imaging. *European Journal of Nuclear Medicine*, **26**(3): 253–259.

Sadato, N., Okada, T., Honda, M., & Yonekura, Y. 2002. Critical period for cross-modal plasticity in blind humans: a functional MRI study. *NeuroImage*, **16**(2): 389–400.

Schlaggar, B., & O'Leary, D. 1991. Potential of visual cortex to develop an array of functional units unique to somatosensory cortex. *Science*, **252:** 1556–1560.

Schmahmann, J. D., & Pandya, D. N. 2006. *Fiber pathways of the brain*. Oxford: Oxford University Press.

Schultz, R. T., Gauthier, I., Klin, A., Fulbright, R. K., Anderson, A. W., Volkmar, F., *et al*. 2000. Abnormal ventral temporal cortical activity during face discrimination among individuals with autism and Asperger syndrome [see comments]. *Archives of General Psychiatry*, **57**(4): 331–340.

Schumann, C. M., & Amaral, D. G. 2006. Stereological analysis of amygdala neuron number in autism. *Journal of Neuroscience*, **26**(29): 7674–7679.

Sears, L. L., Vest, C., Mohamed, S., Bailey, J., Ranson, B. J., & Piven, J. 1999. An MRI study of the basal ganglia in autism. *Progress in Neuro-Psychopharmacology and Biological Psychiatry*, **23**(4): 613–624.

Schlaggar *et al*. 1991

Shallice, T. 1988. *From neuropsychology to mental structure*. Cambridge: Cambridge University Press.

Sherman, S. M., & Guillery, R. W. 2001. *Exploring the thalamus*. San Diego: Academic Press.

Signoret, J. L., Castaigne, P., Lhermitte, F., Abelanet, R., & Lavorel, P. 1984. Rediscovery of Leborgne's brain: anatomical description with CT scan. *Brain and Language*, **22**(2): 303–319.

Sparks, B. F., Friedman, S. D., Shaw, D. W., Aylward, E. H., Echelard, D., Artru, A. A., *et al*. 2002. Brain structural abnormalities in young children with autism spectrum disorder. *Neurology*, **59**(2): 184–192.

Starkstein, S. E., Vazquez, S., Vrancic, D., Nanclares, V., Manes, F., Piven, J., *et al*. 2000. SPECT findings in mentally retarded autistic individuals. *Journal of Neuropsychiatry and Clinical Neurosciences*, **12**(3): 370–375.

Sur, M., & Leamey, C. A. 2001. Development and plasticity of cortical areas and networks. *Nature Reviews. Neuroscience*, **2**(4): 251–262.

Sur, M., Pallas, S. L., & Roe, A. W. 1990. Cross-modal plasticity in cortical development: differentiation and specification of sensory neocortex. *Trends in Neuroscience*, **13:** 227–233.

Sur, M., Schummers, J., & Dragoi, V. 2002. Cortical plasticity: time for a change. *Current Biology*, **12**(5): R168–R170.

Thakkar, K. N., Polli, F. E., Joseph, R. M., Tuch, D. S., Hadjikhani, N., & Barton, J. J., *et al*. 2008. Response monitoring, repetitive behaviour and anterior cingulate abnormalities in ASD. *Brain*. E-pub ahead of print.

Thatcher, R. W., Walker, R. A., & Giudice, S. 1987. Human cerebral hemispheres develop at different rates and ages. *Science*, **236:** 1110–1113.

Thomas, M., & Karmiloff-Smith, A. 2002. Are developmental disorders like cases of adult brain damage? Implications from connectionist modeling. *Behavioral and Brain Sciences*, **25**(6): 727–750.

Tsatsanis, K. D., Rourke, B. P., Klin, A., Volkmar, F. R., Cicchetti, D., & Schultz, R. T. 2003. Reduced thalamic volume in high-functioning individuals with autism. *Biological Psychiatry*, **53**(2): 121–129.

Turner, K. C., Frost, L., Linsenbardt, D., McIlroy, J. R., & Müller, R.-A. 2006. Atypically diffuse functional connectivity between caudate nuclei and cerebral cortex in autism. *Behavioral and Brain Functions*, **2**: 34–45.

Uhlhaas, P. J., & Singer, W. 2006. Neural synchrony in brain disorders: relevance for cognitive dysfunctions and pathophysiology. *Neuron*, **52**(1): 155–168.

Vidal, C. N., Nicolson, R., Devito, T. J., Hayashi, K. M., Geaga, J. A., Drost, D. J., *et al.* 2006. Mapping corpus callosum deficits in autism: an index of aberrant cortical connectivity. *Biological Psychiatry*, **60**(3): 218–225.

Villalobos, M. E., Mizuno, A., Dahl, B. C., Kemmotsu, N., & Müller, R.-A. 2005. Reduced functional connectivity between V1 and inferior frontal cortex associated with visuomotor performance in autism. *NeuroImage*, **25**: 916–925.

von Melchner, L., Pallas, S. L., & Sur, M. 2000. Visual behaviour mediated by retinal projections directed to the auditory pathway. *Nature*, **404**(6780): 871–876.

Waiter, G. D., Williams, J. H., Murray, A. D., Gilchrist, A., Perrett, D. I., & Whiten, A. 2005. Structural white matter deficits in high-functioning individuals with autistic spectrum disorder: a voxel-based investigation. *NeuroImage*, **24**(2): 455–461.

Welchew, D. E., Ashwin, C., Berkouk, K., Salvador, R., Suckling, J., Baron-Cohen, S., *et al.* 2005. Functional disconnectivity of the medial temporal lobe in Asperger's syndrome. *Biological Psychiatry*, **57**(9): 991–998.

Wernicke, C. 1874. *Der aphasische Symptomenkomplex* (repr. 1974 ed.). Berlin: Springer.

Williams, J. H., Whiten, A., Suddendorf, T., & Perrett, D. I. 2001. Imitation, mirror neurons and autism. *Neuroscience and Biobehavioral Review*, **25**(4): 287–295.

Wilson, T. W., Rojas, D. C., Reite, M. L., Teale, P. D., & Rogers, S. J. 2007. Children and adolescents with autism exhibit reduced MEG steady-state gamma responses. *Biological Psychiatry*, **62**(3): 192–197.

Xiong, J., Parsons, L. M., Gao, J. H., & Fox, P. T. 1999. Interregional connectivity to primary motor cortex revealed using MRI resting state images. *Human Brain Mapping*, **8**(2–3): 151–156.

ADHD and Developmental Dyslexia

Two Pathways Leading to Impaired Learning

Guinevere F. Eden[a] and Chandan J. Vaidya[b]

Center for the Study of Learning, Departments of [a]Pediatrics and [b]Psychology, Georgetown University, Washington, DC, USA

Academic success and occupational outcome rely on a person's ability to attend to and learn from their surroundings. The cognitive mechanisms underlying these respective skills are impaired in individuals with attention deficit hyperactivity disorder (ADHD) and learning disability (LD). The high co-occurrence between ADHD and the learning disability developmental dyslexia has raised the possibility of a common etiology. We propose that studying the functional anatomy of disordered executive control and reading-related skills using carefully selected paradigms, coupled with rigorous studies of intervention efficacy, provide the most promising avenue for ameliorating these two commonly encountered impediments to learning.

Key words: **ADHD; dyslexia; learning disability**

Introduction

Dyslexia is the most common learning disability (LD), accounting for about 80% of all LDs and affecting between 8–12% of the population. It manifests as a failure to acquire accurate and fluent reading at the level expected by the child's age and in relation to his or her capacities in other cognitive domains (Lyon, Shaywitz, & Shaywitz, 2003). Like other forms of LD, dyslexia prevents acquisition of specific cognitive skills, in this case impeding decoding of print and comprehension of written language. Behavioral intervention strategies are commonly employed to target phonological and orthographic processes by using explicit, intensive, and repetitive tutoring methods aimed at reinforcing these skills (Alexander & Slinger-Constant, 2004). The diagnostic criteria for ADHD, on the other hand, are formulated by the inclusion of a set of behaviors: signs of inattention, hyperactivity, and impulsivity prior to 7 years of age, expression of these in at least two settings (e.g., home and school) and a pervasiveness of these behaviors leading to the impairment of daily functioning (American Psychiatric Association, 1994). Between 3 and 17% of children are estimated to have ADHD (Barbaresi *et al.*, 2002; Goldman, Genel, Bezman, & Slanetz, 1998). Pharmacological approaches to the treatment of ADHD are more widely practiced than any available therapeutic methods (Barkley, 1990) and target dopaminergic neurotransmitter systems underlying frontal lobe and basal ganglia function. Pharmacokinetic systems have not been identified in dyslexia or in the context of skills that support reading. Special education services that address dyslexia do not assist children with ADHD, and medication is not used to treat dyslexia. Treatment approaches for ADHD are generally prescribed by a physician, whereas reading interventions are planned and conducted within the field of special education.

Although dyslexia and ADHD each require proper identification and specific treatment, both conditions, which by definition require the ruling out of other medical and psychiatric conditions, share some important features that

Address for correspondence: Guinevere Eden, D.Phil., Center for the Study of Learning, Georgetown University Medical Center, Box 571406, Suite 150, Building D, 4000 Reservoir Road, NW, Washington, DC 20057. edeng@georgetown.edu provide the basis for the perspective put forward here. Firstly, behaviors characterizing ADHD or dyslexia are exhibited by all children and are considered problematic only when expressed in an age- or context-inappropriate manner. Inability to control impulsive behaviors and attend to relevant cues prevents adapting to social and professional settings. Likewise, reading skills are required to navigate an increasingly literate society. Failure to become agile with print will prevent a person from accessing resources that support communication and vocational practices. Secondly, behaviors characterizing ADHD and dyslexia in typical children are plastic and follow a protracted period of development (Ehri, 1999; Rueda *et al.*, 2004). In fact, symptoms of dyslexia and ADHD cannot be discerned accurately prior to school entry (usually at 6 to 7 years of age). Further, executive function and reading-related skills in ADHD and dyslexia can be enhanced through training. This training can result in improved attention (Sohlberg & Mateer, 2001) and working memory (Klingberg, Forssberg, & Westerberg, 2002) in individuals with ADHD, and phonological awareness in those with dyslexia (Torgesen *et al.*, 2001). Intervention is more beneficial if provided early. However, this does not preclude later intervention: both ADHD (Sohlberg & Mateer, 2001) and dyslexia (Eden *et al.*, 2004) have been successfully treated in adulthood. Thirdly, both conditions are highly heritable (Faraone & Doyle, 2000; Fisher & DeFries, 2002), and diagnoses of either is more prevalent in boys than girls (Rutter *et al.*, 2004; Willcutt *et al.*, 2003b). Fourthly, when left untreated, dyslexia and ADHD pose significant barriers for school success and later adaptation in a variety of settings (Cornwall & Bawden, 1992; Mannuzza, Klein, Bessler, Malloy, & Hynes, 1997). These problems are greatly compounded in individuals with comorbidity and these numbers are surprisingly high: it is estimated that 15–40% of children with dyslexia are also diagnosed with ADHD and 25–40% of children with ADHD also have dyslexia (Semrud-Clikeman *et al.*, 1992;

Willcutt & Pennington, 2000). Lastly, research efforts in the fields of ADHD and dyslexia have independently aspired to identify a core deficit that would provide an explanation encompassing all of the signs and symptoms exhibited within these groups and would offer a clear avenue for intervention. However, these attempts have not been fruitful in either case, and recent models have moved away from the single cognitive deficit approach and have instead embraced the idea of subtypes and multiple phenotypes (Pennington, 2005).

In this review, we argue that there is a substantial body of evidence indicating the involvement of multiple brain regions and the impairment of multiple skills in both ADHD and dyslexia. Dyslexia is associated with sensory and cognitive deficits that are the direct derivative of perturbations at the cortical and subcortical level, usually involving perisylvian cortex and thalamus (Galaburda & Livingstone, 1993). ADHD, on the other hand, is the consequence of a failure to invoke brain systems that would normally provide intermediary mechanisms to facilitate sensation and cognition. These mechanisms may be attentional or motivational, serving to regulate goal-driven behavior and are subserved by basal ganglia and frontal cortex. Of importance, these mechanisms dismantle normal behavior directly or indirectly, with the resultant deficits exhibiting both commonalities and dissociations. Rather than trying to account for the exact cascade by which these problems of learning arise (from genes to behavior), it may be more useful to identify the brain correlates of successful treatment. In view of recent advances in noninvasive functional brain imaging, we propose that it is necessary (1) to obtain insights into the neural underpinnings of the behaviors that are disordered in ADHD and dyslexia in populations that exhibit one or both of these conditions using process-pure, cognitive probes that evoke the affected behaviors; and (2) to conduct these neuroimaging studies in the context of treatments that have been scientifically proven to be effective. Only in this way can it be demonstrated whether the best treatment approaches involve targeting the deficits (e.g., phonological awareness or reading comprehension in the case of dyslexia) or whether intermediary systems (e.g., attention) pose better options for intervention in these conditions. Successful interventions can then be evaluated for plasticity at the neuronal level, and a relationship between brain changes and transfer-of-learning inferred. That is, does an intervention targeting one skill generalize to improving other skills, and what is the neural signature of this altered behavior? The outcome of this approach could lead to a better understanding of common obstacles to classroom-based learning and provide a positive influence on the future of clinical practice and educational policy.

What Do ADHD and Dyslexia Look Like?

Cognitive theories of dyslexia and ADHD try to explain how biological factors (e.g., gene and brain function) influence behavior, as behavior is the primary measure used for diagnostic purposes. Current models of ADHD conceptualize it as a disorder of executive function that is defined broadly as the ability to constrain attention and actions in a goal-directed manner. Executive function can be assessed neuropsychologically with a variety of measures that require children to exert inhibitory control either by suppressing a prepotent response (termed *response inhibition* and measured by Go/No-Go and Stop signal tasks) or irrelevant response (termed *interference control* and measured by paradigms such as the Stroop task), shift attentional set flexibly (measured by tasks such Tower of London or Intra- and Extra-dimensional shifting), and temporarily holding task-relevant information in mind (termed *working memory* and measured by tasks such as memory search). A large body of research suggests that response inhibition and working memory are reduced in children with ADHD relative to control chil-

dren. Attention shifting and interference control, however, show less consistent differences between ADHD and control children across studies (Willcutt *et al.*, 2003a). Further, sensorimotor processes that contribute to executive function such as timing, processing speed, and motor skills (fine and gross) are impaired in ADHD children (Castellanos, Sonuga-Barke, Milham, & Tannock, 2006). While an executive function deficit is considered to be a core cognitive deficit in ADHD, it is important to note that it is neither a necessary nor a sufficient cause of ADHD (Willcutt, Doyle, Nigg, Faraone, & Pennington, 2005). Effect sizes of executive function measures are small ($d = .4-.6$) in light of the wide overlap in the group distributions. Further, almost all other developmental disorders also exhibit some level of problems with executive function (e.g., autism and conduct disorder), suggesting that executive dysfunction is a pervasive outcome of multiple pathological developmental processes, much as a fever is to multiple infectious agents.

Like ADHD, dyslexia is characterized by numerous manifestations, although not all contribute to the formal definition (Lyon *et al.*, 2003). These include poor phonological awareness (Bradley & Bryant, 1983; Snowling, 1995; Wagner, 1986), rapid retrieval of phonological codes (Denckla & Rudel, 1976), and verbal working memory (Torgesen, Wagner, Simmons, & Laughon, 1990). Deficits in visual processing (Lovegrove, 1993), auditory discrimination (Tallal, 1980), and motor control (Nicolson & Fawcett, 1994) have also been reported. In the face of this behavioral complexity, it is not surprising that identifying a single theory that can account for the myriad problems related to dyslexia has been challenging. The most widely accepted explanation for dyslexic reading difficulties involves poor phonological awareness (PA). PA is a broad class of skills that involve attending to, thinking about, and intentionally manipulating the phonological aspects of spoken language (Scarborough & Brady, 2002). Measures of PA have been implicated as the best predictor of children's future reading ability (Wagner & Torgesen, 1987) and poor PA persists into adulthood (Eden *et al.*, 2004). Importantly, PA is the only skill domain in which strong evidence exists for a causal role in dyslexia: children with poor PA are likely to go on to become poor readers, and teaching programs that emphasize PA often facilitates reading acquisition (Vellutino, Fletcher, Snowling, & Scanlon, 2004). However, while most therapies for the remediation of dyslexia have tended to target PA, the "phonological core deficit hypothesis" has failed to address all deficits exhibited by individuals with dyslexia. Other models, reviewed elsewhere (Eden & Zeffiro, 1998), have tried to fill this void by viewing dyslexia either in terms of temporal integration (Stein, 1993), or a "double deficit," taking into account rapid phonological retrieval (Wolf & Obregon, 1992); others have considered the role of automaticity (Nicolson, Fawcett, & Dean, 2001) and language impairment (Catts, 1996).

Co-morbidity of ADHD and Developmental Dyslexia

The causal pathways leading to co-morbidity between ADHD and dyslexia are not well understood, but researchers agree that their coexistence is not artifactual because associations have been observed in different epidemiological samples and across diverse settings (Semrud-Clikeman *et al.*, 1992; Willcutt & Pennington, 2000). Furthermore, the two conditions do not share diagnostic criteria and each is evaluated by different methods: ADHD by parent and teacher ratings of behavior and dyslexia by direct tests of reading performance. Hypotheses explaining the co-morbidity of dyslexia and ADHD fall into two broad classes. One is an association in the absence of any etiological factors, termed the "phenocopy hypothesis." This model proposes a bi-directional influence such that behavioral problems associated with ADHD disrupt learning to read, hence making the child appear dyslexic or, by the same logic, frustrations due to reading problems making the dyslexic child appear inattentive (Hinshaw, 1992; Pennington, Groisser, & Welsh, 1993). The other school of thought, termed the "cognitive subtype hypothesis," makes an association with etiological factors and posits that co-morbid groups in fact represent a third disorder that is due to either etiological factors that are distinct relative to those related to each disorder alone (Rucklidge & Tannock, 2002) or to common factors that increase susceptibility to both disorders (Willcutt *et al.*, 2003a). The cognitive subtype hypothesis is strongly favored (Nigg, Hinshaw, Carte, & Treuting, 1998) and has spurred the search for genetic factors that increase susceptibility to both disorders. Studies in twins indicate that both disorders are highly heritable (Faraone & Doyle, 2000; Fisher & DeFries, 2002), and bivariate genome-wide analyses indicate that common chromosomal loci (e.g., 14q32, 13q32, 20q11) increase susceptibility to both ADHD and dyslexia (Gayan *et al.*, 2005). There is wide agreement that both disorders are likely to be polygenic, with some loci increasing shared susceptibility and others exerting unique influences on each disorder; this is reviewed in detail elsewhere (Fisher & DeFries, 2002). However, mechanisms by which these chromosomal differences alter developmental trajectories of neurocognitive processes that are faulty in ADHD and reading disability remain elusive.

What Do Dyslexia and ADHD Share?

Systematic studies of executive functions that have included well-controlled samples of ADHD, dyslexia, and co-morbid groups (ADHD plus dyslexia) indicate that while each disorder exhibits the deficits characteristic for each disorder (e.g., poor response inhibition in ADHD, phonological coding deficits in dyslexia, and both in the co-morbid groups), all groups also exhibit abnormalities with processing speed (Rucklidge & Tannock, 2002) and verbal working memory (Willcutt *et al.*, 2001). While common causes may underlie these similarities in cognitive deficits, it is equally likely that different causes may lead to the same deficit. Thus verbal working memory spans may be reduced either because interference control is poor (e.g., in ADHD) or because phonological representations are impoverished (i.e., in dyslexia). A specific example is processing speed, which may be slower in either condition because of greater intra-individual variability (Castellanos & Tannock, 2002; Rubia *et al.*, 1999) or because of poor temporal integration (Nicolson *et al.*, 2001). An anatomical candidate for this impaired behavior is the cerebellum (Nicolson *et al.*, 2001). This approach also takes into account that a single perturbation at the level of the brain might give rise to multiple cognitive deficits, and each cognitive deficit in turn could give rise to a multitude of behavioral impairments (Gilger & Kaplan, 2001).

Brain-Basis for ADHD and Dyslexia

Characteristics of brain anatomy and brain function that distinguish ADHD and dyslexia from typical controls are shared in part across the two conditions. As discussed above, one would expect such overlap in the pathophysiology regardless of whether there is a common or separate etiology of ADHD and dyslexia (and hence a tendency for co-morbidity) because similar brain anomalies may arise from different genetic or environment sources. That is, although some of the morphological differences observed in these conditions appear to relate to a nongenetic etiological factor (because they are observed in the affected proband of monozygotic twins discordant for the condition), they may still be of importance to the question of intervention. No landmark brain malformation characterizes either condition, and the anatomical and functional differences are subtle. Here we only provide a brief description of the findings and refer elsewhere for

summaries for ADHD (Bush, Valera, & Seidman, 2005; Sowell *et al.*, 2003) and dyslexia (Eckert, 2004).

Anatomical studies of ADHD subjects relative to controls have reported smaller volumes of the right frontal lobe (Castellanos *et al.*, 1996; Filipek *et al.*, 1997; Semrud-Clikeman *et al.*, 2000) and the left orbitofrontal regions (Hesslinger *et al.*, 2002). Abnormalities of basal ganglia structures have also been noted, but the details vary in terms of laterality of the reduction. These differences could be attributed to developmental factors as caudate volumes are initially smaller in ADHD children but do not differ by adolescence because of reductions in growth trajectories of typical development (Castellanos *et al.*, 2002). Differences in posterior structures have also been associated with ADHD. Posterior portions of the corpus callosum (connecting white matter fibers from the posterior frontal, parietal, and temporal lobes of the two hemispheres) is smaller in ADHD than in control subjects (Hynd *et al.*, 1991; Semrud-Clikeman *et al.*, 1994). Studies of the size of the corpus callosum in dyslexia have produced conflicting findings, usually complicated by co-morbidity in the sample under study. The cerebellum, which boasts extensive anatomical connections to frontal cortex and basal ganglia, is smaller in ADHD subjects (Berquin, Giedd, Jacobsen *et al.*, 1998; Castellanos *et al.*, 2001; Castellanos *et al.*, 2002; Mostofsky, Reiss, Lockhart, & Denckla, 1998) and shows a reduction of right grey matter in dyslexic subjects (Nicolson *et al.*, 2001). In ADHD, measurements of cortical surface have shown reduced grey matter in bilateral inferior prefrontal cortex and anterior temporal lobes and increased grey matter in posterior temporal cortices and inferior parietal cortex (Sowell *et al.*, 2003). In dyslexia, the most common cortical findings distinguishing good and poor readers involve left hemisphere occipito-temporal, parietal, and inferior frontal measures (Eckert, 2004).

Studies examining brain activation with cognitive challenges in ADHD have focused on executive functions such as working memory, inhibition, and selective attention. Early SPECT and PET studies employing auditory attention tasks demonstrated low metabolic activity in the frontal (premotor and pre-frontal) and striatal (caudate, putamen) regions of ADHD patients (Lou, Henriksen, & Bruhn, 1984; Lou, Henrikson, Bruhn, Berner, & Nielsen, 1989; Zametkin, Liebenauer, Fitzger-ald *et al.*, 1993; Zametkin *et al.*, 1990). Func-tional MRI studies of inhibitory processing also showed reduced activation in ADHD com-pared to controls in the anterior cingulate in adults during the performance of a Stroop task (Bush *et al.*, 1999) and in children during a mo-tor inhibition task (Tamm, Menon, Ringel, & Reiss, 2004). Activation is also reduced in pre-frontal and striatal regions during interference suppression (Vaidya *et al.*, 2005) and during mo-tor inhibition (Booth *et al.*, 2005; Rubia *et al.*, 1999; Vaidya *et al.*, 1998) in pediatric popu-lations with ADHD. Parietal cortex shows hy-poactivity bilaterally during visual selective at-tention in ADHD children relative to controls (Booth *et al.*, 2005). Across studies, then, frontal, temporal, and parietal cortical lobes and sub-cortical striatal structures demonstrate hypoac-tivity in ADHD when compared to controls.

Brain imaging studies have also character-ized the anomalous patterns of neural activa-tion associated with reading and phonological representation in adults with persistent or com-pensated developmental dyslexia (Brunswick, McCrory, Price, Frith, & Frith, 1999; Eden *et al.*, 2004; Paulesu *et al.*, 1996; Rumsey *et al.*, 1997). Employing various experimental ap-proaches and paradigms (e.g., the detection or judgment of rhymes, nonword reading, and implicit reading), these studies have localized dysfunctional phonological representations in dyslexia when compared to controls, specif-ically in left-hemisphere temporo-parietal and occipito-temporal cortices. Relative hypoactiv-ity in the parietal cortex has been reported for tasks necessitating phonological represen-tation and reading in pediatric (Shaywitz *et al.*, 2002; Temple *et al.*, 2001) and adult dyslexic populations (Brunswick *et al.*, 1999; Eden *et al.*,

2004; Paulesu *et al.*, 1996; Rumsey *et al.*, 1997; Shaywitz *et al.*, 1998). In addition, there are reports of hypoactivity in the left occipito-temporal junction (Brunswick *et al.*, 1999; Paulesu *et al.*, 2001; Rumsey *et al.*, 1997; Shay-witz *et al.*, 1998). The left inferior frontal gyrus has been shown to be underactivated during some tasks (Brunswick *et al.*, 1999; Shaywitz *et al.*, 1998) but not others (Brunswick *et al.*, 1999; Eden *et al.*, 2004; Paulesu *et al.*, 1996; Rumsey *et al.*, 1997; Rumsey *et al.*, 1994).

Functional abnormalities in ADHD and dyslexia are not limited to reductions in ac-tivation, but also include increases in activa-tion relative to controls. For example, ADHD subjects show increased activation in primary sensory cortices during tasks of attention (Lou *et al.*, 1984; Lou *et al.*, 1989) and working memory (Schweitzer *et al.*, 2000). During mo-tor inhibition, however, ADHD children show hyperactivity in left temporal (Tamm *et al.*, 2004) and ventral prefrontal cortices (Schulz *et al.*, 2004; Schulz, Newcorn, Fan, Tang, & Halperin, 2005; Vaidya *et al.*, 1998). In dyslexia it has been proposed that overactivity of the left inferior frontal gyrus serves as a compensatory mechanism for the hypoactivity expressed in posterior regions (Shaywitz *et al.*, 2002). In sum-mary, structural and functional abnormalities in ADHD are primarily found bilaterally in frontal, striatal, and parietal areas as well as cerebellum whereas those in dyslexia are lo-cated in the inferior frontal, temporal, and parietal cortices of the left hemisphere and cerebellum.

Intervention Studies in Dyslexia and ADHD Employing Brain Imaging

Behavioral plasticity after treatment of indi-viduals with learning disorders could be accom-panied by neuronal changes of the following type: (1) increased engagement of the normal network found in nonimpaired individuals; (2) a compensatory mechanism wherein new areas are recruited (as has been reported as a mechanism supporting the functional recovery of stroke patients); or (3) some combination of the two. Brain imaging studies investigating neural plasticity after phonologically based intervention in children with dyslexia have reported intervention-induced increases in left hemisphere regions that are initially hypoactive in dyslexics when contrasted to controls (Aylward *et al.*, 2003; Shaywitz *et al.*, 2004; Simos *et al.*, 2002). However, the results are not limited to the same regions, some showing changes in parietal cortex (Aylward *et al.*, 2003; Simos *et al.*, 2002) and others in extrastriate visual cortex (Shaywitz *et al.*, 2004). The mechanisms for reading recovery in adults with developmental dyslexia seems to involve a combination of "compensation" and "normalization," with increases observed in left-hemisphere regions engaged by normal readers (parietal and frontal cortices) and additional compensatory activity found in the right perisylvian cortex (Eden *et al.*, 2004).

In contrast to treatment effects on reading ability that are relatively permanent, symptoms are alleviated temporarily (4 to 8 hours) after pharmacological treatment with stimulant medications (e.g., methylphenidate and amphetamines) in ADHD. Functional MRI studies of pharmacological treatment in children with ADHD have shown that stimulant medications "normalize" brain activation during executive task performance, increase engagement of fronto-striatal regions (Kim, Lee, Cho, & Lee, 2001; Lou *et al.*, 1984; Lou *et al.*, 1989; Shafritz, Marchione, Gore, Shaywitz, & Shaywitz, 2004; Vaidya *et al.*, 1998), and decrease engagement of sensorimotor (Lee *et al.*, 2005; Lou *et al.*, 1984) and parietal (Szobot *et al.*, 2003) regions. Methylphenidate-related changes are often rate-dependant, such that increases were greater in those with higher rather than lower hyperactivity in the putamen (Teicher *et al.*, 2000), cerebellar vermis (Anderson, Polcari, Lowen, Renshaw, & Teicher, 2002), and striatum (Vaidya *et al.*, 1998). A study in adolescents with both ADHD and dyslexia found no dif-

ferences in methylphenidate-related changes in the co-morbid or dyslexic group (Shafritz *et al.*, 2004). Pharmacological effects on regional activation appear to be selective because not all atypically activated regions were modulated by medication (Shafritz *et al.*, 2004), yet some variations in findings may relate to the fact that pharmacological response varied across individuals. Overall, however, these findings suggest that differences in fronto-striatal function are central to ADHD and to the efficacy of pharmacological treatment.

Conclusions

Because of the complexity of the phenotypes of ADHD and dyslexia, the etiology of these disorders of learning remains unknown. It has been proposed that greater attention needs to be paid to the neurocognitive heterogeneity of these conditions and that, further, there is a need to identify endophenotypes or phenotypes that are more closely linked to the neurobiological substrate of a disorder (Pennington, 2005). Here we propose that these approaches will be complemented by assessing the functional anatomy of successful treatment. Specifically, behavioral plasticity has been shown for performance on executive function and reading-related tasks (either pharmacologically or behaviorally), and the neural correlates of these changes can be determined using functional brain imaging technology. This approach places less emphasis on determining *why* specific brain areas may differ between impaired learners and typically developing children, the reasons for which may differ between, as well as within, diagnostic groups. Instead, determining which brain regions support successful intervention will shed a new light on the problem of addressing the underlying pathophysiology. Specifically, this approach entails the identification of common endophenotypes for ADHD and dyslexia. For example, disturbances of processing speed characterize both disorders and may relate to dysfunction of sensorimotor systems. If phenotypes (e.g., brain imaging data) suggest that problems arising in both ADHD and dyslexia stem from this fundamental disability, then treatment approaches would have to confirm this hypothesis by demonstrating behavioral and neural plasticity in sensorimotor systems and examine whether they also generalize to other domains that are important to learning. In this process, targeting populations suffering from both ADHD and dyslexia will provide valuable information, as they can confirm or deny whether treatments target the same brain regions as those observed in either condition alone.

Acknowledgments

The authors are grateful for their support from the National Institute of Child Health and Human Development (Grants HD40095 and HD37890 to G.F.E.) and the National Institute of Mental Health (Grant MH065395 to C.J.V.).

Conflicts of Interest

The authors declare no conflicts of interest.

References

Alexander, A. W. & Slinger-Constant, A. M. 2004. Current status of treatments for dyslexia: critical review. *Journal of Child Neurology* **19**(10): 44–758.

American Psychiatric Association. 2000. *Diagnostic and statistical manual of mental disorders* (4th ed., text rev.). Washington, DC: Author.

Anderson, C. M., Polcari, A., Lowen, S. B., Renshaw, P. F., & Teicher, M. H. 2002. Effects of methylphenidate on functional magnetic resonance relaxometry of the cerebellar vermis in boys with ADHD. *American Journal of Psychiatry* **159**(8): 1322–1328.

Aylward, E. H., Richards, T. L., Berninger, V. W., Nagy, W. E., Field, K. M., Grimme, A. C., *et al.* 2003. Instructional treatment associated with changes in brain activation in children with dyslexia. *Neurology* **61**(2): 212–219.

Barbaresi, W. J., Katusic, S. K., Colligan, R. C., Pankratz, V. S., Weaver, A. L., Weber, K. J., *et al.* 2002. How common is attention-deficit/hyperactivity disorder? Incidence in a population-based birth cohort in Rochester, Minn. *Archives of Pediatrics and Adolescent Medicine* **156**(3): 217–224.

Barkley, R. A. 1990. *Attention deficit hyperactivity disorder: A handbook for diagnosis and treatment*. New York: Guilford Press.

Berquin, P. C., Giedd, J. N., Jacobsen, L. K., *et al.* 1998. Cerebellum in attention deficit hyperactivity disorder: a morphometric MRI study. *Neurology* **50**: 1087–1093.

Booth, J. R., Burman, D. D., Meyer, J. R., Lei, Z., Trommer, B. L., Davenport, N. D., *et al.* 2005. Larger deficits in brain networks for response inhibition than for visual selective attention in attention deficit hyperactivity disorder (ADHD). *Journal of Child Psychology and Psychiatry* **46**(1): 94–111.

Bradley, L., & Bryant, P. 1983. Categorizing sounds and learning to read: a causal connection. *Nature* **301**: 419–421.

Brunswick, N., McCrory, E., Price, C. J., Frith, C. D., & Frith, U. 1999. Explicit and implicit processing of words and pseudowords by adult developmental dyslexics: a search for Wernicke's Wortschatz? *Brain* **122**(Pt 10): 1901–1917.

Bush, G., Frazier, J. A., Rauch, S. L., Seidman, L. J., Whalen, P. J., Jenike, M. A., *et al.* 1999. Anterior cingulate cortex dysfunction in attention-deficit/hyperactivity disorder revealed by fMRI and the Counting Stroop. *Biological Psychiatry* **45**(12): 1542–1552.

Bush, G., Valera, E. M., & Seidman, L. J. 2005. Functional neuroimaging of attention-deficit/hyperactivity disorder: a review and suggested future directions. *Biological Psychiatry* **57**(11): 1273–1284.

Castellanos, F. X., Giedd, J. N., Berquin, P. C., Walter, J. M., Sharp, W., Tran, T., *et al.* 2001. Quantitative brain magnetic resonance imaging in girls with attention-deficit/hyperactivity disorder. *Archives of General Psychiatry* **58**(3): 289–295.

Castellanos, F. X., Giedd, J. N., Marsh, W. L., Hamburger, S. D., Vaituzis, A. C., Dickstein, D. P., *et al.* 1996. Quantitative brain magnetic resonance imaging in attention-deficit hyperactivity disorder. *Archives of General Psychiatry* **53**: 607–616.

Castellanos, F. X., Lee, P. P., Sharp, W., Jeffries, N. O., Greenstein, D. K., Clasen, L. S., *et al.* 2002. Developmental trajectories of brain volume abnormalities in children and adolescents with attention-deficit/hyperactivity disorder. *Journal of the American Medical Association* **288**(14): 1740–1748.

Castellanos, F. X., Sonuga-Barke, E. J., Milham, M. P., & Tannock, R. 2006. Characterizing cognition in ADHD: beyond executive dysfunction. *Trends in Cognitive Sciences* **10**(3): 117–123.

Castellanos, F. X., & Tannock, R. 2002. Neuroscience of attention-deficit/hyperactivity disorder: the search for endophenotypes. *Nature Reviews. Neuroscience* **3**(8): 617–628.

Catts, H. W. 1996. Defining dyslexia as a developmental language disorder: an expanded view. *Topics in Language Disorders* **16**: 14–29.

Cornwall, A., & Bawden, H. N. 1992. Reading disabilities and aggression: a critical review. *Journal of Learning Disabilities* **25**(5): 281–288.

Denckla, M. B., & Rudel, R. G. 1976. Naming of object-drawings by dyslexic and other learning disabled children. *Brain and Language* **3**(1): 1–15.

Eckert, M. 2004. Neuroanatomical markers for dyslexia: a review of dyslexia structural imaging studies. *Neuroscientist* **10**(4): 362–371.

Eden, G. F., Jones, K. M., Cappell, K., Gareau, L., Wood, F. B., Zeffiro, T. A., *et al.* 2004. Neural changes following remediation in adult developmental dyslexia. *Neuron* **44**(3): 411–422.

Eden, G. F., & Zeffiro, T. A. 1998. Neural systems affected in developmental dyslexia revealed by functional neuroimaging. *Neuron* **21**(2): 279–282.

Ehri, L. C. 1999. Phases of development in learning to read words. In J. Oakhill & R. Beard (Eds.), *Reading development and the teaching of reading* (pp. 79–108). Oxford: Blackwell.

Faraone, S. V., & Doyle, A. E. 2000. Genetic influences on attention deficit hyperactivity disorder. *Current Psychiatry Reports* **2**(2): 143–146.

Filipek, P. A., Semrud-Clikeman, M., Steingard, R. J., Renshaw, P. F., Kennedy, D. N., & Biederman, J. 1997. Volumetric MRI analysis comparing subjects having attention-deficit hyperactivity disorder with normal controls. *Neurology* **48**: 589–601.

Fisher, S. E., & DeFries, J. C. 2002. Developmental dyslexia: genetic dissection of a complex cognitive trait. *Nature Reviews Neuroscience* **3**(10): 767–780.

Galaburda, A., & Livingstone, M. 1993. Evidence for a magnocellular defect in developmental dyslexia. *Annals of the New York Academy of Sciences* **682**: 70–82.

Gayan, J., Willcutt, E. G., Fisher, S. E., Francks, C., Cardon, L. R., Olson, R. K., *et al.* 2005. Bivariate linkage scan for reading disability and attention-deficit/hyperactivity disorder localizes pleiotropic loci. *Journal of Child Psychology and Psychiatry* **46**(10): 1045–1056.

Gilger, J. W., & Kaplan, B. J. 2001. Atypical brain development: a conceptual framework for understanding developmental learning disabilities. *Developmental Neuropsychology* **20**(2): 465–481.

Goldman, L. S., Genel, M., Bezman, R. J., & Slanetz, P. J. 1998. Diagnosis and treatment of attention-deficit/hyperactivity disorder in children and adolescents. Council on Scientific Affairs, American Medical Association. *Journal of the American Medical Association* **279**(14): 1100–1107.

Hesslinger, B., Tebartz van Elst, L., Thiel, T., Haegele, K., Hennig, J., & Ebert, D. 2002. Frontoorbital volume reductions in adult patients with attention deficit hyperactivity disorder. *Neuroscience Letters* **328**(3): 319–321.

Hinshaw, S. P. 1992. Externalizing behavior problems and academic underachievement in childhood and adolescence: causal relationships and underlying mechanisms. *Psychological Bulletin* **111**(1): 127–155.

Hynd, G. W., Semrud-Clikeman, M., Lorys, A. R., Novey, E. S., Eliopulos, D., & Lyytinen, H. 1991. Corpus callosum morphology in attention deficit-hyperactivity disorder: morphometric analysis of MRI. *Journal of Learning Disabilities* **24**(3): 141–146.

Kim, B. N., Lee, J. S., Cho, S. C., & Lee, D. S. 2001. Methylphenidate increased regional cerebral blood flow in subjects with attention deficit/hyperactivity disorder. *Yonsei Medical Journal* **42**(1): 19–29.

Klingberg, T., Forssberg, H., & Westerberg, H. 2002. Training of working memory in children with ADHD. *Journal of Clinical and Experimental Neuropsychology* **24**(6): 781–791.

Lee, J. S., Kim, B. N., Kang, E., Lee, D. S., Kim, Y. K., Chung, J. K., *et al*. 2005. Regional cerebral blood flow in children with attention deficit hyperactivity disorder: comparison before and after methylphenidate treatment. *Human Brain Mapping* **24**(3): 157–164.

Lou, H. C., Henriksen, L., & Bruhn, P. 1984. Focal cerebral hypoperfusion in children with dysphasia and/or attention deficit disorder. **41**: 825–829.

Lou, H. C., Henrikson, L., Bruhn, P., Berner, H., & Nielsen, J. B. 1989. Striatal dysfunction in attention deficit and hyperkinetic disorder **46**: 48–52.

Lovegrove, W. 1993. Weakness in transient visual system: a causal factor in dyslexia? In P. Tallal, A. M. Galaburda, R. R. Llinas, & C. von Euler (Eds.), *Temporal information processing in the nervous system: Special reference to dyslexia and dysphasia* (Vol. 682 of the *Annals of the New York Academy of Sciences*, pp. 57–69). New York: New York Academy of Sciences.

Lyon, G. R., Shaywitz, S. E., & Shaywitz, B. A. 2003. A definition of dyslexia. *Annals of Dyslexia* **53**: 1–14.

Mannuzza, S., Klein, R. G., Bessler, A., Malloy, P., & Hynes, M. E. 1997. Educational and occupational outcome of hyperactive boys grown up. *Journal of the American Academy of Child and Adolescent Psychiatry* **36**: 1222–1227.

Mostofsky, S. H., Reiss, A. L., Lockhart, P., & Denckla, M. B. 1998. Evaluation of cerebellar size in attention-deficit hyperactivity disorder. *Journal of Child Neurology* **13**: 434–439.

Nicolson, R. I., & Fawcett, A. J. 1994. Comparisons of deficits in cognitive and motor skills among children with dyselxia. *Annals of Dyslexia* **44:** 147–164.

Nicolson, R. I., Fawcett, A. J., & Dean, P. 2001. Developmental dyslexia: the cerebellar deficit hypothesis. *Trends in Neuroscience* **24**(9): 508–511.

Nigg, J. T., Hinshaw, S. P., Carte, E. T., & Treuting, J. J. 1998. Neuropsychological correlates of childhood attention-deficit/hyperactivity disorder: explainable by comorbid disruptive behavior or reading problems? *Journal of Abnormal Psychology* **107**(3): 468–480.

Paulesu, E., Demonet, J.-F., Fazio, F., McCrory, E., Chanoine, V., Brunswick, N., *et al.* 2001. Dyslexia: cultural diversity and biological unity. *Science* **291:** 2165.

Paulesu, E., Frith, C., Snowling, M., Gallagher, A., Morton, J., Frackowiak, R. S. J., *et al.* 1996. Is developmental dyslexia a disconnection syndrome? Evidence from PET scanning. *Brain* **119:** 143–157.

Pennington, B., Groisser, D., & Welsh, M. 1993. Contrasting cognitive deficits in attention deficit hyperactivity disorder versus reading disability. *Developmental Psychology* **29:** 511–523.

Pennington, B. F. 2005. Toward a new neuropsychological model of attention-deficit/hyperactivity disorder: subtypes and multiple deficits. *Biological Psychiatry* **57**(11): 1221–1223.

Rubia, K., Overmeyer, S., Taylor, E., Brammer, M., Williams, S. C., Simmons, A., *et al.* 1999. Hypofrontality in attention deficit hyperactivity disorder during higher-order motor control: a study with functional MRI. *American Journal of Psychiatry* **156**(6): 891–896.

Rucklidge, J. J., & Tannock, R. 2002. Neuropsychological profiles of adolescents with ADHD: effects of reading difficulties and gender. *Journal of Child Psychology and Psychiatry* **43**(8): 988–1003.

Rueda, M. R., Fan, J., McCandliss, B. D., Halparin, J. D., Gruber, D. B., Lercari, L. P., *et al.* 2004. Development of attentional networks in childhood. *Neuropsychologia* **42**(8): 1029–1040.

Rumsey, J. M., Nace, K., Donohue, B., Wise, D., Maisog, J. M., & Andreason, P. 1997. A positron emission tomographic study of impaired word recognition and phonological processing in dyslexic men. *Archives of Neurology* **54**(5): 562–573.

Rumsey, J. M., Zametkin, A. J., Andreason, P., Hanahan, A. P., Hamburger, S. D., Aquino, T., *et al.* 1994. Normal activation of frontotemporal language cortex in dyslexia, as measured with oxygen 15 positron emission tomography. *Archives of Neurology* **51**(1): 27–38.

Rutter, M., Caspi, A., Fergusson, D., Horwood, L. J., Goodman, R., Maughan, B., *et al.* 2004. Sex differences in developmental reading disability: new findings from 4 epidemiological studies. *Journal of the American Medical Association* **291**(16): 2007–2012.

Scarborough, H. S., & Brady, S. A. 2002. Toward a common terminology for talking about speech and reading: a glossary of the ŎphonŎ words and some related terms. *Journal of Literacy Research* **34:** 299–334.

Schulz, K. P., Fan, J., Tang, C. Y., Newcorn, J. H., Buchsbaum, M. S., Cheung, A. M., *et al.* 2004. Response inhibition in adolescents diagnosed with attention deficit hyperactivity disorder during childhood: an event-related FMRI study. *American Journal of Psychiatry* **161**(9): 1650–1657.

Schulz, K. P., Newcorn, J. H., Fan, J., Tang, C. Y., & Halperin, J. M. 2005. Brain activation gradients in ventrolateral prefrontal cortex related to persistence of ADHD in adolescent boys. *Joural of the American Academy of Child and Adolescent Psychiatry* **44**(1): 47–54.

Schweitzer, J. B., Faber, T. L., Grafton, S. T., Tune, L. E., Hoffman, J. M., & Kilts, C. D. 2000. Alterations in the functional anatomy of working memory in adult attention deficit hyperactivity disorder. *American Journal of Psychiatry* **157**(2): 278–280.

Semrud-Clikeman, M., Biederman, J., Sprich-Buckminster, S., Lehman, B. K., Faraone, S. V., & Norman, D. 1992. Comorbidity between ADDH and learning disability: a review and report in a clinically referred sample. *Journal of the American Academy of Child and Adolescent Psychiatry* **31**(3): 439–448.

Semrud-Clikeman, M., Filipek, P. A., Biederman, J., Steingard, R., Kennedy, D., Renshaw, P., *et al.* 1994. Attention-deficit hyperactivity disorder: magnetic resonance imaging morphometric analysis of the corpus callosum. *Journal of the American Academy of Child and Adolescent Psychiatry* **33**(6): 875–881.

Semrud-Clikeman, M., Steingard, R. J., Filipek, P., Biederman, J., Bekken, K., & Renshaw, P. F. 2000. Using MRI to examine brain-behavior relationships in males with attention deficit disorder with hyperactivity. *Journal of the American Academy of Child and Adolescent Psychiatry* **39**(4): 477–484.

Shafritz, K. M., Marchione, K. E., Gore, J. C., Shaywitz, S. E., & Shaywitz, B. A. 2004. The effects of methylphenidate on neural systems of attention in attention deficit hyperactivity disorder. *American Journal of Psychiatry* **161**(11): 1990–1997.

Shaywitz, B. A., Shaywitz, S. E., Blachman, B. A., Pugh, K. R., Fulbright, R. K., Skudlarski, P., *et al.* 2004. Development of left occipitotemporal systems for skilled reading in children after a phonologically-based intervention. *Biological Psychiatry* **55**(9): 926–933.

Shaywitz, B. A., Shaywitz, S. E., Pugh, K. R., Mencl, W. E., Fulbright, R. K., Skudlarski, P., *et al.* 2002.

Disruption of posterior brain systems for reading in children with developmental dyslexia. *Biological Psychiatry* **52**(2): 101–110.

Shaywitz, S. E., Shaywitz, B. A., Pugh, K. R., Fulbright, R. K., Constable, R. T., Mencl, W. E., et al. 1998. Functional disruption in the organization of the brain for reading in dyslexia. *Proceedings of the National Academy of Sciences of the United States of America* **95**(5): 2636–2641.

Simos, P. G., Fletcher, J. M., Bergman, E., Breier, J. I., Foorman, B. R., Castillo, E. M., et al. 2002. Dyslexia-specific brain activation profile becomes normal following successful remedial training. *Neurology* **58**(8): 1203–1213.

Snowling, M. J. 1995. Phonological processing and developmental dyslexia. *Journal of Research in Reading* **18**(2): 132–138.

Sohlberg, M. M., & Mateer, C. A. 2001. Improving attention and managing attentional problems: adapting rehabilitation techniques to adults with ADD. *Annals of the New York Academy of Sciences* **931:** 359–375.

Sowell, E. R., Thompson, P. M., Welcome, S. E., Henkenius, A. L., Toga, A. W., & Peterson, B. S. 2003. Cortical abnormalities in children and adolescents with attention-deficit hyperactivity disorder. *Lancet*, 1699–1707.

Stein, J. F. 1993. Dyslexia: impaired temporal information processing? *Annals of the New York Academy of Sciences* **682:** 83–86.

Szobot, C. M., Ketzer, C., Cunha, R. D., Parente, M. A., Langleben, D. D., Acton, P. D., et al. (2003. The acute effect of methylphenidate on cerebral blood flow in boys with attention-deficit/hyperactivity disorder. *European Journal of Nuclear Medicine and Molecular Imaging* **30**(3): 423–426.

Tallal, P. 1980. Auditory temporal perception, phonics, and reading disabilities in children. *Brain and Language* **9:** 182–198.

Tamm, L., Menon, V., Ringel, J., & Reiss, A. L. 2004. Event-related FMRI evidence of frontotemporal involvement in aberrant response inhibition and task switching in attention-deficit/hyperactivity disorder. *Journal of the American Academy of Child and Adolescent Psychiatry* **43**(11): 1430–1440.

Teicher, M. H., Anderson, C. M., Polcari, A., Glod, C. A., Maas, L. C., & Renshaw, P. F. 2000. Functional deficits in basal ganglia of children with attention-deficit/hyperactivity disorder shown with functional magnetic resonance imaging relaxometry. *Nature Medicine* **6**(4): 470–473.

Temple, E., Poldrack, R. A., Salidis, J., Deutsch, G. K., Tallal, P., Merzenich, M. M., et al. 2001. Disrupted neural responses to phonological and orthographic processing in dyslexic children: an fMRI study. *Neuroreport* **12**(2): 299–307.

Torgesen, J. K., Alexander, A. W., Wagner, R. K., Rashotte, C. A., Voeller, K. K. S., & Conway, T. 2001. Intensive remedial instruction for children with severe reading disabilities: immediate and long-term outcomes from two instructional approaches. *Journal of Learning Disabilities* **34**(1): 33–58, 78.

Torgesen, J. K., Wagner, R. K., Simmons, K., & Laughon, P. 1990. Identifying phonological coding problems in disabled readers: naming, counting, or span measures? *Learning Disability Quarterly* **13**(Fall): 236–243.

Vaidya, C. J., Austin, G., Kirkorian, G., Ridlehuber, H. W., Desmond, J. E., Glover, G. H., et al. 1998. Selective effects of methylphenidate in attention deficit hyperactivity disorder: a functional magnetic resonance study. *Proceedings of the National Academy of Sciences of the United States of America* **95**(24): 14494–14499.

Vaidya, C. J., Bunge, S. A., Dudukovic, N. M., Zalecki, C. A., Elliott, G. R., & Gabrieli, J. D. 2005. Altered neural substrates of cognitive control in childhood ADHD: evidence from functional magnetic resonance imaging. *American Journal of Psychiatry* **162**(9): 1605–1613.

Vellutino, F. R., Fletcher, J. M., Snowling, M. J., & Scanlon, D. M. 2004. Specific reading disability (dyslexia): what have we learned in the past four decades? *Journal of Child Psychology and Psychiatry* **45**(1): 2–40.

Wagner, R. K. 1986. Phonological processing abilities and reading: implications for disabled readers. *Journal of Learning Disabilities* **19**(10): 623–631.

Wagner, R. K., & Torgesen, J. K. 1987. The nature of phonological processing and its causal role in the acquisition of reading skills. *Psychological Bulletin* **101**(2): 192–212.

Willcutt, E. G., DeFries, J. C., Pennington, B. F., Olson, R. K., Smith, S. D., & Cardon, L. R. 2003a. Genetic etiology of comorbid reading difficulties and ADHD. In R. Plomin, J. C. DeFries, P. McGuffin, & I. Craig (Eds.), *Behavioral genetics in a postgenomic era* (pp. 227–246). Washington, DC: APA.

Willcutt, E. G., DeFries, J. C., Pennington, B. F., Olson, R. K., Smith, S. D., & Cardon, L. R. 2003b. *Genetic etiology of comorbid reading difficulties and ADHD*. Washington, DC: APA.

Willcutt, E. G., Doyle, A. E., Nigg, J. T., Faraone, S. V., & Pennington, B. F. 2005. Validity of the executive function theory of attention-deficit/hyperactivity disorder: a meta-analytic review. *Biological Psychiatry* **57**(11): 1336–1346.

Willcutt, E. G., & Pennington, B. F. 2000. Comorbidity of reading disability and attention-deficit/hyperactivity disorder: differences by gender and subtype. *Journal of Learning Disabilities* **33**(2): 179–191.

Willcutt, E. G., Pennington, B. F., Boada, R., Ogline, J. S., Tunick, R. A., Chhabildas, N. A., *et al*. 2001. A comparison of the cognitive deficits in reading disability and attention-deficit/hyperactivity disorder. *Journal of Abnormal Psychology* **110**(1): 157–172.

Wolf, M., & Obregon, M. 1992. Early naming deficits, developmental dyslexia, and a specific deficit hypothesis. *Brain and Language* **42**(3): 219–247.

Zametkin, A. J., Liebenauer, L. L., Fitzgerald, G. A., *et al*. 1993. Brain metabolism in teenagers with attention deficit hyperactivity disorder. *Archives of General Psychiatry* **50:** 333–340.

Zametkin, A. J., Nordahl, T. E., Gross, M., King, A. C., Semple, W. E., Rumsey, J., *et al*. 1990. Cerebral glucose metabolism in adults with hyperactivity of childhood onset. *New England Journal of Medicine* **323:** 1361–1366.

Index of Contributors

Bavelier, D., 71–82
Ben-Yehudah, G., 260–274
Bennett, I.J., 184–198
Bozzali, M., 212–221

Caltagirone, C., 212–221
Carter, E.J., 283–299
Chan, A.H.D., 30–40
Conway, C.M., 113–131
Corina, D.P., 100–112
Crain, K., 83–99

Darwent, G., 222–236
Doyon, J., 151–172
Dye, M.W.G., 71–82

Eden, G.F., ix–xii, 13–29, 83–99,
     237–259, 316–327
Einbinder, E.R., 237–259

Fawcett, A.J., 222–236
Fiez, J.A., 260–274
Flowers, D.L., ix–xii, 13–29, 237–259
Folia, V., 132–150
Forkstam, C., 132–150

Goebel, C., 199–211
Goertz, R., 199–211
Goswami, U., 1–12
Griffiths, P.D., 222–236

Hagberg, G.E., 212–221
Hagoort, P., 132–150
Hansen, P.C., 41–55
Hauser, P.C., 71–82
Howard, D.V., 184–198
Howard, Jr., J.H., 184–198

Ingvar, M., 132–150

Jack, A., 173–183

Kaushanskaya, M., 56–70
Knapp, H.P., 100–112
Koo, D., 83–99
Koyama, M.S., 41–55

LaSasso, C., 83–99
Laycock, S.K., 222–236
Li, G., 30–40
Li, P., 30–40
Luke, K.-K., 30–40
Lungu, O., 151–172
Lyon, L.G., 13–29

Macaluso, E., 212–221
Maisog, J.M., 237–259
Marian, V., 56–70
Menghini, D., 212–221
Mortimer, J., 275–282
Müller, R.-A., 300–315

Nalewajko, M., 199–211
Nicolson, R.I., 222–236

Orban, P., 151–172

Pelphrey, K.A., 283–299
Petersson, K.M., 132–150
Petrosini, L., 212–221
Pisoni, D.B., 113–131

Ray, N.J., 173–183
Romano, J.C., 184–198
Rvachew, S., 275–282

Sireteanu, R., 199–211
Stein, J.F., 41–55, 173–183
Stoodley, C.J., 173–183

Tan, L.H., 30–40
Thiel, A., 199–211
Turkeltaub, P.E., 13–29, 237–259

Uddén, J., 132–150

Vaidya, C.J., 316–327
Vicari, S., 212–221

Wallis, L.I., 222–236
Weekes, B., 30–40

Werner, I., 199–211
Wilkinson, I.D., 222–236
Wonders, S.H., 222–236

Yip, V., 30–40